Operative Strategy in General Surgery

An Expositive Atlas

Volume II

Operative Strategy in General Surgery

An Expositive Atlas

Volume II

Jameson L. Chassin

Professor of Clinical Surgery
New York University School of Medicine

Director of Surgery
Booth Memorial Medical Center

Illustrated by Caspar Henselmann
With 440 illustrations

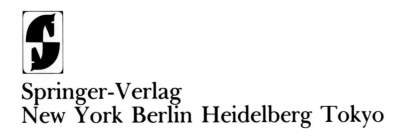

Springer-Verlag
New York Berlin Heidelberg Tokyo

Jameson L. Chassin, M.D.
Professor of Clinical Surgery
New York University School of Medicine

Director of Surgery
Booth Memorial Medical Center
Flushing, New York 11355 U.S.A.
(*Use this address for correspondence.*)

Visiting Surgeon
University Hospital, New York University Medical Center
and
Consulting Surgeon
New York Veterans Administration Hospital

Attending Surgeon
Bellevue Hospital

Library of Congress Cataloging in Publication Data
(Revised for vol. II)
Chassin, Jameson L.
  Operative strategy in general surgery.
  Includes index.
  1. Surgery, Operative—Atlases. I. Title.
[DNLM: 1. Surgery, Operative—Atlases. WO 517 C488o
1980]
RD32.C42   617′.91′00222   79-29758

Typeset by Kingsport Press, Kingsport, Tennessee.
Printed and bound by Halliday Lithograph, West Hanover, Massachu-
setts.
Printed in the United States of America.

9 8 7 6 5 4 3 2 1

ISBN 0-387-90984-2
Springer-Verlag New York Berlin Heidelberg Tokyo
ISBN 3-540-90984-2
Springer-Verlag Berlin Heidelberg New York Tokyo

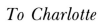

To Charlotte

Contents

Breast

44 Concept: Which Operation for Breast Cancer 15

45 Modified Radical Mastectomy (Patey) 23

48 Cholecystectomy   59

49 Cholecystostomy   79

56   Periampullary Diverticulectomy   138

57   Operations for Carcinoma of Hepatic Duct Bifurcation   144

Pancreas

58   Concept: Which Operations for Pancreatic Cancer   157

59   Partial Pancreatoduodenectomy (Whipple)   161

60   Total Pancreatoduodenectomy   189

61   Distal Pancreatectomy   206

62 Operations for Pancreatic Cyst   214

63 Pancreaticojejunostomy (Puestow) for Chronic Pancreatitis   224

Spleen

Esophagus

66   Concept: Operations for Reflux Esophagitis, Stricture, Short Esophagus, and Paraesophageal Hernia   255

67 Transabdominal Fundoplication (Nissen) 264

68 Posterior Gastropexy (Hill) 276

Abdominal Wall

Anus and Rectum

85   Lateral Internal Sphincterotomy for Chronic Anal Fissure   466

86   Anoplasty for Anal Stenosis   470

Head and Neck

Miscellaneous

96   Drainage of Subphrenic Abscess   571

Appendix

Contents of Volume I

Appendixes

Index

Foreword

This surgical atlas should be of great value to all clinical surgeons, both those in training and those in surgical practice, and Dr. Chassin is superbly qualified to author this work. During more than three decades as a member of the faculty of the New York University School of Medicine, he has taught countless residents many aspects of the art of surgical technique. One measure of Dr. Chassin's unusual teaching ability is that he is both Professor of Clinical Surgery at New York University and Director of Surgery at Booth Memorial Hospital, where our fourth-year surgical residents have rotated regularly for the past 12 years. Booth Memorial is the only hospital outside the New York University Medical Center to which New York University residents rotate. This simple fact well underlines Dr. Chassin's remarkable capability for teaching.

When a surgical complication develops after an operation, two or three possibilities should be considered. First, of course, was the diagnosis correct? If it was, then the cause of the complication is usually either an inadequate operative technique or a flawed concept underlying the selection of the operative procedure. When the surgical technique seems faultless, a postoperative complication would strongly indicate that the concept was erroneous, albeit cherished perhaps for decades.

Unlike any other atlas on operative technique, this book specifically discusses the conceptual basis of the operation as well as the strategy that will help the surgeon avoid common pitfalls. The operative technique is then described step by step.

I am confident that in the years ahead this atlas will be regarded as one of the major contributions to our literature of surgical technique.

Frank C. Spencer, M.D.
George David Stewart Professor and Chairman
Department of Surgery
New York University School of Medicine

Preface to Volume II

In writing the second volume of this atlas of *Operative Strategy in General Surgery*, I have tried to follow the same precepts that formed the foundation for Volume I. Each chapter starts with a review of the concept underlying the selection of the proper operation. The next important step in a surgeon's preparation for a major operation is his formulation of an operative strategy. It is the detailed discussion of the operative strategy of each operation that makes this atlas unique. My definition of the term operative strategy is the advance plan that the surgeon develops to anticipate and avoid all the technical pitfalls and danger points inherent in the operation under study. The ultimate goal is to make each operation safe and free of complications.

Following discussion of the concept and the operative strategy in each chapter is a detailed description of each step in the operation by the technique that I use, as illustrated by the detailed drawings of Mr. Caspar Henselmann whose illustrations for Volume I were cited for their excellence by the Association of Medical Illustrators.

In selecting operations to be included in this work, I planned to include all those operations in general surgery whose safety and efficacy I was able to evaluate on the basis of adequate personal experience and expertise. Volume I included most of the operations of the gastrointestinal tract, while Volume II covers the remaining general surgical procedures with a few exceptions. Operations for morbid obesity have been omitted from this book because, in my opinion, this area of surgery has not yet emerged from the stage of experimental research; no single operative procedure for morbid obesity seems ready for general application at this time. Some operations upon the endocrine glands and the liver have not been included in this work for another reason. The *Manual of Endocrine Surgery,* 2nd edition by Edis, Grant, and Egdahl and the *Manual of Liver Surgery* by Longmire are recently published (Springer-Verlag, N.Y., 1984 and 1981) atlases by outstanding authorities who have covered their fields far better than I could have done.

Special attention has been devoted to certain newer operations that I have found valuable. These include repair of the traumatized spleen, pancreatoduodenectomy with pylorus preservation, total pancreatectomy, choledochoscopy, hiatus herniorrhaphy with Collis-Nissen gastroplasty, Shouldice repair of inguinal hernia, mesh repair of recurrent inguinal and ventral hernias, ileoanal anastomosis with ileal reservoir after total colectomy and mucosal proctectomy, esophagectomy and gastric pull-up without thoracotomy, bile-diverting operations or colon (jejunum) interposition for recurrent reflux esophagitis, and operations for infected abdominal wound dehiscence.

At the end of Volume I is a glossary (Appendix D) which defines or illustrates terms, products, and instruments cited in the text. The items of this type that are cited in Volume II, but that were not included in Appendix D, will be found in Appendix E at the end of Volume II.

Finally, I would like to express my gratitude for the complimentary reviews of Volume I that have been published both in the U.S.A. and in Europe.

Breast

43 Operations for Benign Breast Diseases

Fibroadenoma

Concept: Management of Fibroadenoma

Most fibroadenomas are small, round, freely movable, well-encapsulated nodules that are easily diagnosed on physical examination and occur most often in women aged 15 to 30. Operation is indicated because some of these tumors will continue to grow, especially during pregnancy. Occasionally, carcinoma may masquerade as a fibroadenoma.

Operative Strategy

Although most fibroadenomas are completely surrounded by a smooth fibrous capsule, occasionally a fibroadenoma of the pericanalicular type may at some point be fixed to surrounding breast tissue. Whenever this is the case, include a narrow rim of normal adjacent breast in the specimen that is being excised. Otherwise, a local recurrence of the tumor is possible.

Among the errors encountered in surgery for a fibroadenoma is the failure to locate the lesion. This can occur when a deep-seated tumor is being excised under local anesthesia. Unless the tumor is easily palpable and is superficial, it may not be easy to localize, especially when the operation is being performed under local anesthesia through a cosmetic type of circumareolar incision at a distance from the lesion.

A more important consideration, especially in cases of fibroadenomas that are large in size, is the possibility of overlooking the diagnosis of cystosarcoma phyllodes. This latter tumor, which may be malignant, often resembles a large fibroadenoma on physical examination. The most important characteristic of the cystosarcoma is a strong predilection for local recurrence. With each local recurrence, there is an increase in the risk of malignancy. Therefore, whenever a fibroadenoma exceeds 4–5 cm in diameter, suspect the existence of a cystosarcoma and include a 1-cm shell of normal breast tissue in the specimen around its entire circumference.

Another pitfall to be avoided is postoperative bleeding. Following any breast excision, *do not depend on the presence of a small latex drain to compensate for inadequate hemostasis.* A large hematoma may develop despite the use of a drain. It is essential that hemostasis be complete. This is generally a simple matter with careful dissection and electrocoagulation.

Operative Technique

Incision

Superior cosmetic results follow the use of a circumareolar incision or an incision made in the inframammary fold. However,

3

it is not advisable to dissect through a large distance of breast when trying to extract a fibroadenoma via one of these incisions. For tumors more than 2–3 cm away from the areola, make an incision in the line of Langer directly over the tumor. These lines are essentially circular in nature in the skin overlying the breast, each circle being concentric with the areola.

Dissection

After opening the skin, use a scalpel to carry the incision through the subcutaneous fat down to breast tissue. Then, using electrocautery, incise the breast tissue down to the lesion. Electrocoagulate each bleeding point so that the field remains bloodless.

When the capsule of the fibroadenoma appears, incise it with a scalpel. If the fibroadenoma then shells out with no further attachment, the capsule may be left behind. If there are any attachments between the fibroadenoma and the surrounding tissue, excise the capsule and a small rim of breast tissue with it.

Repair

If the dissection has created a deep defect in the breast, use PG sutures on cutting-edged needles to repair only the deepest portion of the defect. Otherwise, make no attempt to resuture the defect in the breast, as these sutures will often create a mass at the site of the repair. In the months and years following surgery, evaluation of the patient's breast on physical examination can be made extremely difficult by the presence of a firm mass at the site of the previous excision. For this reason, we generally leave most small defects unsutured.

Close the skin with interrupted sutures of 6–0 nylon. If hemostasis has been complete, no drain is necessary.

Postoperative Care

In order to apply even pressure on the operative site, request that the patient wear a supportive bra continuously for the first few postoperative days.

Remove the drain, if any, in one or two days.

Postoperative Complications

Hematoma

Infection

Fibrocystic Disease

Concept: Operation versus Aspiration

Solitary Mass

A solitary cyst of the breast differs from a fibroadenoma in that it is not as freely movable with respect to the surrounding breast tissue, although the overlying skin does move freely. Also, cystic disease occurs at a later age than does fibroadenoma, the age incidence extending from 30 to the menopause. Some breast cysts give a sense of fluctuation when palpated, confirming the diagnosis. A breast mass, suspected of containing a cyst, should be aspirated using a syringe and needle. While a gauge No. 22 needle is adequate in many cases, using a larger needle, such as a No. 18, has been reported to be followed by fewer cyst recurrences. If the mass disappears *completely* after the cyst has been emptied, no biopsy is necessary. However, if the cyst should refill within 3–4 weeks after aspiration, a biopsy is indicated. If the cyst recurs at a later date, repeat aspiration is acceptable treatment. Another positive indication for biopsy is the presence of old blood in the aspirate. Occasionally, a bloody tap will yield bright red blood together with the clear yellow fluid in the cyst. This event may be followed by a small ecchymosis in the region of the needle puncture. Further observation is indicated in this situation.

If the patient has several isolated cysts, aspirate each of them and follow the same guidelines as above. Rarely will surgery be indicated if a cystic mass disappears after aspiration.

Studying the cyst aspirate for cell cytology has not proved to be fruitful in finding cases of breast cancer; we do not perform this test in the usual case of cyst aspiration.

Multiple Areas of Induration

More commonly, patients with fibrocystic disease present with multiple areas of induration, often in the upper outer quadrant and the axillary tail of Spence. These are often bilateral, but one breast may demonstrate much more induration than the other. Deciding which of these patients needs a biopsy can be a vexing problem to the surgeon. Generally, patients in this category require repeated physical examinations at 3–6 month intervals. Whenever a "dominant lump" appears, one that has not been noted on previous examinations, prompt biopsy is indicated. Otherwise, make a sketch of the findings on each physical examination so that new areas of suspicion will be identified early. While the accuracy of mammography is impaired by the dense breast of women in their early thirties, this X-ray study can be quite helpful in identifying malignant areas in a dysplastic breast of an older woman.

Nonoperative Treatment

Although the prime consideration in following patients with fibrocystic disease is to avoid overlooking an early carcinoma, other manifestations of the disease also merit attention. Patients may complain of pain in the breasts especially around the time of their menstrual periods. Frequently, the anxiety related to this complaint is the result of the patient's conviction that she is suffering from cancer. Strong reassurance, that there is no evidence of malignancy, is often the only treatment required. Otherwise, supporting the breast with a good bra and treatment with a mild analgesic may be necessary.

Hormonal therapy with danazol, aimed at reducing estrogen levels, has been suggested (Humphrey and Estes) for the relief of these symptoms. Insufficient experience has been gathered to determine whether there are significant risks associated with altering the patient's hormonal balance with these medications. It does not seem advisable to prescribe them until enough time has elapsed for the unfavorable side effects to be made known.

Prophylactic Bilateral Subcutaneous Mastectomy with Prosthetic Implant

In patients, who have a strong family history of breast cancer as well as multiple areas of induration in the breast, some surgeons advocate bilateral mastectomy with preservation of the nipples and the areolas followed by prosthetic implants in the hope of preventing the occurrence of breast cancer. Unfortunately, this operation does not remove all of the breast tissue and we are aware of at least one patient in whom cancer occured in a 1-cm area of residual breast following prophylatic mastectomy. For patients who are conscientious about returning to an experienced physician for regular followup examinations and for annual mammography (after age 40), prophylactic mastectomy is not indicated for fibrocystic disease.

Indications

In patients with fibrocystic disease, the only indication for surgery is the suspicion of cancer, no matter how lumpy the breasts may be.

Preoperative Care

Preoperative mammography is advisable to determine whether there are any additional suspicious areas identifiable by roentgenography that the surgeon was unable to identify earlier. Once the decision is made that an area in the breast is suspicious for carcinoma on physical examination, a negative finding on mammography does not constitute a reason to cancel the operation.

Although breast sonography can contribute information in some cases, we do not consider it worthwhile as a routine procedure.

Operative Strategy

Local Excision versus Segmental Resection

In a thin-breasted woman a well-localized mass is easily removed by local excision. On the other hand, in many cases a suspicious thickening of the breast may be due to a scirrhus tumor. Except for the patient with thin breasts, the core of a scirrhus carcinoma may be 3 cm or more deep to the area of thickening. It is these tumors that the unsophisticated surgeon may fail to reach during his attempt at local excision. Removing the overlying breast may result in a negative biopsy when, in fact, the carcinoma remains behind. For this reason, when the suspicious area is not clearly defined and well localized, it is preferable to excise a segment of breast extending from the subcutaneous fat down to the pectoral fascia in order to be sure that in performing an excision the cancer has not been missed.

If the area of suspicion is in the upper outer quadrant of the breast, the most common site of fibrocystic disease, the segmental excision will include the axillary tail of Spence together with the area of suspicion, as described below.

After excising a segment of breast, we prefer to omit closing the defect by suturing so that a new mass will not be created by the sutures. Postoperatively, palpating a gap in the continuity of the breast tissue is easier to interpret than palpating a mass.

Operative Technique—Upper Quadrant Tylectomy

Incision

Make the incision along the skin lines of Langer (**Fig. 43–1**) directly over the lesion with consideration of the anticipated location of the skin incision that will be made in case a mastectomy becomes necessary. Make the incision long enough to provide adequate exposure for the procedure.

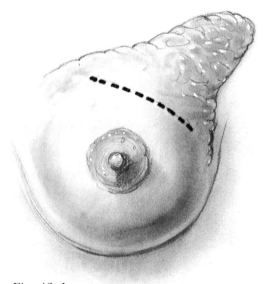

Fig. 43–1

Dissection

Carry the scalpel incision through the sub-cutaneous fat down to the surface of the breast. Then dissect the subcutaneous fat off the breast over the entire area to be excised (**Fig. 43–2**). Expose the axillary tail of Spence.

Whenever a blood vessel is encountered use the coagulating current to achieve complete hemostasis. When the entire area of induration in the upper outer quadrant has been identified, insert the left index finger between the pectoral fascia and the overlying breast to be excised. Now, with the finger as a guide, complete the incision through the full thickness of the breast (**Fig. 43–3**) and remove the specimen.

Achieving complete hemostasis is much more efficient if each bleeding point is electrocoagulated as soon as it is encountered rather than leaving it until the specimen has been removed. Close the overlying skin with interrupted 6–0 nylon sutures. A drain is not necessary if hemostasis is perfect.

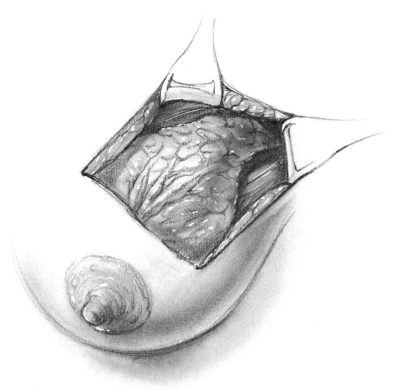

Fig. 43–2

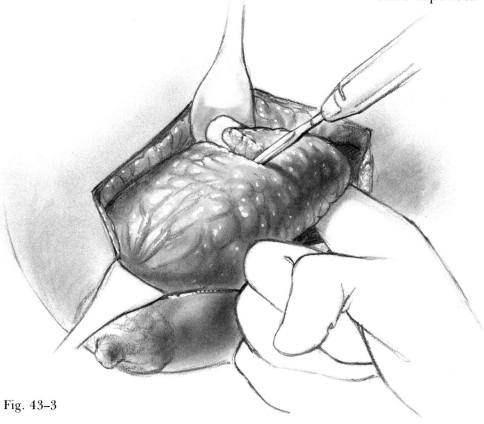

Fig. 43–3

7

Postoperative Care

If a drain has been used, remove it in 1–2 days.

Instruct the patient to wear a supportive bra, around the clock, for the first 2–4 days.

Postoperative Complications

Hematoma
Infection

Excision of Mammary Ducts

Concept: Management of Nipple Discharge

Presence or Absence of Mass

When a patient has a nipple discharge, the presence of a mass is a positive indication for the excision and biopsy of this lesion. The combination of a mass with a bloody nipple discharge indicates a high incidence of carcinoma.

In the *absence of a palpable mass*, nipple discharge was accompanied by a 12% incidence of carcinoma in the study of Urban and Egeli while Seltzer, Perloff, Kelley, and Fitts noted that 8% of their patients who underwent surgery for nipple discharge without a palpable mass had breast cancer. Nipple discharge, that is physiological, does not require biopsy. This type of discharge is almost always bilateral and can be seen to arise from multiple ducts in the nipples. This is common during pregnancy but may also be initiated by the administration of estrogens, chlorpromazine, and other drugs. Birth control pills may occasionally produce a clear serous or milky discharge from a single duct, although it more commonly produces secretion from multiple ducts. According to Urban and Egeli, "true pathologic nipple discharge is spontaneous, persistent, intermittent and usually secondary to pathologic lesions of the intraductal epithelium. It typically arises from a single duct opening in the nipple, and is most often unilateral, but occasionally bilateral." It should be remembered that each of the dozen or so mammary ducts has its individual orifice in the nipple so that secretion from a single diseased duct will always exude from the same nipple orifice. Persistent, spontaneous discharge from a single nipple duct is an indication for surgery.

Nature of Discharge

Bloody
On rare occasions a bloody discharge may appear from a single nipple duct during pregnancy owing to vascular engorgement of the breast. However, in 16% of cases bloody nipple discharge is due to malignant disease of the ducts; in most of the remaining cases, bloody nipple discharge is caused by benign intraductal papilloma, either single or multiple.

Serous
Although a clear serous discharge from the nipple is almost always caused by a benign process, 2% of Urban's cases had cancer, and Haagensen noted an even higher incidence of malignancy. Serous discharge from multiple nipple ducts, especially if bilateral, may be treated expectantly if there is no mass and if mammography is negative. Persistent, single-duct serous discharge requires duct excision.

Cloudy, Purulent, Multicolored
Most patients with turbid nipple discharge suffer from duct ectasia and stasis, although 3.8% of Urban's series of 435 lesions had cancer. For this reason, this type of discharge also requires duct excision.

Cytology

Surprisingly, attempts to detect cancer by studying the cytology of the nipple discharge have not been successful (Urban and Egeli).

Indications

Nipple discharge with palpable mass. The combination of a single-duct discharge, especially if bloody in nature, with a palpable mass indicates a high incidence of breast cancer and requires prompt operation.

Single-duct discharge without a palpable mass, if persistent and spontaneous, is accompanied by 11.8% incidence of cancer. It is an indication for surgery.

Multiple-duct discharge, especially if bilateral, is not, by itself, an indication for operation.

Preoperative Care

Localize the diseased duct. If the surgeon anticipates the excision of a single diseased duct, it is important to localize this duct preoperatively. This may be accomplished by applying finger pressure at varying points along the outer margin of the areola in order to determine which segment of the breast contains the offending duct, as the finger pressure will induce discharge from this duct. If this is not accomplished at a single examination, apply collodion to the surface of the nipple in order temporarily to occlude all of the ducts and prevent any discharge. At a subsequent examination a week later, remove the collodion and repeat the attempt to localize the offending duct. Also, collodion may be applied to the surface of the nipple one week prior to operation in order to cause distention of the diseased duct.

Perform mammography prior to operation on the ductal system.

Obtain radiological ductograms by inserting a tiny catheter into the duct orifice and injecting a small amount of aqueous radiopaque medium. This is a difficult procedure and many radiologists have no experience with it. If the entire ductal system of the breast is to be excised, a ductogram will be of no value and need not be done.

Operative Strategy

Single-Duct Excision versus Total Duct Excision

When the indication for surgery is a bloody nipple discharge, the diagnosis is generally carcinoma or intraductal papilloma. In the latter case, the lesions are often multiple, and excision of a single duct may overlook an intraductal carcinoma. For this reason, we agree with Urban (1963) that total excision of the mammary ducts is preferable to a single-duct excision. With other types of discharge, where the incidence of carcinoma is much lower, excision of a single duct is satisfactory, once the offending duct has been accurately localized by repeated preoperative examination.

Prevention of Skin Necrosis

Total excision of the mammary ducts requires elevation of the entire areola. This may impair the vascularity of the distal tip of the skin flap unless careful dissection is performed. Do not make the circumareolar incision greater than 40%–50% of the circumference of the areola. Also, be sure that the breast defect beneath the areola is reconstructed so that the resutured skin flap may have an opportunity to derive a blood supply from underlying soft tissue.

Operative Technique—Single-Duct Excision

Incision

A single duct may be excised either through a radial incision or an incision around the circumference of the areola. Use a sharp scalpel and obtain hemostasis with accurate electrocoagulation.

Identification and Excision

If collodion has been used to occlude the surface of the nipple for a week prior to surgery, the diseased duct will by now be distended. If it contains blood, its surface will display a purplish hue. In this case, gently dissect the duct from surrounding tissue. Divide it between hemostats at its junction with the nipple and dissect it out to a point about 1–2 cm beyond the circumareolar incision. Submit it for frozen section histological examination.

   If the duct cannot be clearly identified, it will be necessary to excise an area of the ductal system beginning at the nipple and proceeding in a peripheral direction. Then have the pathologist examine the specimen to ascertain that the pathology has indeed been excised.

Closure

In many cases it is necessary only to close the skin incision with interrupted 6–0 nylon sutures. In some cases a few PG sutures may be placed if there is a significant defect in the underlying breast. If hemostasis is perfect, drainage is not necessary. Otherwise, a 6-mm wide latex drain may be brought out through the incision.

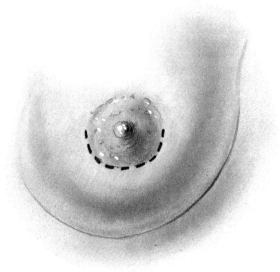

Fig. 43–4

Operative Technique—Total Duct Excision

Incision

Make an incision along the circumference of the areola at the exact margin between the areola and skin **(Fig. 43–4)**. The length of the incision should encompass 50% of the areola's circumference. Insert sutures in the edge of the incised areola temporarily and apply a hemostat to each suture. These will be used to apply traction while the areola is being dissected off the breast **(Figs. 43–5a and 43–5b)**. Use scalpel or scissors dissection to elevate the areola with a thin layer of fat. This dissection must be continued beyond the nipple so that the entire skin of the areola has been elevated. Do not detach the nipple from its ducts at this stage of the operation.

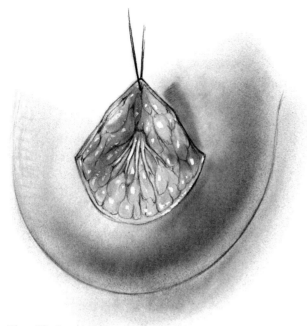

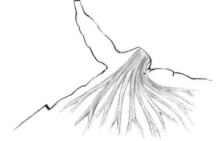

Fig. 43–5a   Fig. 43–5b

Excising the Ductal System

After the skin has been elevated, it will be noted that the 12 or so ducts constitute the only attachment between the nipple and the underlying breast. Apply a ligature to these ducts and make an incision that will detach them flush with the nipple **(Figs. 43–6a and 43–6b).**

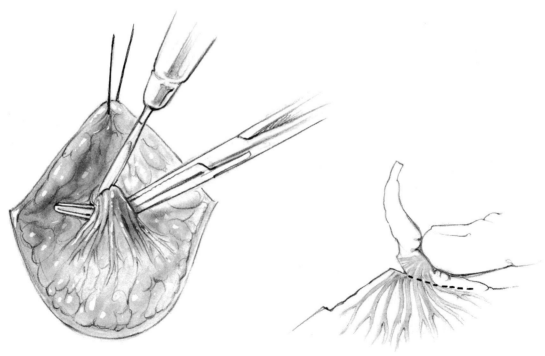

Fig. 43–6a   Fig. 43–6b

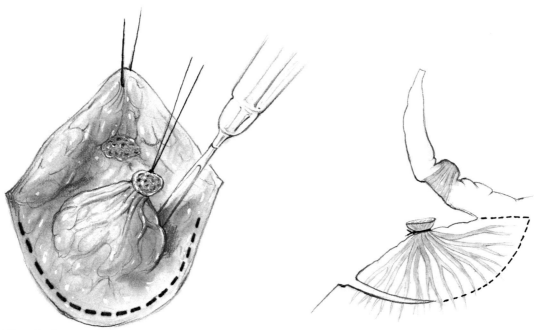

Fig. 43–7a   Fig. 43–7b

Now, dissect the ducts for a distance of 3–5 cm. Using the electrocoagulator, excise the circle of ducts and breast tissue **(Figs. 43–7a and 43–7b).** The circular mass of tissue will have a radius of 3–5 cm and a thickness of 1–2 cm. If any of the diseased ducts is dilated and extends beyond 5 cm, follow this duct and remove a further section until it disappears into the breast tissue. Occasionally a diseased duct involves a section of the nipple, which may be inverted. In this case a tiny segment of nipple may be removed. Obtain complete hemostasis with the electrocoagulator.

Reconstruction

In the patient with a large breast, the resulting defect may be relatively shallow so that the reconstructed areola will rest on a solid base of breast tissue. In this case no further reconstruction is necessary. In many cases, however, there will be a significant defect beneath the areola. Since the blood supply of the areola is somewhat tenuous, it requires a firm base of breast tissue for optimal healing. In this case, close the defect in the breast in layers with interrupted small sutures of catgut or PG material.

If detaching the areola results in a tendency for the nipple to invert, corrective measures must be taken. Before closing the

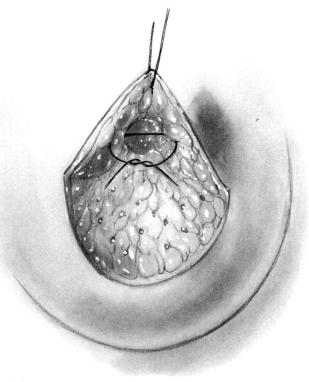

Fig. 43–8

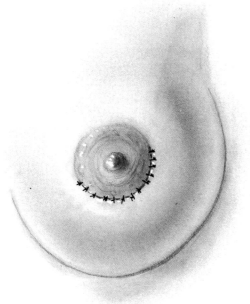

Fig. 43–9

skin incision, insert a 5–0 PG purse-string suture in the subcuticular tissues at the base of the nipple in order to maintain it in the erect position **(Fig. 43–8).** Then close the skin incision with interrupted 6–0 nylon sutures **(Fig. 43–9).**

Postoperative Care

If a latex drain has been used, remove it after 1–2 days.

Instruct the patient to wear a supportive bra over a moderately bulky dressing to apply even pressure for the first 7 days and nights after surgery.

Postoperative Complications

Hematoma
Occasionally following a total duct excision, elevation of the entire areola in a plane too close to the subcutis results in an area of *skin necrosis.*

Breast Abscess

Breast abscess is most often seen in a nursing mother. It is generally the result of the introduction of bacteria by a break in the skin of the nipple. In a lactating woman, treatment requires incision along a radial direction in order to produce as little damage as possible to the breast ducts. The pus is evacuated and a gauze packing is loosely inserted until the cavity heals.

In the nonlactating woman, an abscess may appear without very much surrounding inflammation and induration. In some of these cases, an attempt may be made to aspirate the pus with a large needle under local anesthesia. This, together with antibiotic treatment, may avoid the necessity for operation in occasional cases.

Para-Areolar Abscess or Fistula

An abscess in the region of the areola or just adjacent to the areola often originates in an obstructed mammary duct, termed duct ectasia. This may result either in a recurring abscess at the same location or in a chronic draining fistula. In either case, proper treatment requires a radial elliptical incision **(Fig. 43–10)** overlying the duct, which can usually be palpated as a thick-

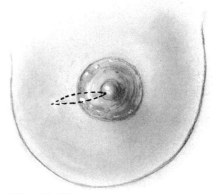

Fig. 43–10

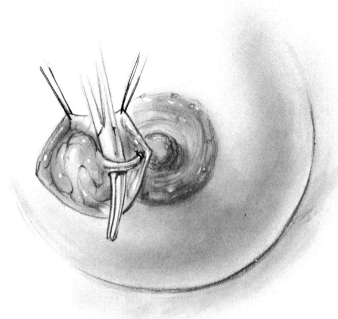

Fig. 43–11

ened cord running from the nipple towards the periphery of the breast. A small ellipse of skin and surrounding breast tissue are removed. Identify the duct **(Fig. 43–11)** and excise it together with the diseased tissue **(Fig. 43–12).** If the incision has not

been greatly contaminated, close the skin loosely around a latex drain. If the area is grossly contaminated, it may be wiser to insert the skin sutures for delayed primary closure 4–6 days later.

If the diseased duct is not removed, the abscess or fistula will recur.

References

Haagensen DD (1971) Diseases of the breast, Saunders, Philadelphia

Humphrey LJ, Estes NC (1979) Aspects of fibrocystic disease of the breast; treatment with danazol. Postgrad Med J 55:48

Seltzer MH, Perloff LJ, Kelley RL, Fitts WT Jr (1970) The significance of age in patients with nipple discharge. Surg Gynecol Obstet 131:519

Urban JA (1963) Excision of the major duct system of the breast. Cancer 16:516

Urban JA, Egeli RA (1978) Non-lactational nipple discharge. CA 28:130

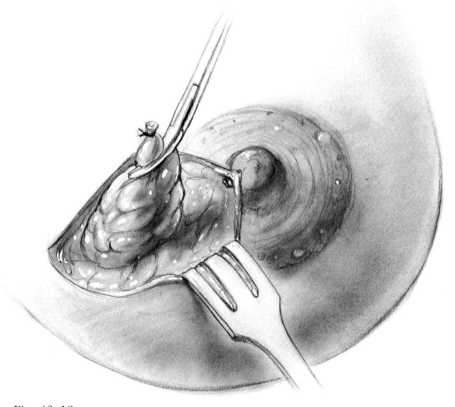

Fig. 43–12

44 Concept: Which Operation for Breast Cancer

Introduction

The past decade or two has witnessed the adoption of a large number of new therapies for breast cancer ranging from biopsy-plus-radiotherapy all the way to super-radical mastectomy. It is important to distinguish fact from fancy in addressing this controversy.

First, Rosen, Fracchia, Urban, and Schottenfeld have shown that local excision of breast cancer, including removal of an entire quadrant of breast, leaves residual microscopic malignancy in the remaining three quadrants or in the axillary nodes in 56% of patients who have small primary lesions and in 69% of those who have tumors greater than 2 cm in diameter. It is clear that *local excision alone is poor therapy for breast cancer.* A number of prominent radiotherapists (Calle, Pilleron, Schlienger, and Vilcoq; Harris, Levene, and Hellman; Montague, Gutierrez, Barker, Tapley, et al.) feel that application of 5,000 rads or more will eliminate small foci of cancer in the breast and in the axillary nodes. Although local excision of breast cancer standing alone is an obviously inadequate procedure, the combination of tylectomy (quadrantectomy) and adequate radiotherapy is indeed a legitimate subject for experimental study for patients with clinical Stage I cancer.

Second, it is fallacious to compare the results of lumpectomy–radiotherapy studied in France (Calle) with the survival figures noted after radical mastectomy at Memorial Hospital in New York City, because the two investigations studied entirely different patient populations. Not only is a prospective randomized study necessary to establish fact in this field, but the survival data must be accumulated for a period of 10–20 years. It is not rare to identify a distant metastasis or a local recurrence 15–20 years after mastectomy for breast cancer. The fact that a given study shows no significant difference in survival or recurrence rates at the end of 5 years *does not mean that a difference does not indeed exist. It simply means that the particular study failed to detect such a difference.* Prolonging the study for another decade may elicit such data. Urban (1980) cites Rissanen and Holsti's studies of Stage I and II breast cancer in Finland between 1936 and 1973. They compared radical mastectomy with wide local excision, followed in each case by conservative dosages of radiation. Five-year survival was similar in the two groups. At 10 years there was a definite advantage for mastectomy in the T2 tumors, but not for the T1 lesions. At 15 years the T1 patients had a survival of 63% following radical mastectomy but only 49% following local excision. The T2 patients experienced a 45% 15-year survival following radical mastectomy but only 29% with conservative surgery. Similarly, Atkins, Hayward, Klugman, and Wayte randomized a group of patients in which radical mastectomy was compared with wide local excision, both being followed by conservative doses of radiation therapy. After 5 years there was no significant difference in the survival rates of the two groups. After 10 years, survival studies showed no significant difference between the two procedures in Stage I patients, but 67% of Stage II cases survived following radical mastectomy and only 23% following conservative treatment. This difference was statistically significant. It is true that modern radiotherapy uses dosages and techniques that are more advanced than those used by Rissanen and Holsti or by Atkins and colleagues. The point is that after 5 years there was no difference between tylectomy and mastectomy for either Stage I or II cases. It required the passage of 15 years (Rissanen and Holsti as quoted by Urban, 1980) and 10 years (Atkins et al.) to demonstrate the differences in the survival rates between the two procedures. The 5-year results were of no value in this respect. In the case of early cancer, identifying the best primary treatment requires not only a randomized prospective study but also a 15–20-year followup.

Another randomized clinical trial by Langlands, Prescott, and Hamilton compared radical mastectomy with simple mastectomy plus modern radiotherapy (2 MeV Van de Graaff generator, 4,500 rads). After 10 years, 68% of Stage I patients survived after radical mastectomy and 52% after simple mastectomy–radiotherapy. For Stage II patients the corresponding figures are 58% and 49% (Welch).

Table 44–1. Clinical-Diagnostic Staging System of the American Joint Committee for Cancer Staging and End-Results Reporting: TNM Classification

Primary tumor (T)

TX	Tumor cannot be assessed
TO	No evidence of primary tumor
TIS	Paget's disease of the nipple with no demonstrable tumor
	NOTE: Paget's disease with a demonstrable tumor is classified according to the size of the tumor.
T1*	Tumor 2 cm or less in greatest dimension
	T1a No fixation to pectoral fascia or muscle
	T1b Fixation to pectoral fascia, muscle, or both
T2*	Tumor more than 2 cm but not more than 5 cm in greatest dimension
	T2a No fixation to pectoral fascia or muscle
	T2b Fixation to pectoral fascia, muscle, or both
T3*	Tumor more than 5 cm in greatest dimension
	T3a No fixation to pectoral fascia or muscle
	T3b Fixation to pectoral fascia, muscle, or both
T4	Tumor of any size with direct extension to chest wall or skin
	NOTE: Chest wall includes ribs, intercostal muscles, and serratus anterior muscle but not pectoral muscle.
	T4a Fixation to chest wall
	T4b Edema (including peau d'orange), ulceration of the skin of the breast, or satellite skin nodules confined to the same breast
	T4c Both of above
	T4d Inflammatory carcinoma

Nodal involvement (N)

NX	Regional lymph nodes cannot be assessed clinically
NO	No palpable homolateral axillary nodes
N1	Movable homolateral axillary nodes only
	N1a Nodes not considered to contain growth
	N1b Nodes considered to contain growth
N2	Homolateral axillary nodes considered to contain growth and fixed to one another or to other structures
N3	Homolateral supraclavicular or infraclavicular nodes considered to contain growth, or edema of arm
	NOTE: Edema of the arm may be caused by lymphatic obstruction and lymph nodes may not then be palpable.

Distant metastases (M)

MX	Not assessed
MO	No (known) distant metastasis
M1	Distant metastasis present

* Dimpling of the skin, nipple retraction, or any other skin changes except those in T4 may occur in T1, T2, or T3 without affecting the classification.

Third, at this point in time the two modalities of treatment that effectively improve survival in patients with breast cancer are surgical removal of the breast and axillary lymph nodes and, in selected cases, adjuvant chemotherapy. There are as yet no randomized studies with adequate long-term followup to demonstrate that tylectomy or simple mastectomy, with or without radiotherapy, are optimal treatments for potentially curable breast cancer. While conservative surgical excision combined with *high dosage* radiotherapy deserves a randomized clinical trial, this form of treatment *cannot* yet be offered to the patient as the method of choice.

Recognizing that new data will require new judgments in the future, we treat breast cancer at this time according to the policies described in the remainder of this chapter.

Preinvasive Cancer

Lobular carcinoma in situ is a slow-growing premalignant lesion that predicts the development of an invasive cancer in 11%–22% of patients observed for 10 years. Urban believes that these patients should undergo total mastectomy with conservative lateral axillary lymph node dissection, but Haagensen, Bodian, and Haagensen feel

Table 44–2. Stage Groupings, Clinical-Diagnostic and Postsurgical Treatment-Pathologic, According to the American Joint Committee for Cancer Staging and End-Results Reporting

Stage TIS	TIS	N0	M0			
Stage I	T1a	N0,	N1a	M0		
	T1b	N0,	N1a	M0		
Stage II	T0	N1b	M0			
	T1a,	T1b	N1b	M0		
	T2a,	T2b	N0,	N1a,	N1b	M0
Stage III	T3	N0,	N1,	N2	M0	
	T2a,	T2b	N2	M0		
Stage IV	T4	any N	any M			
	any T	N3	any M			
	any T	any N	M1			
Stage X	Not stageable (TX or NX)					

Table 44–3. Histopathology of Breast Cancer[a]

Noninfiltrating Carcinoma (CA)
Paget's disease with intraductal CA
In situ ductal (intraductal) CA
In situ lobular CA

Infiltrating Carcinoma (CA)
Paget's disease with infiltrating CA
Ductal CA
Infiltrating but not otherwise specified CA
Adenoid cystic CA
Comedo CA
Medullary CA
Mucinous (colloid) CA
Papillary CA
Lobular CA

Other Neoplasms
Cystosarcoma phyllodes, malignant
Sarcoma

[a] Inflammatory carcinoma of the breast is a *clinicopathologic entity* characterized by diffuse brawny induration of the skin of the breast with erysipeloid edge, usually without an underlying palpable mass. *Histologically*, inflammatory carcinoma consists of infiltrating mammary carcinoma that diffusely permeates dermal lymphatics. Inflamed cancers that are clinically similar to the above due to inflammation, infection, or necrosis but lack microscopic dermal lymphatic permeation are not classified as inflammatory carcinoma.

that lifelong, careful, periodic examinations will detect the malignancy in sufficient time to achieve a long-term cure. A complicating feature of this disease is its high incidence of bilaterality. The cancer may occur in the *opposite* breast and is usually of the duct-cell type.

Intraductal carcinoma in situ should be treated by total mastectomy, including removal of the pectoralis fascia, as well as the lateral third of the axillary lymph nodes, because this condition is frequently accompanied by areas of invasive carcinoma in the same breast.

Stage I and Stage II

Currently accepted worldwide is the TNM (see Table 44–1) staging classification of breast cancer developed by the Union Internationale Centre de Cancer (UICC) as amended in 1978 by the American Joint Committee (AJC) for cancer staging and end-results reporting. This classification is given in Tables 44–1, 44–2, and 44–3.

For the Stage I and II categories of breast cancer, the Patey operation (total mastectomy with excision of the pectoralis fascia, the minor pectoral muscle, and *all* of the axillary nodes) is claimed by Handley to have the same 10-year survival as the radical mastectomy. We agree with Handley.

Stage III

T3 N0 or N1

It is important not to adopt a defeatist attitude in the surgery of Stage III breast cancer. Fracchia, Evans, and Eisenberg have demonstrated that T3 patients with negative axillary nodes (12% of their 430 cases) had an 82% 5-year and a 75% 10-year survival following radical mastectomy! In fact, even the presence of skin edema or malignant skin infiltration did not adversely affect 10-year survival in T3 patients whose lymph nodes were negative. Fracchia and associates classified T4a and T4b tumors as Stage III and included them in their study, although the 1978 AJC system placed T4a and T4b tumors in Stage IV. In spite of this policy, their 5-year survival for all the Stage III cases was 41% and the 10-year rate, 21%. Fifty percent of patients having less than four involved axillary nodes lived 5 years. Finding nodes that were matted or fixed (N2) did not influence either survival or recurrence rates. Invasion of the pectoral muscle did not affect survival rates in patients with positive lymph nodes undergoing radical mastectomy. Postoperative radiotherapy (4,000–5,500 rads), as administered to these patients, did not improve either their survival or the incidence of local recurrence. Because this study was not randomized, it is possible that the most advanced cases received radiotherapy. Nevertheless, it seems clear that radical mastectomy is the basic treatment for Stage III breast cancer. Surgery should be followed by adjuvant chemotherapy.

T2 or T3 N2

In patients with some degree of fixation of their axillary nodes (N2), perform a radical mastectomy unless the degree of fixation seems so advanced as to rule out adequate surgical resection. In cases of advanced matting, one should probably precede surgery by a course of either chemotherapy (Perloff and Lesnick; Aisner, Morris, Elias, and Wiernik) or radiotherapy in the hope that this treatment will shrink these lymph nodes so that they become resectable. Whether radiation or chemotherapy is the preferred choice is a problem currently under study. The answer is not yet available.

Whichever preoperative adjuvant is employed, these patients should have a full course of chemotherapy following surgery because many of them have undetected metastatic deposits away from the field of surgery.

Stage IV

T4 N1 M0

In the absence of distant metastases, the problem in the T4-N1 patient is to eradicate the disease from the chest wall. In some cases, preoperative radiotherapy (Pollak and Getzen) or chemotherapy may help reduce the size of the primary tumor and make surgery feasible. In other cases, radical mastectomy with resection of a small portion of the chest wall may be necessary for the complete removal of a tumor that invades the thoracic cage. We do not believe that radiotherapy alone is the method of choice for the management of large T4 lesions.

Any T N3 M0

In the N3 situation surgery cannot eradicate the metastatic lymph nodes completely. Therefore perform a total mastectomy. Whether the metastatic lymph nodes should be treated by radiotherapy or chemotherapy or some combination of the two, is a question regarding which there is no data. We would follow the mastectomy by intensive chemotherapy. If this modality did not control the metastatic lymph nodes, radiotherapy would be added. Alternatively, radiotherapy and chemotherapy may be given simultaneously.

T3 or T4 Any N M1

In patients with distant metastases, treatment of the primary lesion is palliative. If the distant metastases are not advanced and the primary tumor is large but resectable, a palliative debulking partial mastectomy may be indicated. Otherwise the brunt of treatment falls in the realm of chemotherapy.

Management of Recurrent Carcinoma

Local Recurrence

A small solitary recurrence may appear at the site of operation 5–10 years following mastectomy. In this situation, local excision of the recurrence may be adequate therapy because the patient obviously has had an excellent immune response to the tumor. On the other hand, most local recurrences appear relatively soon after mastectomy and are often indicative of widespread malignant disease. In such cases, biopsy or excise the local lesion and initiate chemotherapy. Sometimes local radiotherapy is also helpful in controlling disease in the chest wall.

Bone Metastases

If a bone metastasis appears to be symptomatic and solitary, local radiotherapy is indicated. Otherwise, systemic therapy (chemotherapy or hormonal alteration) is preferred.

Visceral Metastases

With advanced hepatic or pulmonary metastases, intensive chemotherapy offers the best means of palliation.

Estrogen Receptor Status

If a tumor is rich in estrogen receptors (estrogen receptor-positive), it is likely that altering the patient's hormonal status by oophorectomy or administering an anti-estrogen drug like tamoxifen is likely to produce palliation in 60%–70% of cases. A favorable response to hormonal therapy requires a number of weeks or months before reaching its maximal effectiveness. For this reason it is not a suitable method of treating patients who have advanced metastases that are distressingly symptomatic. However, for tumors that appear to be advancing slowly, patients, in whom the estrogen receptor determination has been positive, either in the primary tumor or in a biopsy of a metastasis, will very likely benefit from hormonal alteration.

It is not clear at this time whether such patients should have oophorectomy or treatment with tamoxifen. In a patient who has had a favorable response to oophorectomy or tamoxifen and then has a relapse, adrenalectomy may offer further palliation. However, the indications for each of these therapies, including chemotherapy, is constantly being refined by the accumulation of additional data. Consequently, statements made at this time must be tentative.

The Medial Lesion

It has been demonstrated that lesions in the medial half of the breast or in the areola have a significant incidence of metastases to the lymph nodes along the internal mammary vessels. Urban (1978) has had excellent results in a large series of patients of this type upon who he has performed an extended radical mastectomy that includes removal of a narrow segment of chest wall together with the underlying internal mammary vessels and lymph nodes. Unfortunately, his cases were not selected on a randomized prospective basis, which makes the information difficult to interpret. Other surgeons routinely prescribe a course of postoperative radiotherapy to the internal mammary nodes for all patients with medial lesions. Here, also, no randomized prospective study has been reported. While radiotherapy has been demonstrated to reduce the incidence of local recurrence of tumor, patient survival has not been improved thereby.

Another question that has not been investigated is whether adjuvant chemotherapy, which has been shown to improve 5-year survival in premenopausal patients with positive axillary lymph nodes, does or does not control metastases to the internal mammary chain. Lacking conclusive data makes the choice of management difficult.

In patients who will receive adjuvant chemotherapy because of positive axillary nodes, we do not believe that the initiation of chemotherapy should be delayed by a course of radiotherapy to the internal mammary glands. Patients with medial lesions, who do not have obviously metastatic axillary nodes, should probably undergo biopsy of the internal mammary nodes in the second and third interspaces unless the primary tumor is 1.5 cm or less in diameter. If the internal mammary nodes prove to be harboring tumor, adjuvant chemotherapy is indicated. Without biopsy, patients with medial lesions, who have negative axillary lymph nodes, would not ordinarily receive chemotherapy because the internal mammary metastasis would have gone unnoticed. The prognosis for patients with involved internal mammary nodes that go untreated is not good. Alternatively, postoperative radiotherapy may be prescribed.

Frozen-Section or Two-Stage Procedure?

Currently in the lay press there is a strident demand that any patient suspected of breast cancer should have her biopsy performed at one stage and then be permitted to discuss the results of the biopsy with her surgeon prior to deciding on the ultimate therapy. If there is the slightest doubt about the competence of the pathologist who will be interpreting the frozen-section biopsy, then it is certainly wise to delay a decision until further consultation may be obtained concerning the histological diagnosis. This is also true when a competent pathologist has any doubt about the presence of cancer.

However, when an experienced pathologist is competent to make a positive diagnosis of cancer on a frozen-section examination, and the patient has confidence in her surgeon, there is no good reason to submit her to a second anesthesia and a second operation. Of course, this will require that the surgeon and the patient have a detailed discussion in advance of the biopsy regarding the options available if the diagnosis turns out to be cancer. This approach demands that the surgeon discuss the options with some patients in whom the suspicion of cancer will not be confirmed as well as with those who turn out to have malignancy. Although this requires more time on the part of the surgeon, it does spare the patient the emotional and physical strain of the second operation.

Some superficial tumors can be biopsied safely under local anesthesia as an outpatient procedure. In this case the two-stage sequence is acceptable. However, many tumors are deep in the breast tissue. Other tumors are scirrhus in nature. In this category of tumor the overlying induration of the breast represents mostly fibrosis and may not yield a positive biopsy unless the central core of tumor is identified. This requires the deep excision of a segment of breast. Other lesions, which are manifested by an area of vague induration, also require the excision of a full thickness segment of the breast in order to avoid missing the tumor. All of these patients, in whom the tumor is not superficial or obvious, require general anesthesia if one is not to risk missing the pathology. If general anesthesia is required for the biopsy, we believe that a positive frozen section should be followed by a definitive operation at one stage.

Positive Mammography in the Absence of Palpable Tumor

When the signs of a localized carcinoma are seen on the mammogram and the patient has no palpable lesion, localizing the area for biopsy may be difficult. One option is to measure the location of the area of suspicion on the craniocaudal and the mediolateral X-ray views. Then, excise a full thickness segment of the breast in the area of suspicion. Once the specimen is removed, perform a mammogram on it. If the area of suspicion is identified on the mammogram of the specimen, transport it to the pathologist for a frozen section. Some pathologists prefer to slice the specimen in many narrow segments, then to lay each section flat on the X-ray plate for specimen mammography. In this fashion it is possible to determine which slice contains the area of suspicion.

Another method that has proven successful is for the mammographer, an hour or two prior to biopsy, to insert a needle into the breast under X-ray control until the tip of the needle lies in the area of suspicion. Through the needle, he inserts a hooked wire (available as a "Kopans Breast Locator" from Cook Inc., P.O. Box 489, Bloomington, Indiana, 47402, U.S.A.). This wire is inserted into the lesion under X-ray control. The wire acts as a harpoon and will stay in place if cov-

ered with a sterile dressing until surgery is begun. The surgeon proceeds to excise the area of breast that is located near the tip of the wire. The operation should be done within a few hours after the needle has been inserted. When the specimen has been removed, tissue mammography should confirm that it contains the area of suspicion, unless it is obvious to the surgeon and the pathologist that the specimen contains cancer.

References

Aisner J, Morris D, Elias EG, Wiernik PH (1982) Mastectomy as an adjuvant to chemotherapy for locally advanced or metastatic breast cancer. Arch Surg 117:882

Atkins Sir H, Hayward JL, Klugman DJ, Wayte AB (1972) Treatment of early breast cancer: a report after ten years of a clinical trial. Br Med J 2:423

Calle R, Pilleron JP, Schlienger P, Vilcoq JR (1978) Conservative management of operable breast cancer: ten years experience at the Foundation Curie. Cancer 42:2045

Fracchia AA, Evans JF, Eisenberg BL, (1980) Stage III carcinoma of the breast, a detailed analysis. Ann Surg 192:705

Haagensen CD, Bodian C and Haagensen D (1981) Breast carcinoma, risk and detection, Saunders, Philadelphia

Handley RS (1976) The conservative radical mastectomy of Patey: 10-year results in 425 patients. Breast 2:16

Harris JR, Levene MB, Hellman S (1978) Role of radiation therapy in the primary treatment of carcinoma of the breast. Sem Oncol 5:403

Langlands AO, Prescott RJ, Hamilton T (1980) A clinical trial in the management of operable cancer of the breast. Br J Surg 67:170

Montague ED, Gutierrez AE, Barker JL, Tapley ND, et al. (1979) Conservation surgery and irradiation for treatment of favorable breast cancer. Cancer 43:1058

Perloff M, Lesnick GJ (1982) Chemotherapy before and after mastectomy in stage III breast cancer. Arch Surg 117:879

Pollak EW, Getzen LC (1978) Inflammatory carcinoma of the breast, a therapeutic approach followed by improved survival. Am J Surg 136:722

Rosen PP, Fracchia AA, Urban JA, Schottenfeld D (1975) Residual mammary carcinoma following simulated partial mastectomy. Cancer 35:735

Urban JA (1978) Selective radical surgical treatment for primary breast cancer. In: Gallager HS, Leis HP Jr, Snyderman RK, Urban JA (eds) The breast, Mosby, St. Louis

Urban JA (1980) Surgical management of palpable breast cancer. Cancer 46:983

Welch CE (1982) Cancer of the breast. J Clin Surg 1:425

45 Modified Radical Mastectomy (Patey)

Concept: Defining the Modified Radical Mastectomy

The term modified radical mastectomy has come to mean removal of the breast together with a variable number of axillary lymph nodes. Some surgeons take a few outer lymph nodes, some do a complete excision of the lateral third of the axillary nodes using the pectoralis minor muscle as the upper boundary for their dissection, some elevate the pectoralis minor and take a few lymph nodes deep to this muscle, while others do a complete axillary lymph node dissection to the level of the clavicle. Patey described an operation removing all of the breast tissue together with the underlying fascia of the pectoralis major in continuity with a total axillary lymphadenectomy. The pectoralis minor muscle also was excised.

Without removing or dividing the pectoralis minor muscle, it is not possible in most cases to achieve more than a limited lymphadenectomy. Furthermore, Durkin and Haagensen demonstrated that after chemically treating the axillary specimen to dissolve the fat, but preserving all the lymph nodes, that they could identify as many as 12 Rotter's nodes in the area between the minor and major pectoral muscles. When Handley showed that the 10-year survival following modified radical mastectomy was equal to that following the radical operation, it was the Patey operation that he had performed. In the treatment of infiltrating breast cancer, complete axillary lymphadenectomy is indicated because 25% of patients with clinically negative lymph nodes harbor microscopic metastases in the axillary nodes.

Indications

The Patey modified radical mastectomy is the operation of choice for an infiltrating T1 or T2 carcinoma of the breast that does not involve the fascia of the pectoralis major. Otherwise, radical mastectomy is preferred.

Preoperative Care

Perform mammography not only to study the area already under suspicion but to identify any possible additional sites of malignancy away from the primary area of suspicion.

Only in Stage III and suspected Stage IV breast cancer is it necessary to perform a bone scan and a chemical profile for liver dysfunction. For Stage I and II breast cancer, scanning the bones or the liver is counterproductive because the incidence of false positive results will outweigh the few cases of proven metastases that these studies will detect.

Pitfalls and Danger Points

Performing an inadequate biopsy that fails to detect the cancer

Ischemia of skin flaps

Injury to axillary vein or artery

Injury to brachial plexus

Injury to chest wall resulting in pneumothorax

Injury to lateral pectoral nerve resulting in atrophy of the pectoralis major muscle

Operative Strategy

Biopsy

Incision
Before making the *biopsy* incision, be sure to plan the direction of the incision that will be made for the *mastectomy* in case the biopsy is malignant. If the biopsy incision is made in a vertical direction and then it is decided to perform the mastectomy through a transverse incision, it will be difficult to excise the entire field of the biopsy procedure. If a transverse mastectomy incision is anticipated, make a transverse biopsy incision.

Incisional Wedge Biopsy, Total Excision of the Tumor, or Segmental Mastectomy?
When the primary tumor is larger than 3–4 cm in diameter, perform the biopsy simply by excising a wedge of the tumor, but leave the bulk of the tumor behind. Otherwise, such a large defect is made in the breast that it is difficult to avoid entering the field of the biopsy procedure when doing the mastectomy. When the tumor is smaller than 3–4 cm, excise the entire lesion for the biopsy and the estrogen receptor determmination. This has the advantage that manipulating the breast will not dislodge additional tumor emboli into the lymphatic and blood streams. When the breast is large, a larger primary cancer can be excised for the biopsy without difficulty, as compared with patients who have a small breast.

In many situations the surgeon will undertake to biopsy an area of breast that is the site of suspicious thickening as, for instance, in early scirrhus carcinoma. In these cases there may be no discrete tumor mass. It is important, therefore, that a sufficient sample of breast tissue be excised for the pathologist. Given an inadequate sample, the pathologist will not identify the malignancy. In such cases the aim of the biopsy should be to excise a segment of the breast, rather than to try to localize a mass. This often requires that the dissection be carried down to a plane just superficial to the pectoral fascia. Then insert the left index finger into this plane and excise a segment of overlying breast containing the entire area of suspicion.

Use of Electrocautery for the Biopsy
Rapid and effective in accomplishing hemostasis during breast surgery, the electrocautery device nevertheless has one disadvantage. If excessive heat is applied to the breast tumor during electrocoagulation, this may render the determination of estrogen receptors inaccurate. Consequently, use only the cutting current when incising the breast tissues surrounding the tumor. This does not result in excessive heat. When a bleeding point is encountered, use the electrocoagulating current only for the bleeding point. If the tumor is small, use the electrocoagulating current with great caution to avoid overheating the specimen.

Incision and Skin Flaps

Thickness of Skin Flap
While Halsted emphasized the importance of removing almost all of the skin of the

breast and employing very thin skin flaps, subsequent experience has shown that these precepts were necessitated by the advanced stage of cancer encountered by Halsted. How thin to make the skin flap depends on how much subcutaneous fat exists between the skin and the breast. Obese patients may have 1–2 cm of subcutaneous fat, while thin patients may have only a few millimeters of fat in this location. The important strategy is to remove all of the breast tissue. Leaving behind a layer of subcutaneous fat on the skin flap does not increase the incidence of local tumor recurrence. On the other hand, it does help assure the viability of the skin flap and facilitates the reconstruction of the breast at a subsequent operation for those patients who desire this procedure.

Cooper's ligaments extend from the breast to the subcutis and form a discontinuous layer of thin white fibrous tissue, visible against the background of yellow fat. Incising this fibrous layer where it joins the subcutaneous fat is one good method of assuring complete removal of the breast tissue while at the same time preserving an even layer of subcutaneous fat. This technique is described below.

Alternative Incisions for Mastectomy

Placing the incision in a horizontal direction gives the best cosmetic result because the scar will not be visible when the patient wears a low-cut gown. While the horizontal incision is easy to apply to tumors in the 3 or 9 o'clock positions **(Figs. 45–1 and 45–2)**, some modifications are necessary for tumors in the upper or lower portions of the breast. A good basic approach is to draw a circle around the tumor leaving a margin of 4 cm on all sides. Then plan the remainder of the incision so that the entire areola will be included in the specimen. If possible, accomplish this in a horizontal direction. After having drawn the circle around the tumor, preserve as much of the remaining skin as possible. This will avoid tension on the skin suture line. The redundant skin can be excised after the specimen has been removed. At that time an accurate judgment as to the proper tension can be formulated. Also, the redundant skin that has been excised at the end of the operation can be converted into a full-thickness skin graft by excising the underlying fat. By planning ahead in this fashion, it is almost never necessary to obtain a dermatome split-thickness skin graft

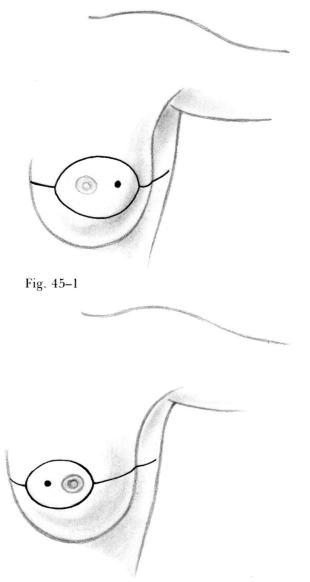

Fig. 45–1

Fig. 45–2

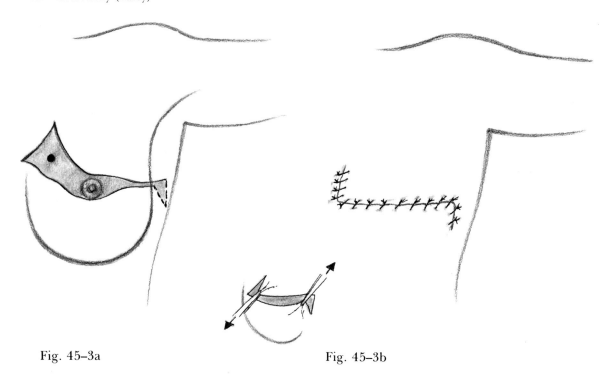

Fig. 45–3a   Fig. 45–3b

from another part of the body. Not only does this technique save operating time, but it also avoids a graft donor site wound that is often painful. Furthermore, the full-thickness graft provides a far superior cosmetic and functional result as compared with the split-thickness graft. Properly performed, one can expect a 100% "take" of the full-thickness graft.

If any defatted surplus skin remains, wrap it in gauze and store it in a small bottle of sterile saline solution in a refrigerator. At any time in the next 10–14 days, if the patient should require a skin graft, remove the skin from the refrigerator and use it.

There are a number of alternative incisions for tumors in various locations of the breast. **Fig. 45–3a** illustrates a difficult horizontal incision for a lesion at 10 o'clock. **Fig. 45–3b** illustrates the resultant scar after the redundant triangle of skin has been removed.

Cosmetic Considerations

Following the lead of the two originators of the radical mastectomy, William Stewart Halsted and Willy Meyer, surgeons have for many decades used incisions for the

mastectomy that were made generally in a vertical direction. A significant portion of the scar extended above the clavicle or over the shoulder and was exposed when the patients wore any type of sleeveless gown. Also, complete removal of the major pectoral muscle left a marked hollow beneath the clavicle.

Without detracting from the efficacy of the mastectomy, modern techniques can avoid many of these cosmetic deficiencies. During a radical mastectomy, it is advisable to leave the clavicular head of the major pectoral muscle. This improves the cosmetic appearance and does not interfere with performing a complete lymphadenectomy.

In performing either a radical or the Patey modification of the radical mastectomy, it is far preferable from the cosmetic viewpoint to make an incision that is horizontal rather than vertical. For tumors in the upper outer quadrant of the breast, it may be necessary to make the incision in an oblique direction as shown in **Fig. 45–4**; it is almost never necessary to carry the incision over the shoulder. Complete

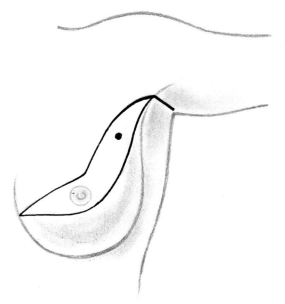

Fig. 45–4

exposure of the axilla can be obtained with an incision that crosses the upper axilla in a transverse direction rather than one that passes along the anterior aspect of the upper arm.

Tranverse incisions also have the advantage of enhancing the cosmetic appearance following the insertion of a silicone implant at a later date in an effort to reconstruct the breast following mastectomy.

Combining a total mastectomy with a later plastic reconstruction is a procedure much to be preferred over local excision and radiotherapy.

Another cosmetic defect, that should be avoided, is the "dog-ear" deformity that can result at either end of the incision following mastectomy. This bunching together of skin is interpreted by many women as a residual tumor and is a cause for great anxiety. It is easily prevented by excising an additional triangle of skin until the incision lies flat on the chest wall (**Figs. 45–5a and 45–5b**).

Skin Grafts

Although Halsted advocated excision of most of the skin of the breast followed by an extensive split-thickness skin graft, most of our patients in the modern era come for treatment with disease at a much earlier stage than did those in Halsted's time. Extensive excision of the skin is designed to minimize the incidence of local tumor recurrence on the chest wall. Skin recurrences in the parasternal region are usually the result of tumor in the internal mammary lymph nodes rather than residual tu-

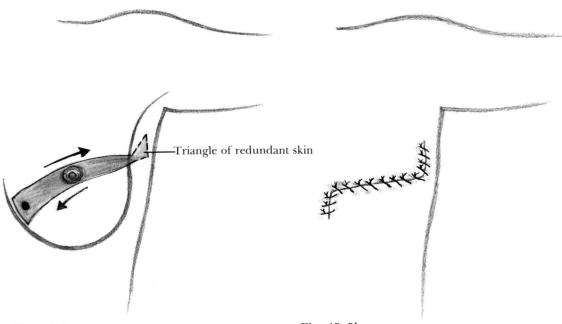

Triangle of redundant skin

Fig. 45–5a   Fig. 45–5b

mor in the subcutaneous tissues. Parasternal recurrences will not be eliminated simply by removing more skin. In general, removing all of the skin over the tumor plus an additional 4 cm seems to allow for an adequate margin and a low recurrence rate.

Traditionally, surgeons have used the dermatone to obtain a split-thickness graft from the skin of the thigh to replace a deficit on the chest wall following mastectomy. A full-thickness graft is preferable both from the functional and the cosmetic point of view. In planning the skin incision for the mastectomy most surgeons outline an incision that is symmetrical and elliptical. In so doing, they do not leave any surplus skin on the chest wall, but rather they remove the surplus with the specimen. This can be avoided by drawing a circle with the skin marking pen and measuring 4 cm from the outer perimeter of the tumor. Only the skin of this circle plus that of the areola need be removed for the purpose of avoiding local recurrence. The remainder of the skin of the breast temporarily may be left behind on the chest wall. If this strategy is followed and a skin graft is necessary, then this graft may be obtained by trimming the skin from that portion of the chest wall where it is in surplus. This patch of skin is then defatted by pinning it to a sterile board and removing all of the subcutaneous fat. This will convert the patch of skin into a full-thickness skin graft. In our experience a properly defatted full-thickness skin graft has resulted in approximately as many as 100% "takes" as can be expected following split-thickness grafts. By following this strategy over a period of many years we have had to perform split-thickness grafts only in thin patients with small breasts or in patients with unusually large tumors. Not only is the functional and cosmetic result superior following full-thickness grafts, but the painful second wound at the donor site is avoided.

Pros and Cons of Electrocautery

For the past decade or two we have used an electrocautery technique both for the sharp dissection involved in elevating the skin flap and for hemostasis. Although the use of the coagulating current for incising subcutaneous fat creates an intense amount of heat (and sometimes actually boils the fat), using the cutting current avoids producing much heat. In fact, dissecting with the cutting current does not seem to have an effect on the tissue very much different from that of the cold scalpel blade. In other words, there does not appear to be any significant heating of the local tissues; nor does there seem to be a considerable hemostatic effect. Why, then, do we dissect with a cutting current? In this portion of the operation, using the cutting current will not produce instant hemostasis. However, we use an electrocautery instrument that has a fingertip control that can very easily be switched from cutting to coagulating current. By making an incision with a cutting current, the switch can instantly be changed to the coagulating current when one encounters a bleeding point. Thus, the local vessel may be coagulated without interposing the step of grasping it with a hemostat and then ligating it or applying electrocoagulation to the hemostat. Once the technique is mastered, it encourages the development of rapid and efficient surgery with minimal blood loss.

Achieving hemostasis in a fatty layer requires considerably more skill than coagulating a bleeding point in muscle. Coagulating the fat in the general vicinity of a bleeding point creates tissue damage and little hemostasis. Try to see the actual blood vessel from which the bleeding is coming. Touch the blood vessel at a point proximal to its cut end using the flat part of the electrocoagulator's electrode.

After many years of using electrocoagulation for virtually all of the bleeding points in the radical or modified radical mastectomy, except for the axillary artery and vein branches, we have not noticed any increase in wound complications, nor in the incidence and severity of serum accumulations under the skin flaps. The incidence of serum accumulation seems to be related more to the degree of obesity than to the method of obtaining hemostasis.

Operative Technique

Biopsy

Determine the direction that the mastectomy incision will take and make the biopsy incision directly over the tumor in the same direction as the anticipated mastectomy incision. If the tumor is 2–3 cm in diameter, make the biopsy incision 3–4 cm in length. Then carry this incision through the subcutaneous fat down to the level of breast tissue. Apply sharp rake retractors to the subcutaneous fat. Use the cutting current of the electrocautery to dissect in the plane between the fat and the breast tissue until an area of breast about 3–4 cm in diameter has been exposed.

If the tumor is easily identified, use the cutting current to incise the breast tissue around the perimeter of the tumor until the lesion has been removed. Now use a coagulating current to achieve complete hemostasis in the wound, while the pathologist is performing a cryostat frozen-section examination of the specimen. Be sure that a portion of the specimen is submitted for the estrogen receptor determination.

It is generally not necessary to apply sutures in the attempt to close the defect left in the breast following the biopsy excision. Closing the defect in layers with sutures will produce an area of induration in the breast that may well resemble a tumor. If the lesion is benign, this area of induration may persist for months or years and cause great consternation to the patient and her personal physician. Leaving the defect unsutured makes postoperative evaluation of the breast on physical examination more accurate.

When the area to be biopsied consists of nondiscrete thickening, excise the entire area down to pectoral fascia (see Figs 43–1 to 43–3).

If the lesion is benign, close the skin with interrupted 6–0 nylon sutures. If the specimen is reported to be malignant, close the incision with continuous heavy silk. Change gowns, gloves, and instruments, and redrape the patient.

Incision and Elevation of Skin Flaps

Position the patient so that the arm is abducted 90° on an arm board and place a folded sheet, about 5 cm thick, underneath the patient's scapula and posterior hemithorax. Prepare the area of the breast, upper abdomen, shoulder, and upper arm with an iodophor solution. Enclose the entire arm in a double layer of sterile orthopedic stockinette to maintain sterility of the entire extremity because the arm must be flexed during the dissection of the upper axilla. We prefer to place a sterile Mayo instrument stand over the patient's head. This will be used for extra hemostats and gauze pads for the assistant as well as to support the arm during the period of the operation that requires it to be flexed.

Using a sterile marking pen, draw a circle 4 cm away from the perimeter of the primary tumor. Depending on the location of the tumor, mark the medial and lateral extensions of the incision as discussed above. In addition to the area of skin outlined by the circle drawn around the tumor, include the entire areola and nipple in the patch of skin left on the specimen (**Fig.**

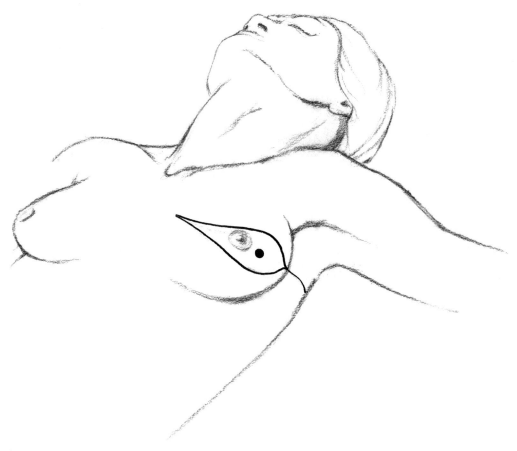

Fig. 45–6

45–6). Then use a scalpel to make the incision through all the layers of the skin. Attain hemostasis by applying electrocoagulation to each bleeding point. We then generally cover the skin of the specimen with four layers of sterile gauze that are fixed in place by applying multiple Adair clamps to attach the gauze to the cut edge of the skin along the perimeter of the specimen.

Now apply additional Adair clamps, about 2–3 cm apart, to the cut edge of the skin on the lower flap. Have the assistant elevate the skin flap by drawing the Adair clamps in an anterior direction. Apply countertraction by depressing the breast posteriorly. Then use the electrocautery set on a medium cutting current to incise Cooper's ligaments, which attach the subcutaneous tissues to the surface of the breast **(Fig. 45–7).** Leave no breast tissue on the skin flap. When any significant bleeding is encountered, change the switch on the handle of the electrocautery device from the "cutting" to the "coagulating" setting. By using the cutting current for dissecting the fat off the breast not much heat is generated nor is the tissue trauma significantly greater than that imposed by the cold steel scalpel. Whenever a blood vessel is encountered, the surgeon has in his hand the electrocoagulating device and need only move the switch from one setting to the other. This technique facilitates performing a radical mastectomy with minimal trauma and excellent hemostasis. Continue elevating the inferior skin flap until the dissection is beyond the breast.

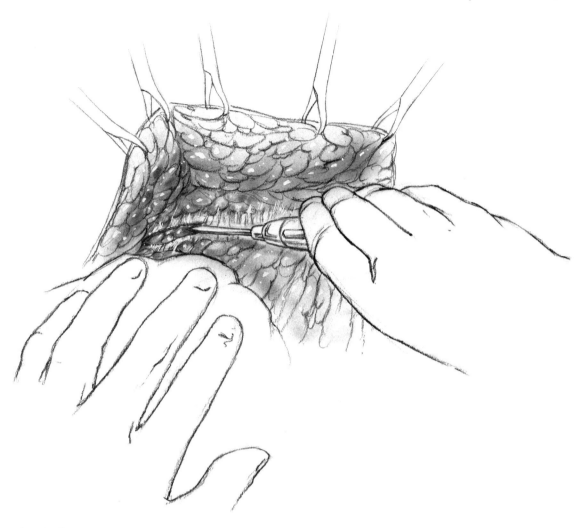

Fig. 45–7

The medial margin for the dissection is the sternum. The lateral margin is the anterior border of the latissimus dorsi muscle, which is exposed for the first time during this phase of the operation. Apply a moist gauze pad to the operative site. Remove the Adair clamps from the lower skin flap and apply them now to the upper skin flap.

Use the same technique to elevate the upper skin flap to a point about 2 cm below the clavicle. Whichever skin incision has been selected, it should permit wide exposure of the axillary contents from the clavicle to the point where the axillary vein crosses over the latissimus muscle. The final step in achieving exposure consists of clearing the fat from the anterior border of the latissimus muscle with a scalpel so that the entire lateral margin of the dissection has been identified.

Clearing the Pectoral Fascia

After checking to ascertain that complete hemostasis has been achieved, use a scalpel to incise the fascia overlying the major pectoral muscle. Begin near the medial margin of this muscle and proceed with the scalpel dissection going from the medial to the

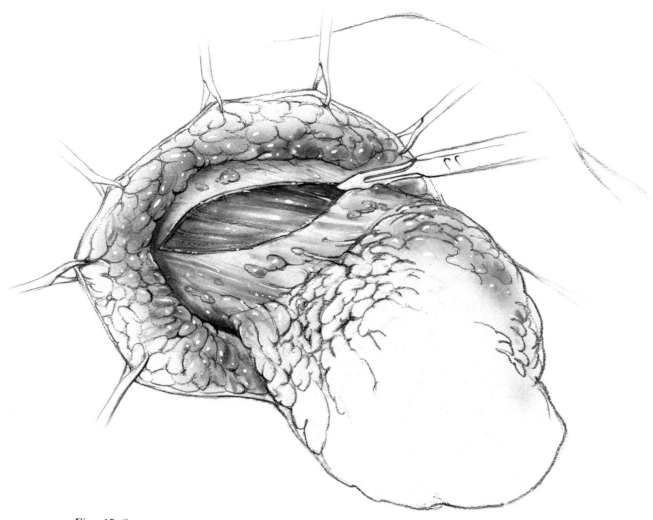

Fig. 45–8

lateral margin **(Fig. 45–8).** Simultaneous hemostasis will be achieved if the first assistant will electrocoagulate each of the branches of the mammary vessels as they are exposed or divided by the dissection. Whether you use either electrocautery or hemostats, exercise caution in pursuing a vessel that has retracted into the chest wall after being divided. We have on a few occasions, especially in thin patients, observed pneumothorax following this step. When the vessel is not easily controlled by electrocoagulation or a hemostat, simply apply a suture-ligature to control it.

When the lateral margin of the pectoralis major has been reached, use a combination of blunt and sharp dissection to elevate the edge of the pectoral muscle from its investing fascia. This will maintain continuity between the breast, the pectoral fascia, and the lymph nodes of the axilla.

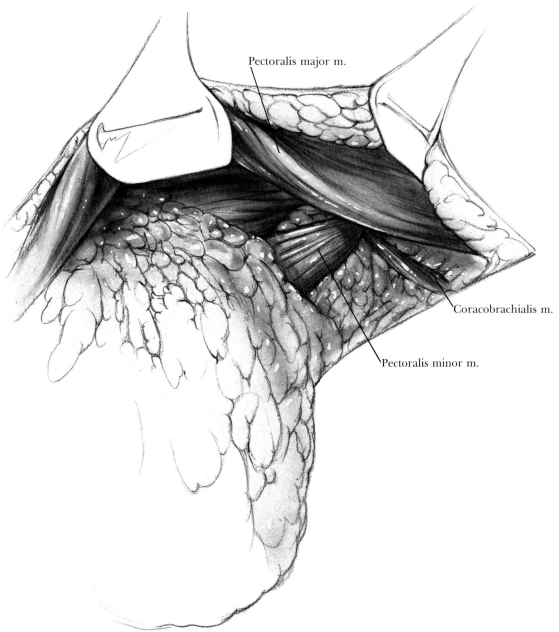

Pectoralis major m.

Coracobrachialis m.

Pectoralis minor m.

Fig. 45–9

Unroofing the Axillary Vein

Use a Richardson retractor to elevate the major pectoral muscle. Identify the pectoralis minor muscle **(Fig. 45–9).** Branches of the medial pectoral nerve will be seen lateral to the origin of the pectoralis minor. These may be divided without serious consequence, but be sure to identify and preserve the major branch of the lateral pectoral nerve that emerges just *medial* to the origin of the pectoralis minor and travels along the undersurface of the major pectoral muscle. Division of this nerve may result in paralysis, atrophy, and contraction of the pectoralis major.

Dissect the fat and fascia off the anterior-inferior edge of the coracobrachialis muscle using the scalpel. Directly inferior

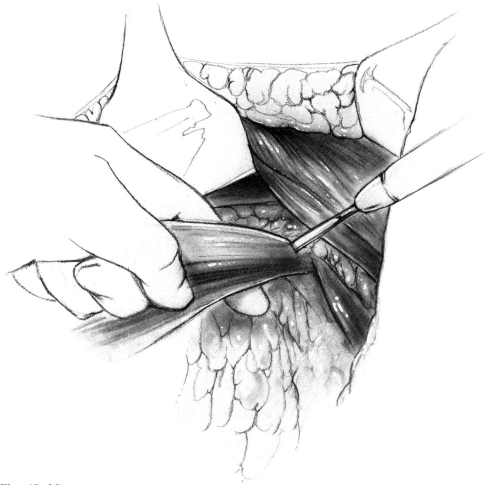

Fig. 45–10

to this muscle will be found the brachial plexus and the axillary vessels. Continuing the dissection of the inferior border of the coracobrachialis in a medial direction will lead to the coracoid process upon which the pectoralis minor inserts. Divide the pectoralis minor muscle near its insertion using the electrocoagulator **(Fig. 45–10)**. Free up enough of the divided muscle to provide complete exposure of the axillary vein. Deep to the point where the pectoralis minor muscle was divided will be found a well-defined fat pad overlying the junction of the cephalic and axillary veins. Gentle blunt dissection will generally succeed in elevating this fat pad and drawing it in a caudal direction to expose the anterior surface of the axillary vein.

Now incise the adventitial sheath of the axillary vein **(Fig. 45–11)**. Although light dissection with the belly of the scapel can accomplish this, most surgeons prefer to use a Metzenbaum scissors. A few branches of the lateral anterior thoracic artery, vein, and nerve will cross over the anterior wall of the axillary vein. Divide these branches between Hemoclips. In order to complete the division of the sheath

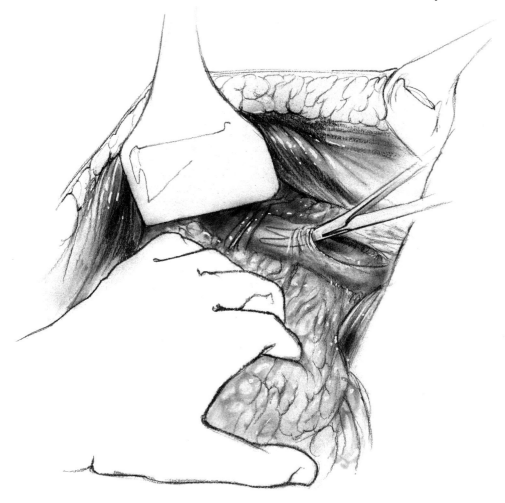

Fig. 45–11

of the axillary vein from the region of the latissimus muscle to the clavicle, it will be necessary to flex the upper arm. This will relax the major pectoral muscle, which is then elevated with a Richardson retractor.

Axillary Vein Dissection

Axillary lymphadenectomy aims at removing all of the lymph glands anterior and inferior to the axillary vein. Only when these glands are replaced by metastases will tumors spread to the nodes cephalad to the axillary vein and to the neck. Not only is it unnecessary to strip all of the fat from the brachial plexus, but this maneuver may produce a lifelong painful neuritis in some patients.

Now identify all the branches entering the axillary vein from below. Clear each of the branches of adventitia, and divide

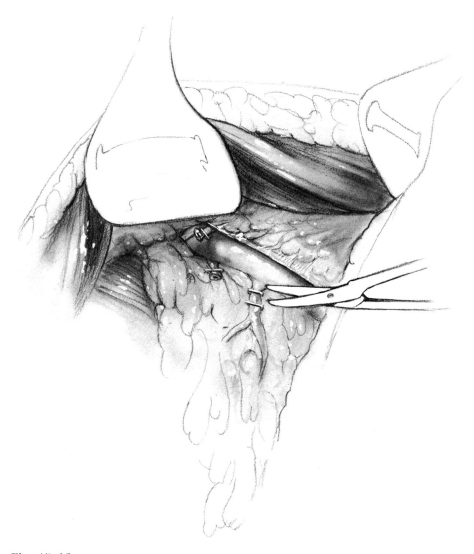

Fig. 45–12

each between Hemoclips **(Fig. 45–12).** The subscapular vein, which enters the axillary from behind, need not be divided.

At this point, it is essential to label the apex and the lateral margin of the axillary specimen. Many pathologists prefer that a third label be attached at the point where the pectoralis minor muscle crosses the axillary specimen. It is important that the pathologist be able to tell the surgeon

which nodes are involved as a metastasis to the apical node has a worse prognosis than one to the lateral node group.

The upper boundary of the axillary dissection is the crossing of the clavicle over the axillary vein. Detach the lymphatic and areolar tissue at this point with the electrocoagulator. Now make a scalpel incision in the clavipectoral fascia on a line parallel to and 1 cm below the axillary vein. Do not retract the axillary vein in a cephalad direction as this may expose the underlying axillary artery to injury during this step.

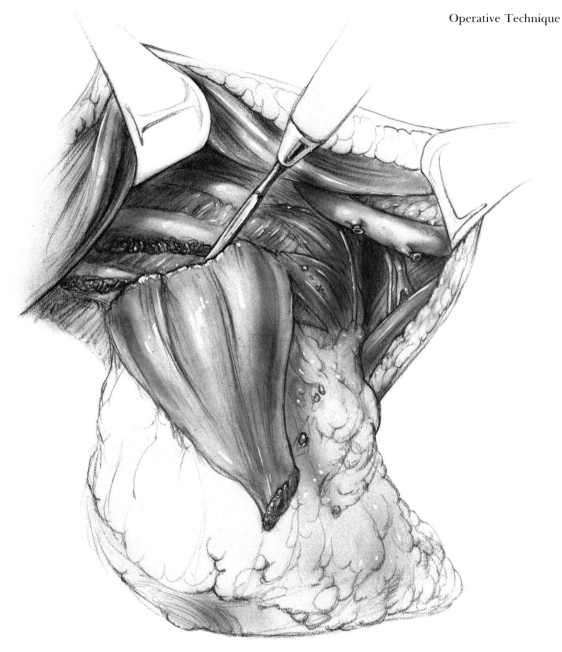

Fig. 45–13

Dissect the areolar and lymphatic tissues off the intercostal muscles and ribs going from medial to lateral. When the minor pectoral muscle is encountered, divide it 2–3 cm from its origin with the electrocoagulator **(Fig. 45–13)** and leave the excised muscle attached to the specimen.

This will insure removal of all of Rotter's lymph nodes. Now restore the arm to its previous position of 90° abduction. As the chest wall is cleared laterally, one or two intercostobrachial nerves will be seen emerging from the intercostal muscle on their way to innervate the skin of the upper inner arm. Since these nerves penetrate the specimen, divide them even though this

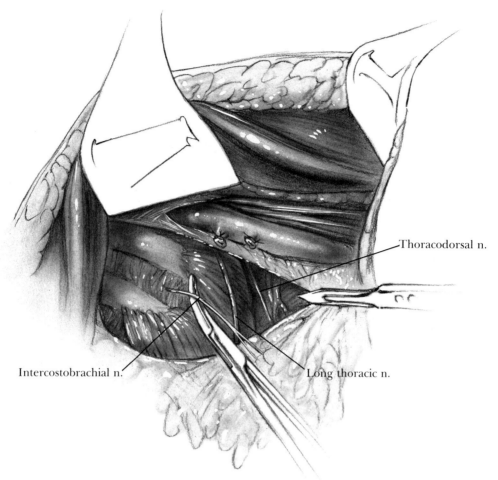

Thoracodorsal n.

Intercostobrachial n.

Long thoracic n.

Fig. 45–14

will result in a sensory deficit in the upper arm **(Fig. 45–14).**

Then use a sterile gauze pad to wipe the loose fat out of the subscapular space going from above downward. This maneuver will expose the long thoracic nerve that runs along the rib cage in the anterior axillary line in a vertical direction from above downwards to innervate the anterior serratus muscle. The thoracodorsal nerve can be identified as it leaves the area of the subscapular vein and runs both laterally and downward together with the thoracodorsal artery and vein to innervate the latissimus dorsi muscle. Since these two nerves run close to the peripheral boundary of the dissection, they may be preserved when no metastatic lymph nodes are seen in their vicinity.

Detach the lymphatic tissue inferior to that portion of the axillary vein that crosses over the latissimus muscle. Preserving the long thoracic nerve is complicated by the fact that a number of small veins cross over the nerve in its distal portion. Circumvent this difficulty by moving the partly detached breast in a medial direction so that it rests on the patient's chest after freeing the specimen from the anterior border of the latissimus muscle. Then make an incision in the fascia of the serratus muscle 1 cm medial to the long thoracic nerve. Dissecting this fascia a few centimeters in a medial direction will detach the entire specimen from the chest wall **(Fig. 45–15).**

Irrigation and Closure

Thoroughly irrigate the operative field with sterile water, a solution that has a can-

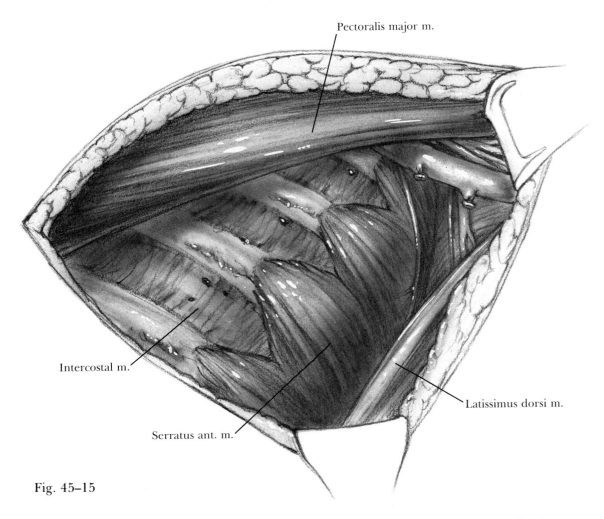

Pectoralis major m.

Intercostal m.

Serratus ant. m.

Latissimus dorsi m.

Fig. 45–15

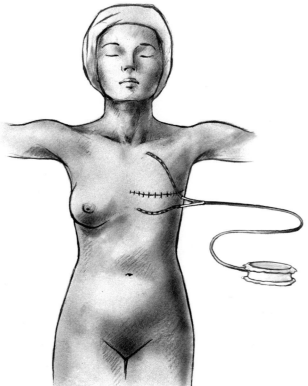

Fig. 45–16

ceridal effect on loose tumor cells that may have been dispersed into the operative field. Check the entire field to be sure that *complete* hemostasis has been achieved.

Then insert two multiperforated catheters, each about 4mm in diameter, through puncture wounds in the lower axilla. Bring one catheter deep to the axillary vein where it may be sutured with some fine catgut. Bring the other catheter across the thoracic wall from the puncture wound to the region of the sternum. Suture each catheter to the skin at the site of the puncture wounds and attach to closed-suction drainage (Hemovac) **(Fig. 45–16).**

Then close the skin with interrupted fine nylon sutures or skin staples. Be certain that there is no significant tension on the incision or else postoperative necrosis of the skin flap may be anticipated. Often

39

shifting the skin flaps in a medial or lateral direction will relieve tension. Do not permit either of the skin flaps at the lateral margin of the incision to become bunched up in such a fashion that a "dog ear" will form. Many patients are convinced that this represents residual tumor. The "dog ear" deformity can be eliminated by excising a triangular wedge of skin as noted in Figs. 45–3 and 45–5.

When closed-suction drainage is used postoperatively, it is not necessary to apply bulky pressure dressing.

Postoperative Care

Leave the two closed-suction drainage catheters in place until the daily drainage diminishes to 30–40 ml/day or about 5–7 days.

Encourage early ambulation but do not permit the patient to abduct the arm on the side of the operation for 5–7 days, as this activity prevents the skin flaps from adhering to the chest wall and encourages prolonged drainage of serum. Permit the patient to use this arm for ordinary activities not requiring abduction. Do not initiate active abduction exercises until the 10th postoperative day. This delay will not interfere with the patient's ability to regain a complete range of motion of the arm, as demonstrated by the study of Lotze, Duncan, Gerber, Woltering, and colleagues.

Take appropriate steps throughout postoperative treatment to assure the patient's emotional as well as her physical rehabilitation.

Do not remove the skin sutures for 2 weeks because the operation has separated the skin flaps from much of their blood supply. This slows down the rate of healing.

Aspirate any significant collections of serum beneath the skin flaps with a sterile syringe and needle as necessary.

Administer adjuvant treatment with chemotherapy as soon as the incision is healed in all premenopausal women with axillary lymph node metastases. Although supporting data as yet are not complete, chemotherapy should be given also to postmenopausal women with positive axillary nodes. The role of radiotherapy as an adjuvant agent in the treatment of breast cancer is not clear at this time and requires further study.

Conduct follow-up examinations every 3 or 4 months for the first 5 years and then every 6 months for life. These examinations, combined with annual mammography, are an integral part of the treatment of breast cancer. Aside from the search for local recurrence and distant metastases, the opposite breast must be carefully followed because 10% of patients will develop a new primary tumor in the opposite breast following mastectomy for cancer.

Also, carefully inspect the arm for the development of lymphedema, which can become a disabling complication if not detected and treated early. Warn the patient to avoid trauma, including sunburn, to the arm and forearm of the operated side. If at any time the hand should be traumatized or any evidence of infection should appear in the hand or arm, prompt treatment with antibiotics (dicloxacillin) for a period of 7–10 days, followed by the application of a specially fitted elastic sleeve of the Jobst type, may prevent the development of permanent arm edema.

Postoperative Complications

Ischemia of Skin Flap

This complication is preventable by avoiding tension on the suture line as well as excessive devascularization of the skin flaps. It is a serious complication. When ischemia is permitted to develop into gangrene of the skin, a process that takes 2 or more weeks, some degree of cellulitis invariably follows. This process occludes many residual collateral lymphatic channels through which the lymph fluid from the arm manages to return to the general circulation. Blocking these channels increases the incidence and severity of permanent lymphedema of the arm. Consequently, skin necrosis should be anticipated when purple discoloration appears in the skin flap on the 5th or 6th day following mastectomy. If this purple discoloration cannot be blanched by finger pressure, it represents devitalization of the skin and is not cyanosis.

Once this skin change has been observed, the patient should promptly be returned to the operating room. With a minimal amount of local anesthesia, excise the devitalized skin and replace it with a skin graft. At this early date infection will not yet have ensued, and primary healing of the skin graft may be anticipated. This prompt action will eliminate weeks of morbidity as well as damage to the collateral lymphatic channels. It is, of course, far preferable to prevent skin necrosis in the first place by utilizing a skin graft during the primary operation whenever excessive tension is observed during the skin closure.

Wound Infection

Wound infection is uncommon in the absence of skin necrosis.

Seromas

Seromas, collections of serum beneath the skin flap, occur in the first few weeks following mastectomy when there has been failure of the skin flap to become adherent to the chest wall. This appears to be more common in obese patients. Treatment consists of aspirating the serum every 3–5 days. On rare occasions this process may continue for several months. In such a case, it is preferable to make an incision with local anesthesia and insert a latex drain. Repeated aspiration over a period of many weeks may result in infection of the seroma.

Lymphedema

Lymphedema of the arm is more common in obese patients, in those who have had radiotherapy to the axilla, and in those who have experienced skin necrosis, wound infection, or cellulitis of the arm. Treat cellulitis of the arm promptly with antibiotics. Lymphedema in the absence of any sign of infection is treated as soon as it is detected by the application of a Jobst elastic sleeve, which applies a pressure of 50 mm of mercury over the course of the forearm and arm. These sleeves should be changed whenever they lose their elasticity, generally after 6 weeks. This kind of treatment should be instituted whenever one detects an increase in circumference of the arm 2 cm or more. Generally, elastic compression will keep the condition under control if it has not already been long neglected. Once the edema has been permitted to remain for many months, subcutaneous fibrosis replaces the edema and makes it irreversible. Intermittent pneumatic compression has been recommended, but few patients will tolerate the many hours a day of intermittent compression which are necessary before significant progress is demonstrated in long-standing edema. Prompt treatment of the hand or arm with antibiotics and early application of elastic compression is helpful in preventing and controlling edema.

References

Durkin K, Haagensen CD (1980) An improved technique for the study of lymph nodes in surgical specimens. Ann Surg 191:419

Handley RS (1976) The conservative radical mastectomy of Patey: 10-year results in 425 patients. Breast 2:16

Lotze MT, Duncan MA, Gerber LH, Woltering EA, et al. (1981) Early versus delayed shoulder motion following axillary dissection, a randomized prospective study. Ann Surg 193:288

41

46 Radical Mastectomy

Indications

Radical mastectomy is preferable to the Patey modification in patients who have relatively large tumors, especially when they are close to or when they invade the pectoral fascia.

Preoperative Care

Same as for the Patey operation (see Chap. 45).

Pitfalls and Danger Points

Same as for the Patey operation (see Chap. 45).

Operative Strategy

After elevating the skin flaps by the usual technique, the radical mastectomy can be accomplished in one of two sequences. In the technique described below, the axillary lymphadenectomy precedes removal of the breast from the chest wall. It is also feasible to remove the breast and the major pectoral muscle from the chest wall prior to doing the axillary dissection, a sequence that is observed in the Patey operation. Proponents of the latter sequence feel that it reduces the incidence of tumor emboli caused by traction applied to the specimen.

When the breast is removed going from medial to lateral, gravity provides sufficient retraction. Since there are no data available comparing these two sequences, each surgeon will base his choice on personal preference.

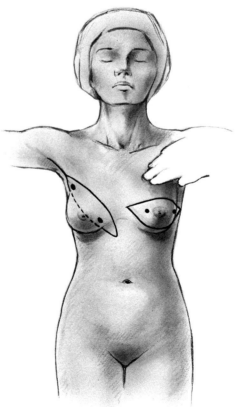

Fig. 46–1

Operative Technique

Incision

The principles underlying the choice of an incision for radical mastectomy are the same as those for the Patey operation (**Fig. 46–1**). Also, see Figs. 45–1 to 45–5.

Elevation of Skin Flaps

Same as for the Patey operation (see Chap. 45).

Exposing the Axilla

To perform a complete axillary lymphadenectomy, it is not necessary to remove that portion of the major pectoral muscle which arises from the clavicle. On the other hand, preservation of the clavicular head of this muscle improves the cosmetic appearance of the upper chest wall. Consequently, develop a line of separation by blunt dissection between the sternal and clavicular heads of the pectoral muscle. Continue this separation to the point where the major pectoral muscle inserts upon the humerus. Place the left index finger underneath the sternal head of the muscle near its insertion and divide the muscle from its insertion with the electrocoagulating current (**Fig. 46–2**). Complete the line of division between the two heads of the muscle going in a medial direction until the sternum is reached. A number of lateral anterior tho-

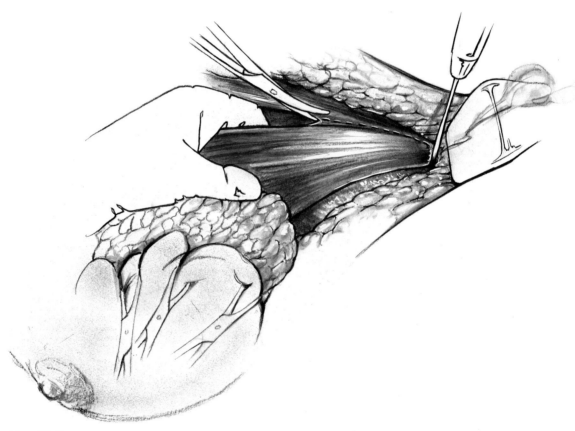

Fig. 46–2

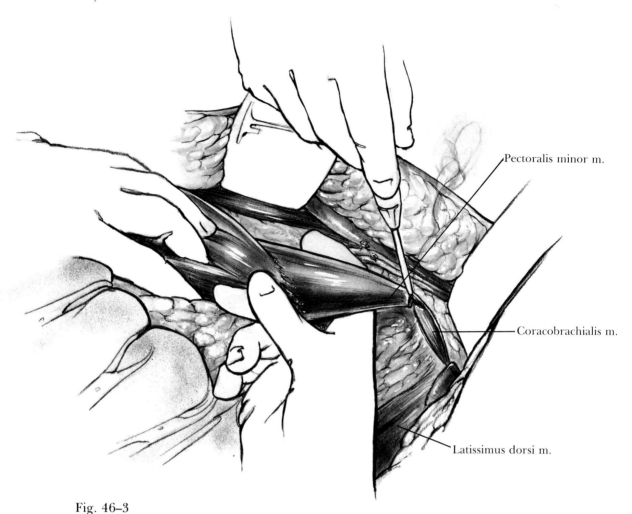

Pectoralis minor m.

Coracobrachialis m.

Latissimus dorsi m.

Fig. 46–3

racic arteries, veins, and nerves will be divided between Hemoclips during this dissection. Also detach the upper 2–3 cm of the major pectoral muscle from the upper sternal region.

Incise the areolar tissue and fascia over the surface of the coracobrachial muscle and continue in a medial direction until the coracoid process is reached. This will expose where the junction is between the coracobrachial muscle and the insertion of the minor pectoral muscle **(Fig. 46–3)**. Just caudal to the coracobrachial muscle are the structures contained in the axilla, namely, the brachial plexus and the axillary artery and vein. They are covered not only by fat and lymphatic tissue, but also by a thin

layer of costocoracoid fascia. Clearing the fascia away from the inferior border of the coracobrachial muscle serves to unroof the axilla as well as to expose the insertion of the minor pectoral muscle. Detach this muscle from its insertion after isolating it by encircling it with the index finger; use the coagulating current to divide the muscle near the coracoid process **(Fig. 46–3)**. A pad of fat overlying the axillary vein near the entrance of the cephalic branch can be swept downward by blunt dissection, exposing the axillary vein.

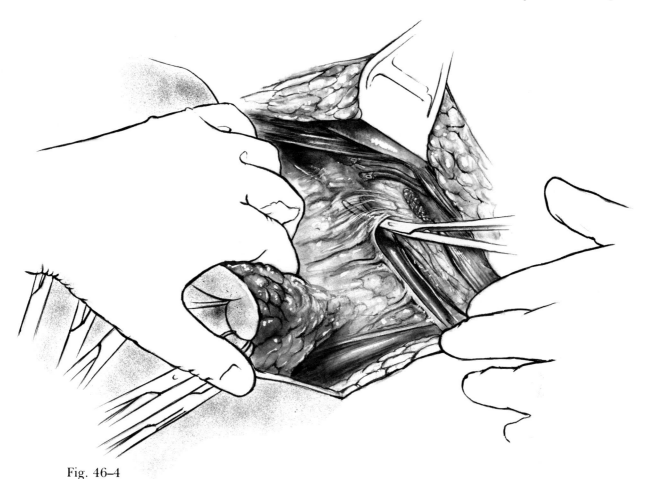

Fig. 46–4

Dissecting the Axillary Vein

It is not necessary to clean all of the fat off the brachial plexus or to remove tissue cephalad to the axillary vein. Pick up the sheath of the axillary vein with a Brown-Adson or DeBakey forceps and use a Metzenbaum scissors to separate the adventitia from underlying vein **(Fig. 46–4).** Once the unopened scissors has been inserted underneath the adventitia to establish the plane, remove the scissors and then insert one blade of the scissors under this tissue. Close the scissors, dividing the adventitia. Continue this dissection along the anterior wall of the axillary vein from the region of the latissimus muscle to the clavicle. The only structures crossing anterior to the axillary vein will be some thoracoacromial, lateral anterior thoracic, and pectoral blood vessels and nerves. Divide these structures between ligatures or Hemoclips. At the conclusion of this step, the branches of the axillary vein will have been fairly well skeletonized. Now divide each of the branches of the axillary vein that comes

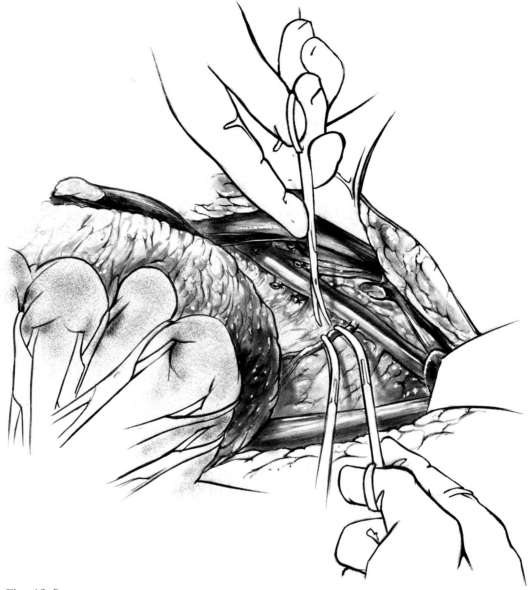

Fig. 46–5

from below, using Hemoclips or 3–0 PG ligatures **(Fig. 46–5).**

At this point use some silk sutures to apply labels to mark the apex and the lateral portion of the lymphadenectomy specimen.

Dissecting the Chest Wall

Make a scalpel incision through the clavipectoral fascia just inferior to the medial portion of the axillary vein **(Fig. 46–6).** This will clear fat and lymphatic tissue from the upper chest wall. Continue this dissec-

tion laterally until the subscapular space has been reached. Then clear the areolar tissue from the subscapular space by using a gauze pad, bluntly dissecting from above downward. This maneuver will reveal the location of the long thoracic nerve descending from the brachial plexus in apposition to the lateral aspect of the thoracic cage. Preserve this nerve. Identify the thoracodorsal nerve that crosses the subscapular vein and travels 2 or 3 cm laterally to-

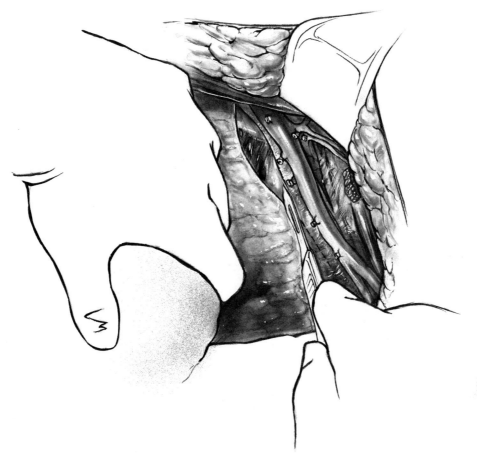

Fig. 46–6

gether with the artery and vein supplying the latissimus dorsi muscle (**Fig. 46–7**). In the absence of obvious lymph node metastases in this area, dissect out the thoracodorsal nerve down to its junction with the serratus muscle.

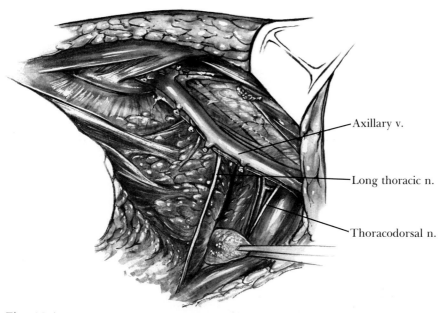

Axillary v.

Long thoracic n.

Thoracodorsal n.

Fig. 46–7

47

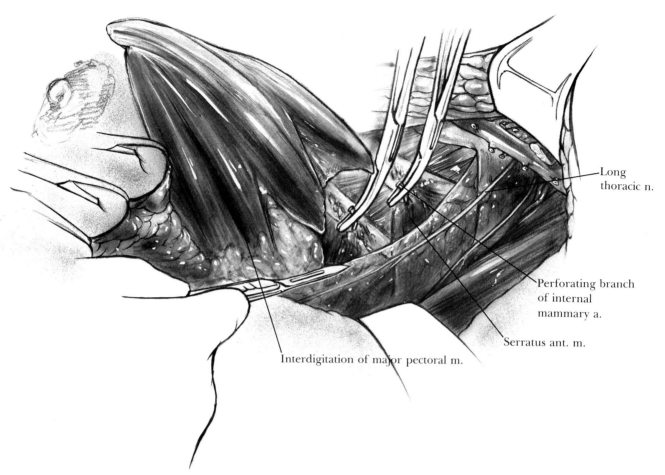

Long
thoracic n.

Perforating branch
of internal
mammary a.

Serratus ant. m.

Interdigitation of major pectoral m.

Fig. 46–8

If the anterior border of the latissimus muscle has not yet been thoroughly exposed, complete this maneuver now. The entire lymphadenectomy specimen should be freed from the axillary vein, the upper anterior chest wall, and the anterior border of the latissimus muscle.

Detaching the Specimen

Keeping the long thoracic nerve in view, make an incision in the fascia of the anterior serratus muscle on a line parallel to and 1 cm medial to this nerve. Elevate the fascia by dissecting in a medial direction exposing the underlying muscle until the interdigitations of the pectoral muscles are encountered **(Fig. 46–8).** Detach these muscles from their points of origin with the electrocautery. Apply small hemostats to each bleeding vessel. Try to avoid including any extraneous tissue in the hemostat other than the blood vessel. If this is accomplished, each of the blood vessels on the chest wall may be occluded by applying the coagulating current to each hemostat at the conclusion of the dissection. As the pectoral muscles are divided, leave about 0.5 cm of muscle tissue on the rib cage as this will facilitate applying the hemostats to the perforating branches of the internal mammary vessel. If these are divided flush with their point of emergence from the chest wall, they will often retract into the chest, which makes hemostasis difficult and increases the risk of pneumothorax. Continue the retraction in a medial direction of the pectoral muscles and the attached breast, proceeding until all of the internal mammary branches have been clamped and divided and the dissection has been completed at the border of the ster-

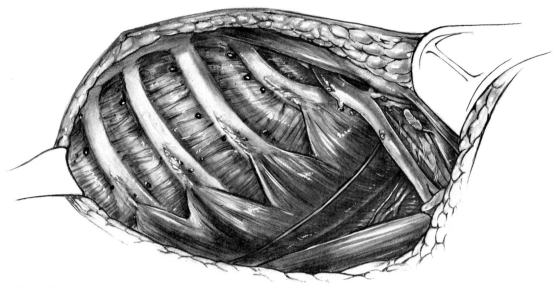

Fig. 46–9

num. Then remove the specimen and electrocoagulate each of the hemostats. Ascertain that hemostasis is complete. Then irrigate the entire operative field with ster-

ile water in the attempt to wash out detached tissue and malignant cells. (**Fig. 46–9**).

Closure of Incision and Insertion of Drains

Same as for the Patey operation (**Fig. 46–10**).

Full-thickness Skin Graft

Whenever an area of excessive tension is encountered during the closure of the skin wound by means of suturing, leave this portion of the incision unsutured. Measure the defect and determine if there is sufficient redundant skin in other areas of the skin flaps which may be excised, defatted, and transplanted into the defect. In order to expedite the defatting of skin to be grafted, it is helpful to pin one edge of the skin patch down to a sterile board. Then grasp the fat with the forceps and use a large scalpel blade to dissect all of the fat off the skin. Sometimes a few remaining bits of fat may be excised with a curved Metzenbaum scissors. When a patch of skin has been sufficiently defatted to convert it into a full-thickness graft, the undersurface of the skin assumes a characteristic pitted appearance. Then place the

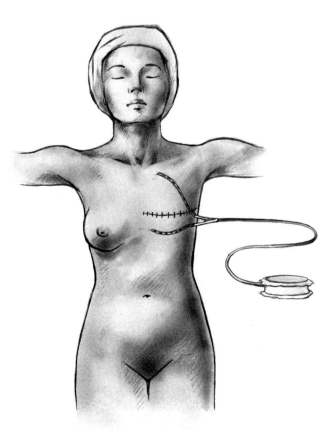

Fig. 46–10

49

full-thickness skin graft into the defect and tailor its dimensions so that there is mild tension on the graft after it is sutured into place.

First suture the edges of the skin down to the chest wall musculature with interrupted 3–0 silk. Use about six such sutures to fix the skin edges down to the chest wall to stabilize the perimeter of the defect. Then insert a continuous over-and-over suture of atraumatic 5–0 nylon to attach the skin graft to the edges of the skin defect using small bites. Skin staples are another good method of fixing the graft in place.

Make multiple puncture wounds in the skin graft with a No. 10 scalpel blade to permit seepage of serum from the wound through the graft. Over the skin graft apply a single layer of iodophor gauze. Over this, place a small mass of gauze fluffs. Then tie the long ends of the previously placed silk sutures over the gauze stent in order to fix the skin graft in position with some pressure.

This step may be accelerated by omitting sutures entirely and fixing the skin graft in place either with Steristrip adhesive tapes or skin staples. Then the gauze fluffs are taped into place over the graft.

Split-Thickness Skin Graft

When there is no surplus of skin on the chest wall to be harvested for a skin graft, use an electric dermatome to obtain a split-thickness graft from the anterolateral portion of the upper thigh. After this area has been cleansed with soap and an iodophor solution has been applied, dry the area and apply a sterile lubricating solution of mineral oil. Then have the assistants stretch the skin by applying traction in opposite directions with wooden tongue depressors. Set the electric dermatome so that the graft will be 0.015 inches in thickness. Apply the dermatome to the surface of the skin with firm pressure and start the motor. Apply even pressure and move the dermatome in a cephalad direction. It may be helpful for the scrub nurse to pick up the cut edge of the graft with two forceps while the sur-

geon continues to operate the dermatome until an adequate patch of skin has been obtained. Place the skin graft in a normal saline solution temporarily. Apply a single layer of coarse gauze anointed in iodophor ointment to the donor site over which apply a moist sterile gauze laparotomy pad.

Suture the skin graft into the defect as described above.

Postoperative Care

With reference to the skin graft, unless there are signs of infection, do not remove the gauze stent for 5–7 days. After this, the healing skin graft may be left exposed or covered with a loose dry dressing.

Remove the dressing from the donor site, with the exception of the single layer of iodophor gauze, on the day following operation. We prefer to leave this area exposed to the air. Use an electric hair dryer on the donor site intermittently to accelerate the formation of a solid crust over this area. As this crust begins to loosen around its periphery at the end of about 3 weeks, gradually trim that portion of the crust and the attached layer of gauze with a scissors.

See also the section on postoperative care following the Patey operation (Chap. 45).

Postoperative Complications

See discussion of postoperative complications following the Patey operation (Chap. 45).

With reference to the skin graft, complications include infection of the grafted area and occasionally of the donor site. Failure of a complete "take" is generally due to hematoma or serum collecting underneath the graft and separating it from its bed. This can be prevented by careful hemostasis at the time of surgery and also by making several perforations with a scalpel blade to permit the seepage of serum.

Biliary Tract

47 Concept: When to Remove the Gallbladder

Mortality Following Cholecystectomy

Despite the potential risk of surgical errors, which may produce complications of a horrendous nature, cholecystectomy in the hands of a skilled surgical team is followed by a remarkably low mortality rate. In a review of 1,100 cholecystectomies without common bile duct (CBD) exploration performed (1969–1980) for nonmalignant gallbladder disease, including acute cholecystitis, by the residents and staff of the Booth Memorial Medical Center in Flushing, New York, the hospital mortality was 0.25%. Martin and van Heerden reported a 0.3% rate for 586 cholecystectomies for chronic cholecystitis and 2.1% for acute cholecystitis. McSherry and Glenn found a 0.5% hospital mortality rate following cholecystectomy for chronic disease of the biliary tract; in patients under age 50 the mortality rate was 0.1%, while those over age 50 experienced a rate of 0.9%. In studying cholecystectomy for acute cholecystitis, the same authors found a mortality rate of 1.3% for the entire group of 1,643 cases: under age 50, 0.4% died while over age 50 the rate was 2.2%. These authors surveyed 11,808 patients who underwent surgery from 1932 to 1978. It is our experience that in the modern era improved monitoring of cardiorespiratory dynamics has markedly reduced the risk of elective surgery in the aged population, and we did not find a significant increase in the fatality rate after cholecystectomy in the patients over 50 as compared to those under the age of 50.

More important in its influence on surgical mortality is the addition of choledocholithotomy to simple cholecystectomy. The Booth Memorial Medical Center mortality for the latter operation was 2.5%, a tenfold increase over the risk of simple cholecystectomy. One third of the deaths were due to acute pancreatitis following manipulation of the common bile duct for the extraction of calculi. In municipal hospitals, where the patient population contains a higher percentage of patients with acute suppurative cholangitis or other types of advanced sepsis than are to be found in voluntary hospitals, the mortality rate of CBD explorations is often much higher than 2.5%.

Not only is the magnitude of choledocholithotomy considerably greater than that of cholecystectomy but the patient suffering from CBD stones tends to be much older and to have had biliary tract disease for a longer period of time. Also, virulent bacteria are found in the bile much more frequently when stones are present in the CBD. The striking increase in mortality for choledocholithotomy as compared with cholecystectomy is one of the strongest arguments for the early removal of gallbladders that contain calculi.

Symptomatic Cholelithiasis

Symptoms Produced by Gallstones

When a gallbladder stone becomes impacted in the orifice of the cystic duct, the classical symptoms of "gallbladder colic" are produced. This symptom complex consists of intermittent colicky pain, generally of sudden onset, located most frequently in the high epigastrium and radiating directly to the back or to the right scapula. The initial episode of pain may last 1–8 hours to be followed by a period of respite. The cycle may be repeated several times. Often, a single injection of Demerol will terminate the attack of biliary colic. Most episodes of biliary colic terminate within 12 hours either because the stone passes through the cystic duct or because the stone falls back out of the cystic duct into the gallbladder.

Other symptoms, that have long been attributed to gallbladder disease, such as fatty food intolerance, belching, excessive flatus, or flatulent dyspepsia, *are not due to gallstones or to cholecystitis.* Because removal of the gallbladder cannot be expected to relieve these symptoms, the patient will generally be disappointed following cholecystectomy if he has been told something to the contrary. On the other hand, cholecystectomy does relieve gallbladder colic.

Diagnosis of Cholelithiasis

An oral cholecystogram X ray can confirm the diagnosis of cholelithiasis by demonstrating the calculi. When the cholecystogram shows no gallbladder visualization after a second dose of dye, this, too, confirms the diagnosis of gallstones unless the radiographic contrast tablets have been lost by vomiting or diarrhea, or unless the patient has a significant bilirubin elevation. We do not consider it necessary to perform either a sonogram or an intravenous cholangiogram in cases of nonvisualization if the patient has symptoms characteristic of gallbladder colic.

In the hands of experienced technical personnel, sonography also can confirm the diagnosis of gallstones in 95% of cases. If the technician operating the sonographic equipment is not highly skilled, then this procedure is less accurate than the oral cholecystogram.

Use of the computerized tomographic (CT) scan is not indicated for the diagnosis of gallstones because calculi that do not contain calcium will not be detected by this device.

Biliary Colic with Negative Cholecystogram and Sonogram; the Cholecystoses

About 3%–5% of patients with normal cholecystograms and an equal number with normal sonograms do indeed have gallstones, generally of small size. Consequently, the surgeon will occasionally encounter a patient with classical symptoms of biliary colic, who nevertheless has normal X rays and sonograms. While some of these patients are suffering from undetected gallstones, others may be experiencing their symptoms due to one of the "cholecytoses," noncalculous diseases of the gallbladder such as cholesterosis or cholecystitis glandularis proliferans. In this group of patients, if they suffer repeated episodes of typical gallbladder colic, cholecystectomy is indicated even in the presence of normal X ray and sonographic studies.

Atypical Pain with Negative Cholecystogram

When a patient has chronic, recurrent, ill-defined upper abdominal pain, and the X ray and sonographic studies are normal, cholecystectomy is not indicated. These patients require careful gastroenterological studies, including upper gastrointestinal and barium colon enema X rays, gastroscopy, and liver function tests. The symptoms in most of these patients will be found to be functional in origin, although in a few cases the symptoms may be atypical manifestations of biliary tract calculi. Occasionally an endoscopic radiographic cholangiopancreatogram (ERCP) will disclose calculi in the CBD or even in the gallbladder when previously the cholecystogram and the sonogram were normal. Some surgeons believe that symptomatic noncalculous cholecystitis can be detected by the use of cholecystokinin cholangiogram X ray because the hormone cholecystokinin, by inducing contraction of the gallbladder, will reproduce the patient's symptoms. We do not believe that the data reported in support of this procedure are convincing.

Asymptomatic Cholelithiasis

Occasionally the diagnosis of gallstones will be made by X ray or sonogram in a patient who has no symptoms. There has been considerable debate concerning whether such a patient should have a "prophylactic" cholecystectomy under these conditions. It is our opinion that many of these patients will develop serious complications from their biliary calculi over a period of years and that a healthy patient should undergo cholecystectomy if he has gallstones, providing that the surgeon can perform this procedure with minimal risk. A contrary opinion is expressed by Gracie and Ranshoff after studying 123 male university faculty members; in this group the probability of developing biliary pain was 18% after 20 years.

Acute Obstructive Cholecystitis

Pathogenesis and Diagnosis

In 95% of cases, acute obstructive cholecystitis results from impaction of a calculus in the cystic duct. At first, this impaction produces the classical picture of biliary colic. When the stone remains impacted for a period of 24–48 hours, acute inflammation of the gallbladder wall develops. After a few days, the gallbladder bile be-

comes infected, presumably by migration of intestinal bacteria through the biliary lymphatics. Occasionally necrosis of the gallbladder wall produces perforation. This is generally walled off by adjacent colon or omentum. In about 2% of cases, a free perforation of the gallbladder occurs, causing a generalized bile peritonitis. This complication has a high mortality rate.

A typical patient with acute cholecystitis will present with fever, leukocytosis, and a tender globular mass in the right upper quadrant. The most rapid confirmatory procedure is a Technetium Tc 99m dimethyl acetanilid imine diacetic acid (HIDA) or similar nuclear scan. This study should demonstrate radioactivity in the CBD but none in the gallbladder. Under these conditions, one can diagnose complete cystic duct obstruction, which confirms the diagnosis of acute cholecystitis.

Sonography may demonstrate gallstones and even thickening of the gallbladder wall. In many patients, an oral cholecystogram may be performed even in the presence of acute cholecystitis, providing the patient is not nauseated and is able to take the contrast medium by mouth. Failure of the gallbladder to visualize is confirmatory evidence of gallbladder disease. An intravenous cholangiogram (IVC) that demonstrates dye in the CBD but fails to visualize the gallbladder is also confirmatory evidence of acute cholecystitis, but the IVC X-ray procedure is quite cumbersome to perform, especially in a patient who is obese or distended. The PIPIDA or HIDA nuclear scan is by far the best method of confirming the diagnosis of acute cholecystitis.

Early versus Late Operation for Acute Cholecystitis

When to operate on patients with acute cholecystitis has long been a point of controversy. Some surgeons believe in treating the acute episode conservatively with nasogastric suction and antibiotics, postponing cholecystectomy for 4–6 weeks in the expectation that the operation will be both technically simpler and safer after the delay. On the other hand, we have found that cholecystectomy, performed 24–48 hours after hospital admission, permits adequate time for diagnostic study, fluid replacement, diabetic regulation, and fine tuning of the cardiovascular function, while at the same time eliminating a long period of convalescence from the episode of acute cholecystitis and then a second period of convalescence a month or two later following the delayed operation. Our mortality rate for early cholecystectomy has been identical with that following elective cholecystectomy. Operations in the early period following the onset of acute cholecystitis are in fact not technically difficult in most cases. Some patients do indeed have marked inflammation, fibrosis, or localized perforation, which makes the operation difficult. However, this type of pathology is not always improved by a delay of even 6–8 weeks.

We agree with Jarvinen and Hastbacka that not only is early operation safe if done by a surgeon experienced in this type of surgery but such an operation also markedly shortens the period of illness experienced by the patient. These authors, in a prospective randomized clinical trial comparing early cholecystectomy versus operation delayed for 2–4 months, found no significant difference in 1) the operative mortality or 2) the incidence of technical difficulty. Postoperative morbidity was significantly greater after delayed operation. Also, 13% of patients assigned to the delayed group required emergency operations for spreading peritonitis, cholangitis, or unresolving gallbladder empyema. An additional 15% of the patients undergoing delayed cholecystectomy suffered attacks of recurrent acute cholecystitis, pancreatitis, or biliary colic while awaiting surgery. Finally, patients in the delayed group required an average of 7.5 days of increased

hospitalization and lost 14.4 additional days of employment compared to those undergoing early cholecystectomy. In 100 consecutive cholecystectomies for acute cholecystitis, which we have performed within 1–5 days of admission no fatalities nor any CBD injuries occurred.

Indications for Cholecystostomy

Although experienced surgeons may find it necessary to perform a cholecystostomy in only 1%–2% of operations for acute cholecystitis, there should be no hesitation on the part of any surgeon to perform a cholecystostomy when he feels that, for technical reasons, there will be a risk of damage to the bile ducts or any other vital structures if he attempts to perform a cholecystectomy. On rare occasions one will encounter a patient with advanced cardiac or other systemic disease in whom the surgeon may decide preoperatively that cholecystostomy is the operation of choice. A liberal incision and general anesthesia will be necessary if one desires to remove all of the calculi from the gallbladder and the cystic duct; this is difficult to accomplish through a small incision made with local anesthesia.

In summary, we believe a cholecystectomy should be performed on a patient diagnosed as having acute cholecystitis within a few days of hospital admission rather than delayed in the hope of making the operation easier at a later date.

Hyperamylasemia

Some patients with acute obstructive cholecystitis present with marked elevations of the serum amylase level. In most cases there will be no clinical signs of acute pancreatitis. For instance, there will be no epigastric or left upper quadrant tenderness and rigidity; there will be no hypotension or oliguria or other signs of a large shift of extracellular fluid into the "third space"; there will be no hypocalcemia and hyperglycemia. When the clinical diagnosis of acute obstructive cholecystitis has been confirmed by one of the tests mentioned above in patients without symptoms of acute pancreatitis, the elevation in serum amylase should not be a contraindication to early cholecystectomy, since most of the patients with these manifestations do not, in fact, have evidence of acute pancreatitis when the pancreas is observed at laparotomy.

If, on the other hand, one observes at operation a *normal* gallbladder with an acutely inflamed pancreas, the proper procedure is simply to close the abdomen without any further dissection. Do not drain the gallbladder, the CBD, the lesser sac, or the retropancreatic space. The inflamed pancreas should neither be disturbed nor drained. If the patient has more than three grave signs (Ranson, Rifkind, Roses, Fink, et al.), then a peritoneal dialysis catheter can be inserted at operation prior to closing the abdomen without any other drains. Inserting a drain in a patient, mistakenly operated on early in the course of acute pancreatitis, serves only to increase the incidence of pancreatic abscess, and there are no data to suggest that the drain has any beneficial effect.

Acalculous Acute Cholecystitis

There is a group of patients who suffer from acalculous acute cholecystitis, often following major surgery unrelated to the biliary tract, or following trauma, burns, or other serious illnesses. Because of the antecedent illness, the diagnosis of acute cholecystitis is often overlooked or not even considered by the attending physician. Another instance where this type of acute cholecystitis occurs is in a patient who has been fed parenterally for a prolonged period of time and who then begins to eat. The pathogenesis of this disease

is not clear. In some instances it may be related to the "low flow" state combined with the stasis of bile.

In any case, a high index of suspicion is necessary for early diagnosis in this group of patients. There is a high incidence of gangrene or free perforation of the gallbladder because the progress of the disease in acalculous acute cholecystitis appears to be much more rapid than in acute obstructive cholecystitis. Conservative treatment is *not* indicated in these patients. Prompt cholecystectomy is mandatory. Otherwise the mortality rate will be exceedingly high. It is not at this time clear whether the HIDA scan or the sonogram are of great diagnostic value in these patients. Operation must be performed, in general, on the clinical findings.

Gallstone Pancreatitis

Acute pancreatitis in the nonalcoholic patient generally follows the passage of a relatively small calculus through the CBD and ampulla. This hypothesis has been supported by the finding of gallstones in the stool of patients admitted with nonalcoholic acute pancreatitis. In almost all of these cases there are additional calculi in the gallbladder. However, it is the *exceptional* patient with acute gallstone pancreatitis who also suffers from an impacted CBD stone. Traditional management of acute gallstone pancreatitis consisted of the usual treatment of acute pancreatitis by means of intravenous fluids, nasogastric suction, and antibiotics until all signs of the acute process had subsided. Then the patient was generally discharged from the hospital with instructions to return in 4–6 weeks for cholecystectomy.

In our experience and in the experience of others "20–30% of these patients would develop recurrent acute pancreatitis during this period of delay" (Paloyan, Simonowitz, and Skinner). Studies by Ranson and by Tondelli, Stutz, Harder, Shupisser, and colleagues also agree with this concept. Consequently, as soon as the acute pancreatitis has subsided and after the diagnosis of cholelithiasis has been confirmed, either by oral cholecystogram X rays or by a gallbladder sonogram, cholecystectomy and cystic duct cholangiography are performed. This is about 2 weeks from the date of admission in the average case. Of course, there are some cases of gallstone pancreatitis that may be extremely severe, even life threatening. These patients may take a number of weeks before all the signs of acute pancreatitis subside, and in these cases cholecystectomy should be delayed. This type of patient will generally have three or more of the grave signs listed by Ranson and colleagues.

Incidental Cholecystectomy

A patient undergoing surgery for hiatus hernia, duodenal ulcer, or colon cancer, who also has symptomatic gallstones, should have his gallbladder removed if the primary surgery has gone smoothly and if the patient is a good risk. When gallstones are discovered during the course of another operation and there has been no history of gallbladder symptoms, the decision whether or not to perform incidental cholecystectomy is more controversial. In general, in a good-risk patient, whose primary operation has gone smoothly without significant contamination, we remove the gallbladder as a prophylactic measure if the incision for the primary operation provides excellent exposure as well for the cholecystectomy. We have not found that this adds to the risk or the morbidity of the primary operation. In the patient with nonsymptomatic gallstones, we do not perform routine cholangiography during incidental cholecystectomy.

References

Gracie WA, Ranshoff DF (1982) The natural history of silent gallstones. N Eng J Med 307:798

Jarvinen HJ, Hastbacka J (1980) Early cholecystectomy for acute cholecystitis. Ann Surg 191:501

Martin JK Jr, van Heerden JA (1980) Surgery of the liver, biliary tract, and pancreas. Mayo Clin Proc 55:333

McSherry CK, Glenn F (1980) The incidence and causes of death following surgery for non-malignant biliary tract disease. Ann Surg 191:271

Paloyan D, Simonowitz D, Skinner DB (1975) The timing of biliary tract operations in patients with pancreatitis associated with gallstones. Surg Gynecol Obstet 141:737

Ranson JHC, Rifkind KM, Roses DF, Fink SD, et al. (1974) Prognostic signs and the role of operative management in acute pancreatitis. Surg Gynecol Obstet 139:69

Ranson JHC (1974) The timing of biliary surgery in acute pancreatitis. Ann Surg 189:654

Tondelli P, Stutz K, Harder F, Shupisser J-P, et al. (1982) Acute gallstone pancreatitis: best timing for biliary surgery. Br J Surg 69:709

48 Cholecystectomy

Indications

(See Chap. 47.)

Gallbladder calculi

Acute cholecystitis, both calculous and noncalculous

Chronic noncalculous cholecystoses and cholesterosis, when accompanied by symptoms of gallbladder colic

Carcinoma of gallbladder

Preoperative Care

Diagnostic confirmation of gallbladder disease as discussed above in Chap. 47

Perioperative antibiotics in patients suspected of having acute cholecystitis or choledocholithiasis and in patients undergoing simple cholecystectomy, if over age 70

Nasogastric tube for patients with acute cholecystitis or coledocholithiasis

Pitfalls and Danger Points

Injury to bile ducts

Injury to hepatic artery or portal vein

Hemorrhage from cystic or hepatic artery, or from liver bed

Injury to duodenum or colon

Operative Strategy

Anomalies of the Extrahepatic Bile Ducts

Anomalies, major and minor, of the extrahepatic bile ducts are quite common. A surgeon who is not aware of the variational anatomy of these ducts is much more prone to injure them during biliary surgery. The most common anomaly is a right segmental hepatic duct that drains the dorsal caudal segment of the right lobe. This segmental duct may drain into the right hepatic duct, the common hepatic duct **(Fig. 48–1a),** the cystic duct **(Fig. 48–1b),** or into the common bile duct **(Fig. 48–1c).** Division of this segmental duct may result in a postoperative bile fistula that drains

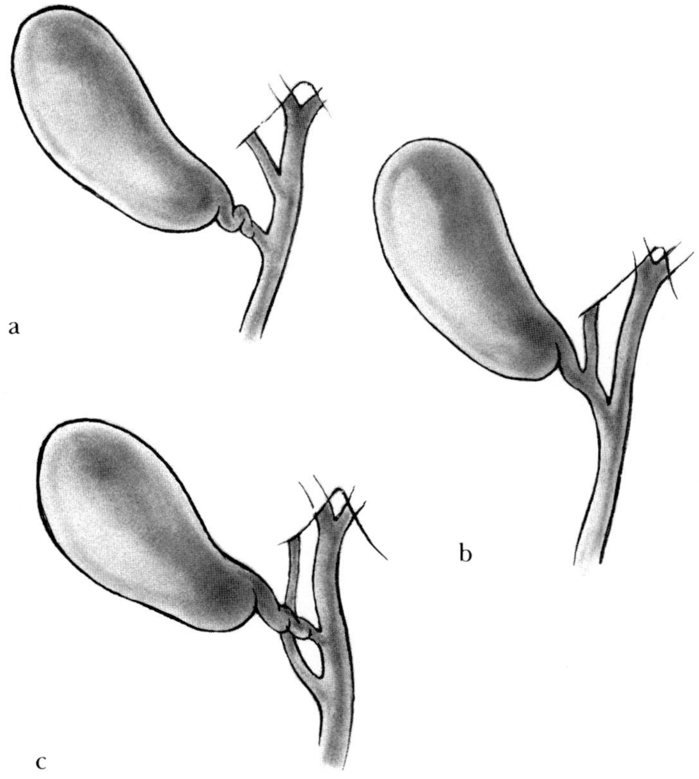

Fig. 48–1   Anomalous segmental right hepatic ducts

as much as 500 ml of bile per day. Long-mire and Tompkins advocate ligating a damaged segmental duct rather than attempting an anastomosis because, "unless unobstructed, uninfected biliary flow can be achieved through a segmental or lobar duct, it is better that the duct be completely obstructed and the affected liver parenchyma allowed to atrophy, provided there is normal biliary flow from the residual 50% of liver." If a small duct of this type is anastomosed and if the anastomosis becomes stenotic, cholangitis and liver abscess are apt to develop. Longmire and Tompkins assert that the same policy may be applied to either the right or the left main lobar duct. If such a duct is damaged in the operating room and there is no infection, it may be safely ligated because, "unobstructed drainage of 50% of an otherwise normal liver through either the right

or left uninfected hepatic duct is adequate to restore normal liver function, even if the obstructed lobe remains in place." In some of the cases that these authors reported, a bile fistula nevertheless ensued following deliberate ligature of a segmental duct. However, bile drainage eventually ceased, presumably owing to fibrotic obstruction of the duct, and no infection developed. It is, of course, far preferable to identify these anomalies in the operating room and to avoid injuring the ducts.

Important cystic duct anomalies (**Fig. 48–2**) include the entrance of the cystic duct into the right hepatic duct (**Fig. 24–2e**) a low entrance of the cystic duct which occasionally joins the CBD rather close to the ampulla (**Fig. 48–2c**) and a cystic duct that enters the left side of the CBD (**Fig. 48–2f**).

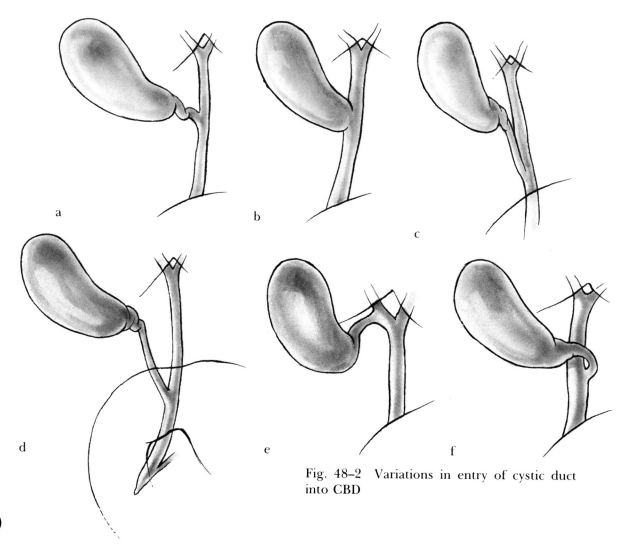

Fig. 48–2 Variations in entry of cystic duct into CBD

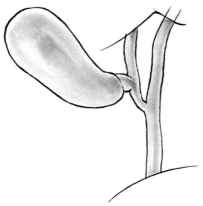

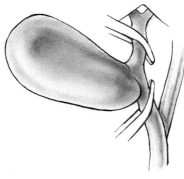

Fig. 48–4

Fig. 48–3 Anomalous entry of right hepatic duct into cystic duct

Another extremely important anomaly of which the surgeon should be aware is the apparent entrance of the right main hepatic duct into the cystic duct. The latter duct, in turn, joins the left hepatic duct to form the CBD. This is illustrated in **Fig. 48–3.** In this case, dividing and ligating the cystic duct at its apparent point of origin early in the operation will result in occluding the right hepatic duct. If the technique that is described in the next section is carefully followed, this accident can be avoided.

Avoiding Injury to the Bile Ducts

Most serious injuries of the bile ducts are not caused by congenital anomalies or by unusually severe pathological changes. In most cases iatrogenic trauma results because the surgeon who mistakenly ligates and divides the CBD thinks that it is the cystic duct. It is important to remember that the diameter of the normal CBD may vary from 2 to 15 mm (Longmire). It is easy to clamp, divide, and ligate a small CBD as the first step in cholecystectomy under the erroneous impression that it is the cystic duct. The surgeon who makes this mistake will also have to divide the common hepatic duct before the gallbladder is freed from all its attachments. This will leave a 2–4 cm segment of common and hepatic duct attached to the specimen

(Fig. 48–4). Because this is the most common cause of serious duct injury, *we never permit the cystic duct to be either clamped or divided until the entire gallbladder has been dissected free down to its junction with the cystic duct.* Division of the cystic duct is always the very last step in the cholecystectomy. When the back wall of the gallbladder is being dissected away from the liver, it is important to carefully dissect out each structure that may enter the gallbladder from the liver. Generally, there are only a few minor blood vessels that may be divided by sharp dissection and then occluded by electrocoagulation. Any structure that resembles a bile duct must be carefully delineated by sharp dissection. In no case should the surgeon apply a hemostat to a large wad of tissue running from the liver to the gallbladder, as this may contain the common hepatic duct.

Although it has often been stated that there are anomalous bile ducts that enter the gallbladder directly from the liver bed, we have rarely in our experience encountered any such duct.

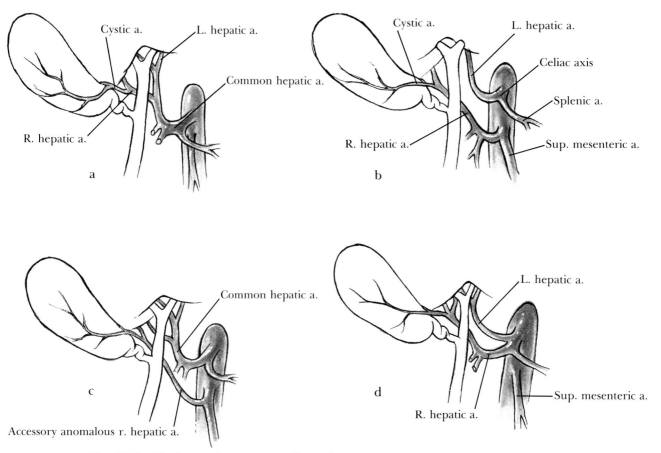

Fig. 48–5   Variations in anatomy of hepatic arteries

Ligating the Hepatic Artery Inadvertently

Careful dissection will prevent injury or inadvertent ligature of one of the hepatic arteries. However, in case one of these vessels should be ligated accidently, this complication is not ordinarily fatal because hepatic viability can usually be maintained by the remaining portal venous flow and by arterial collaterals, such as those from the under surface of the diaphragm. This is true only if the patient has normal hepatic function and there has been no jaundice, hemorrhage, shock, trauma, or sepsis. Generally, based on findings from experimental work on animals, antibiotics are administered in cases of this type. However, the necessity for antibiotic therapy has not been firmly established in humans.

In some of the reports on hepatic dearterialization for the treatment of metastatic cancer to the liver, there has not been a high mortality rate. On the other hand, neither has the mortality rate been 0%. Consequently, if a major lobar hepatic or the common hepatic artery has been inadvertently divided or ligated, an end-to-end arterial reconstruction may be performed if local factors are favorable. For other branches of the hepatic artery, arterial reconstruction is not necessary (Brittain, Marchioro, Hermann, Waddell, and associates). Variations in the anatomy of the hepatic arteries are shown in **Fig. 48–5.**

Avoiding Hemorrhage

In most cases, hemorrhage during the course of cholecystectomy is due to inadvertent laceration of the cystic artery. Often the stump of the bleeding vessel will retract into the fat in the vicinity of the hepatic duct and make accurate clamping difficult. If the bleeding artery is not distinctly visible, do not apply any hemostats. Rather, grasp the hepatoduodenal ligament between the index finger and thumb of the left hand and compress the common hepatic artery. This will stop the bleeding temporarily. Now check whether the exposure is adequate and whether the anesthesiologist has provided good muscle relaxation. If necessary, have the first assistant enlarge the incision appropriately. After adequate exposure has been achieved, it is generally possible to identify the bleeding vessel, which is then clamped and ligated. Occasionally the cystic artery has been torn off flush with the right hepatic artery. This will require that the defect in the right hepatic artery be closed with a continuous vascular suture such as 6–0 Tevdek. On rare occasions it may be helpful to occlude the hepatoduodenal ligament by the application of a noncrushing vascular clamp. It is safe to perform this maneuver for as long as 15–20 minutes.

The second major cause of bleeding during the course of performing a cholecystectomy is hemorrhage from the gallbladder bed in the liver. Bleeding occurs when the plane of dissection is too deep. This complication may be prevented if the plane is kept between the submucosa and the "serosa" of the gallbladder. If this layer of fibrous tissue is left behind on the liver, there will be no problem in controlling bleeding. With this plane intact, it is easy to see the individual bleeding points and to control them by electrocoagulation. Occasionally, a small artery requires a suture-ligature or a Hemoclip for hemostasis. With proper exposure, hemostasis should be perfect. On the other hand, when this fibrous plane has been removed with the gallbladder, and liver parenchyma is exposed, the surface is irregular and the blood vessels retract into the liver substance making electrocoagulation less effective. Blood may ooze from a large area. In this case, apply a layer of Surgicel or Avitene to the bleeding surface and cover it with a dry gauze pad; use a retractor to apply pressure to the gauze pad. After a period of 15 minutes, remove the gauze pad carefully. In most cases, it will also be possible carefully to remove the layer of Surgicel, if desired, although leaving a flat layer of oxidized cellulose over the liver bed has not proved harmful in our experience.

Cystic Duct Cholangiography

For the past 20 years the proper role of cystic duct cholangiography has been subject to considerable controversy. Most instances in which stones were left behind in the CBD following biliary tract surgery have occurred in patients who have had many calculi removed from the CBD. Consequently, all patients who have undergone choledocholithotomy should have a *completion* cholangiogram through the T-tube. Because instrumentation produces spasm of the ampulla, about one-quarter of these cases will not show passage of the dye into the duodenum on a *completion* cholangiogram. For this reason, we always perform a cystic duct cholangiogram *prior to* exploring the CBD. Failure of the dye to enter the duodenum in the course of a cystic duct cholangiogram, done *prior to* opening the CBD, indicates obstruction owing to a calculus.

Studies by Jolly, Baker, Schmidt, Walker, and Holm and by Schulenberg disclose that in 4%–6% of cases routine cystic duct cholangiography will reveal CBD stones in patients who have no other indication of choledocholithiasis. It is probable that some of these nonsymptomatic CBD stones would have passed spontaneously, but perhaps half of them would have required secondary cholecholithotomy during the course of the next 5–10 years. Counterbalancing the discovery of these nonsymptomatic common duct stones is a 2%–4% incidence of false positive cystic duct cholangiograms that may lead to an unnecessary CBD exploration.

A major advantage of cystic duct cholangiography is that the percentage of patients undergoing CBD exploration has been reduced from 40% to 20%. Patients having palpable stones in the CBD, a markedly dilated and thickened duct, a recent history of chills, fever, and a bilirubin over 5 mg/dl, should probably have CBD explorations. Other cases (e.g., patients with small calculi in the gallbladder and a large cystic duct, a history of pancreatitis, or moderate enlargement of the CBD) do not require CBD exploration if the cystic duct cholangiogram is normal. Thus, routine cystic duct cholangiography has eliminated the need for CBD exploration in about half the cases. Because the addition of a CBD exploration to a simple cholecystectomy results in a higher mortality rate, the use of routine cystic duct cholangiography appears to be valuable. It has the additional virtue of dilineating the anatomy of the bile ducts, which will help prevent inadvertent injury. When cholangiography is used routinely, it requires only 5–10 minutes of additional operating time, and the surgical and radiological team gains expertise with the technique, making the results more accurate.

Modifications in Operative Strategy Owing to Acute Cholecystitis

Decompressing the Gallbladder

Often there is a marked tense enlargement of the gallbladder owing to an obstruction of the cystic duct. This interferes with exposure of the vital structures around the gallbladder ampulla. For this reason, it is generally necessary to insert a trocar or an 18-gauge needle attached to suction in order to aspirate the bile or pus from the gallbladder and to permit the organ to collapse. After the trocar has been removed, apply a large hemostat to the wound in the gallbladder.

Sequence of Dissection

Although there is sometimes so much edema and fibrosis around the cystic and common ducts that the gallbladder must be dissected from the fundus down, in most patients an incision in the peritoneum overlying the cystic duct near its junction with the CBD will reveal that these two structures are not intimately involved in the acute inflammatory process. When this is the case, identify and encircle—but do not ligate—the cystic duct with 4–0 cotton and then dissect out the cystic artery.

If the cystic artery is not readily seen, make a window in the peritoneum overlying Calot's triangle just cephalad to the cystic duct. Next, insert the tip of a Mixter right-angle clamp into this window and elevate the tissue between the window and the liver, on the tip of this clamp. This will improve the exposure of this area. By carefully dissecting out the contents of this tissue, one can generally identify the cystic artery. Ligate it with 2–0 cotton and divide the artery. When this can be done early in the operation, there will be less bleeding during the liberation of the fundus of the gallbladder.

Dissecting the Gallbladder Away from the Liver

Use a scalpel incision on the back wall of the gallbladder. Carry it down to the mucosal layer of the gallbladder. If part of the mucosa is necrotic, then dissect around the necrotic area in order not to lose the proper plane. If it has not been possible to delineate the proper plane and the dissection inadvertently is between the outer layer of the gallbladder and the hepatic parenchyma, complete the dissection quickly and apply either Surgicel or Avitene to the oozing liver bed. Then apply a moist gauze pad and use a retractor over the gauze pad to maintain exposure while the dissection is being completed.

If the cystic artery has not been ligated in the previous step, it will be identifiable as it crosses from the region of the common hepatic duct toward the back wall of the gallbladder.

Management of the Cystic Duct;

Cholangiography

Cholangiography is performed in patients with acute obstructive cholecystitis, even in the absence of significant jaundice, because the incidence of CBD stones in this group approaches 20%. If the cystic duct is not patent, perform a cholangiogram through a small scalp vein needle inserted directly into the CBD.

Occasionally, the cystic duct is so inflamed that it is easily avulsed from its junction with the CBD. If this accident occurs, suture the resulting defect in the CBD with a continuous 5–0 Vicryl suture. If the cystic duct has been avulsed and its orifice in the CBD cannot be located, simply insert a sump or closed suction catheter down to a point deep to the CBD in the right renal fossa after accomplishing a cholangiogram.

When to Abandon Cholecystectomy and Perform Cholecystostomy

If at any time during the course of dissecting the gallbladder such an advanced state of fibrosis or inflammation is encountered that continued dissection may endanger the bile ducts or other vital structures, all plans for completing the cholecystectomy should be abandoned. Convert the operation to cholecystostomy. If a portion of the gallbladder has already been mobilized or removed, it is possible to perform a partial cholecystectomy and to insert a catheter into the gallbladder remnant. Then sew the remaining gallbladder wall around the

catheter. Place additional drains into the renal fossa. Remove the gallbladder remnant at a later date, after the inflammation has subsided. Meanwhile, the pus has been drained out of the gallbladder. The technique of cholecystostomy is illustrated in Chap. 49.

The necessity for abandoning cholecystectomy for a lesser procedure will occur in no more than 1% of all cases of acute cholecystitis if the surgeon is experienced in this type of surgery. The less-experienced surgeon should have no hesitation to perform a cholecystostomy when he feels that removing the gallbladder may damage a vital structure.

Summary

By strictly following this strategy and the technique described below in the course of performing personally a series of 1,300 cholecystectomies, I have encountered no known case of transection, ligation, or significant operative trauma to the bile ducts, either during elective or emergency operations.

Operative Technique

Incision

We prefer to make a subcostal incision in almost all cases of cholecystectomy because of the excellent exposure afforded in the region of the gallbladder bed and cystic duct. It is important to start the incision at least one centimeter to the left of the linea alba. Then incise in a lateral direction roughly parallel to and 4 cm below

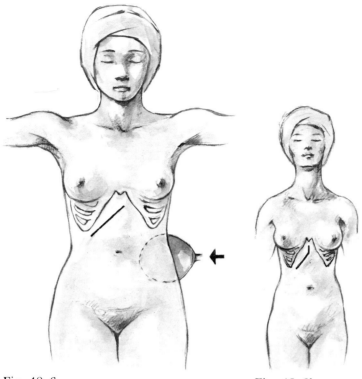

Fig. 48–6a   Fig. 48–6b

the costal margin, (**Fig. 48–6a**). Continue for a variable distance depending on the patient's body build. This incision will divide the 9th intercostal nerve, which emerges just lateral to the border of the rectus muscle. Cutting one intercostal nerve will produce a small area of hypoesthesia of the skin but no muscle weakness. If more than one intercostal nerve is divided, a bulge in the abdominal musculature sometimes occurs.

In a thin patient with a narrow costal arch, a Kehr hockey-stick modification is useful (**Fig. 48–6b**). This incision starts at the tip of the xiphoid and goes down the midline for 3–4 cm and then curves laterally in a direction parallel to the costal margin until the width of the right belly of the rectus muscle has been encompassed. If a midline incision in utilized, excellent exposure will often require that the incision be continued 3–6 cm below the umbilicus.

When the liver and gallbladder are high under the costal arch and this anatomical configuration interferes with exposure or when necessary in obese patients, add a Kehr extension (up the midline to the xiphoid) to a long subcostal incision and divide the falciform ligament. This vertical extension of the incision often improves exposure to a remarkable degree. Also, apply an Upper Hand or "chain" retractor to the costal arch and draw it upward.

After the incision has been made, thorough exploration of the entire abdomen is carried out. Then direct attention to the gallbladder, confirming the presence of stones by palpatation. Check the pancreas for pancreatitis or carcinoma and palpate the descending duodenum for a possible ampullary cancer.

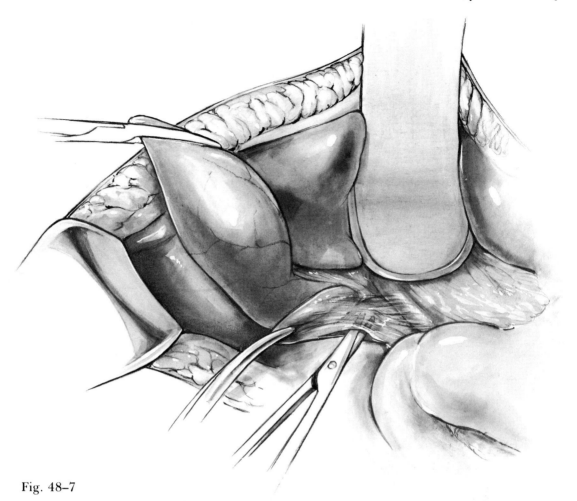

Fig. 48–7

Dissecting the Cystic Duct

Expose the gallbladder field by applying a Foss retractor to the inferior surface of the liver just medial to the gallbladder as well as a Richardson or a Balfour self-retaining retractor to the costal margin. Alternatively, affix an Upper Hand retractor (Vol. I, Fig. D–22) to the operating table. Then attach a blade to the Upper Hand and use it to elevate and to pull the right costal margin in a cephalad direction. Then apply a gauze pad over the hepatic flexure and another over the duodenum. Occasionally adhesions between omentum, colon, or duodenum and the gallbladder must be divided prior to placing the gauze pads. Then, have the first assistant retract the duodenum away from the gallbladder with his left hand. This will place the common bile duct on stretch.

Place a Kelly hemostat on the ampulla of the gallbladder. With traction on the ampulla of the gallbladder, slide a Metzenbaum scissors beneath the peritoneum that covers the area between the wall of the gallbladder ampulla and the CBD **Fig. 48–7).** By alternately sliding the Metzenbaum beneath the peritoneum to define the plane and then cutting along the gallbladder wall, expose the cystic duct. If the inferior surface of the gallbladder ampulla is dissected free and elevated, this plane of dissection must lead the surgeon to the cystic duct, provided that the plane hugs the surface of the ampulla. By inserting a right-angle Mixter clamp behind the gallbladder, the cystic duct can be easily delineated. Apply a temporary ligature of 4–0 cotton to the cystic duct with a single throw in order to avoid inadvertently milking calculi from the gallbladder into the CBD. The cystic duct should not be injured by strangulating it with this ligature because this structure will, on occasion, prove to be a small-size CBD and not the cystic duct. If you do not elect to do a cholangiogram, proceed to the step of ligating and dividing the cystic artery. Otherwise, at this point in the operation perform a cystic duct cholangiogram.

Cystic Duct Cholangiography

For reasons discussed in the previous chapter, we routinely perform a cholangiogram during cholecystectomy. There are two major impediments to catheterizing the cystic duct. First, the internal diameter may be too small for the catheter. Second, the valves of Heister will frequently prevent the passage of the catheter or needle even for the 4–5 mm that are necessary to properly secure the catheter tip with a ligature. Although the valves may be disrupted by the insertion of the silver probe or a pointed hemostat, this maneuver will sometimes result in shredding the cystic duct. One method that will facilitate intubating the cystic duct is to isolate the proximal portion of the duct, including its junction with the gallbladder ampulla. Here the duct is large enough to permit introduction of the catheter at a point *proximal* to the valves of Heister, simplifying the entire task.

After the cystic duct has been isolated, continue the dissection proximally until the mouth of the gallbladder ampulla has been freed. The diameter at this point should be 4–5 mm. Then milk any stones up out of the cystic duct into the gallbladder, ligate the ampulla with a 2–0 cotton

ligature. **(Fig. 48–8a).** Pass another 2–0 ligature loosely around the cystic duct. Make a small transverse scalpel incision in the ampulla of the gallbladder near the entrance of the cystic duct.

At this point attach a 2 meter length of plastic tubing to a 50 ml syringe that has been filled with a solution of half Conray and half saline. Then check to see that the entire system, including syringe, 2 meters of plastic tubing, and the cholangiogram catheter are *absolutely free of air bubbles.* Pass the catheter into the incision in the ampulla and for a distance of 5 mm into the cystic duct **(Fig. 8–8b).** Tie the previously placed 2–0 ligature just above the bead at the termination of the cholangiogram catheter **(Fig. 48–8c).** Under no condition should the surgeon consider confirming the position of the catheter by attempting to aspirate bile into the system because this maneuver will often result in aspirating air bubbles into the tubing. Some surgeons prefer a ureteral or an intravenous catheter over the Taut cholangiogram catheter to intubate the cystic duct.

The left side of the patient should be elevated about 10 cm above the horizontal table in order to prevent the image of the CBD from being superimposed upon the vertebral column with its confusing shadows. This is done either by having the anesthesiologist inflate a previously positioned rubber balloon under the left hip and flank (see Fig. 48–6a) or, alternatively, two folded sheets may be placed beneath the patients left hip and flank.

The surgeon now takes his place behind a portable lead shield covered with a sterile sheet. After the film and X-ray tube have been positioned, the surgeon slowly injects no more than 4 ml of contrast medium for the first exposure. A second X-ray film is then put into position and a second exposure taken after an additional injection of 4–6 ml. When X-raying a hugely dilated bile duct, as much as 30–40 ml may be required in *fractional* doses. On rare occasions, spasm in the region of the ampulla of Vater will not permit pas-

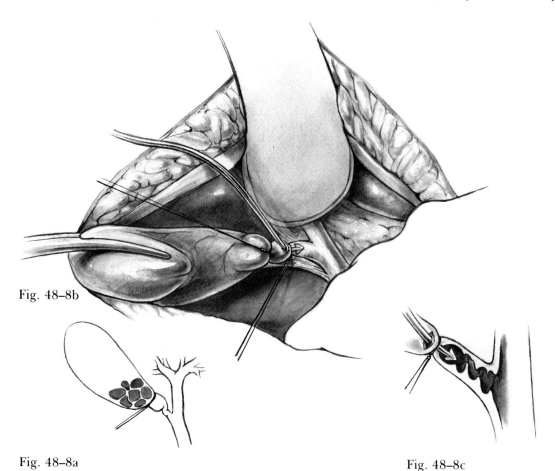

Fig. 48–8b

Fig. 48–8a

Fig. 48–8c

sage of contrast medium into the duodenum unless 1 mg of nitroglycerine, dissolved in 2–3 ml of water, is administered into the patient's nose. This medication is absorbed rapidly (1–2 minutes) from the nasal mucosa. We have found it to be superior to intravenous glucagon (1 mg) in relieving sphincter spasm. If, after this is done, the duodenum is still not visualized, choledochotomy and exploration are indicated.

While waiting for the films to be developed, the surgeon continues with the next step in the operation, ligating and dividing the cystic artery, without removing the cannula from the cystic duct. In order to insure objectivity, interpretation of the cholangiographic films should be made *by a radiologist* rather than exclusively by the operating surgeon.

When cystic duct cholangiography is performed prior to instrumentation of the CBD and ampulla, dye will almost always enter the duodenum if there is no CBD or ampullary pathology. When T-tube cholangiography is performed after completing the bile duct exploration, spasm will often prevent visualization of the terminal CBD and ampulla. This problem can be averted by routine cholangiography prior to choledochotomy, even if CBD exploration has already been decided upon.

Common Errors of Operative Cholangiography

Injecting too much contrast material. When a large dose of contrast material is injected into the ductal system, the duodenum is frequently flooded with dye. This may obscure stones in the distal CBD.

69

Dye too concentrated. Especially when the CBD is somewhat enlarged, the injection of concentrated contrast material can mask the presence of small radiolucent calculi. Consequently, dilute the contrast material 1:2 with normal saline solution when the CBD is large.

Air bubbles. Compulsive attention is necessary to eliminate air bubbles from the syringe and the plastic tubing leading to the cystic duct. Also, never try to aspirate bile into this tubing since the ligature fixing the cystic duct around the cholangiogram cannula may not be airtight and thus air may often be sucked into the system and later injected into the CBD; then it may be impossible to differentiate between air bubble and calculus.

Poor technical quality. If the radiograph is not of excellent quality, there is a greater chance of achieving a false negative interpretation. It is useless to try to interpret a film that is not technically satisfactory. One technical error is easily avoided by elevating the left flank of the patient for a distance of about 8–10 cm in order that the image of the bile ducts is not superimposed on the patient's vertebral column (see Fig. 48–6a). Especially in obese patients it is important to be sure that all the exposure factors are correct by using a scout film prior to starting the operation. Using an image-enhancing film holder with a proper grid also improves technical quality. If the *hepatic ducts* have not been filled with the contrast material, repeat the X ray after injecting another dose into the cystic duct. Otherwise hepatic duct stones will not be visualized. It is sometimes helpful to administer morphine sulfate. This drug will induce sphincter spasm. Then, dye injected into the cystic duct will fill the hepatic ducts.

Performing cystic duct cholangiograms routinely serves to familiarize the technicians and the surgical team with all of the details necessary to provide superior films. It also serves to shorten the time requirement for this step to 5–10 minutes.

Sphincter spasm. Spasm of the sphincter of Oddi sometimes prevents the passage of the contrast medium into the duodenum. Although this outcome is far more frequent after CBD exploration with instrumentation of the ampulla, it also does occur on rare occasions during a cystic duct cholangiogram. We have found that instilling into the patient's nostril a solution of nitroglycerine (1 mg dissolved in 2–3 ml of water) seems to be more effective than using glucagon intravenously to relax the sphincter. Simultaneous with sphincter relaxation, there is generally a mild drop in the patient's blood pressure. At this time inject the contrast medium into the CBD. This medication is also useful when performing a completion cholangiogram after the CBD exploration has been completed.

Failing to consult with the radiologist. It is not reasonable for the operating surgeon to be the only physician responsible for interpreting the cholangiographic films. The surgeon tends to be overoptimistic, tends to accept poor technical quality, and is responsible for an excessive number of false negative interpretations. Always have a consultation with a radiologist familiar with this procedure before forming a final conclusion concerning the cholangiogram.

Ligating the Cystic Artery

Gentle dissection in the triangle of Calot will reveal the cystic artery, which may cross over or under the common or right hepatic duct on its way to the gallbladder. It frequently divides into two branches,

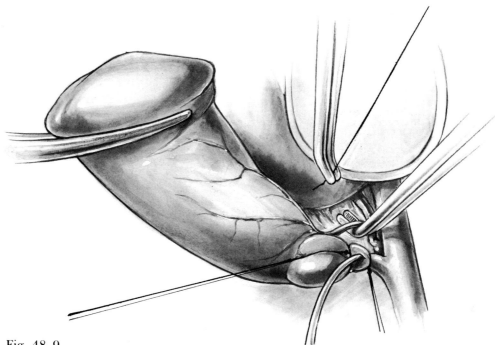

Fig. 48–9

one anterior, one posterior. Confirmation of the identity of this structure is obtained by tracing the artery up along the gallbladder wall and demonstrating the lack of any sizeable branch going to the liver. Often the anterior branch of the cystic artery can be seen running up the medial surface of the gallbladder. By tracing this branch from above down, its point of origin will lead to the location of the cystic artery. Ligate this artery in continuity after passing a 2–0 cotton ligature around it with a Mixter right-angle hemostat (**Fig. 48–9**). Apply a Hemoclip to the gallbladder side of the vessel and transect the cystic artery, preferably leaving a 1 cm stump of artery distal to the cotton ligature (**Fig. 48–10**).

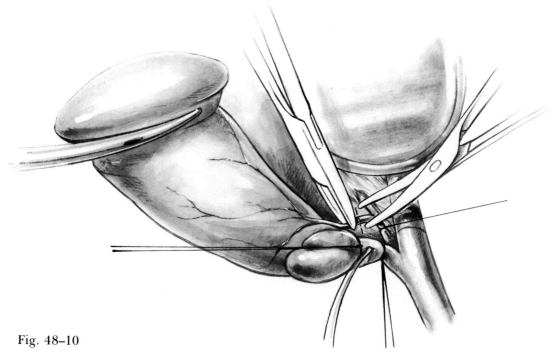

Fig. 48–10

If there is fibrosis in Calot's triangle and the artery is not evident, pass a Mixter clamp beneath these fibrotic structures. While the first assistant exposes the structures by elevating the Mixter clamp, the surgeon can more easily dissect out the artery from the surrounding scar tissue. In case the cystic artery is torn and hemorrhage results, this is easily controlled by inserting the left index finger into the foramen of Winslow and then compressing the hepatic artery between the thumb and forefinger until the exact source of bleeding is controlled by a clamp or a suture.

Dissecting the Gallbladder Bed

In no case of cholecystectomy is the cystic duct transected or clamped prior to complete mobilization of the gallbladder. This mobilization may be done by taking advantage of the incision in the peritoneum overlying Calot's triangle as described above and simply continuing this peritoneal dissection from below upward along the medial border of the gallbladder. Insert a Mixter clamp beneath the peritoneum while the first assistant makes an incision, or incise the peritoneum with a right-angle scissors from below upward. Alternatively, make a scalpel incision in the superficial layer of the gallbladder wall across its fundus (**Fig. 48–11**). Use the scalpel and scissors to dissect the mucosal layer of the gallbladder away from the serosal layer, *leaving as much tissue as possible on the liver side.* This leaves a shiny layer of submucosa on the gallbladder. Tiny vessels coming from the liver to the gallbladder can be identified and individually occluded with electrocautery. When the plane of dissection is deep to the serosa, raw liver parenchyma presents itself. Oozing from raw liver is difficult to control with electrocoagulation. In this case, either prolonged pressure with moist gauze or the application of a small sheet of Surgicel or powdered Avitene to

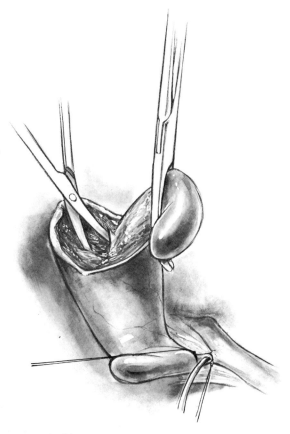

Fig. 48–11

the area of raw liver surface can provide excellent hemostasis after 10–15 minutes of local compression.

As the dissection proceeds down along the liver, do not apply any hemostats as the vessels in this plane are small. Near the termination of this dissection along the posterior wall of the gallbladder, a bridge of tissue will be found connecting the gallbladder ampulla with the liver bed. Instruct the assistant to pass a Mixter clamp through the opening in Calot's triangle that was previously made when the cystic artery was ligated (**Fig. 48–12**). This clamp will elevate the bridge of tissue and the surgeon will dissect out is contents by carefully nibbling away at it with his Metzenbaum scissors in order to rule out the pos-

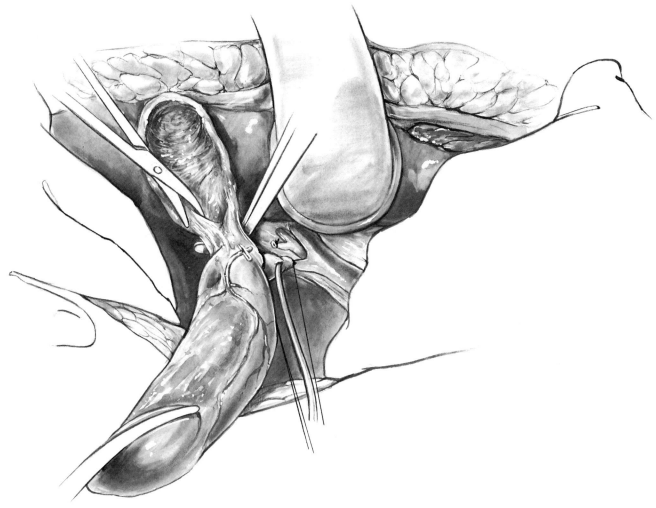

Fig. 48–12

sibility that it contains the common hepatic duct. In cases where excessive fibrosis has prevented the prior identification and ligature of the cystic artery, there is generally, at this stage of dissection, no great problem in identifying this vessel coming from the area near the hilus of the liver toward the back wall of the gallbladder.

With the gallbladder hanging suspended only by the cystic duct, dissect the duct down to its junction with the common hepatic duct. Exact determination of the junction between the cystic and the hepatic ducts is usually not difficult after electrocoagulating one or two tiny vessels that cross over the acute angle between the two

ducts. Rarely, a lengthy cystic duct continues distally towards the duodenum for several centimeters.

The cystic duct may even enter the CBD on its *medial* aspect near the ampulla of Vater. In these cases, it is hazardous to dissect the cystic duct down into the groove between the duodenum and pancreas; thus, it is preferable to leave a few centimeters of duct behind. Confirmation of the anatomy may be accomplished by cholangiography. In general, the cystic duct is clamped at a point about 5 mm

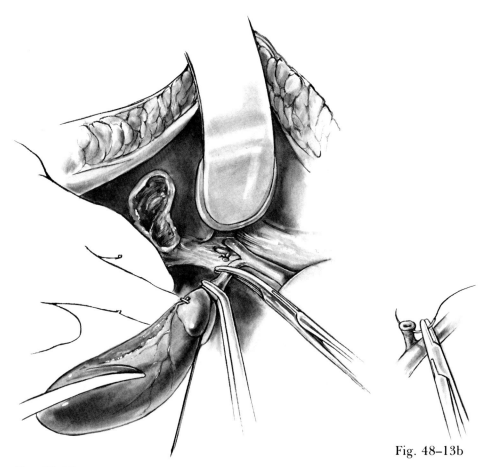

Fig. 48–13b

Fig. 48–13a

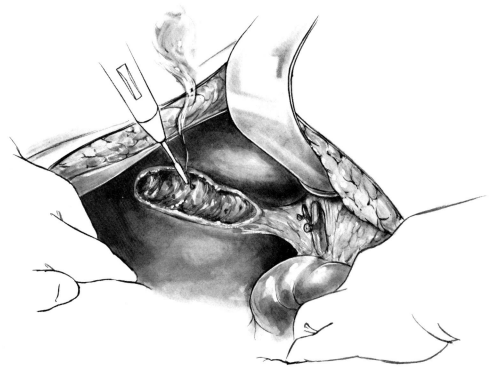

Fig. 48–14

from its termination and divided (**Fig. 48–13a**). Transfix the cystic duct stump with a 3–0 PG suture-ligature (**Fig. 48–13b**). *Never is the cystic duct clamped or divided except as the last step in a cholecystectomy.*

Achieve complete hemostasis of the liver bed with the electrocoagulator (**Fig. 48–14**). If necessary, use suture-ligatures; in unusual cases, leave a sheet of Surgicel in the liver bed to control venous oozing.

Palpating the CBD

Prior to terminating the operation, especially if cholangiography has not been performed, it is essential to properly palpate the CBD in order to reduce the possibility of overlooked calculi. This is done by inserting the index finger into the foramen of Winslow and palpating the entire duct between the left index finger and thumb. Since a portion of the distal CBD is situated between the posterior wall of the duode-

num and the pancreas, *it is necessary to insert the index finger into the potential space posterior to the pancreas and behind the second portion of the duodenum.* It is not necessary to perform a complete Kocher maneuver. If the surgeon will gently insinuate the left index finger behind the CBD and continue in a caudal direction behind the pancreas and the duodenum, he will not encounter bleeding unless he is too rough. In this fashion, with the index finger behind the second portion of the duodenum and the thumb on its anterior wall, carcinomas of the ampulla and calculi in the distal CBD may be detected (**Fig. 48–15**). If this maneuver is not successful, perform a formal Kocher maneuver.

Drainage and Closure

We prefer a flat Silastic Jackson-Pratt closed-suction catheter following cholecystectomy because it has eliminated the occasional staphylococcal drain-tract infection that we used to see when we used latex drains. Bring the catheter out from the renal fossa through a puncture wound just lateral to the right termination of the subcostal incision. Some surgeons prefer to bring the drain out through the incision

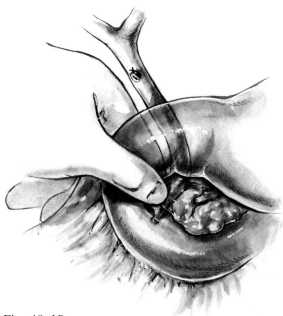

Fig. 48–15

(**Fig. 48–16**) but this pathway, when used for drains, has been reported to result in an increased incidence of wound infections. If a latex drain is used, place a 1.5 cm wide latex rubber drain down into the deepest portion of the renal fossa with its tip at the foramen of Winslow. Bring the drain out through a stab wound near the lateral margin of the subcostal incision. Avoid wrinkles in the drain, which should lie flat and in a straight line. In the absence of sepsis, leave the drain in place for 3–4 days. Then, if there is no bile drainage, remove it without prior shortening.

There is now abundant evidence that a patient who has undergone a technically precise and uncomplicated simple cholecystectomy does not require the insertion of any type of drain (Budd, Cochran, and Fouty; also Elboim, Goldman, Hann, Palestrant et al.).

Do not reperitonealize the liver bed since this step serves no useful purpose. Close the abdominal wall in routine fashion (see Chap. 5). We now use 1 PDS suture material for this step.

Postoperative Care

After an uncomplicated cholecystectomy, nasogastric suction is not necessary. In patients with acute cholecystitis, paralytic ileus is not uncommon; thus nasogastric suction will be necessary for 1–3 days.

After uncomplicated cholecystectomy, antibiotics are not necessary except in the older age group (over 70). The elderly patients have a high incidence of bacteria in the gallbladder bile and should have perioperative antibiotics prior to and for 2–3 doses after operation. Following cholecystectomy for acute cholecystitis, administer antibiotics for 4–5 days, depending on the Gram stain of the gallbladder bile sampled in the operating room.

Unless there is a significant amount of bilious drainage, remove the drain on approximately the 4th postoperative day.

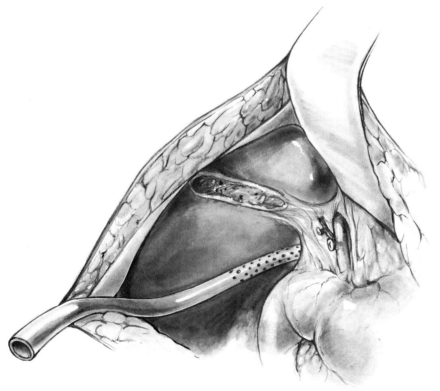

Fig. 48–16

Postoperative Complications

"Drain fever" drain-tract sepsis. Occasionally after the use of the usual latex drain, shortening the drain during the postoperative period will result in a temperature spike of 1°–3°C. This phenomenon also occurs sometimes following the removal of this drain. In most cases the cause of this complication is the accumulation of serum or bile around a wrinkled portion of the latex. When the drain is mobilized, this material is diffused and produces the fever. It can be prevented if the latex drain is brought out in a straight line with no wrinkles. This complication can also be prevented by using a closed-suction catheter instead of the latex drain. Another advantage of the closed-suction drain is the virtual elimination of sepsis that results when skin bacteria invade the drain tract, generally producing a staphylococcal drain-tract abscess. This complication has not been seen following properly managed closed-suction drainage through a puncture wound in the abdominal wall. The puncture wound should be treated with local application daily of iodophor ointment and a small sterile dressing.

Bile leak. Minor drainage of bile may follow the interruption of some small branches of the bile ducts in the liver bed. This does not occur if the outer layer of the gallbladder serosa is left behind on the liver bed. On very rare occasions a duct of significant size may enter the gallbladder, but we have never encountered such an instance. Bile drainage of 100–200 ml will occur if the surgeon has inadvertently transected an anomalous duct draining the dorsal caudal segment of the right lobe. If this complication is diagnosed by a sinogram X ray, expectant therapy may result in gradual diminution of drainage as the tract becomes stenotic. However, if there is any infection in the area drained by the duct, recurrent cholangitis or liver abscess may occur. In this case, permanent relief may eventually necessitate resecting the segment of the liver drained by the transected duct.

If the volume of bile drainage exceeds 400 ml/day, transection of the hepatic or the common bile duct may be suspected. After waiting until the 7th or 8th postoperative day for a tract to form, request the radiologist to perform a sinogram by injecting sterile aqueous contrast material into the tract. This will generally identify the point of leakage in the ductal system. If the common hepatic duct has been transected, reconstructive surgery will be required.

Jaundice. Postcholecystectomy jaundice is usually due either to ligature of the CBD or an overlooked CBD stone. If other causes, such as halothane hepatitis are ruled out, an ERCP is indicated to identify the obstruction.

Hemorrhage. If the cystic artery has been accurately ligated, postoperative bleeding is an extremely rare complication. Occasionally oozing from the liver bed may continue postoperatively and may require relaparotomy for control.

Subhepatic abscess; hepatic abscess. Following cholecystectomy these two complications are seen primarily in cases of acute cholecystitis. Postoperative abscesses are extremely rare in patients whose surgery was for chronic cholecystitis unless a bile leak occurs. Treatment requires relaparotomy for drainage.

References

Brittain RS, Marchioro TL, Hermann, G, Waddell WR, et al. (1964) Accidental hepatic artery ligation. Am J Surg 107:822

Budd DC, Cochran RC, Fouty WJ Jr (1982) Cholecystectomy with and without drainage: a randomized prospective study of 300 patients. Am J Surg 143:307

Elboim CM, Goldman L, Hann L, Palestrant AM, et al. (1983) Significance of post-cholecystectomy subhepatic collections. Ann Surg 198:137

Jolly PC, Baker JW, Schmidt HM, Walker JH, Holm JC (1968) Operative cholangiography: a case for its routine use. Ann Surg 168:551

Longmire WP Jr, Tompkins RK (1975) Lesions of the segmental and lobar hepatic ducts. Ann Surg 182:478

Longmire WP Jr (1977) The diverse causes of biliary obstruction and their remedies. Curr Probl Surg 14:1

Schulenberg CAR (1969) Operative cholaniography: 1,000 cases. Surgery 65:723

49 Cholecystostomy

Indications

Patients suffering from acute cholecystitis when cholecystectomy may be hazardous for technical reasons, especially if the surgeon is inexperienced in operating on acute cholecystitis, or if the patient is a very poor risk

Cholecystostomy sometimes serves as a first-stage operation for obstructive jaundice owing to a tumor of the pancreas with serum bilirubin over 20 mg/dl.

Contraindication

Patients who have acute cholangitis owing to common bile duct obstruction

Preoperative Care

Appropriate antibiotics
Vitamin K for jaundiced patients

Pitfalls and Danger Points

Overlooking acute purulent cholangitis
Overlooking gangrene of gallbladder
Postoperative bile leak

Operative Strategy

When Is Cholecystostomy an Inadequate Operation?

Gagic and Frey reported an operative mortality of 27% in 22 cases of cholecystostomy for acute cholecystitis. Most of the deaths were due to suppurative cholangitis and septicemia. This group of patients had chills, fever, upper abdominal pain, and serum bilirubin levels averaging 12 mg/dl. Whenever the serum bilirubin rises above 6–7 mg/dl, the patient is probably suffering from common bile duct (CBD) obstruction secondary to calculi. Either eliminate this possibility by means of an operative cholangiogram, or drain the CBD with a T-tube. Cholecystostomy does *not* provide adequate drainage for an infected bile duct.

In most cases it is not difficult to differentiate acute cholecystitis from acute cholangitis. In acute cholecystitis there is usually marked localized tenderness and muscle spasm in the right upper quadrant and only slight elevation of the serum bilirubin. The patient with acute cholangitis is generally more acutely ill and suffers from pain, chills, fever, and jaundice. In most cases, right upper quadrant tenderness is not a prominent part of the clinical picture, and a tender mass is not palpable except in the very unusual case where the patient has both acute cholecystitis and acute cholangitis.

When a patient with acute cholangitis does not respond immediately to antibiotic treatment, prompt drainage of the CBD is lifesaving. This must be accomplished

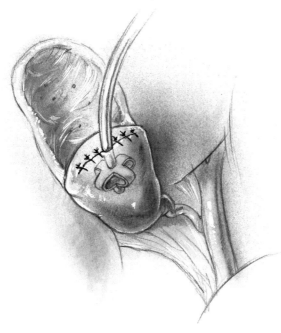

Fig. 49–1

by laparotomy and choledochostomy although in the poor-risk patient endoscopic radiographic cholangiopancreatographic (ERCP)-catheterization of the CBD has proved successful in achieving drainage of an infected bile duct. Undrained acute purulent cholangitis is often rapidly fatal. In performing cholecystostomy, one must be alert not to overlook this disease of the bile duct.

Another complication of acute cholecystitis, for which cholecystostomy is an inadequate operation, is gangrene of the gallbladder. This may occur in the deep portion of the gallbladder fundus, where it may be hidden by adherent omentum or bowel. Performing a cholecystostomy through a small incision under local anesthesia, where only the tip of the gallbladder is exposed, could easily result in overlooking this patch of necrosis. When a necrotic area is found in the gallbladder, it is preferable to perform a cholecystectomy, either complete, or, if this is impossible for technical reasons, a partial cholecystectomy around a catheter with removal of the gangrenous patch (**Fig. 49–1**).

Choice of Anesthesia

Because of the danger of overlooking disease of the CBD as well as gangrene or perforation of the gallbladder, it is preferable to perform the cholecystostomy through an adequate incision under general anesthesia. By using modern anesthesia techniques, including monitoring of the pulmonary artery pressure and cardiac output during the operation, and pharmacological manipulation to maintain homeostasis, it is safer for most bad-risk patients to undergo a biliary operation under general rather than local anesthesia.

Preventing Bile Leaks

One distressing complication that occasionally follows cholecystostomy is leakage of bile around the catheter into the free peritoneal cavity resulting in bile peritonitis. This complication may generally be avoided by using a large-size catheter and suturing the gallbladder around the catheter (**Fig. 49–2**). It is important also to su-

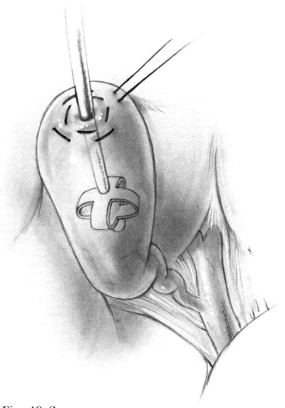

Fig. 49–2

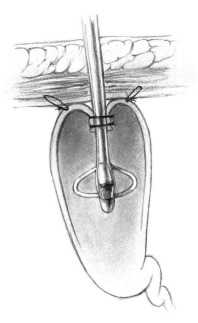

Fig. 49–3

ture the fundus of the gallbladder to the peritoneum around the exit wound of the drainage catheter **(Fig. 49–3).** In addition, adequate drainage in the vicinity of the gallbladder is necessary.

Operative Technique

Incision

Under general anesthesia, make a subcostal incision at least 12–15 cm in length. Find the plane between the adherent omentum and the inflamed gallbladder. Once this plane is entered, the omentum may generally be freed by gentle blunt dissection from the gallbladder wall. Continuing in this plane, inspect the gallbladder and its ampulla.

Emptying the Gallbladder

After ascertaining that there is no perforation of the gallbladder nor any patch of gangrene, empty the gallbladder either with a No. 16 needle or a suction-trocar that is inserted into the tip of the gallbladder. Also, order an immediate Gram stain. Enlarge the stab wound in the gallbladder. Attempt to remove the gallbladder calculi

with pituitary scoops and Randall stone forceps. It may be necessary to compress the gallbladder ampulla manually to milk stones up toward the fundus. After flushing the gallbladder with saline, insert a 2OF straight or Pezzar catheter 3–4 cm into the gallbladder. Close the defect in the gallbladder wall with two inverting purse-string sutures of 2–0 chromic catgut or PG suture material (Fig. 49–2). If the gallbladder wall is unusually thick, it may be necessary to close the gallbladder around the catheter with interrupted Lembert sutures.

If the patient is in satisfactory condition, a cholangiogram through the gallbladder catheter may be attempted. On the other hand, it is not always possible to extract a stone that is impacted in the cystic duct. This will eliminate the possibility of obtaining a cholangiogram by this route. Alternatively, a cholangiogram may be obtained by inserting an intravenous-type catheter or scalp vein needle directly into the CBD. On the other hand, since cholecystostomy is often performed because the patient is a very poor risk, it requires sophisticated judgment on the part of the surgeon to decide whether a cholangiogram is necessary to rule out the presence of cholangitis. In many cases it will not be necessary because most patients undergoing cholecystostomy will require a second operation at a later date anyhow. The object of the immediate procedure is to tide the patient over the septic process in the gallbladder.

Now make a stab wound to exit the catheter through the abdominal wall close to the fundus of the gallbladder. Draw the catheter through the abdominal wall and then suture the fundus of the gallbladder to the peritoneum alongside the stab wound (Fig. 49–3). Make a stab wound and insert either latex drains or sump-suction catheters or both. These drains should be placed as follows: one in the vicinity of the cholecystostomy and one in the right renal fossa.

Then close the abdominal incision in routine fashion as described in Chap. 5. We now use 1 PDS sutures for this closure.

Postoperative Care

Connect the cholecystostomy catheter to a sterile plastic collecting bag for gravity drainage.

Continue antibiotic treatment for the next 7–10 days. Until bacterial culture and sensitivity studies have been reported on the gallbladder bile, use antibiotics that are effective against the Gram-negative bacteria, the enterococcus, and the anaerobes.

Employ nasogastric suction until bowel function has resumed.

Measure the daily output of bile and replace with an appropriate dose of sodium.

Do not remove the gallbladder drainage catheter for 12–14 days. Perform a cholangiogram before removing the catheter.

Postoperative Complications

Bile peritonitis

Subhepatic, subphrenic, or intrahepatic abscess

Septicemia

Patients with acute cholecystitis generally respond promptly to adequate drainage of the infection. If the patient shows persistent signs of sepsis and bacteremia, it is likely that this complication stems from an undrained focus of infection. This may be an obstructed CBD with cholangitis or a subhepatic, *intrahepatic*, or subphrenic abscess. ERCP and CT scanning may be helpful in detecting these complications.

References

Gagic N, Frey CF (1975) The results of cholecystostomy for the treatment of acute cholecystitis. Surg Gynecol Obstet 140:255

50 Common Bile Duct Exploration

Concept: When to Explore the Common Bile Duct (CBD)

As pointed out by Way, Admirand, and Dunphy, the true incidence of CBD stones in patients undergoing surgery for gallstones is probably between 12% and 15% in the United States. By using indications essentially identical to those stated below and by performing routine preexploratory cystic duct cholangiography, Way performed CBD explorations in only 21% of 952 cholecystectomies. These explorations were positive for calculi in 65% of the patients explored. Of the 952 cholecystectomy cases, 14% had CBD stones. In 6 additional reports collected by Way in which routine cystic duct cholangiography was employed, the results were similar. On the other hand, the same author cited 3 other reports from the Lahey Clinic of cases in which preexploratory cholangiography was not performed. Here, of 33% of patients undergoing CBD exploration only 30% of the ducts contained stones. Whereas the use of routine cystic duct cholangiograms resulted in the recovery of CBD stones in over 14% of the cholecystectomies reported by Way and colleagues, the authors who omitted preexploratory cholangiography were able to discover CBD stones in only 10% of their cholecystectomy cases. In other words, *routine preexploratory cholangiography markedly reduces the number of CBD explorations performed yet achieves a higher recovery rate of CBD stones* (see Table 50–1).

In the absence of cystic duct cholangiography, opening the CBD for the indication that the duct is dilated or that the gallbladder contains many small stones will yield no more than 10%–14% positive explorations. The presence of jaundice, with serum bilirubin below 7 mg/dl as the *only* indication for exploring the CBD yielded, in Way's series, positive results in 35% of explorations. Consequently, we do not consider the presence of many small stones, of mild jaundice, or of a dilated CBD to be an absolute indication for duct exploration if the preexploratory cystic duct cholangiogram is negative.

Counterbalancing the advantage of a greater yield of CBD calculi for a smaller number of duct exploration is the fact that cholangiography does produce an occasional false positive result. Most often this is due to inexperience on the part of the surgeon in that air bubbles are permitted to enter the system causing the false positive interpretation. With increasing experience, the incidence of false positives should be no more than 2%–3%.

TABLE 50–1 Detection of CBD Stones during Routine Cholecystectomy

Routine Cholecystectomy	Cases	
	CBD Stones Retrieved (%)	CBD Explorations Undertaken (%)
With preexploratory cholangiogram (N = 952)	14	21
Without preexploratory cholangiogram (N = 4,187)	10	33

Source: Adapted from Way et al., 1972

Even when there is an absolute indication for CBD exploration, we prefer to do preexploratory cystic duct cholangiography. Not only does this delineate the anatomy and anomalies of the ductal system but also it may provide the only opportunity to visualize radiographically the distal CBD and ampulla. Often, following instrumentation of the CBD, sphincter spasm prevents the passage of dye into the distal CBD and the duodenum during the postexploratory T-tube cholangiogram. Preexploratory cholangiography is omitted in patients suffering acute suppurative cholangitis.

Patients presenting with signs of suppurative cholangitis often will require emergency surgery after only a few hours or preoperative preparation because without CBD drainage the disease is often fatal within 24 hours. In the classical case, the patient will experience chills, fever, jaundice, some degree of mental confusion and septic shock due to Gram-negative bacteremia. Occasionally, a *Clostridium* is involved. After inserting a central venous or pulmonary artery pressure monitor, pursue vigorous fluid replacement and antibiotic therapy.

At operation, the typical case will demonstrate purulent material in a dilated CBD obstructed by calculi. The most important feature of surgery is to drain the CBD with a large T-tube. Remove all of the calculi if this step can be accomplished safely. In some cases satisfactory drainage can be accomplished by the percutaneous transhepatic or the ERCP approach.

Concept: How to Manage Multiple and "Primary" CBD Stones

Multiple CBD Stones

Some surgeons advocate performance of either choledochoduodenostomy or sphincteroplasty in patients who have multiple calculi in the bile ducts. They reason that the surgeon who has removed 10 stones from the bile ducts has a high likelihood of having overlooked 1 or 2 additional calculi. On this basis, these enthusiasts advocate biliary-intestinal bypass or sphincteroplasty so that the residual stones may pass into the duodenum without obstructing the bile ducts. It is true that the patients who suffer from retained CBD calculi are most often those who have had a large number of stones removed from their CBDs rather than those who have had a negative CBD exploration or whose CBD was not explored at all.

Nevertheless, we are not convinced that there is sufficient data to mandate that every patient who has more than, say, 8 or 10 stones should automatically have a bypass or a sphincteroplasty. Neither of these operations is free of complications. Even though experts with a large experience, like Madden and Jones, can perform choledochoduodenostomy or sphincteroplasty with a mortality rate of 1%–2%, such favorable results as these will not be achieved by a large number of surgeons. Furthermore, with the aid of cholangiography and choledochoscopy in the operating room, it is possible to reduce the incidence of retained bile stones to 0–2%. It does not seem logical to perform bypass surgery or sphincteroplasty for the 2% of patients who will have retained bile stones if the other 98% do not require this additional surgery.

On the other hand, when there is evidence of one or more retained stones in the bile ducts that cannot be retrieved in the operating room, bypass or sphincteroplasty may be indicated. This is so even though it is sometimes simple to remove some of these stones by ERCP-papillotomy or by instrumentation through the T-tube tract 6 weeks after the operation. In patients with Caroli's hepatic duct lithiasis, where intrahepatic stones are present, bypass is indicated.

"Primary" CBD Stones

Madden has emphasized the concept that many CBD stones are formed in the bile duct, hence the term "primary" stones. Most surgeons believe that the vast majority of stones found in the CBD originated in the gallbladder, Madden contends that, in his experience, careful observation of the morphology of CBD stones has disclosed that over 60% of these calculi are primary stones, even in patients who have not had previous cholecystectomy and who in fact also may have stones in their gallbladders.

Madden describes the morphology of a primary CBD stone as follows:

> Characteristically, the primary bile duct stone is ovoid, conforming in shape to the common duct, and easily morcellated between the thumb and fingers to give the "earthy" appearance so aptly described by Aschoff. On cross-section, it is laminated and commonly has a yellow nidus with a brownish-yellow periphery. Some primary stones have laminated rings of variegated colors or simply a symmetrical brownish-yellow pigmentation. When multiple, they may be faceted and appear like secondary or gallbladder stones, but the ease with which they are crushed is the differentiating feature.

Since many of these characteristics can be noted in stones contained in the gallbladder, there is some skepticism whether morphological considerations alone can determine that a stone found in the CBD is indeed a primary stone. The reason that this differentiation assumes importance is Madden's insistence that even at the patient's first exploration, the presence of a primary CBD stone is a definite indication for choledochoduodenostomy. Saharia, Zuidema, and Cameron found that clearing the CBD of all the primary stones with insertion of a T-tube had excellent long-term results in 82% of their patients who had primary CBD stones. In commenting on Saharia's paper, Warren and Sandblom both vigorously opposed the routine use of choledochoduodenostomy for primary CBD stones. Thomas, Nicholson, and Owen as well as Rutledge both strongly favored routine sphincterosplasty for primary CBD stones on the basis that these calculi are the result of bile stasis, even where there is no apparent mechanical obstruction at the ampulla. Pending further study, we remain conservative in this situation and simply remove all of the calculi as well as the gallbladder. If soft calculi and sludge reappear in later years after once having been completely removed, then biliary-intestinal bypass or a sphincteroplasty is indicated (Allen, Shapiro, and Way).

Although primary stones may be caused by bile stasis and the CBD may be markedly enlarged, *ampullary stenosis in these cases is rare.* Indeed, Saharia and colleagues mentioned that in many of their operations for primary stones, the ampulla was widely patent despite the presence of a very large CBD, which suggested that the stasis of bile might be due to an "abnormal functional dilation" of the duct. Only 1 in 30 of their patients had a significant ampullary stenosis. It is difficult to comprehend how sphincteroplasty will help most of the patients who suffer from primary CBD stones but do not have ampullary stenosis.

Indications

Positive Indications

Chills, fever, and jaundice prior to operation indicates that in over 90% of cases CBD exploration will reveal calculi.

Palpation of calculus in CBD

Acute suppurative cholangitis

Positive finding of calculus on routine cystic duct cholangiography or preoperative ERCP, or percutaneous transhepatic cholangiogram

Relative Indications

Moderate elevation of the serum bilirubin (4–6 mg/dl), especially in the presence of acute cholecystitis, is *not by itself* a positive indication for choledochotomy since the ampulla of a distended gallbladder may compress the CBD, thereby producing jaundice in the absence of choledocholithiasis. In these cases, negative cholangiography avoids the necessity for opening the CBD, provided the films are of proper quality.

Some surgeons feel that the presence of a thick-walled, CBD with an external diameter of over 1.6 cm requires duct exploration even in the presence of apparently normal cholangiography, since small calculi may be obscured in the radiography of a large duct. If the contrast medium is properly diluted, one need not explore a large duct if the cholangiogram is normal.

A recent history of acute pancreatitis in the absence of alcoholism requires either CBD exploration or a normal cystic duct cholangiogram.

The presence of multiple small calculi in the gallbladder by itself does not constitute an indication for choledochotomy, even if the cystic duct is large in diameter. Adequate cholangiography will detect calculi of a size sufficient to require choledochotomy. Although this may on occasion result in overlooking a stone 1–2 mm in diameter, this policy will also avoid the performance of a large number of unnecessary CBD explorations. A tiny calculus will almost always spontaneously pass into the duodenum. On the other hand, the addition of an unnecessary CBD exploration to a cholecystectomy may increase the mortality rate.

Failure of contrast medium to enter the duodenum during preexploratory cystic duct cholangiography requires choledochotomy to rule out the presence of a stone at the ampulla.

Patients with biliary colic who have no *gallbladder* stones at laparotomy require a cholangiogram because many of these patients do have *common bile duct* calculi.

Preoperative Care

Order a sonogram of the bile ducts and pancreas as the initial diagnostic test in the jaundiced patient. If a CBD stone is demonstrated, no further diagnostic studies are indicated. If the sonogram shows dilated bile ducts right down to the ampulla, but no stones, then an endoscopic radiographic cholangiopancreatogram (ERCP) will help by providing a picture of the biliary and pancreatic ducts as well as a biopsy of any periampullary tumor. When the intrahepatic ducts are large on the sonogram, but not the CBD, then a percutaneous transhepatic cholangiogram (PTC) will identify intrahepatic tumors of the bile ducts and other unusual lesions. In the absence of the expertise to accomplish an excellent PTC or ERCP, good cystic duct cholangiography and careful choledochoscopy will generally accomplish the same results. Whenever either PTC or ERCP is to be performed, give the patient parenteral antibiotics before these procedures to protect against the bacteremia that they often induce.

Abnormalities of the serum prothrombin should be corrected preoperatively with injections of vitamin K1 oxide. When CBD exploration is planned, the patient should receive perioperative intravenous antibiotics beginning 1 hour prior to operation. In order to assure an adequate antibacterial blood level, repeat the dose in 3 hours, during the operation. We use either cephazolin or a penicillin–aminoglycoside combination.

Pitfalls and Danger Points

Injuring the bile ducts

Creating a false passage into the duodenum when probing the CBD; damaging the amupulla or pancreas; inducing postoperative pancreatitis.

Perforating a periampullary duodenal diverticulum

Sepsis

Failing to remove all of the biliary calculi

Operative Strategy

Avoiding Postoperative Pancreatitis

With reference to the decision for or against adding choledochotomy to simple cholecystectomy, it should be noted that the mortality rate at the author's hospital increased from 0.25% to about 2.5% when a CBD exploration was added to a simple cholecystectomy. Although many of these deaths were due to sepsis accompanying neglected choledocholithiasis in aged patients, we have witnessed fatalities after negative CBD explorations on rare occasions. These deaths were generally caused by postoperative acute pancreatitis. Consequently, all manipulations carried out in the distal CBD and ampulla must be done with great delicacy in order to avoid this potentially fatal complication. Due to the increased operative risk of choledochotomy, use routine cholangiography in order to minimize the number of unnecessary CBD explorations. When CBD exploration is necessary, execute the procedure with meticulous care to avoid trauma to the ampulla or pancreas, which may induce pancreatitis.

CBD Perforations

Another *serious and often fatal* error is to perforate the distal CBD and penetrate the pancreas with an instrument such as the metal Bakes dilator. When the surgeon ex- periences any difficulty in negotiating the ampulla with an instrument, duodenotomy and direct exposure of the ampulla is preferable to repeated blunt trauma from above. Using either the olive-tip (Coudé) woven or a 10F whistle-tip rubber catheter rather than a metal dilator lessens the risk of ampullary trauma and of postoperative acute pancreatitis. Never employ forcible dilatation of the sphincter of Oddi; this procedure serves no useful purpose, and the trauma to the ampulla not only increases the risk of postoperative acute pancreatitis but also produces lacerations and hematomas of the ampulla.

If an instrument has perforated the distal CBD and the head of the pancreas, this may be detected when the CBD is irrigated with saline by noting a leak of saline from the posterior surface of the pancreas. The perforation may also be detected by cholangiography. This type of trauma, which leads to a flow of bile directly into the head of the pancreas, often causes a fatal pancreatitis. For this reason, when this complication is identified, divide the CBD just above its entry into the pancreaticoduodenal sulcus; transfix the distal end of the duct with a suture and anastomose the proximal cut end of the CBD to a Roux-Y segment of jejunum. When this procedure is carried out, diverting the bile from the traumatized pancreas may prove life-saving.

If the CBD has been perforated at a point proximal to the head of the pancreas, suture the laceration with a 5–0 Vicryl suture if the laceration is accessible. If the laceration is not accessible, simply insert a large caliber T-tube into the CBD for decompression proximal to the laceration. Then place a closed-suction catheter drain down to the region of the laceration.

Locating and Removing Biliary Calculi

In order to avoid overlooking biliary calculi, it is important to perform a cystic duct cholangiogram before exploring the CBD.

Be sure that the X ray clearly shows both the hepatic ducts and the distal CBD. If the hepatic ducts cannot be seen because the dye runs into duodenum, either administer morphine to induce spasm of the ampulla or open the CBD, insert an 8F Foley catheter into the proximal CBD, and use this device to obtain an X ray of the intrahepatic radicals.

Once the CBD has been opened, the safest and most effective device for extracting stones is the pituitary scoop with a malleable handle. Available with various size cups, this device can bend in the exact direction required to pass through the CBD down to the ampulla. By delicate maneuvering, the surgeon can remove most stones with the scoop. Also, it is often easy to palpate a stone against this metallic instrument.

Always perform a Kocher maneuver before exploring the CBD. This permits the surgeon to place the fingers of his left hand behind the ampullary region with the thumb on top of the anterior wall of the duodenum. In this fashion he can more accurately direct the manipulation of the instrument while he is palpating its distal tip.

Other methods that are helpful in retrieving stones are the Randall stone forceps, the Fogarty balloon, and thorough saline irrigation. On rare occasions a Dormia basket may retrieve a stone that is otherwise inaccessible.

Choledochoscopy, which is discussed below, is another excellent means of helping to identify residual biliary calculi in the operating room.

When the ampullary region contains an impacted stone that cannot be removed with minimal trauma by the usual methods, *there must be no hesitation to perform a sphincteroplasty for the purpose of extracting the stone* under direct vision. Otherwise, excessively traumatizing the ampullary region may cause a serious postoperative acute pancreatitis.

A completion cholangiogram through the T-tube after the exploration has been concluded is an essential part of the maneuvers required to minimize the number of stones overlooked at operation. Several authors, notably White and Harrison, have accumulated data supporting the use of manometry and studies of the rate at which saline flows through the CBD as two methods of identifying caculi and other pathological obstructions to the CBD. Thus far, we have had no experience with this technique.

It is important to use a T-tube that is size 16F or larger following choledocholithotomy. Otherwise, the tract remaining when the T-tube is removed may not be large enough to admit the instruments required for removal of residual stones by the technique of Burhenne. Since Burhenne's method has a success rate of over 90%, it is important that the T-tube tract be large enough to retrieve a stone that has been left behind. Even small ducts will admit a 16F T-tube if the tube is trimmed by the technique described below (see Fig. 50–5).

Operative Technique—CBD Exploration Simultaneous with Cholecystectomy

Cholangiogram

If for some reason the cystic duct was not a suitable route for cholangiography by the technique described in Chap. 48, then perform this procedure by inserting a 21-gauge scalp vein needle into the CBD. Aspirate in order to confirm that the needle is in the duct lumen. Use a suture to fix the needle to the CBD. Attach a 2-meter length of sterile plastic tubing filled with the proper contrast medium. The remaining details of cholangiography are the same as those described in Chap. 48.

Kocher Maneuver

After the gallbladder has been removed and it is determined that a CBD exploration is indicated, perform a Kocher maneuver (see Figs 7–14, 7–15, and 7–16) by incising the lateral peritoneal attachments along the descending duodenum. Then incise the layer of avascular fibrous tissue that attaches the posterior duodenum to Gerota's fascia and to the foramen of Winslow. With the left index and the middle fingers situated behind the pancreas and duodenum and the thumb applied to the anterior wall of the duodenum, palpate the distal CBD and the ampulla. Pay special attention to the ampullary region in order not to overlook a small ampullary carcinoma, which may often be felt as a hard protrusion into the lumen from the back wall of the duodenum.

Choledochotomy Incision

Incise the peritoneum overlying the CBD in order to identify accurately the duct's anterior wall. Select an area for the choledochotomy preferably distal to the entrance of the cystic duct. Insert 2 guy sutures of 4–0 chromic catgut, one opposite the other on the anterior wall of the duct. If there are any obvious blood vessels located in this area, either transfix them with 5–0 Vicryl suture-ligatures or apply careful electrocoagulation. Use a No. 15 scalpel blade to make a short incision in the anterior wall of the CBD while the assistant holds up the guy sutures. Then use a Potts angled scissors to enlarge the incision in both directions. Pay attention to the possibility that the cystic duct may share a common wall with the CBD for a distance of 2 cm or more. If the incision is made in the vicinity of this common wall, it is possible to open the cystic duct instead of the CBD. This will produce considerable confusion. It is even possible to make an incision along the common wall and not encounter the lumen of either the cystic duct or the CBD and to expose the portal vein.

If the anteromedial aspect of the CBD is used for the choledochotomy incision, this problem will be avoided.

Exploring the CBD

As soon as the CBD has been opened, take a sample of the bile for a bacteriological culture and make a Gram stain for prompt identification of the bacteria that are frequently present.

Using the left thumb and index finger, milk down any possible stones from the common hepatic duct into the choledochotomy incision. Perform the same maneuver on the distal CBD. This maneuver will often deliver several calculi into the choledochotomy.

Pass a pituitary scoop of the appropriate size up into the right and the left main hepatic ducts for the removal of any possible calculi (**Fig. 50–1**). Then, with the left

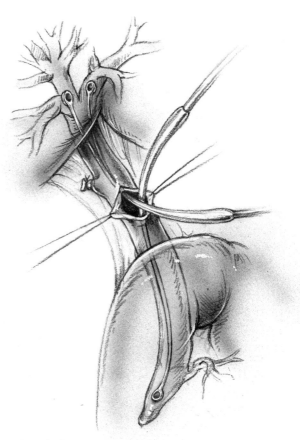

Fig. 50–1

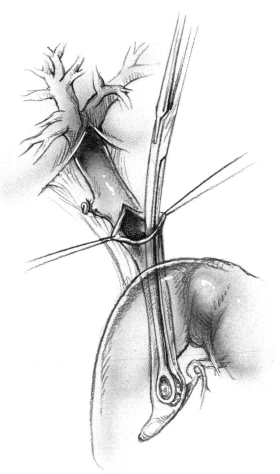

Fig. 50–2

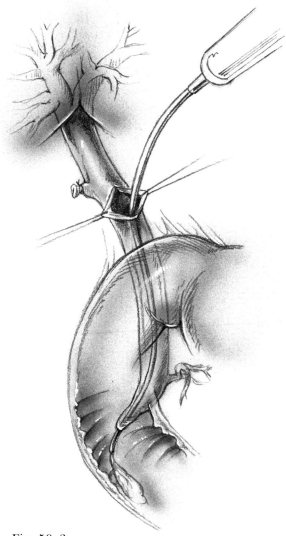

Fig. 50–3

index finger placed behind the ampulla, use the right hand to pass a pituitary scoop down to the region of the ampulla and remove any calculi encountered in this maneuver. It is helpful simultaneously to palpate with the left index finger behind the distal CBD while the scoop is being passed. Avoid excessive trauma to the ampulla. A Randall stone forceps (**Fig. 50–2**) may be inserted into the CBD for the purpose of removing stones, but we have not found this instrument to be particularly valuable as compared to the pituitary scoop. Following these maneuvers, use a small straight catheter to irrigate both the hepatic ducts and the distal CBD with normal saline solution (**Fig. 50–3**).

Now try to pass a 10F olive-tip (Coudé) catheter, preferably of the silk-woven type, through the ampulla. Injecting the catheter with saline will confirm its presence in the duodenum if the saline enters the duodenum without washing back through the choledochotomy incision. If the surgeon prefers to use the metal Bakes dilators to determine the patency of the ampulla, he should perform this maneuver with great delicacy as it is easy to perforate the distal CBD and to make a false passage through the head of the pancreas. It is not necessary to pass any instrument larger than a No. 3 Bakes dilator through the ampulla. Some surgeons feel that if the No. 3 dilator cannot pass, this is diagnostic of ampullary stenosis and is an indication for sphincteroplasty. *We do not agree with this concept,* as we explain in Chap. 53.

If there appears to be a calculus in the distal end of the CBD and it is not easily removed by means of the scoop, insert a Fogarty biliary catheter down the CBD into the duodenum. Blow up the balloon; this will help identify the ampulla. Gradually decompress the balloon as the catheter is withdrawn. As soon as the balloon is inside the CBD, reinflate it and withdraw. This will occasionally remove a stone that has been overlooked. Repeat the same maneuver in the right and left hepatic ducts. It is in the retrieval of the hepatic duct stones that the Fogarty catheter has its greatest usefulness.

Another maneuver that occasionally will successfully remove a stone is to use a 16F rubber catheter. Cut most of the flared proximal end of the catheter off and insert this end down the CBD to make contact with the stone. Amputate the tip of the catheter and attach a syringe to the distal tip of the catheter; apply suction while simultaneously withdrawing the catheter. The suction sometimes traps the calculus in the end of the catheter, after which it is easily removed.

If an impacted stone in the distal CBD cannot be removed in a nontraumatic fashion by these various maneuvers, do not hesitate to perform a sphincteroplasty, the technique for which is described below (Chap. 53). Sphincteroplasty is safer than traumatizing the ampulla.

Choledochoscopy

An intregal part of the CBD exploration is, we believe, choledochoscopy. This procedure can detect and retrieve stones or detect and biopsy ductal tumors, in some cases when all other methods have failed. Of the instruments currently available for endoscopy of the bile ducts, the rigid right-angle choledochoscope manufactured by Storz-Endoscopy, which contains a Hopkins rod-lens system that is illuminated by a fiberoptic channel, gives the best image quality. It is simpler to operate and much less expensive than the flexible fiberoptic endoscopes. The Storz choledochoscope shares with the flexible scopes the disadvantage that they require ethylene oxide gas sterilization, which precludes repeated utilization of the same scope on the same day. Only the Wolf choledochoscope is alleged to withstand steam autoclaving without damage. Flexible fiberoptic choledochoscopes are manufactured by ACM, Olympus, Fuji, and Machida. Although these flexible instruments have a much higher initial cost, more expensive upkeep, shorter lifespan, much greater susceptibility to damage, and somewhat inferior optical properties, they do indeed have one important advantage over the rigid scopes. The flexible scope can be passed for greater distances up along the hepatic radicals for the extraction of an otherwise inaccessible stone in this location. Similarly, the flexible scope can be passed right down to the ampulla and in about one-third of cases into the duodenum to rule out the presence of stones in the distal ampulla. Even if the scope does not enter the duodenum, when it is passed down to the ampullary orifice and the flow of saline enters the duodenum without refluxing back up into the CBD, this constitutes good evidence that the distal duct is free of calculi. The rigid scopes are not generally of sufficient length to accomplish this mission. Another area, in which the flexible scope is occasionally useful, is to extract retained calculi via the T-tube tract subsequent to CBD exploration.

Because of their lower cost and greater durability, the rigid scopes have been adopted more widely than have the flexible, despite the handicap mentioned above.

The horizontal arm of the Storz choledochoscope comes in two lengths: 40 mm and 60 mm. The vertical limbs of both models are identical. The cross section of the horizontal limb, which has to pass into the bile duct, is 5 by 3 mm, approximately the diameter of a No. 5 Bakes dilator. If the CBD will not admit a No. 5 dilator, choledochoscopy by this technique is contraindicated.

The choledochoscope operates in a liquid medium. This requires that a continuous stream of sterile saline under pressure be injected into the sidearm of the scope. The saline will then flow into the bile ducts. By crossing the two guy sutures over the choledochotomy incision, the CBD can be maintained in a state of distension by the flow of saline, providing optimal visualization. If the CBD is large enough, a metal instrument channel can be attached to the choledochoscope. Through this channel can be passed a flexible biopsy punch, a flexible forceps (7F size), a Dormia stone basket, or a Fogarty biliary catheter (5F caliber).

To use the choledochoscope, stand on the left side of the patient. Make the choledochotomy incision as far distal in the CBD as possible. Insert the choledochoscope toward the hepatic duct **(Fig. 50–4).** Initiate the flow of saline and cross over the two guy sutures to reduce the loss of saline from the choledochotomy incision.

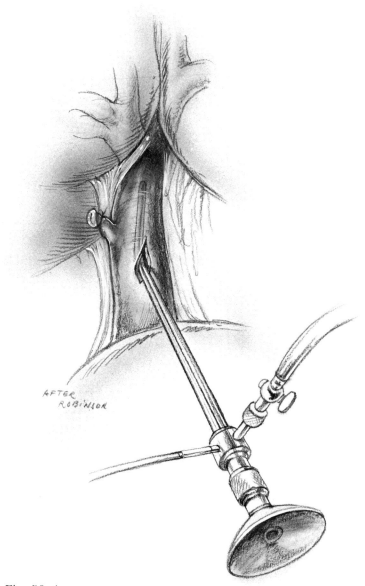

Fig. 50–4.

Enclose the 1-liter bag of sterile saline in a pressure pump (Fenwall) and use sterile intravenous tubing to connect the bag of saline to a 3-way stopcock. Insert the stopcock into the saline channel on the side of the choledochoscope.

Pass the horizontal limb of the scope up the common hepatic duct. Very soon the bifurcation of the right and left ducts will be seen. Occasionally the first branch of the right main duct will open into the bifurcation so that it resembles a trifurcation. Generally the left duct appears to be somewhat larger and easier to enter than the right. By properly directing the scope, it is possible to see into the orifices of many of the secondary and tertiary ducts. Withdraw the scope until the bifurcation is again seen and then pass the instrument into the right main duct using the same technique.

Before passing the scope down into the distal CBD, be sure that the duodenum has been completely Kocherized. By placing slight traction with the left hand on the region of the ampulla, the surgeon will help elongate and straighten the course of the CBD. This is important because the scope visualizes the duct with clear focus to infinity. What the surgeon really wants to learn from the choledochoscopy is whether there are any residual calculi between the scope and the ampulla. This requires an exact knowledge of the appearance of the ampulla, which has been described as an inverted cone with a small orifice that opens and closes intermittently to permit the passage of saline. However, we have found that using these landmarks as the only criterion for identifying the ampulla may lead to error. Occasionally, this type of error will permit a stone in the distal CBD to go undetected. Consequently, we believe there are only two positive methods of identifying the distal termination of the CBD. One is the passage of the 60-mm choledochoscope through a patulous ampulla (rarely possible). When this step can be accomplished, if the duodenum is inflated with saline, one can see quite clearly the duodenal mucosa that is markedly different from the smooth epithelium of the CBD. If the duodenum is not filled with saline, the mucosa will not be seen. If the scope does not pass into the duodenum spontaneously, make *no* attempt to pass it forcibly. A second method of positively identifying the termination of the CBD is to pass a Fogarty balloon catheter alongside the choledochoscope into the duodenum. Then inflate the balloon and draw back on the catheter. By following the catheter with a choledochoscope down to the region of the balloon one can be more certain that the entire CBD has been visualized and that no residual calculi remain in the CBD.

Occasionally, the view of the distal CBD is impeded by what appear to be shreds of either fibrin or ductal mucosa that may hang as a partially obscuring curtain across the lumen of the duct. Despite some of these difficulties in interpreting choledochoscopic observations, this procedure does indeed detect stones that have been missed by all other methods. In the hands of an experienced observer, choledochoscopy is probably the most accurate single method of detecting CBD stones. Calculi are easily identified. It may at first be confusing to find that a calculus 3 mm in diameter looks as big as a chunk of coal through the magnifying lens system. It is important to note that the Storz type of choledochoscope achieves a clear focus at distances from about 5 mm to infinity, and that any object within 0–5 mm from the tip of the scope will not be in focus.

If stones are seen, remove the choledochoscope and extract the stones by the usual means. If this is not possible, reinsert the choledochoscope and use a flexible alligator forceps, the Fogarty catheter, or the Dormia stone basket, *all under the direct visual control of the choledochoscope.*

If any lesion of the mucosa which is suspicious of carcinoma is identified, insert a flexible biopsy punch and obtain a sample. Sometimes an ampullary carcinoma can be identified and biopsied in this manner. Occasionally patients with ampullary carcinoma will have a second carcinoma in either the common or the hepatic duct. Under direct visual control, accurate biopsy is not difficult through the choledochoscope.

Results reported by Berci, Shore, Morgenstern, and Hamlin and by Nora, Berci, Dorazzio, Kirschenbaum, and others indicate that routine CBD exploration and removal of calculi is accompanied by a 5% incidence of retained stones and that, following choledochoscopy, the incidence of residual stones can be reduced to 0–2%.

Using choledochoscopy routinely during CBD exploration adds no more than 10 minutes to the procedure and, in our experience, does occasionally detect a stone that has been missed by all other modalities. Because it appears to be devoid of dangerous complications, we have adopted choledochoscopy as a part of routine CBD exploration. We have seen one complication that was possibly related to the saline flush under pressure during choledochoscopy, namely, a mild case of postoperative pancreatitis. However, we have no data to indicate that the incidence of postoperative pancreatitis is indeed increased by the use of choledochoscopy.

Sphincterotomy for Impacted Stones

Perform a complete Kocher maneuver down to the third part of the duodenum and insert a folded gauze pad behind the duodenum and the head of the pancreas. Pass a stiff catheter or a No. 4 Bakes dilator into the choledochotomy incision and down to the distal CBD. Do not pass it into the duodenum. By palpating the tip of the catheter or the Bakes instrument through the anterior wall of the duodenum, ascertain the location of the ampulla. Make a 4 cm incision in the lateral wall of the duodenum opposite the ampulla. In-

sert small Richardson retractors to expose the ampulla. Often the impacted stone is not in the lumen of the CBD but partially buried in the duct wall. This permits the Bakes dilator to pass beyond the stone and to distend the ampulla. If this is the case, make a 10-mm incision with a scalpel through the anterior wall of the ampulla down to the metal instrument at 11 o'clock, a location far away from the entrance of the pancreatic duct. A 10 mm incision will allow the dilator to enter the duodenum. Remove the Bakes dilator through the choledochotomy incision, and explore the distal CBD through the sphincterotomy incision. Use the smallest size pituitary scoop. Often the stone can be easily removed in this fashion. If the papillotomy incision has to be extended a significant distance to provide adequate exposure, then a complete sphincteroplasty should be undertaken. This technique is described in Chap. 53. If the sphincterotomy is only 10 mm in length, it is generally not necessary to suture the mucosa of the CBD to that of the duodenum. Rather, if there is no bleeding, leave the papillotomy undisturbed after the impacted stone has been removed. Repair the duodenotomy by the same technique as described following spincteroplasty (see Chap. 53). Then insert the T-tube into the CBD incision.

Checking for Ampullary Stenosis

Before completing the CBD exploration, the diameter of the ampulla of Vater may be calibrated by passing either a catheter or a Bakes dilator. If a 10F rubber catheter passes through the ampulla, no further calibration is necessary. If this device is too soft, use a Coudé olive-tip silk-woven catheter, borrowed from the urologist. The Coudé catheter is stiffer than rubber but softer than metal. Unfortunately, these catheters require gas sterilization, but they are a safer means of examining the ampulla than are Bakes dilators. If a 10F Coudé catheter passes into the duodenum, the diagnosis of ampullary stenosis can be eliminated. The presence of the catheter in the duodenum can be confirmed by injecting saline through the catheter. If the catheters fail to pass, insert the left hand behind the region of the ampulla and pass a No. 3 Bakes dilator gently through the ampulla. Failure to pass through the ampulla with ease is more often due to pushing the instrument in the wrong direction than to ampullary stenosis. In the absence of malignancy, we have found it to be indeed rare that we were unable to pass a catheter or dilator through the ampulla using manipulation. If the preexploration cystic duct cholangiogram showed dye passing through the duodenum, then failing to pass a 3-mm instrument through the ampulla is not by itself an indication for sphincteroplasty or biliary-intestinal bypass. We are not convinced that ampullary stenosis is a cause of clinical symptoms, save for the exceptional patient.

In any case, never use excessive force in passing these instruments because penetration of the intrapancreatic portion of the CBD may produce fatal complications, es-

pecially if the damage is not recognized during the operation.

Insertion of the T-Tube

Although it may be possible in some cases to avoid draining the CBD following the removal of stones, we believe that a T-tube should routinely be inserted to decompress the CBD and also to facilitate a cholangiogram 7–8 days following surgery. Do not use a silicone T-tube, as this substance is nonreactive. Consequently, there may be no well-organized tract from the CBD to the outside. When the silicone tube is removed, bile peritonitis will follow. Use a 16F rubber tube. If a smaller size is used, it may not be possible to extract a residual stone postoperatively through the T-tube tract. A 16F tube can almost always be used, even in a small CBD, if half the circumference is excised from the horizontal limb as illustrated in **Figs. 50–5a and 5b.** After inserting the T-tube, close the choledochotomy incision with a continuous

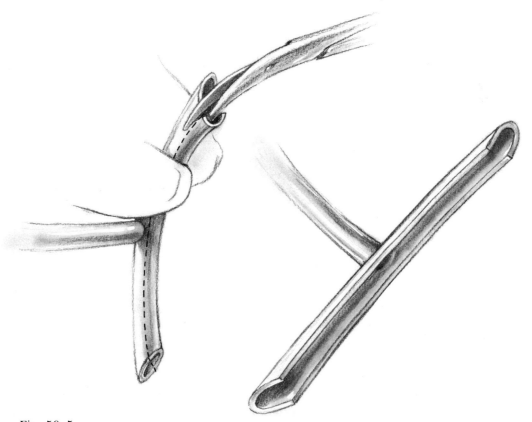

Fig. 50–5

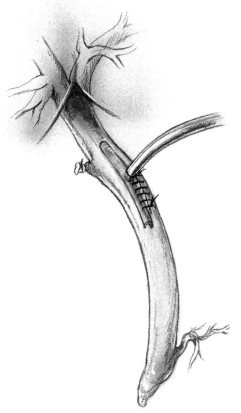

Fig. 50–6

5–0 atraumatic Vicryl suture **(Fig. 50–6).** Make this closure snug around the T-tube to avoid leakage during cholangiography.

Completion Cholangiogram

Eliminate the air in the long limb of the T-tube by inserting the long cholangiogram catheter that was used for the cystic duct cholangiogram down into the vertical limb of the T-tube for its full distance. Then, gradually inject the contrast medium into this limb while simultaneously removing the plastic catheter. This will fill the vertical limb with contrast material and displace the air. Then, attach the T-tube directly to a long plastic connecting tube that is in turn attached to a 30 ml syringe.

Elevate the left flank about 10 cm above the horizontal operating table. Stand behind a lead screen covered with sterile sheets and perform the cholangiogram by injecting 4 ml of diluted contrast medium for the first radiograph and an equal amount for the second and third pic-

tures. We use a mixture of 1 part Conray and 1 or 2 parts saline. The larger the duct, the more dilute the solution.

If the contrast material has not entered the duodenum, repeat the sequence after 1 mg of nitroglycerine in 3 ml of water has been instilled into the patient's nose by the anesthesiologist. If the contrast material still does not enter the duodenum but the X ray is otherwise negative, discontinue the study. Severe sphincter spasm often follows ampullary instrumentation and cannot be overcome during the completion cholangiogram.

Drainage and Closure

Bring the T-tube out through a stab wound near the anterior axillary line together with a radiopaque latex drain. The stab wound should be large enough to admit the surgeon's fingertip. Suture the T-tube to the skin, leaving enough slack between the CBD and the abdominal wall to allow for some abdominal distension.

Close the abdominal wall by the Smead-Jones technique utilizing No. 1 PDS by the technique described in Chap. 5.

Postoperative Care

Attach the T-tube to a sterile plastic bag. Permit it to drain freely by gravity until a cholangiogram is performed through the T-tube in the X ray department on the 7th or 8th postoperative day. Do not permit any contrast material to be injected into the T-tube under pressure since this may produce pancreatitis or bacteremia. Injection by gravity flow is preferable. If the cholangiogram is negative and shows free flow into the duodenum, clamp the T-tube for the next few days. Unclamp it if the patient experiences any abdominal pain, nausea, vomiting, shoulder pain, or leakage of bile around the T-tube. Remove the T-tube on the 10th to 14th postoperative day. Although we generally prefer to remove the tube on the 10th postoperative day, we have indeed experienced a 1%–2% incidence of localized bile peritonitis because the T-tube tract was not sufficiently well walled off and thus permitted leakage of bile into the peritoneal cavity. It is possible that leaving the tube in for a few more days may reduce the incidence of this complication. White and Harrison suggest that the T-tube be withdrawn only sufficiently to be removed from the CBD. They then permit the tube to remain in place for 1–2 days with the T just outside the bile duct so that it acts as a drain for any possible bile leakage.

Following choledocholithotomy, continue antibiotics for at least 3 days, depending on the nature of the Gram stain, the bacteriological studies, and the patient's clinical response.

Continue nasogastric suction for 1–3 days, or until the patient shows evidence of bowel activity.

Remove the latex drain 4–7 days following surgery unless there has been significant bilious drainage.

Observe the patient carefully for the possible development of a postoperative acute pancreatitis by obtaining serum amylase determinations every 2 days. If there is significant elevation, continue nasogastric suction and intravenous fluids. Some patients with postoperative acute pancreatitis do not have pain or significant elevations of the serum amylase, but they do have intolerance for food with frequent vomiting after nasogastric suction has been discontinued. In these cases a sonogram showing an enlarged pancreas is enough to confirm the diagnosis. In general, do not feed the patient following biliary tract surgery if his serum amylase is significantly elevated or if there is any other strong suspicion of acute pancreatitis; for this complication may be serious.

Postoperative Complications

Bile Leak and Bile Peritonitis

T-Tube Displaced

The T-tube is fixed at two points: (1) the CBD and (2) the point on the skin where the T-tube is sutured in position. Enough slack must be left in the long limb of the T-tube between the CBD and the skin so that an increase in abdominal distension will not result in the tube being drawn out of the CBD. Occasionally, the T-tube is inadvertently partially withdrawn from the CBD even before the abdominal incision is closed. When bile leaks around the choledochotomy incision, bilious drainage will be noted from the drain tract alongside the T-tube. If this leak occurs during the first few days following the operation, upper abdominal pain and tenderness may appear, indicating bile peritonitis. While a localized leak of bile is fairly well tolerated in the postoperative patient who has adequate drainage, the spreading of bile diffusely over a large part of the abdominal cavity may produce a generalized bile peritonitis if the bile is infected. Diffuse abdominal tenderness generally demands immediate laparotomy for replacement of the T-tube.

Duct Injury

When a completion cholangiogram through the T-tube has been accomplished in the operating room, a *major* duct injury will be apparent on the film. However, the cholangiogram may not disclose an injury to an *accessory* duct. If this becomes manifest by the continuous drainage of small to moderate amounts of bile along the drain tract and the cholangiogram is persistently normal, remove the T-tube and insert a small Foley catheter into the drain tract. Perform a cholangiogram through this catheter after the balloon has been inflated. Do this procedure 2 weeks following surgery. The most frequently injured anomalous bile duct is that which drains the dorsal caudal segment of the right lobe.

Postoperative Acute Pancreatitis

Acute pancreatitis following choledocholithotomy accounts for about half the postoperative fatalities. It is often caused by instrumental trauma to the ampullary region owing to excessive zeal either in dilating the ampulla or in extracting an impacted stone. In the case of the impacted stone, if it cannot be removed with ease through the choledochotomy incision, approach it via a duodenotomy and papillotomy. Treatment of acute pancreatitis calls for prolonged nasogastric suction, fluid replacement, and respiratory support when indicated. Antibiotics are probably also indicated.

Frequent determination of the serum amylase in patients following choledocholithotomy is necessary because some patients with postoperative pancreatitis do not complain of an unusual degree of pain. Their only symptom may be abdominal distension and vomiting, unless shock and hypoxia supervene. The mortality rate following postoperative acute pancreatitis is reported to be quite high, approaching 30%–50%. Total parenteral nutrition is indicated because many of these patients require from 3–6 weeks of nasogastric suction before the amylase returns to normal, at which time food may be given by mouth. Premature feeding in these cases may cause a severe and even fatal exacerbation.

Another cause of postoperative pancreatitis is the use of an indwelling catheter or a long-armed T-tube, which transverses the ampulla and tends to obstruct the orifice of the pancreatic duct. No indwelling tube should be permitted to remain in the ampulla unless a sphincteroplasty has been performed.

Increasing Jaundice

After choledocholithotomy in the jaundiced patient, it is common for the serum bilirubin concentration to increase by 4–6 mg/dl in the first postoperative week. This does not mean that the patient necessarily has a CBD obstruction. Rather, the imposition of major surgery and anesthesia upon the liver, already damaged by a period of duct obstruction, temporarily aggravates the hepatic dysfunction. By the 10th–12th postoperative day, the bilirubin will have peaked and have started on its way down toward normal, unless the patient does indeed have another cause for his postoperative jaundice. This may be a halothane hepatitis, a blood clot, or an overlooked carcinoma in the main hepatic duct. Obstruction of the distal CBD by a retained stone will not produce postoperative jaundice if the T-tube is functioning properly. Obtain a routine cholangiogram through the T-tube by the 10th postoperative day. This will clarify the cause of persistent jaundice.

Hemorrhage

Intra-Abdominal Hemorrhage
Intra-abdominal hemorrage is often manifested by red blood coming through the drain tract. If this is not accompanied by any systemic symptoms or abdominal signs, one may suspect that the bleeding arises from a blood vessel in the skin or the abdominal wound. Bleeding of sufficient magnitude to require one or more blood transfusions invariably originates from the operative area. The cause may be a defective ligature on the cystic artery or oozing from the liver or from some other intra-abdominal blood vessel. These patients require prompt reexploration through the same incision, complete evacuation of the blood clots, and identification of the bleeding point.

Hemobilia

Bleeding through the T-tube indicates hemobilia. This may arise from intrahepatic trauma during attempts to extract an intrahepatic calculus. Generally, expectant therapy is sufficient if any vitamin K deficiency has been corrected preoperatively. In case of persistent hemobilia, perform both a T-tube cholangiogram and a hepatic arteriogram as iatrogenic trauma to a specific branch of the hepatic artery during the hepatic duct exploration may be the source of bleeding. This type of complication occurred in less than 1 in 1,000 cases of CBD exploration (White and Harrison). Treatment consists of ligating the proper branch of hepatic artery, as identified on the arteriogram, or of occluding the vessel by transcatheter embolization in the angiography suite.

The Residual CBD Stone

Early Postoperative Treatment

Most often a residual CBD stone will be detected when the postoperative T-tube cholangiogram is performed. When this study is read as positive for calculi by the radiologist, carefully review the films. Request a repeat study to rule out the possibility that the shadow may be due to an air bubble. Shadows that are odd in shape may not be calculi but may be due to residual blood clot or debris. There is no necessity for early operative intervention aimed at removing a residual CBD stone, so long as the T-tube is draining well. This is true because the nonoperative methods of extracting calculi are extremely effective and have a low complication rate. Also, some of the radiographic shadows, interpreted as calculi, may indeed be artifacts that will disappear without treatment.

If the radiographic evidence is convincing and a stone less than 1 cm in diameter is seen in the lower portion of the CBD, an attempt at a saline flush with or without heparin solution may be indicated, if tolerated by the patient. This is performed not before the 12th postoperative day. Infuse 1,000 ml of normal saline with 5,000 units of heparin through the T-tube over a 24-hour period, provided this does not produce excessive pain. If the calculus completely obstructs the distal CBD, this technique is contraindicated. Repeat this therapy every day for 4–5 days if tolerated. Then repeat the cholangiogram. If the radiographic appearance of the stone shows reduction in size, repeat the series of saline flushes again the following week. Otherwise, send the patient home with the T-tube in place. If the stone is not obstructing and the patient tolerates clamping of the T-tube, keep the tube clamped. Prescribe a choleretic like Decholin in order to dilute the bile. Otherwise, have the patient inject 30–60 ml of sterile saline into the T-tube daily. Ask the patient to return to the hospital about 6 weeks following operation.

Subsequent Postoperative Treatment

When the patient returns for examination 6 weeks after the operation, repeat the T-tube cholangiogram in order to confirm the persistence of the residual stone, since in a number of cases there may be spontaneous passage of the calculus into the duodenum. The simplest and safest method of extracting residual calculi is that described by Burhenne. In this method, it is necessary that the long arm of the T-tube be at least the size of a 14F–16F catheter. After the cholangiogram is completed and does indeed confirm the presence of stones, remove the T-tube and insert a flexible catheter that can be manipulated, like the one available from Medi-Tech. With a continuous flow of contrast medium through the catheter, insert the device down the T-tube tract until the CBD has been entered. Then, directing the tip of the catheter toward the calculus, insert a Dormia stone basket device through the Medi-Tech catheter. Under fluoroscopic control, trap the stone in the stone basket and withdraw the basket, the stone, and the catheter through the T-tube tract. Experienced radiologists, like Burhenne, have reported a success rate better than 90% with this technique. If the stone is quite large, it may not fit into the T-tube tract. However, really large stones are not commonly left behind by competent surgeons. For this reason, almost all residual stones can be removed by this technique. It is even possible to cannulate the right and left hepatic ducts to remove stones.

Another method of accomplishing the same end is to pass a flexible fiberoptic choledochoscope into the CBD via the T-tube tract.

If these methods have failed, endoscopic papillotomy by ERCP technique should be tried *if an expert is available.* Experienced endoscopists have reported performing ERCP–papillotomy and extraction of retained stones with 1%–2% mortality. If expertise with this technique is not available, a stone that is blocking the flow of bile to the CBD will require relaparotomy and choledochotomy for removal. A CBD stone that is not symptomatic when the T-tube is clamped presents a more difficult problem. Some surgeons may elect to remove the T-tube, continue to observe the patient, and reserve reoperation for those patients who later become symptomatic. Alternatively, it may well be argued that it is safer to perform an elective operation for removal of the stone rather than an urgent procedure in the presence of cholangitis. In most cases elective choledocholithotomy is indicated (see Chap. 51).

References

Allen B, Shapiro H, Way LW (1981) Management of recurrent and residual common duct stones. Am J Surg 142:41

Berci G, Shore JM, Morgenstern L, Hamlin JA (1978) Choledochoscopy and operative flourocholangiography in the prevention of retained bile duct stones. World J Surg 2:411

Burhenne HJ (1976) Complications of nonoperative extraction of retained common duct stones. Am J Surg 131:260

Jones SA (1978) The prevention and treatment of recurrent bile duct stones by transduodenal sphincteroplasty. World J Surg 2:473

Madden JL (1978) Primary common bile duct stones. World J Surg 2:265

Nora PF, Berci G, Dorazzio RA, Kirschenbaum G, et al. (1977) Operative choledochoscopy. Am J Surg 44:105

Rutledge RH (1976) Sphincteroplasty and choledochoduodenostomy for benign biliary obstructions. Ann Surg 183:476

Saharia PC, Zuidema GD, Cameron JL (1977) Primary common duct stones. Ann Surg 185:598

Thomas CG Jr, Nicholson CP, Owen J (1971) Effectiveness of choledochoduodenostomy and transduodenal sphincteroplasty in the treatment of benign obstruction of the common duct. Ann Surg 173:845

Way LW, Admirand WH, Dunphy JE (1972) Management of choledocholithiasis. Ann Surg 176:347

White TT, Harrison RC (1973) Reoperative gastrointestinal surgery. Little Brown, Boston

51 Concept: When to Perform Other Operations on the Common Bile Duct (CBD)

Operations for Retained or Recurrent CBD Stones

Choice of Operative Procedure

When stones are found in the bile ducts long after the first CBD operation has been done, the T-tube tract is healed and Burhenne's method of retrieval cannot be applied. The options then available to the surgeon are: endoscopic radiographic cholangiopancreatogram (ERCP)-papillotomy, transabdominal choledocholithotomy, biliary-intestinal bypass, or sphincteroplasty. The pros and cons of these procedures are discussed below.

ERCP-Papillotomy

Experienced operators have reported performing a large number of ERCP-papillotomies with a mortality rate of 1.5% (Reiter, Bayer, Mennicken, and Manegold). With increasing experience, this rate may undergo further improvement. Consequently, if an expert with this technique is available, this may well be the procedure of choice especially in the poor-risk patient. In patients, who have previously undergone Billroth II gastrectomy or who have unusually large calculi (over 2.5 cm in diameter), ERCP-papillotomy is contraindicated. ERCP-papillotomy has, on occasion, provided a brilliant solution to the problem of a recurrent CBD stone in the patient with disabling cardiac disease. However, when the ERCP-papillotomy is performed by an endoscopist lacking experience and expertise, the results may be disastrous, just as one may expect disastrous results when a secondary choledocholithotomy is performed by a poorly trained surgeon. Whether the ERCP-papillotomy performed by an expert is superior to secondary choledocholithotomy also performed by an expert is a question that cannot be answered with precision at this time because of inadequate data. Because most hospitals around the world have not yet developed real expertise with the ERCP-papillotomy, laparotomy and choledocholithotomy are the treatment of choice in most cases for recurrent or residual calculi. The poor-risk patient, however, should be referred to a center where expertise in ERCP-papillotomy is available.

Laparotomy for Secondary Choledocholithotomy; Bypass; Sphincteroplasty

Reexploring the CBD for residual stones during the first month following primary choledocholithotomy has a mortality rate of 10.7%, according to Bergdahl and Holmlund. Relaparotomy for retained stones is rarely indicated during the first 4–6 weeks after the primary operation for several reasons. First, small stones often pass spontaneously. Second, by using Burhenne's method, one can extract 80%–90% of the stones through the T-tube tract if the T-tube is 14–16F or larger in size. Third, relaparotomy is safer when it is performed after a delay of 4–6 weeks. In our experience, a secondary choledocholithotomy performed after the 6th week is not more dangerous than an elective primary choledocholithotomy. Girard and Legros confirm this observation. There should be no hesitation about operating to remove stones from the CBD, once they have been detected either by sonogram, intravenous cholangiogram, PTC, or ERCP, especially if the stones produce symptoms. In the good-risk patient, the operation for removal of the stones should be performed even if the patient is nonsymptomatic, unless the stone is so small (less than 1.0 cm) that it is likely to pass spontaneously.

The major controversy in this area centers about the question whether a biliary-intestinal bypass or a sphincteroplasty should be added to the choledocholithotomy procedure.

When to Perform Bypass or Sphincteroplasty for Secondary Choledocholithiasis

There is a wide variety of opinion concerning when a biliary-intestinal bypass or sphincteroplasty should be performed in patients with common duct stones. For instance, Schein and Gliedman advocate doing a choledochoduodenostomy whenever a CBD is encountred that is 1.4 cm or more in diameter during the performance of either a primary or a secondary choledocholithotomy. They also routinely perform a choledochoduodenostomy whenever they open a CBD for retained or recurrent stones or when a patient suffers from ampullary stenosis. Their operative mortality rate is 3.2%.

In a study of 126 consecutive CBD explorations, Madden diagnosed the presence of "primary" CBD stones in 60% of the cases and performed a choledochoduodenostomy in each to prevent recurrence.

Jones advocates sphincteroplasty during a primary CBD operation:

> when one encounters impacted distal common duct stones, stenosis of Papilla (defined as inability to pass a 3-mm dilator or catheter from above or below and from either side of the table), benign stricture of the distal duct (e.g., from pancreatitis), irremovable hepatic duct stones, ductal mud, sludge, or stasis stones pathogno-

> monic of chronic intermittent distal ductal obstruction, and multiple ductal calculi by which is meant a sufficient number of stones present to make complete clearing of the ducts doubtful . . . When operating for residual stones, sphincteroplasty is indicated when the stones are of the stasis type with mud and sludge present in the bile, and when any of the indications described under primary duct exploration are present. Sphincteroplasty is not advised at primary or secondary choledocholithotomy when the calculi appear to be of gallbladder origin, the bile is clear, only a few large calculi are present, the papilla is 3 mm in diameter or larger, choledochodoscopy shows a clear duct, and the completion cholangiogram is normal. [Emphasis is ours.]

In a series of 312 patients undergoing sphincteroplasty, Jones encountered a mortality rate of 0.96%. This enviably low mortality rate unfortunately will not be duplicated by less-experienced surgeons.

We are in general agreement with the above quotation from Jones's paper. However, together with Longmire, and with White and Harrison, we do not believe that the failure to pass a 3 mm catheter or dilator through the ampulla constitutes proof of a diseased ampulla or, by itself, an indication for bypass or sphincteroplasty. We also disagree with Jones on several other points. When a duodenotomy is required to remove a stone impacted in the ampulla, a simple sphincterotomy about 8–10 mm long will usually release the stone without the necessity of a longer incision in the sphincter of Oddi, the exposure of the duct of Wirsung, or the choledochoduodenal suturing that are required when a long sphincteroplasty is performed. Cases of multiple ductal calculi in which a skilled surgeon is unable to clear the ducts completely with the aid of choledochoscopy and cholangiography are rare. Consequently, the percentage of patients undergoing either primary or secondary choledocholithotomy who will require a bypass or a sphincteroplasty is quite low.

In cases of "primary" CBD stones or sludge, encountered at secondary choledocholithotomy, Saharia, Zuidema, and Cameron found that 82% of their patients who underwent simple *choledocholithotomy* without any additional bypass or sphincteroplasty did well during a followup period that averaged 4 years and 9 months.

There is no data to substantiate the policy advocated by Schein and Gliedman that a choledochoduodenal bypass be performed for every patient who has a large CBD or who has a retained or recurrent CBD stone. The fact that these patients did well during their brief period of postoperative followup observation does not constitute proof that they needed the choledochoduodenostomy in the first place. No prospective study comparing simple choledocholithotomy with bypass procedures has been reported. It is for this reason that this controversy continues.

We perform a bypass or a sphincteroplasty when we believe that we have not cleared the bile ducts of all stones; after one or two previous choledocholithotomy operations for multiple "primary" type CBD stones; and when there is an obstruction of the distal CBD because of a stricture or obstruction of the distal 3–4 cm of the CBD by chronic pancreatitis. Apart from the few exceptions described above, secondary choledocholithotomy followed by negative choledochoscopy and cholangiography, will give results equal to or better than those following bypass procedures or sphincteroplasty, and without the increased risk that these procedures will add to a simple choledocholithotomy when they are executed by surgeons who have *not* performed 100 (Schein and Gliedman), 175 (Degenshein), 138 (Partington), or 312 (Jones) operations. The postoperative mortality rates for choledochoduodenostomy have been reported to be 3.2% (Schein and Gliedman), 3.2% (Degenshein), 3.0% (average of 10 reports summarized by Thomas, Nicholson, and Owen), and 7.8% (Kraus and Wilson). For sphincteroplasty, the mortality rates have been 0.96% (Jones), 2.9% (Partington), and 4.6% (average of 10 reports by Thomas and colleagues). Choledochoduodenostomy and sphincteroplasty are procedures that add to the operative risk; they should be employed only for serious indications.

A more realistic appraisal of the mortality following sphincteroplasty and choledochoduodenostomy may perhaps be obtained by Hutchinson's review of 100 consecutive cases requiring duodenotomy by various staff members at the Swedish Hospital in Seattle. Ninety-three of these cases included either sphincterotomy or sphincteroplasty, often together with choledocholithotomy. Of these 93 patients, 6 (or 6.4%) died of complications directly related to the surgery. Three patients died of pancreatic and duodenal fistula: one from sepsis with cholangitis; one from hepatic necrosis (sepsis); and one from necrotising pancreatitis. Four other patients suffered from a postoperative duodenal fistula following sphincterotomy, but survived. There were two additional postoperative deaths in this series; they followed choledochoduodenostomy and were caused by pancreatic and biliary fistulas and sepsis.

In reviewing 100 contemporaneous cases of cholecystectomy and CBD exploration from the same hospital, Hutchinson found a 4% mortality, but all four of these patients were in their 9th decade of life and died of causes not directly related to the biliary tract or pancreas. These causes included general debility, pulmonary embolus, polycystic kidneys with perirenal abscess, and myocardial insufficiency. Two hundred fifty patients underwent cholecystectomy at the same institution with no deaths and only four complications, while 100 patients undergoing gastric resection encountered no fatalities and only 8% complications. All patients with neoplastic diseases were excluded from Hutchinson's study. One can conclude from this data that opening the duodenum, either for surgery on the sphincter or choledochoduodenostomy, appears to be more hazardous than is generally appreciated. The duodenum and the sphincter of Oddi must be treated with great respect and the most meticulous surgical technique.

Operations for Noncalculous Biliary Tract Disease

Ampullary Stenosis

Papillitis or fibrosis of the papilla of Vater, with concomitant stenosis of the pancreatic duct orifice, as an important cause of abdominal symptoms is a concept that was emphasized by Nardi and Acosta. The clinical signs and symptoms caused by the ampullary stenosis were said to include postcholecystectomy pain, recurrent pancreatitis, jaundice, enlargement and thickening of the CBD, and liver dysfunction. These authors claimed that histological examination of tissue removed from the papilla by operative biopsy proved the presence of inflammation or fibrosis in these patients. Confirmation of the diagnosis of ampullary stenosis was obtained by operative cholangiography or the inability to pass a No. 3 Bakes dilator through the ampulla, or both. We agree with Longmire and with White and Harrison "that passage of dilators at operation to determine the presence of sphincter stenosis is an unreliable indicator." On the basis of cholangiographic studies, the only finding that suggests a diagnosis of ampullary stenosis is a large CBD in the absence of any other organic obstruction.

Concerning recurrent pancreatitis, White (1973) pointed out that sphincteroplasty appears to be of no value in the treatment of *alcoholic* pancreatitis. There are rare instances of recurrent pancreatitis being caused by stenosis of the orifice of the duct of Wirsung. This diagnosis can be made on the basis of either an ERCP or an operative pancreatogram demonstrating a dilatation of the pancreatic duct beginning right at the orifice of the duct of Wirsung. In this case, a sphincteroplasty of the ampulla of Vater as well as a sphincteroplasty of the orifice of Wirsung's duct may be helpful (Bartlett and Nardi; Moody, Berenson, and McCloskey).

In patients suffering postcholecystectomy pain, recommended operative remedies have included relaparotomy for excision of cystic duct remnants or neuromata of the cystic duct stump, papillotomy for biliary dyskinesia, as well as a host of other procedures. It is extremely important to recognize that many patients classified as "postcholecystectomy syndrome" in reality are experiencing pain on the basis of some emotional disorder. Often the initial cholecystectomy was not performed for biliary calculi but for the complaints of epigastric discomfort and flatulence. Careful questioning will frequently disclose very little difference between the symptoms labeled as "postcholecystectomy syndrome" and those symptoms of which the patient complained *prior to* the initial cholecystectomy. Longmire stated, "stenosis of the sphincter of Oddi without demonstable common duct stones or debris is a rare cause of recurrent episodic upper abdominal pain with limited specific physical findings."

Schein felt that the diagnosis of ampullary stenosis could be made with the following criteria:

1) Dilated and thickened CBD

2) Delay of more than 90 minutes in the emptying of the CBD following intravenous cholangiography

3) Elevation of intraductal pressure on CBD manometry

4) Difficulty in passing a No. 3 Bakes dilator through the ampulla

Some of these criteria, such as elevation of the manometric pressure in the CBD and difficulty in passing a No. 3 dilator can both occur in patients who are devoid of symptoms. This discrepancy raises some question about the reliability of Schein's criteria in predicting whether sphincteroplasty is indicated.

At the present time it appears that symptomatic ampullary stenosis is a rare disease that is difficult to diagnose with accuracy. Patients who have a dilated CBD, in the absence of any apparent additional etiology, and pain accompanied by some elevation of the serum bilirubin or liver enzymes may be benefited by sphincteroplasty. The likelihood of successful results following sphincteroplasty is enhanced if the patient also suffers from biliary sludge or primary stones. Otherwise, "sphincteroplasty is a procedure with potentially serious risk that should be used with the utmost discrimination and care" (Longmire).

Recently, Nardi, Michelassi, and Zannini reported a study of 85 cases of transduodenal sphincteroplasty with Wirsung ductoplasty (see Fig. 53–5) with a followup of 1–25 years. Overall, 50% of the patients experienced a successful long-term result. These authors perform the morphine-prostigmin test as follows: 10 mg of morphine and 1 mg of prostigmin methylsulfate are injected intramuscularly. Serum amylase and lipase levels are measured 1, 2, and 4 hours later. The test is considered positive only if enzyme levels rise to three times normal or higher. Sphincteroplasty-ductoplasty has relieved symptoms in 28% of patients when the test is negative. A positive morphine-prostigmin test predicts good long-term results, especially in patients who have never had previous abdominal surgery and who do not suffer from alcoholism, narcotic abuse, or diarrhea. This report suggests that there is indeed a *small* cohort of patients who have recurrent severe abdominal pain secondary to recurrent acute pancreatitis caused by partial obstruction of Wirsung's duct and who may benefit from a ductoplasty.

CBD Obstruction Due to Periductal Chronic Pancreatic Fibrosis

An uncommon cause of obstruction to the distal 3–5 cm of the CBD is a chronic pancreatitis that produces periductal fibrosis and a long stricture-like condition of the distal duct. The degree of obstruction may sometimes be complete. Surgery for this condition requires a biliary-intestinal bypass, as sphincteroplasty is contraindicated in this situation because the length of the constriction is greater than one can encompass with sphincteroplasty. Whether this bypass should consist of a choledochoduodenostomy or a Roux-Y choledochojejunostomy is discussed below.

CBD Obstruction Due to Inoperable Carcinoma of Pancreas

In many hospitals the standard operation aimed at relieving jaundice in an inoperable carcinoma of the pancreas is a side-to-side cholecystojejunostomy or cholecystoduodenostomy (Dayton, Traverso, and Longmire). There are two drawbacks to these operations. One is the fact that the pancreatic carcinoma sometimes grows up along the wall of the CBD and occludes the cystic duct within a matter of a few weeks or months. This causes recurrence of the patient's jaundice and requires a second procedure for palliation. A second drawback is the fact that a leak from either a cholecystoduodenostomy or a side-to-side cholecystojejunostomy constitutes a serious complication with a significant mortality rate.

On the other hand, if a Roux-Y anastomosis is made between the jejunum and the anterior wall of the dilated hepatic duct in these cases, leakage from this anastomosis would consist of pure bile. In the presence of any type of external drainage, this type of leak is harmless. The argument that the Roux-Y technique, which requires a second jejunojejunal anastomosis, is more time consuming can be answered by constructing the jejunojejunostomy with a stapling device. This method takes only 2–3 minutes (see Chap. 55).

Biliary-Intestinal Bypass versus Sphincteroplasty

Once it has been decided that a patient requires some type of bypass procedure or sphincteroplasty for such conditions as recurrent stasis stones of the CBD or ampullary stenosis, which procedure should be chosen? Sphincteroplasty is indicated for patients who require septectomy for stenosis of Wirsung's duct and for patients with ampullary stenosis, especially if the CBD is less than 1.5 cm in diameter. Sphincteroplasty is contraindicated in the presence of some periampullary diverticula of the duodenum, a lengthy stenosis of the distal CBD secondary to pancreatic fibrosis, and Caroli's cholangiohepatitis.

The bypass is preferred by many surgeons in the elderly, poor-risk patient because it can be accomplished with greater speed and perhaps with a reduced risk of postoperative pancreatitis. If for some reason, an exploratory duodenotomy has already been performed, it may be difficult to construct a proper choledochoduodenal anastomosis since the duodenotomy is likely to be in an unfavorable location for this type of anastomosis. In these cases, perform either a sphincteroplasty or close the duodenotomy and create a choledochojejunal Roux-Y bypass.

A summary of the pros and cons of each procedure may be seen in Table 51–1.

Concept: Choledochoduodenostomy versus Roux-Y Choledochojejunostomy

A proper choledochoduodenal anastomosis should be made about 2.5 cm in length so that any food material that passes into the CBD will easily pass back out again. If the surgeon aims at a 2.5 cm anastomosis, cholangitis secondary to intermittent obstruction by food particles will be uncommon. A proper anastomosis requires that the diameter of the CBD be at least 1.5 cm (Kraus and Wilson). When a patient

Table 51–1 Relative Indications for Sphincteroplasty or Biliary-Intestinal Bypass

	Sphincteroplasty	Biliary-Intestinal Bypass
CBD diam. <1.5 cm	Preferred	Yes, if Roux-Y
CBD diam. >2.5 cm	Yes	Yes
Periampullary diverticulum	No	Yes
Poor-risk patient	No	Yes
Stenosis of Wirsung's duct or Vater's papilla	Yes	No
Long stricture of CBD (chronic pancreatitis)	No	Yes
Exploratory duodenotomy already made	Preferred	Yes
Caroli's cholangiohepatitis, hepatic duct stones	No	Yes
Carcinoma, head of pancreas, inoperable	No	Yes
Surgeon lacks experience with sphincteroplasty	Possible	Preferred

has a CBD whose diameter is less than 1.5 cm, either a Roux-Y choledochojejunostomy or sphincteroplasty is indicated. Inflammation of the duodenal wall is another relative contraindication to choledochoduodenostomy, as is fibrosis of the duodenal wall of sufficient severity to make approximation of the CBD and duodenum difficult to achieve. Leakage from the choledochoduodenostomy produces a high mortality rate. The mortality rate of choledochoduodenostomy (3%) is higher than that of the Roux-Y anastomosis. Bismuth, Franco, Corlette, and Hepp reported no hospital deaths following 123 consecutive Roux-Y hepaticojejunostomies.

Another drawback of the choledochoduodenostomy is the possibility of the "sump" syndrome being caused by food particles or calculi lodging in the CBD distal to the anastomosis. Although this complication was frequently observed endoscopically by Akiyama, Ikezawa, and Kameya, it is said to produce adverse symptoms in only a small percentage of cases. (In reviewing a number of reports concerning choledochoduodenostomy, we find that the authors of these reports do not make it clear whether or not they actually observed a high percentage of patients for a period of 5–10 years.) With the Roux-Y anastomosis, there is no opportunity for food to enter the bile duct.

Although the Roux-Y biliary-jejunal anastomosis is safer, most enthusiasts of the choledochoduodenostomy operation reject the Roux-Y operation in poor-risk patients because the second anastomosis (jejunojejunostomy) requires a longer operating time. If the Roux-Y jejunojejunostomy is performed by a stapling technique, the added operating time will occupy only a few minutes. The Roux-Y procedure has virtually no anastomotic failures and is indeed a good choice for the poor-risk elderly patient. We have found it to be particularly useful in bypassing inoperable carcinomas of the head of the pancreas. In these patients we perform a side-to-end sutured hepaticojejunostomy between the side of common hepatic duct and the end of the jejunum. We also perform a stapled side-to-side antecolonic gastrojejunostomy, and an end-to-side stapled Roux-Y jejunojejunostomy.

Of 52 patients with advanced pancreatic carcinoma treated in this fashion, we have had no anastomatic failures and one postoperative death. The fatality was not related to the operation.

It is more important in the elderly, depleted patient to avoid a serious anastomotic complication than to worry about a few minutes of additional operating time, provided that competent physiological support is available from the anesthesiologist.

One complication that may follow the diversion of bile into the jejunum is the development of peptic ulcer in the duodenum. This occurred in only 2% of the patients studied by Bismuth and colleagues over a mean followup of 5.5 years. Nevertheless, patients having a Roux-Y anastomosis should be made aware of the presenting symptoms of duodenal ulcer. The history of peptic ulcer diathesis may constitute a relative contraindication to performing a Roux-Y choledochojejunostomy.

Following resection of bile duct strictures, reconstruction by a Roux-Y hepaticojejunostomy is preferable to hepaticduodenostomy because it eliminates the possibility of food regurgitating into the anastomosis and causing cholangitis.

Table 51–2   Relative Indications for Choledochoduodenostomy or Roux-Y Choledochojejunostomy

	Choledocho-duodenostomy	Roux-Y Choledochojejunostomy
CBD diam. <1.5 cm	No	Yes
CBD diam. >1.5 cm	Yes	Yes
Duodenal inflammation	No	Yes
Fibrosis of duodenum and/or CBD	No	Yes
Active duodenal ulcer	Yes	No
Carcinoma, head of pancreas, inoperable	No	Yes
Poor-risk patient	Yes	Yes
Caroli's cholangiohepatitis, hepatic duct stones	Yes	Preferred
CBD stricture	Yes	Preferred

A summary of the relative indications for choledochoduodenostomy and the Roux-Y operation are listed in Table 51–2.

References

Akiyama H, Ikezawa S, Kameya S, Iwasaki M (1980) Unexpected problems of external choledochoduodenostomy: fiberscopic examination in 15 patients. Am J Surg 140:660

Bartlett MK, Nardi GL (1960) Treatment of recurrent pancreatitis by transduodenal sphincterotomy and exploration of the pancreatic duct. N Eng J Med 262:643

Bergdahl L, Holmlund DEW (1976) Retained bile duct stones. Acta Chir Scand 142:145

Bismuth H, Franco D, Corlette MB, Hepp J (1978) Long term results of Roux-en-y hepaticojejunostomy. Surg Gynecol Obstet 146:161

Burhenne HJ (1973) Nonoperative retained biliary tract stone extraction: a new reontgenologic technique. Am J Roentgenol Radium Ther Nucl Med 117:388

Dayton MT, Traverso LW, Longmire WP Jr (1980) Efficacy of the gallbladder for drainage in biliary obstruction: a comparison of malignant and benign disease. Arch Surg 115:1086

Degenshein GA (1974) Choledochoduodenostomy: an 18 year study of 175 consecutive cases. Surgery 76:319

Girard RM, Legros, G (1981) Retained and recurrent bile duct stones; surgical or non-surgical removal? Ann Surg 193:150

Hutchinson WB (1971) Duodenotomy. Am J Surg 122:777

Jones SA (1978) The prevention and treatment of recurrent bile duct stones by transduodenal sphincteroplasty. World J Surg 2:473

Kraus MA, Wilson SD (1980) Choledochoduodenostomy: importance of common duct size and occurrence of cholangitis. Arch Surg 115:1212

Longmire WP Jr (1977) The diverse causes of biliary obstruction and their remedies. Curr Probl Surg 14:5

Madden LJ (1978) Primary common bile duct stones. World J Surg 2:465

Moody FG, Berenson MM, McCloskey D (1977) Transampullary septectomy for postcholecystectomy pain. Ann Surg 186:415

Nardi GL, Acosta JM (1966) Papillitis as a cause of pancreatitis and abdominal pain: role of evocative test, operative pancreatography and histologic evaluation. Ann Surg 164:611

Nardi GL, Michelassi F, Zanni P (1983) Transduodenal sphincteroplasty Ann Surg 198:453

Partington PF (1977) Twenty-three years experience with sphincterotomy and sphincteroplasty for stenosis of the sphincter of Oddi. Surg Gynecol Obstet 145:161

Reiter JJ, Bayer HP, Mennicken C, Manegold BC (1978) Results of endoscopic papillotomy: a collective experience from nine endoscopic centers in West Germany. World J Surg 2:505

Rolfsmeyer ES, Bubrick MP, Kollitz PR, Onstad GR, et al. (1982) The value of operative cholangiography. Surg Gynecol Obstet 154:369

Saharia PC, Zuidema GD, Cameron JL (1977) Primary common duct stones. Ann Surg 185:598

Schein CJ (1978) Postcholecystectomy syndromes. Harper & Row, New York

Schein CJ, Gliedman ML (1981) Choledochoduodenostomy as an adjunct to choledocholithotomy. Surg Gynecol Obstet 152:797

Thomas CG Jr, Nicholson CP, Owen J (1971) Effectiveness of choledochoduodenostomy and transduodenal sphincterotomy in the treatment of benign obstruction of the common duct. Ann Surg 173:845

White TT (1973) Indications for sphincteroplasty as opposed to choledochoduodenostomy. Am J Surg 126:165

White TT, Harrison RC (1973) Reoperative gastrointestinal surgery. Little, Brown, Boston

52 Secondary Choledocholithotomy

Indications

Retained or recurrent common bile duct (CBD) stones (See also Chap. 51.)

Preoperative Care

When patients present with the classical signs of biliary colic, chills, fever, and jaundice, no special diagnostic studies may be necessary prior to surgery since the diagnosis of choledocholithiasis would be obvious in such cases.

Patients who do not present with these classical symptoms, should undergo sonography. If the bile ducts are dilated and stones are identified by the sonogram, proceed with surgery. If the ducts are dilated and no stones are identified in the common duct, an endoscopic radiographic cholangiopancreatogram (ERCP) or a percutaneous transhepatic cholangiogram (PTC) will be necessary to clarify the diagnosis. Intravenous cholangiography, once the mainstay among diagnostic procedures for the study of the CBD in the nonjaundiced patient, has fallen into disfavor because it is frequently inaccurate or inconclusive and is responsible for a 40% incidence of false negative reports in choledocholithiasis.

Additional preoperative preparation includes the restoration of the patient's normal prothrombin activity with vitamin K as well as the remaining routine measures to prepare a patient for major surgery.

Perioperative antibiotics are indicated.

Pitfalls and Danger Points

Trauma to adherent duodenum, colon, or liver

Trauma to CBD, hepatic artery, or portal vein

Operative Strategy

If the patient's first operation was not followed by any significant collection of bile, blood, or pus in the right upper quadrant, a secondary choledocholithotomy is not generally a difficult dissection. On the other hand, occasionally the right upper quadrant is obliterated by dense adhesions requiring a carefully planned sequential dissection. First, dissect the peritoneum of the anterior abdominal wall completely free from underlying adhesions. Carry this dissection to the right as far as the posterior axillary line. This will expose the lateral portion of the right lobe of the liver and the hepatic flexure of the colon.

The strategy now is to free the inferior surface of the liver from adherent colon and duodenum. Approach this from the lateral edge of the liver and proceed medially. After 5–6 cm of the undersurface of the lateral portion of the liver has been exposed, start to dissect the omentum and colon away from the anterior border of the undersurface of the liver. The dissection now goes both from lateral to medial as well as from anterior to posterior. If this dissection becomes difficult and there is risk of perforating the duodenum or colon, enter the right paracolic gutter and incise the paracolic peritoneum at the hepatic flexure. Placing the left hand behind the colon will give the surgeon entry into a virgin portion of the abdomen. This will aid in freeing the colon from the liver. The maneuver will uncover the descending portion of duodenum, also in virgin territory. Then perform a Kocher maneuver and bring the left hand up behind the duodenum. This will help guide the dissection toward the CBD. If the foramen of Winslow is uncovered, inserting the finger into this foramen will permit the surgeon to palpate the hepatic artery and give him helpful information concerning the probable location of the CBD.

Now, resume the lateral to medial and anterior to posterior dissection until the undersurface of the liver has been cleared down to the CBD and the hepatic artery. It is not necessary to free the undersurface of the liver for a large area medial to the CBD for adequate exposure.

Operative Technique

Incision

When the patient's previous incision for the cholecystectomy was subcostal in location, we prefer a long vertical midline incision. If the patient has previously been operated on here through a vertical incision, then a long subcostal incision, about two fingers breadth below the costal margin, is preferred. Placing the incision in a site away from the previous operative field makes it easier for the surgeon to enter the abdominal cavity expeditiously. Once the peritoneum and falciform ligament have been identified, free the abdominal wall from all underlying adhesions over the entire right side of the upper abdomen.

Freeing Subhepatic Adhesions

In the usual case, initiate the dissection on the right lateral edge of the liver, clearing its undersurface from right to left. If this dissection goes easily, it may be a simple matter to use Metzenbaum scissors to divide filmy adhesions by the techniques described in Chap. 22. When difficulty is encountered in differentiating colon or duodenum from scar tissue, then identify the ascending colon. Incise the paracolic peritoneum and slide the left hand behind the ascending colon. Liberate the hepatic flexure up to the undersurface of the liver. Then free the colon from the liver.

If similar difficulties are encountered in identifying or dissecting the duodenum, perform a Kocher maneuver and slide the left hand behind the duodenum, dissecting this organ away from the renal fascia, vena cava, and aorta.

Now start dissecting the omentum, colon, and duodenum, as necessary, from the undersurface of the liver, going from anterior to posterior until the hepatoduodenal ligament has been reached. The identity of the hepatoduodenal ligament can be confirmed by inserting the left index finger into the foramen of Winslow and palpating the hepatic artery, which should be just to the left of the CBD. Final confirmation may be obtained by aspirating bile with a No. 25 needle and syringe.

Exploring the CBD

After the CBD has been identified, a cholangiogram may be obtained by inserting a No. 22 Angiocath into the duct. Remove the steel needle, leaving the plastic cannula behind. Suture the hub of this cannula to the CBD with 5–0 chromic catgut and obtain a cholangiogram.

The technique of the CBD exploration is not different from that described in Chap. 50. Choledochoscopy and postexploratory cholangiography should be included in the operative procedure.

Draining the CBD

Insert a 16F T-tube trimmed as in Fig. 50–5, and close the choledochotomy with 5–0 Vicryl sutures, continuous or interrupted. The indications for sphincteroplasty or biliary-intestinal bypass are discussed in Chap. 51. That the common duct is thick-walled or dilated does not itself constitute an indication for additional surgery other than choledocholithotomy.

The abdomen is drained and closed as in Chap. 50.

Postoperative care and complications are similar to those discussed on pages 96–100.

53 Sphincteroplasty

Indications

Failed previous surgery for common bile duct (CBD) stasis with sludge, primary or recurrent stones

Doubt that multiple CBD stones have all been removed; hepatic duct stones that cannot be removed

Stenosis of Vater's ampulla and/or the orifice of Wirsung's duct with recurrent pain or recurrent acute pancreatitis (rare) (See also Chap. 52)

Preoperative Care

Perioperative antibiotics

Vitamin K in the jaundiced patient

Endoscopic radiographic cholangio-pancreatogram (ERCP) indicated to identify CBD calculi or ampullary stenosis and to visualize the pancreatic duct

Pitfalls and Danger Points

Trauma to the pancreatic duct or pancreas resulting in postoperative pancreatitis

Postoperative duodenal fistula secondary to a leak from sphincteroplasty or duodenotomy suture line

Postoperative hemorrhage

Operative Strategy

Protecting the Pancreatic Duct

Make the incision in the ampulla on its superior wall at about 10 or 11 o'clock. After making the initial incision about 5–6 mm in length, locate the orifice of the pancreatic duct. In 80% of cases this can be identified at about 5 o'clock where it enters the ampulla just proximal to the ampulla's termination. Wearing telescopic lenses with a magnification of about 2 ½x for this operation will help a great deal. If the orifice of the pancreatic duct cannot be identified, inject secretin. Give an intravenous dose equal to 1 unit per kilogram of body weight. This will stimulate the flow of the watery pancreatic secretion and will facilitate the identification of the ductal orifice. Insert either a lacrimal probe or a No. 2 Bakes dilator into the orifice to confirm that it is indeed the pancreatic duct. Some surgeons prefer to insert a plastic tube, such as an infant (size 6F) feeding tube, into the duct to protect it while suturing the sphincteroplasty. We agree with Jones that keeping a tube in the duct is not necessary if one keeps the ductal orifice in view during the suturing process.

When the indication for the sphincteroplasty is ampullary stenosis, abdominal pain, or recurrent pancreatitis, it is essential to add a "ductoplasty" of the pancreatic ductal orifice by incising the septum that forms the common wall between the distal pancreatic duct and the ampulla of Vater. After the pancreatic duct's orifice has been enlarged, it should freely admit a No. 3 Bakes dilator.

Preventing Hemorrhage

In performing a long sphincterotomy for the sphincteroplasty operation, the incision cuts across the anterior wall of the distal CBD as well as the back wall of the duodenum for a distance of 1.5–2 cm. This requires a "blind" incision. Consequently, if the patient has an anomalous retroduodenal or an anomalous right hepatic artery arising from the superior mesenteric artery and crossing in the area between the distal CBD and the duodenum, then one of these vessels may be lacerated by the sphincterotomy incision. It is important to palpate the area behind the ampulla for the pulsation of an anomalous artery. If such a vessel is behind the ampulla, then sphincteroplasty by the usual technique may be contraindicated. We are aware, by anecdote, of two patients who died, subsequent to a classical sphincteroplasty by the Jones technique, owing to massive postoperative hemorrhage despite reexploration. In one case, autopsy demonstrated laceration of an anomalous right hepatic artery. The laceration had apparently been temporarily controlled by the 5–0 interrupted silk sutures that had been used to fashion the sphincteroplasty.

By Jones's technique, initially small straight hemostats grasp 3–4 mm of tissue on either side of the contemplated ampullary incision. Then the tissue between the hemostats is divided. Next, a 5–0 silk suture is inserted behind each of the two hemostats; two additional hemostats are then inserted, the sphincterotomy incision is lengthened, and silk sutures again are placed behind each hemostat. In this way, it is possible to partially divide a large anomalous vessel and achieve temporary control, first by the hemostat, and then by the 5–0 silk suture. During the postoperative period the artery may escape from the 5–0 stitch and serious hemorrhage may follow. Although hemorrhage is a rare complication, to omit the application of hemostats prior to making a sphincterotomy incision would appear to be a preferable

technique. If the surgeon first makes a 3–4 mm incision with a Potts scissors, he should become immediately aware of any laceration of a major vessel at a time when proper reparative measures can be effectively undertaken. Otherwise, inflammation that occurs 5 or 6 days after the operation may make accurate identification of the anatomy difficult during any relaparotomy for hemorrhage. For this reason, we recommend making the incision first for a short distance, next the inserting of sutures, then the lengthening of the incision and the inserting of additional sutures sequentially until the proper size sphincteroplasty has been achieved.

Avoiding Duodenal Fistula

Leakage from the duodenum can occur from the apex of the sphincteroplasty because at this point the CBD and duodenum no longer share a single common wall. Here accurate suturing is necessary to reapproximate the incised CBD to the back wall of the duodenum.

A second source of leakage is the suture-line closing the duodenotomy. A longitudinal duodenotomy is preferred because it may be extended in either direction if the situation requires more exposure. Close this longitudinal incision in the same direction that the incision was originally made. Otherwise, distortion of the duodenum takes place and linear tension on the suture line may impair successful healing. Precise insertion of sutures, one layer in the mucosa and another layer in the seromuscular layer, can be accomplished without narrowing the duodenum. That the failure of the suture line is a real problem has been demonstrated by Hutchinson, who found that 7% of a series of 100 duodenotomy cases sustained a postoperative duodenal fistula. White reported detecting a number of duodenal leaks when performing T-tube cholangiograms. These leaks occurred a week after CBD exploration and duodenotomy for sphincteroplasty in patients who did not manifest any clinical symptoms. On the other hand, most leaks from incisions in the second portion of the duodenum cause serious if not lethal consequences; take special care in resuturing the duodenotomy incision.

Operative Technique

Incision and Exploration

Make a long right subcostal or midline incision, free adhesions, and perform a routine abdominal exploration. If a satisfactory preoperative ERCP has not been accomplished, perform a cholangiogram.

Kocher Maneuver

Execute a complete Kocher maneuver because this will simplify the performance of a sphincteroplasty by bringing the duodenum up almost to the level of the anterior abdominal wall, thus facilitating exposure of the ampulla. First incise the peritoneum just lateral to the descending duodenum. Then insert the left index finger behind the avascular ligament that attaches the duodenum to the renal capsule (of Gerota). By pinching this ligament between the thumb and index finger, push the areolar and vascular tissue away from this layer and divide the ligament. In some cases it is necessary to free the hepatic flexure of the colon in order to perform a thorough Kocher maneuver, which should be continued to the third portion of the duodenum almost as far as the point where the superior mesenteric vein crosses the anterior wall of the duodenum. In a cephalad direction, divide the ligament up to the foramen of Winslow. After this has been done, place the left hand behind the head of the pancreas and elevate it from the flimsy attachments to the vena cava and posterior abdominal wall. Place a gauze pad behind the pancreatic head.

CBD Exploration

Make an incision in the anterior wall of the CBD as close to the duodenum as possible because, if for some reason sphincteroplasty is not feasible, it may prove desirable to perform a choledochoduodenostomy. For the latter operation, an incision in the distal portion of the CBD allows the surgeon to make an anastomosis to the duodenum under less tension than an incision made at a higher level. If a CBD exploration for calculi is indicated, follow the same procedure as described in Chap. 50. Then pass a No. 4 Bakes dilator into the CBD down to, but not through, the ampulla of Vater. By palpating the tip of the dilator through the anterior duodenal wall, it is possible to place the duodenal incision accurately with reference to the location of the ampulla.

Duodenotomy and Sphincterotomy

Make a 4 cm scalpel incision along the antimesenteric border of the duodenum (**Fig. 53–1**). Center this incision at the estimated location of the ampulla, as judged by pal-

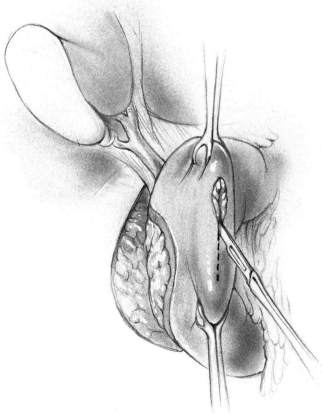

Fig. 53–1

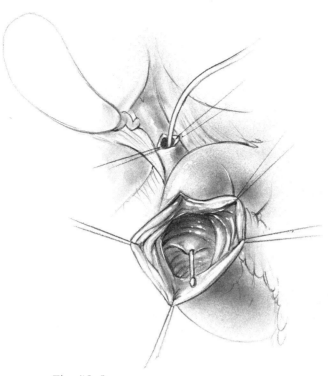

Fig. 53–2

pating the tip of the Bakes dilator **(Fig. 53–2).** Control bleeding points by careful electrocoagulation and an occasional 5–0 PG suture.

Make a 5 mm incision at 10 or 11 o'clock along the anterior wall of the ampulla, using either a scalpel blade against the large Bakes dilator impacted in the ampulla, or a Potts scissors with one blade inside the ampulla **(Fig. 53–3).** Insert one or two 5–0 Vicryl sutures on each side of the partially incised ampulla **(Fig. 53–4).** Leave intact the tails of the tied sutures; they are useful for applying gentle traction by attaching small hemostats.

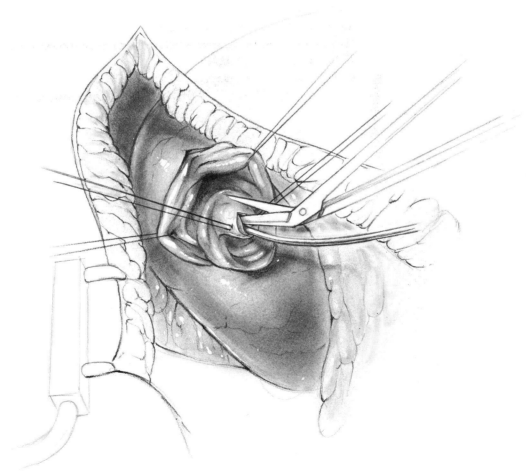

Fig. 53–3

Now identify the orifice of the pancreatic duct, which enters the back wall of the ampulla at about 5 o'clock near its termination. If the exposure of this portion of the ampulla is inadequate, extend the sphincterotomy by another 3–4 mm and insert an additional suture on each side. If the ductal orifice still has not been located, inject secretin (1 unit per kilogram of body weight) intravenously to stimulate the flow of pancreatic juice into the duodenum. Verify the location of the ductal orifice by inserting either a lacrimal probe or a No. 2 Bakes dilator. Then make a mental note to avoid traumatizing this area by inaccurate dissecting or suturing. Continue the sequence of incising the ampulla for about 3 mm at a time and inserting interrupted sutures (**Fig. 53–5**). In order to in-

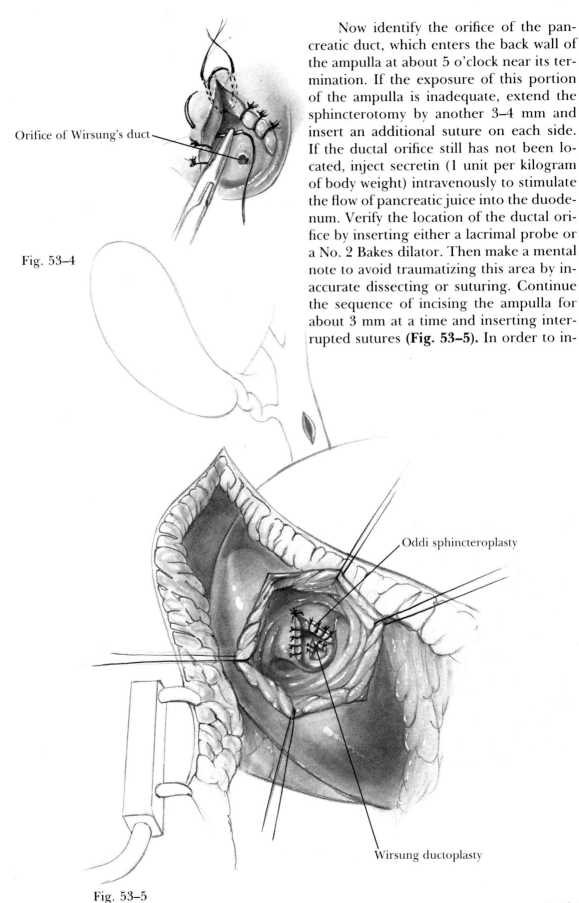

Orifice of Wirsung's duct

Fig. 53–4

Oddi sphincteroplasty

Wirsung ductoplasty

Fig. 53–5

117

cise the entire sphincter of Oddi, the sphincterotomy must be almost 2 cm in length. Additionally, if it is suspected that there are residual calculi and the CBD is large, the length of the sphincterotomy incision should at least equal the diameter of the CBD.

Nardi has reported gaining valuable data confirming the presence of fibrosis by biopsying the ampulla. He obtains the ampullary biopsy before performing the sphincterotomy by inserting a Doubilet sphincterotome into the ampulla. By closing the jaws of this instrument, one can obtain a narrow wedge of tissue for biopsy while simultaneously initiating the sphincterotomy. Other students of this subject have not been able to obtain valuable information concerning fibrosis or inflammation of the sphincter, although it is obvious that any area suspicious of cancer should always be biopsied for frozen-section examination. It is important to insert a figure-of-eight suture at the apex of the sphincterotomy in order to minimize the possibility of leakage. Carefully inspect the sutures at the conclusion of this step. They should be close together, and bleeding should be completely controlled.

When the indication for sphincteroplasty has been recurrent pancreatitis or recurrent abdominal pain, pancreatography is a vital part of the operation unless this step has been done preoperatively by means of ERCP. Pancreatography in the operating room may be accomplished by inserting a suitable plastic tube such as an Angiocath, a ureteral, or a small whistle-tip rubber catheter. Only 2–3 ml of diluted Conray or Hypaque should be used. Make the injection without pressure. Most patients with chronic recurrent pancreatitis will have multiple areas of narrowing and dilatation of the pancreatic duct, making sphincteroplasty a useless therapeutic procedure. If the pancreatic duct is dilated and the ductal orifice is narrowed so that it does not admit a No. 3 Bakes dilator, then the enlarging of this orifice by a ductoplasty

may prove beneficial, although this combination of conditions occurs only rarely. Nardi and Moody, Berenson, and McCloskey have reported good results with ductoplasty for stenosis of the ductal orifice.

Ductoplasty for Stenosis of Orifice of Pancreatic Duct

Magnify the orifice of the pancreatic duct by wearing telescopic lenses. Insert a Potts scissors into the pancreatic duct orifice and incise the septum, which constitutes the common wall between the anterior surface of the pancreatic duct and the posterior wall of the ampulla. Sometimes the orifice is too narrow to admit the blade of the Potts scissors. In this case, insert a metal probe into the ductal orifice and cut the anterior wall of the duct by incising for 3–4 mm using a scalpel against the metal of the probe. Then complete the incision with a Potts scissors. Generally, an 8–10 mm incision will permit the easy passage into the pancreatic duct of a No. 3 Bakes dilator. Insert several 5–0 Vicryl sutures to maintain the approximation of the pancreatic duct to the mucosa of the ampulla (see Fig. 53–5).

After this step, White and Harrison insert an infant size (6F or 8F) polyvinyl feeding tube into the orifice of the pancreatic duct. They next lead the tube through the duodenotomy incision and then through a stab wound in the abdominal wall to drain away the pancreatic secretions in the effort to minimize the ill effects of a possible minor leak of the duodenotomy repair. Jones does not use any drainage tube in the pancreatic duct when he performs a sphincteroplasty. Nor have we adopted this step.

Closing the Duodenotomy

Close the duodenal incision in two layers by the usual method of inverting the mucosa with either a continuous Connell, Cushing, or seromucosal suture and the seromuscular layer by carefully inserting interrupted 4–0 cotton or Tevdek Lembert sutures.

When the diameter of the duodenum appears to be more narrow than usual, include only the protruding mucosa in the first layer; make no attempt to invert the serosa with this suture line. For the second layer, insert interrupted Lembert sutures that take small accurate bites of the seromuscular coat, including submucosa. If this is done with precision, closing the longitudinal incision will not narrow the duodenum.

Cover the duodenotomy with omentum.

Cholecystectomy

If the gallbladder has not been removed at a previous operation, performing a sphincteroplasty will produce increased stasis of gallbladder bile, which may lead to stone formation. Consequently, perform a cholecystectomy.

Abdominal Closure and Drainage

After irrigating the operative site and the incision with a dilute antibiotic solution, drain the area of the sphincteroplasty with one or two closed-suction plastic catheters (4–5 mm diameter) brought out through puncture wounds in the upper abdomen. Be careful to avoid contact between the catheter and the duodenal suture lines. Suture the tips of the catheters in the proper location with fine catgut.

Place an indwelling 14F T-tube into the CBD for drainage.

Then close the abdominal wall by using the modified Smead-Jones technique described in Chap. 5.

Postoperative Care

Continue nasogastric suction for 5 days or until evidence of peristalsis is present with the passage of flatus.

Monitor the serum amylase every 2 days.

Continue perioperative antibiotics for 24 hours. If the bile is infected, continue antibiotics for 7 days.

Perform a cholangiogram on the 10th postoperative day and remove the T-tube on the 10th to 14th postoperative day if the X-ray shows satisfactory flow into the duodenum without leakage.

Remove the closed-suction drain by the 7th postoperative day unless there is bilious or duodenal drainage.

Postoperative Complications

Duodenal Fistula

A suspected duodenal fistula can often be confirmed by giving the patient methylene blue dye by mouth and looking for the blue dye in the closed-suction catheter, or by performing a T-tube cholangiogram. In cases of minor duodenal fistulas where there is neither significant systemic toxicity nor any abdominal tenderness, it is possible that a small leak will heal when managed by continuing the closed-suction drainage, supplemented by systemic antibiotics and intravenous alimentation.

A major leak from the duodenum is a life-threatening complication. If systemic toxicity is not controlled by conservative management, relaparotomy is indicated. Resuturing the duodenum will generally fail because of the local inflammation. In this situation, insert a sump-suction catheter into the duodenal fistula. Isolate the fistula by performing a Billroth II gastrectomy with vagotomy. Divert the bile from the duodenum by dividing the CBD and anastomose the proximal cut end of the duct to a Roux-Y segment of jejunum so that bile drains into the efferent limb of the jejunum distal to the gastrojejunostomy.

119

References

Hutchinson, WB (1971) Duodenotomy. Am J Surg 122:777

Jones SA (1978) The prevention and treatment of recurrent bile duct stones by transduodenal sphincteroplasty. World J Surg 2:473

Moody FG, Berenson MM, McCloskey, D (1977) Transampullary septectomy for postcholecystectomy pain. Ann Surg 186:415

Nardi GL (1973) Papillitis and stenosis of the sphincter of Oddi. Surg Clin North Am 53:1149

Saharia PC, Zuidema GD, Cameron JL (1977) Primary common duct stones. Ann Surg 185:598

White TT, Harrison RC (1979) Reoperative gastrointestinal surgery. Little, Brown, Boston

54 Choledochoduodenostomy

Indications

Common bile duct (CBD) stasis with sludge, primary, or recurrent stones, only if bile duct is more than 1.5 cm in diameter in the poor-risk patient

Doubt that multiple CBD stones have all been removed, only if CBD is more than 1.5 cm in diameter in the poor-risk patient

Constriction of distal CBD because of chronic pancreatitis

(See also Chap. 52)

Contraindications

Diameter of CBD less than 1.5 cm in diameter

Acute inflammation or excessive fibrosis in duodenal wall

Carcinoma of pancreatic head

(Hepaticojejunostomy (Roux-Y) is our preferred bypass procedure for pancreatic carcinoma obstructing the CBD. It is a safer operation; also the anastomosis will not be obstructed by the advancing growth of the malignancy.)

Preoperative Care

Perioperative antibiotics

Vitamin K in jaundiced patients

Nasogastric tube

Pitfalls and Danger Points

Anastomotic stoma too small, resulting in postoperative recurrent cholangitis

Diameter of CBD too small

Anastomotic leak; duodenal fistula

Postoperative "sump" syndrome

Operative Strategy

Size of Anastomotic Stoma

As the anastomotic stoma after choledochoduodenostomy will permit the passage of food from the duodenum into the CBD, it is important that the anastomosis be large enough to permit the food to pass back freely into the duodenum. Otherwise, food particles will partially obstruct the anastomotic stoma and produce recurrent cholangitis. If the surgeon aims at constructing an anastomosis with a stoma 2.5 cm or more in diameter, postoperative cholangitis will be rare. The size of the stoma may be estimated postoperatively by an upper gastrointestinal barium X-ray study.

Obviously, if the diameter of the CBD is small, large anastomotic stoma is difficult to achieve. Kraus and Wilson emphasize that choledochoduodenostomy is contraindicated in a patient whose CBD is less than 1.5 cm in diameter.

Location of the Anastomosis

There are several alternative locations for the incisions in the CBD and the duodenum. If postoperative anastomotic leakage is to be prevented, it is vitally important that these incisions be made in tissues of satisfactory quality and that there be no tension on the anastomosis.

Another problem presents itself when the surgeon has made an incision in CBD in the vicinity of the cystic duct for the CBD exploration; he may also have made a duodenal incision opposite the ampulla for an impacted ampullary calculus. Under these conditions, even with an extensive Kocher maneuver, it may not be possible to approximate these two incisions by suturing because there will be too much tension on the anastomosis. In this situation a Roux-Y choledochojejunostomy or a sphincteroplasty is preferable. When the possibility of a choledochoduodenostomy can be anticipated prior to the CBD exploration, make the incision in the CBD near the point where it enters the sulcus between the pancreas and the duodenum. This will facilitate constructing the anastomosis by the technique described in Figs. 54–1 to 54–5, the method preferred by Schein and Gliedman.

When the incision in CBD has been made in a more proximal location, test the mobility of the duodenum after performing a Kocher maneuver. If the duodenum is easily elevated to the region of the CBD incision, a choledochoduodenostomy by the method illustrated in Figs. 54–6 and 54–7 is also acceptable. There must be no tension on the anastomosis.

Preventing the Sump Syndrome

Sporadic reports have appeared describing the accumulation of food debris or calculi in the terminal portion of the CBD following choledochoduodenostomy. This accumulation produces intermittent cholangitis and has been called the "sump syndrome." Akiyama observed considerable inflammation in the region of the stoma as well as food particles in the distal CBD by endoscopy. Smith, commenting on a paper by White, stated that he had found it necessary to operate on 25 patients with cholangitis caused by the sump syndrome following choledochoduodenostomy performed by other surgeons. McSherry and Fischer in 5 years encountered 6 patients who suffered from cholangitis, acute pancreatitis, or pain and fever owing to calculi in the blind "sump" following side to side choledochoduodenostomy (five cases) or choledochojejunostomy (one case). The symptoms were relieved by endoscopic papillotomy or by laparotomy and choledocholithotomy or sphincteroplasty. These authors state:

> Because of our observation that residual and recurrent common duct calculi are capable of producing symptoms in patients with biliary-intestinal anastomoses, we suggest that the indications for . . . choledochoduodenostomy be re-examined. If the condition of the patient permits, every effort should be made to remove all calculi from the common bile duct at operation . . . Choledochoduodenostomy is best reserved for those patients in the high risk category . . .

Tanaka, Ikeda, and Yoshimoto reported four cases of the sump syndrome following choledochoduodenostomy or side-to-side choledochojejunostomy. All were relieved by endoscopic sphincterotomy.

Enthusiasts of choledochoduodenostomy (Degenshein; Madden; Schein and Gliedman) report that they have not observed the sump syndrome in their cases. However, it is not clear from any of these authors, that they had achieved a comprehensive long-term followup study of all of their patients. Certainly, if the stoma of the choledochoduodenostomy is small, postoperative cholangitis is common. There are no clear data to indicate precisely what is the incidence of postoperative symptoms from the sump syndrome.

White described the technique of dividing the CBD and then performing an

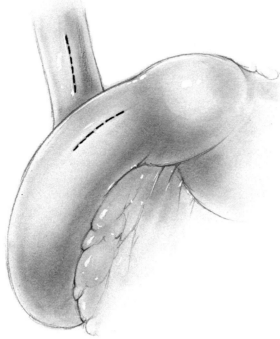

Fig. 54–1

end-to-side choledochoduodenostomy in order to prevent this syndrome. White does not specify what the complication rate of this method is, but he does emphasize that the diameter of the end-to-side choledochoduodenal anastomosis should be over 1.5 cm.

If a choledochojejunostomy by the Roux-Y technique is constructed, then no food will enter the CBD even when the distal CBD has not been divided. However, residual or recurrent calculi in the blind sump may conceivably cause the problems described by McSherry and Fischer. For this reason, Bismuth, Franco, Corlette, and Hepp divide the CBD and implant the proximal cut end into a Roux-Y limb of jejunum. This technique offers the lowest incidence of postoperative symptoms.

Operative Technique

Incision

Either a right subcostal or a midline incision from the xiphoid to a point 5 cm below the umbilicus is suitable for this operation.

Divide any adhesions and explore the abdomen. Perform a complete Kocher maneuver. If the diameter of the CBD is less than 1.5 cm, do *not* perform a choledochoduodenostomy.

Choledochoduodenal Anastomosis

Free the peritoneum over the distal CBD. Make an incision on the anterior wall of the CBD for a distance of at least 2.5 cm. This incision should terminate close to the point where the duodenum crosses the distal CBD. Make another incision of equal size along the long axis of the duodenum at a point close to the CBD (**Fig. 54–1**). Insert the index finger into the duodenum and palpate the ampulla of Vater to be certain that a carcinoma of the ampulla has not been overlooked.

Place guy sutures at the midpoints of both the lateral and medial margins of the CBD incision. Apply traction to these guy sutures in opposite directions to open up the choledochotomy incision (**Fig. 54–2**). One layer of interrupted 4–0 Vicryl sutures will be used for this anastomosis. Insert

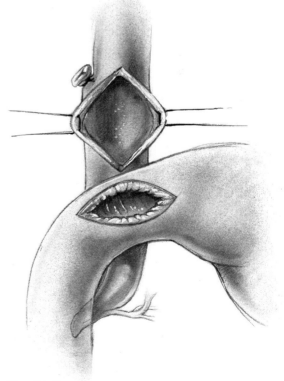

Fig. 54–2

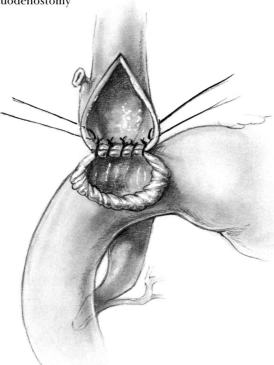

Fig. 54–3

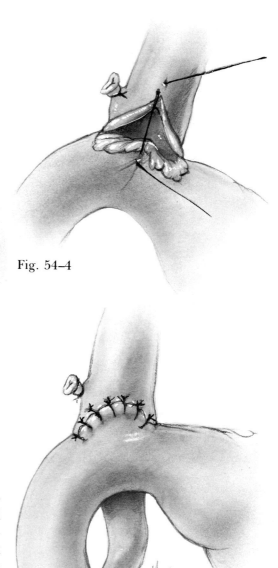

Fig. 54–4

Fig. 54–5

the first stitch of the posterior layer approximating the midpoint of the duodenal incision to the distal margin of the choledochotomy. Tie the stitch with the knot inside the lumen. Insert additional stitches going through the full thickness of the duodenum and of the CBD (**Fig. 54–3**) until the entire posterior layer has been completed. Cut all of the sutures except the most lateral and most medial stitches. Now approximate the proximal margin of the choledochotomy with the same suture material to the midpoint of the anterior layer of duodenum and tie this stitch so as to invert the mucosa of the duodenum (**Fig. 54–4**). Continue to insert interrupted through-and-through sutures until the anterior layer has been completed (**Fig. 54–5**). This anastomosis should be completed without tension.

Alternative Method of Anastomosis

In some cases the surgeon may elect to perform a choledochoduodenal anastomosis after he has already made the choledochotomy incision in a location too far proximal on the CBD to accomplish the anastomosis by the above technique. In this case, enlarge the choledochotomy so that it measures at least 2.5 cm in length.

Next, perform a thorough Kocher maneuver to increase the mobility of the

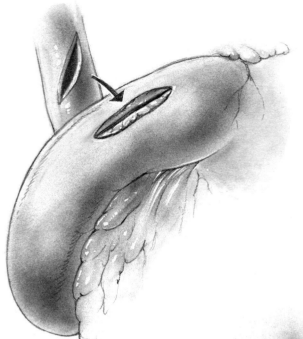

duodenum. Then, move the duodenum toward the choledochotomy incision and determine which portion of the duodenum is most suitable for a side-to-side anastomosis *without tension.* If tension cannot be avoided, perform a Roux-Y anastomosis.

Make an incision in the duodenum that is parallel to the choledochotomy and approximately equal in length **(Fig. 54–6).** Approximate the posterior layer with interrupted sutures and tie them **(Fig. 54–7).** The knots will be inside the lumen. Leave the tails of the most cephalad and most distal sutures long but cut all other sutures.

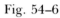

Fig. 54–6

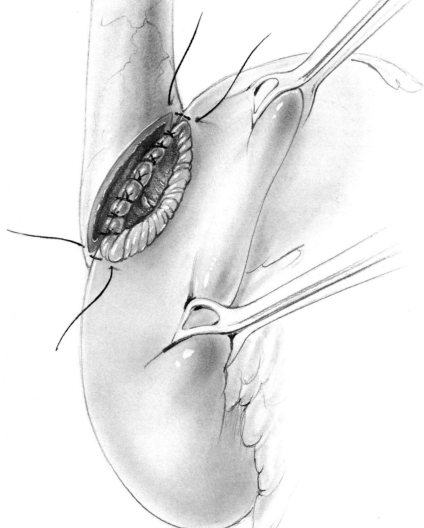

Fig. 54–7

125

Then bisect the anterior layer of the anastomosis and insert a 4–0 PG Lembert suture to approximate the midpoint of the CBD incision to the midpoint of the duodenal incision. Tie this suture so that the duodenal mucosa is inverted. Insert additional sutures of the same type to complete the approximation. The knots will be on the outside surface of the anastomosis for the anterior layer.

Since the CBD is quite large in these cases and the duodenal wall is free of pathology, no T-tube or other stent is necessary.

Drainage and Closure

As bile has an extremely low surface tension, there is a tendency for a small amount of this substance to leak out along the suture holes during the first day or two following a biliary tract anastomosis. For this reason, insert a closed-suction drainage catheter through a puncture wound in the right upper quadrant and bring the catheter to the general vicinity of the anastomosis. Do not use a catheter made of silicone as this material is nonreactive and may not form a tract. In the rare instance of a duodenal fistula complicating this operation, it would be highly desirable to have a well walled-off tract from the duodenum to the outside.

Postoperative Care

Continue nasogastric suction until bowel function resumes.

Do not remove the closed-suction drain for 5–7 days.

Postoperative Complications

Duodenal fistula (see Chap. 53)

Subhepatic abscess

Late development of cholangitis owing to anastomotic stoma being too small.

Late development of "sump" syndrome

References

Akiyama H, Ikezawa H, Kameya S, Iwasaki M (1980) Unexpected problems of external choledochoduodenostomy: fiberscopic examination in 15 patients. Am J Surg 140:660

Bismuth H, Franco D, Corlette MB, Hepp J (1978) Long term results of Roux-en-y hepaticojejunostomy. Surg Gynec Obstet 146:161

Degenshein GA (1974) Choledochoduodenostomy: an 18 year study of 175 consecutive cases. Surgery 76:319

Kraus MA, Wilson SD (1980) Choledochoduodenostomy: importance of common duct size and occurrence of cholangitis. Arch Surg 115:1212

McSherry CK, Fischer MG (1981) Common bile duct stones and biliary-intestinal anastomoses. Surg Gynecol Obstet 153:669

Madden JL (1978) Primary common bile duct stones. World J Surg 2:465

Schein CJ, Gliedman ML (1981) Choledochoduodenostomy as an adjunct to choledocholithotomy. Surg Gynecol Obstet 152:797

Tanaka M, Ikeda S, Yoshimoto H (1983) Endoscopic sphincterotomy for the treatment of biliary sump syndrome. Surgery 93:264

White TT (1973) Indications for sphincteroplasty as opposed to choledochoduodenostomy. Am J Surg 126:165

55 Roux-Y Hepatico- or Choledochojejunostomy

Indications

Common bile duct (CBD) obstruction due to inoperable carcinoma of the distal CBD, duodenum, or head of pancreas

CBD stasis with sludge, primary, or recurrent stones

Doubt that multiple CBD stones have all been removed

Constriction of the distal CBD due to chronic pancreatitis and fibrosis

CBD stricture

Preoperative Care

Perioperative antibiotics

Vitamin K in jaundiced patients

Pitfalls and Danger Points

Devascularizing the jejunal segment by inaccurate division of mesentery

Operative Strategy

If an isoperistalic Roux-Y segment of jejunum was anastomosed to the common hepatic or the CBD, the incidence of postoperative anastomotic failure was zero in the experience of Bismuth, Franco, Corlette, and Hepp, who studied 123 consecutive patients suffering from benign, nonprogressive biliary tract lesions. The postoperative mortality in the first 60 days was also zero. Bismuth and associates feel that the isolated Roux-Y segment should be 70 cm in length to prevent any possibility of food regurgitation into the bile ducts. Many other authors feel that 50 cm is an adequate length. It is clear that a choledochojejunostomy with a Roux-Y construction is probably the safest biliary-intestinal anastomosis yet designed.

When the end of jejunum is anastomosed to the side of the bile duct or when a side-to-side biliary-jejunal anastomosis is constructed by the Roux-Y method, cholangitis will not be produced by the regurgitation of food material. It is conceivable that the blind end of the bypassed CBD may accumulate calculi as they pass down from the hepatic ducts. However, it is much more likely that any material of this type would pass through the large anastomosis into the jejunum rather than collect at the lower end of the CBD. Nevertheless, Bismuth and his colleagues advocate complete division of the CBD, suturing the distal duct closed and then implanting the cut end of the proximal duct into the side of the jejunum. It is not clear that this step is necessary. We prefer to suture the end of the jejunum to the anterior side of the CBD when the CBD is enlarged. Otherwise, a side-to-side biliary-jejunal anastomosis is performed. Although it seems clear that the Roux-Y anastomosis is the safest and also seems to have the fewest long-term complications, most surgeons have been reluctant to abandon choledochoduodenostomy in favor of biliary-jejunal Roux-Y anastmoses because the Roux-Y technique requires a jejunojeunal anastomosis in addition to the choledochojejunostomy. If the jejunojejunostomy is performed by the stapling technique described below, it will take no more than 2–3 minutes of operating time. We have not encountered any complications with this technique of reanastomosing the jejunum.

When the Roux-Y biliary-intestinal bypass is performed for carcinoma of the pancreas, it is necessary to evaluate the root of the small bowel mesentery because some of these tumors can extend deeply into this mesentery, making impossible the proper dissection of the jejunal blood supply for the Roux-Y segment. In these few cases this operation is contraindicated and some other type of bypass must be considered. Under these conditions, anastomosing the gallbladder to the side of a loop of jejunum may prove satisfactory for the short life expectancy characteristic of patients with large pancreatic neoplasms (Dayton, Traverso, and Longmire).

In most cases the marginal artery of the jejunum is divided immediately distal to the artery supplying the second arcade. By dividing only one or two additional arcade vessels, sufficient jejunum can be mobilized to reach the hepatic duct without tension. The jejunum is passed through an incision in the avascular portion of the transverse mesocolon, generally to the right of the middle colic artery. This dissection must be done carefully and will be facilitated by transilluminating the jejunal mesentery by means of a spotlight or a sterilized fiberoptic illuminator.

Operative Technique

Incision and Biopsy

If there has been a previous operation on the biliary tract that utilized a subcostal incision, then make a long midline incision.

If the previous incision was vertical, then make a long subcostal incision and enter the abdomen. In secondary cases, the first effort is to free the peritoneum of the anterior abdominal wall from all its underlying adhesions as far lateral as the midaxillary line. Then continue to free the structures as described in Chap. 51.

In primary operations for carcinoma of the pancreas, make a long midline incision from the xiphoid to a point 6–7 cm below the umbilicus. This will prove to be a good incision either for a bypass or partial or total pancreatectomy. Conduct the usual exploration in order to make an accurate diagnosis. In patients with pancreatic carcinoma that is inoperable, take biopsies from areas of obvious carcinoma with a scalpel or biopsy a metastatic lymph node. When these steps are not possible, we have generally been successful in confirming the diagnosis of carcinoma by inserting a syringe with a 22-gauge needle into the hardest part of the pancreas. As soon as the needle enters the suspicious area, apply suction and plunge the needle for 1 cm distances in two directions. Then, release the plunger of the syringe so that no further suction is being applied. Remove the syringe and the needle. Pass it promptly to the cytopathologist as *immediate* fixation is necessary for an accurate cytological diagnosis. This method has provided us with a higher percentage of positive diagnoses in carcinoma of the pancreas than the tissue techniques. The cytologist's report should not take more than 10–15 minutes.

Creating the Roux-Y Jejunal Limb

Inspect the proximal jejunal mesentery and look for the first two branches from the superior mesenteric artery to the jejunum just beyond the ligament of Treitz. Identify the marginal artery at a point 2 cm beyond its junction with the second je-

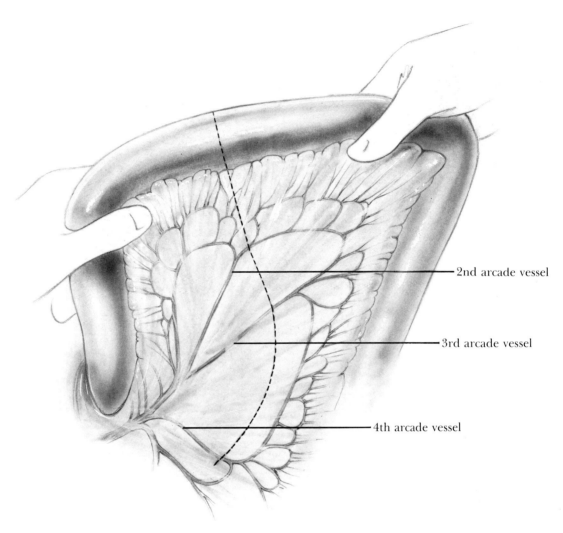

2nd arcade vessel

3rd arcade vessel

4th arcade vessel

Fig. 55–1

junal branch. This is generally about 15 cm from the ligament of Treitz. Make a light scalpel incision over the jejunal mesentery from the jejunum across the marginal artery and into the avascular area of the mesentery. Divide the mesentery in a distal direction until the third vessel is encountered. Divide and ligate this vessel and continue the incision in the mesentery down to the fourth vessel. This most often does not require division **(Fig. 55–1).**

Now clean the mesenteric margin of the jejunum and divide between Allen clamps.

Tentatively pass the liberated limb of jejunum up toward the hepatic duct to determine whether sufficient mesentery has been dissected. If this is so, then expose the right portion of the transverse mesocolon. Find an avascular area, generally to the right of the middle colic vessels and make a 2–3 cm incision through the mesocolon. Pass the liberated limb of jejunum through the incision in the mesocolon. It may be necessary to free some of the omentum from the area of the hepatic flexure

129

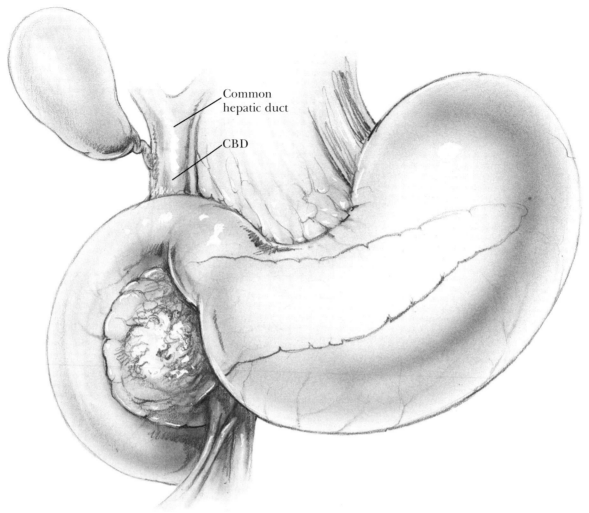

Common
hepatic duct

CBD

Fig. 55–2

in order to permit free passage of the jejunum up to the hepatic duct. The end of the jejunum should reach the proximal portion of the common hepatic duct with no tension whatever.

Hepaticojejunostomy

Remove the Allen clamp by incising the jejunum adjacent to the clamp with the electrocautery. If there is protrusion of more than 2 mm of jejunal mucosa beyond the incised seromuscular layer, then either amputate this excess mucosa flush with the seromuscular incision or else use a continuous suture of 5–0 PG in an over-and-over fashion to approximate the mucosa to the cut end of the seromuscular layer. This step is advisable because the hepaticojejunal anastomosis is performed with one layer of sutures. Clean the mesenteric border of the jejunum for a distance of about 5 mm from its cut end.

In cases of carcinoma, expose the proximal portion of the hepatic duct (**Fig. 55–2)** in order to place the anastomosis as far from the tumor as possible because pancreatic and CBD malignancies grow upward along the wall of the CBD. Placing the anastomsis at a distance will generally avoid occlusion of the anastomosis by further growth of the malignancy. In the case of benign disease, the anastomosis may be made at any convenient location along the dilated hepatic or CBD. Incise the layer of peritoneum overlying the duct. Then make a 2.5–3.5 cm longitudinal incision in the anterior wall of the hepatic duct and evacuate the bile. If the gallbladder is enlarged and interferes with the exposure, gentle compression of the gallbladder should empty its contents after the hepatic duct has been opened. If the cystic duct is already obstructed by tumor and the gallbladder blocks exposure, perform a cholecystectomy. Also, perform a cholecystectomy whenever the hepaticojejunostomy is being performed for benign disease since the bypass anastomosis will produce stasis in the gallbladder and render it functionless.

Only one layer of seromucosal sutures is necessary for this anastomosis (**Fig. 55–3**). Each bite of the suture material should encompass 4 mm of the jejunum and the full thickness of the hepatic duct. Place the sutures about 4 mm apart. Initiate the anastomosis by inserting the first 5–0 Vicryl suture at the caudal end of the anastomosis, which will correspond with the mesenteric border of the jejunum. Tie the suture and tag it with a hemostat. Then insert the most cephalad stitch and tag this with a hemostat. Complete the right side of the anastomosis with interrupted 5–0 sutures by the technique of successive bisection (see Vol. I, Figs. B-22 and B-23). Do not tie any of these sutures but tag each with a hemostat. After all the sutures have been placed, tie

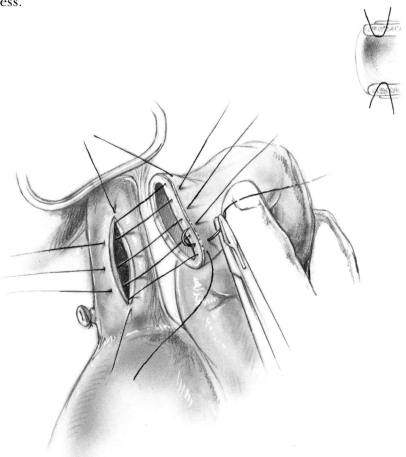

Fig. 55–3

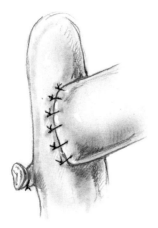

Fig. 55–4

them and complete the right-hand side of the anastomosis **(Fig. 55–4)**. All of the mucosa should have been inverted. If there is any difficulty in inverting this mucosa, it is altogether permissible to use an accurate Lembert type of stitch on the jejunum and a through-and-through stitch on the CBD. Cut all the tails of the sutures except the most proximal and distal stitches, which are retained as guy sutures. Then retract the jejunum somewhat towards the patient's right. Now initiate the left half

of the anastomosis by bisecting the area between the proximal and distal stitches. Insert the first stitch at this point **(Fig. 55–5)**. If the hepatic duct is large, it is permissible to tie these sutures as they are inserted. If the duct is small enough to cause concern that you may catch the opposite wall of the bile duct while inserting stitches, do not tie any of them until all of the sutures have been inserted. Then the bile duct can be easily inspected prior to tying the stitches.

After all the sutures are tied, it will be evident that a quite large end-to-side anastomosis has been accomplished without much difficulty. All the knots will be tied outside the lumen of the anastomosis in this case, although the use of PG synthetic absorbable suture material makes it of no importance whether the knots are inside or outside the lumen. Given the wide availability of the PG materials, we see no indication at this time for the use of nonabsorbable sutures in the bile ducts. We have not used a stent, catheter, or T-tube in any of the Roux-Y biliary-jejunal anastomses, unless they were done for posttraumatic or iatrogenic bile duct strictures.

When a side-to-side hepaticojejunostomy is performed, close the end of the jejunum by applying the TA-55 stapler with 3.5 mm staples. Cut the excess jejunum off flush with the stapler. Lightly coagulate the mucosa. It is not necessary to invert this staple line with sutures. When the side-to-side anastomosis is being done, use the same 5–0 Vicryl suture material, insert through-and-through sutures on the posterior layer, and tie the knots inside the lumen. On the anterior layer of this anastomosis, the knots will be tied outside the lumen with mucosa being inverted. Again, a Lembert suture may be used if necessary because there is not much danger of inverting too much jejunum when only one layer of sutures is used and the duct is large.

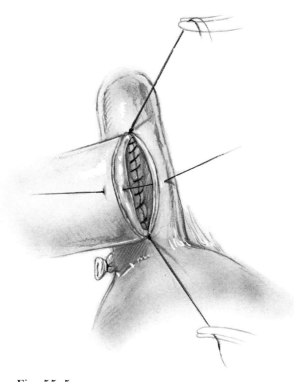

Fig. 55–5

If an anastomosis is contemplated between the divided cut end of the hepatic duct and the side of the jejunum, accomplish an oblique division of the hepatic duct. This will convert the anastomosis from a circular one to an elliptical shape and will have the effect of enlarging the diameter of the anastomotic stoma. In cases of bile duct strictures, try to dissect out and remove that portion of the bile duct that consists largely of scar tissue and has no mucosa. When the diameter of the hepatic duct is 10 mm or less, it is probably wise to introduce a Silastic tube through a puncture wound of the liver into one of the proximal hepatic ducts, (see Figs. 57–7 and 57–8) and then down through the anastomosis. The proximal end of the Silastic tube is brought out through a puncture wound in the abdominal wall. Make an incision on the antimesenteric side of the jejunum. This incision should be a millimeter or two larger than the diameter of the transected hepatic duct. Use 5–0 Vicryl suture material swaged onto atraumatic fine needles. Make the posterior anastomosis first with interrupted sutures. Excise any redundant protruding jejunal mucosa to facilitate a one-layer anastomosis. Take a bite of hepatic duct and then of jejunum, encompassing only 2–3 mm of tissue with each bite, but penetrate the entire wall of the bile duct and of the jejunum. Tie the knots on the inside of the lumen for the posterior half of the anastomosis. Then, for the anterior half of the anastomosis insert the sutures so that the knots are tied outside the lumen. The knots should be spaced 3–4 mm apart. After the anastomsis has been completed, inspect the back side as well as the anterior wall for possible imperfections.

To avoid any linear tension on the anastomosis by gravity, insert a few seromuscular sutures into the jejunum and attach the jejunum to the undersurface of the liver or to adjacent peritoneum.

Gastrojejunostomy

Patients undergoing bypass surgery because of pancreatic carcinoma have a 30% chance of developing duodenal obstruction from growth of the tumor (Blievernicht, Neifeld, Terz, and Lawrence). In order to avoid a secondary operation for duodenal obstruction, it is wise to invest a few minutes in performing a stapled side-to-side gastrojejunostomy. We generally create the anastomosis 50 cm distal to the hepaticojejunostomy and bring the jejunal limb in an antecolonic fashion to the greater curvature of the gastric antrum. In some cases there is enough clear gastric wall to create the stapled side-to-side anastomosis without freeing the omentum from the greater curvature of the stomach. In most cases, divide and ligate the branches of the gastroepiploic arcade along the greater curvature of the antrum so that a 5–7 cm area is free.

Use the electrocautery to make a stab wound on the greater curvature aspect of the stomach and on the antimesenteric side of the jejunum. Insert the GIA stapling device in a position where it will not transect

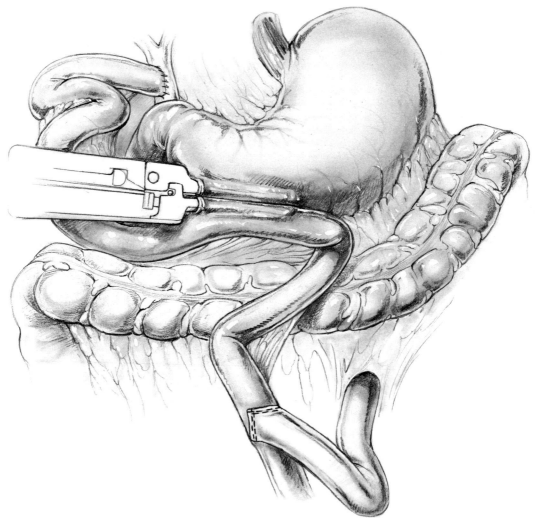

Fig. 55–6

any blood vessels. Lock the device (**Fig. 55–6**). Fire the GIA and remove it. Inspect the suture line for bleeding, which should be controlled either with cautious electrocoagulation or 5–0 PG suture-ligatures. Then grasp the two ends of the GIA staple line with Allis clamps. Apply additional Allis clamps to the gap between stomach and jejunum. Then close this gap with a single application of the TA-55 stapler using 3.5 mm staples. With a Mayo scissors amputate the redundant tissue and lightly electrocoagulate the mucosa. Remove the stapling device and inspect the anastomosis for any possible defects or bleeding (also see Figs. 14–5 to 14–7).

Stapling the Roux-Y Jejunojejunostomy

At a point 10–15 cm distal to the gastrojejunostomy, align the proximal cut end of the jejunum with the descending limb of jejunum, as depicted in Fig. 19–35. It is important to have the cut end of the proximal jejunum facing in a cephalad direction because the construction of the stapled anastomosis is facilitated thereby. Make a 1.5 cm longitudinal incision with the electrocautery on the antimesenteric border of the descending limb of jejunum 10–15 cm distal to the gastrojejunostomy. Now remove the Allen clamp from the proximal end of jejunum and insert the GIA device, one limb into the stab wound and the other limb into the open end of jejunum. Lock the GIA device and fire the stapling device; then remove it. Inspect the staple line for bleeding.

Place a guy suture at the midpoint of the remaining defect approximating the descending limb of jejunum with a proximal open end of jejunum as in Figs. 19–37 and 19–38. Apply an Allis clamp to the anterior termination of the GIA staple line and another Allis clamp to the posterior termination of the GIA staple line. Apply additional Allis clamps to close the remaining defect. Now, perform a stapled closure of this defect by triangulation. Apply a TA-55 stapler with 3.5 mm staples to include the guy suture and the anterior termination of the GIA staple line (Fig. 19–39). Fire the staples and amputate the redundant mucosa. Electrocoagulate lightly.

Next, apply a TA-55 stapler, again including the guy suture and also the Allis clamp on the posterior termination of the GIA staple line. Apply additional Allis clamps as necessary. Fire the TA-55 stapler; amputate the redundant tissue and lightly electrocoagulate the mucosa. Remove the stapler and check for the patency of the anastomosis (Fig. 19–40). This will generally be found to be quite large.

Closure of Mesenteric Gaps

Using 4–0 PG or other suture material, place interrupted sutures to attach the transverse mesocolon to the limb of jejunum, which has been brought up to the incision in the mesocolon. This will eliminate any gaps through which small bowel might herniate. Use the same technique to close the gaps in the mesentery of the jejunum in which the Roux-Y jejunojejunostomy has been constructed.

Abdominal Closure and Drainage

Close the abdomen in routine fashion.

Because bile has an extremely low surface tension, a small amount of bile may escape from the anastomosis in the 1–2 days following the operation. For this reason, insert a closed-suction drainage catheter through a puncture wound in the lateral abdominal wall. Bring the catheter up to the region of the hepaticojejunostomy where it may be sutured with 5-0 chromic catgut.

Postoperative Care

Continue nasogastric suction until evidence of bowel function has resumed.

Administer cimetidine parenterally, 600 mg every 6 hours, until oral intake has been resumed. Then this may be replaced with antacid treatment until the patient is ready to go home.

Remove the closed-suction drain after drainage has essentially ceased.

Postoperative Complications

Bile Leak

Although there is an occasional persistence of bile drainage for as long as 5–7 days, this has invariably ceased in our experience and has never constituted a significant problem following the Roux-Y anastomosis.

Stenosis of the Anastomosis

Late stenosis of the hepaticojejunostomy was reported by Bismuth and associates in only one case of 123. We have not encountered this complication. If a large anastomosis is made with one layer of sutures, this is a rare complication.

Cholangitis

Similarly, cholangitis is quite rare following a Roux-Y hepaticojejunostomy unless the anastomosis has become stenosed. In patients who have had multiple hepatic duct calculi, there may be transient cholangitis while a calculus is in transit from the hepatic duct down to the hepaticojejunostomy.

Postoperative Duodenal Ulcer

We have never encountered a duodenal ulcer when a Roux-Y hepaticojejunostomy has been applied to patients with nonresectable pancreatic cancer. In the patients with nonprogressive biliary tract disease studied by Bismuth and associates, only 2% developed duodenal ulcer over a 5.5 year average followup. McArthur and Longmire noted that as many as 10% of their patients had developed duodenal ulcer. Wheeler and Longmire introduced the concept of interposing a limb of jejunum between the hepatic duct and the duodenum as a possible substitute for the Roux-Y anastomosis in patients with an ulcer diathesis **(Fig. 55–7).** So far, experience with this operation has been limited. However, when a patient has chronic pancreatitis with minimal flow of akaline pancreatic juice into the duodenum and if that patient has all of his bile diverted into the Roux-Y hepaticojejunostomy, there may be an increased tendency for duodenal ulcer formation. These patients should be warned to return for prompt medical attention if they begin to develop symptoms of peptic ulceration. Alternatively, a hepaticojejunoduodenostomy may be performed in a patient known to have an ulcer diathesis.

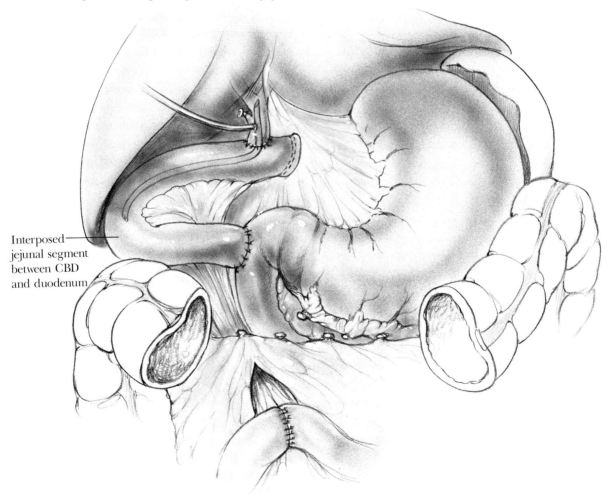

Interposed jejunal segment between CBD and duodenum

Fig. 55–7

Delayed Gastric Emptying

Following choledochojejunostomy, with or without concomitant gastrojejunostomy, 10%–20% of the patients develop delayed gastric emptying. All of our patients responded to a period of nasogastric suction, sometimes with the assistance of bethanecol or metoclopramide.

References

Bismuth H, Franco D, Corlette MB, Hepp J (1978) Long-term results of Roux-en-y hepaticojejunostomy. Surg Gynecol Obstet 146:161

Blievernicht SW, Neifeld JP, Terz JJ, Lawrence W Jr (1980) The role of prophylactic gastrojejunostomy for unresectable periampullary carcinoma. Surg Gynecol Obstet 151:794

Dayton MT, Traverso LW, Longmire WP Jr. (1980) Efficacy of the gallbladder for drainage in bilary obstruction: comparison of malignant and benign disease. Arch Surg 115:1086

McArthur MS, Longmire WP Jr (1971) Peptic ulcer disease after choledochojejunostomy. Am J Surg 122:155

Wheeler ES, Longmire WP Jr (1978) Repair of benign stricture of the common bile duct by jejunal interposition choledochoduodenostomy. Surg Gynecol Obstetet 146:260

56 Periampullary Diverticulectomy

Concept: When a Periampullary Diverticulum Should Be Excised

Complications of Duodenal Diverticula

Although the duodenal diverticulum, which occurs in about 1% of all gastrointestinal X-ray studies, is not an uncommon condition, Whitcomb reported that only one serious complication requiring surgery occurred in a series of 1,064 patients that he studied. More than two-thirds of all duodenal diverticula occur within 2 cm of Vater's ampulla (Eggert, Teichmann, and Wittmann; Thompson). While the pseudo-diverticulum that results from the healing of a duodenal ulcer contains a seromuscular coat as well as mucosa, the periampullary diverticulum, being a true diverticulum, has a sac composed only of mucosa and submucosa. It ranges in size between 0.5 and 6.0 cm, in most cases. Diverticula that have a narrow entrance into the duodenum are more likely to produce symptoms than are widenecked lesions. In the absence of a muscular coat the diverticulum is unable to expel food particles. This sequence of events may lead to ulceration and bleeding into the gastrointestinal tract, compression of the common bile duct (CBD) with episodes of cholangitis, recurrent pancreatitis, as well as perforation of the diverticulum with abscess formation or peritonitis.

Perforation of a duodenal diverticulum produces retroperitoneal sepsis that may resemble acute cholecystitis or acute pancreatitis in its manifestations. Early diagnosis may be enhanced by finding a normal HIDA scan, which rules out acute cholecystitis. Since the serum amylase may be elevated with a perforated duodenal diverticulum, this condition is difficult to differentiate from acute pancreatitis. If the signs and symptoms are localized to the right upper quadrant, acute pancreatitis is less likely than if the patient has pain and tenderness in the epigastrium and the left upper quadrant. Patients with signs and symptoms that are atypical for acute pancreatitis should have a Hypaque gastrointestinal X-ray series. If the abdominal X-ray film demonstrates air in the retroperitoneal tissues of the right upper quadrant, a duodenal perforation is highly likely. Immediate exploration is indicated. The lesion will not be detected in the operating room unless an extensive Kocher maneuver is performed. If operation is performed soon after the perforation, it may be possible to trace the diverticulum to its neck, excise it, and close the seromuscular and mucosal layers of the duodenal wall with interrupted fine sutures. It may be necessary to insert a catheter into the CBD, prior to suturing the orifice of an excised periampullary diverticulum, in order to prevent suture-occlusion of the terminal CBD. If the duodenal wall is markedly inflamed, it is likely that the duodenal suture line will not heal properly. In this case, it may be prudent to isolate the duodenal leak by performing a Billroth II gastrectomy to divert the gastric content to the jejunum and to divide the CBD and transplant its proximal end into a Roux-Y segment of jejunum. Following these procedures, a failure of the duodenal suture line will result in a fistula that releases primarily pancreatic juice. An uncomplicated pancreatic fistula is a relatively benign complication compared to a duodenal fistula that leaks pancreatic juice combined with bile. If the repair of the neck of the excised diverticulum appears to be reasonably secure, place a sump drain down to the vicinity of the repair. If a lateral duodenal fistula appears during the postoperative course, observe the patient carefully. If the patient's defenses appear to be unable to contain the duodenal fistula, do not hesitate to reoperate on the patient to perform a gastrectomy and Roux-Y diversion of bile as described above.

Perforation of a diverticulum involving the third or fourth portions of the duodenum may be exposed by dividing the posterior peritoneal attachments of the right colon and the small bowel mesentery, as described in Chap. 20. After evacuating the abscess and excising the diverticulum, be certain to excise the duodenal wall back to relatively healthy tissue. If this defect is more than 1.5–2.0 cm in diameter, either resect a short segment of duodenum or else anastomose the duodenal defect to the open end of a Roux-Y limb of jejunum. Suturing diseased duodenal wall is doomed to failure.

Iatrogenic Perforation of Periampullary Diverticulum

Another type of perforation occurs when a surgeon passes a Bakes dilator through the CBD into the duodenum during the course of CBD exploration. If the patient is known to have a periampullary diverticulum, this step in the CBD exploration should be omitted and replaced by careful choledochoscopy and cholangiography. When a Bakes dilator passes into the ampulla, it may enter the orifice of a periampullary diverticulum. While the surgeon is passing the probe, thinking it to be in the duodenal lumen, the probe is in fact perfo-

rating not only the sac of the diverticulum but also the head of the pancreas. Although the mortality for operations on the biliary tract was only 0.7% in 806 patients undergoing surgery for gallstone disease, Eggert and associates noticed that the operative mortality in 73 patients who were undergoing surgery for gallstone disease and who also had periampullary diverticula was 7%. Two of their five postoperative deaths were caused by perforation of a periampullary diverticulum during operation. This type of complication may sometimes be detected in the operating room while irrigating the distal CBD with saline; for, this condition is confirmed if the saline appears to leak through the posterior aspect of the pancreas. This leakage can be observed directly if a Kocher maneuver has been performed as part of the CBD exploration, a maneuver that we believe should always be completed prior to opening the CBD. Another method of identifying this complication, is to perform a T-tube completion cholangiogram.

When perforation of a periampullary diverticulum has been caused by passing the Bakes dilator, it is aggravated by the fact that the surgeon, by attempting to palpate the dilator in the lumen of the duodenum, continues to push the dilator through the head of the pancreas. When this damage to the head of the pancreas is accompanied by the leakage of bile through the back wall of the duodenum, an explosive acute pancreatitis occurs, one that is often fatal. In some cases, when a perforation by means of the metal dilator is suspected, it cannot be determined whether the surgeon has perforated the intrapancreatic portion of the CBD or the sac of a periampullary diverticulum. In this situation it is advisable to divide the CBD and implant the proximal end into a Roux-Y limb of jejunum for complete biliary diversion. Then remove the diverticulum and close the orifice as described below. Although complete biliary diversion may seem to constitute excessively radical surgery for this type of perforation, remember that this perforation is often fatal, as indicated by the two fatal cases described by Eggert and associates, the one by Neill and Thompson, and the one experienced in our department. If there has been no damage to the head of the pancreas by the probe, then simply excising the diverticulum and repairing its neck with a catheter in the CBD may constitute adequate treatment. It is these iatrogenic perforations that have led many surgeons to abandon the use of metal instruments in exploring the CBD.

Relationship between Periampullary Diverticulum and Biliary Tract Disease

Increased pressure secondary to the accumulation of food material in a periampullary diverticulum with a narrow neck may produce jaundice, cholangitis, and recurrent acute pancreatitis according to Manny, Muga, and Eyal. Landor and Fulkerson reported that 32% of 163 patients with periampullary diverticula either had concomitant gallstones or previous cholecystectomies. On the other hand, Pinotti, Tacka, Pontes, and Battarello, in studying 491 patients with biliary tract disease or pancreatitis, found that 16 patients (3.2%) had periampullary diverticula that were believed to be contributing to the symptoms of right upper quadrant pain, jaundice, or pancreatitis. Eleven of these patients did well after a primary operation that consisted of cholecystectomy, sphincteroplasty, and diverticulectomy. Five patients did not obtain relief of symptoms from cholecystectomy alone but became asymptomatic after a second operation that included diverticulectomy and sphincteroplasty. Manny and associates reported two patients who underwent cholecystectomy and choledochoduodenostomy for biliary calculi with an enlarged CBD. These patients did not have their periampullary diverticula removed. Both patients required reoperation at a later date for recurrent symptoms at which time a Billroth II gastrectomy was performed in order to divert the passage of food from the area of the diverticulum. Both patients experienced relief of symptoms from this procedure. These authors also reported that out of 12 patients with periampullary diverticula in whom gallstones were found, 3 became asymptomatic after cholecystectomy and diverticulectomy. In the 9 patients who underwent cholecystectomy without diverticulectomy, 3 developed ascending cholangitis and the other 6 continued to have what was described as a "postcholecystectomy syndrome."

Although there is insufficient evidence to believe that a periampullary diverticulum may be the cause of gallstone formation, it is clear that following cholecystectomy and choledocholithotomy without diverticulectomy, a number of patients will have persistent symptoms and recurrent cholangitis, often with enlargement of the CBD. Certainly, in the group of patients with postcholecystectomy complaints, duodenal diverticulectomy is indicated. It is not clear that sphincteroplasty in addition to diverticulectomy, is necessary in these patients, although this is advocated by Pinotti and associates because these authors believe that periampullary inflammation is associated with many of the diverticula. This has not been confirmed by other authors. When diverticulectomy is not feasible owing to local inflammatory changes, it appears that diversion of food by Billroth II gastrectomy will likewise relieve the symptoms caused by the distension of a periampullary diverticulum with food.

Indications

Perforation of diverticulum

Hemorrhage from diverticulum, especially if proved by endoscopic localization of the source of bleeding

Postcholecystectomy patients with intermittent jaundice, pain, cholangitis, or recurrent pancreatitis who have a periampullary diverticulum

It is not clear that a patient undergoing surgery for biliary calculi and/or cholangitis should have concomitant diverticulectomy as a routine procedure, although some data in support of this concept have been accumulating.

Preoperative Care

The diagnostic workup of patients with postcholecystectomy symptoms should include gastrointestinal X-rays and endoscopic radiographic cholangiopancreatography (ERCP) for the detection of periampullary diverticula.

Perioperative antibiotics

Pitfalls and Danger Points

Injury to pancreas, resulting in postoperative acute pancreatitis

Injury to distal CBD

Operative Strategy

The strategy of managing patients operated on because they have perforated a periampullary diverticulum depends on the degree of surrounding inflammation. Neill and Thompson stated that in some cases the neck of the diverticulum may be free of inflammation despite the perforation. In these cases it may be possible to accomplish primary closure of the neck of the sac with interrupted sutures. In many cases leakage of duodenal content through a perforated periampullary diverticulum will produce a violent inflammatory reaction. One cannot expect primary suture of the duodenal wall to be secure under these conditions. Consequently, as a lifesaving measure it may be necessary to divert the gastric content by means of a Billroth II gastrectomy. Divert the bile by dividing the CBD and implanting it into a Roux-Y limb of jejunum. Then insert multiple suction drains to the area of perforation.

In elective cases where the diverticulum is free of inflammation, we prefer the technique described by Iida. This involves inverting the sac of the diverticulum through an incision in the second portion of the duodenum. The diverticulum is excised and the defect in the duodenal wall is closed from inside the lumen.

An alternative technique involves dissecting the duodenal diverticulum from surrounding pancreas and duodenal wall down to its neck near the ampulla. The terminal CBD must be identified as it enters the posterior wall of the duodenum. Place a catheter in the CBD. Then transect the diverticulum at its neck and repair the defect in the duodenal wall. This technique may be facilitated by inflating the duodenal diverticulum with air injected through a nasogastric tube. It requires meticulous dissection of the pancreas away from its attachments to the posterior duodenal wall. As the pancreas is dissected away from the duodenum, the terminal portion of the CBD and the diverticulum may be exposed. This dissection is tedious and sometimes difficult. It carries a greater risk of inducing a postoperative acute pancreatitis than does the transduodenal approach.

Operative Technique— Transduodenal Diverticulectomy

Incision

Make either a midline incision from the xiphoid to a point about 5 cm below the umbilicus or, alternatively, a long subcostal incision.

Kocher Maneuver

Incise the lateral peritoneal attachments of the descending duodenum and mobilize the duodenum and the head of the pancreas as shown in Figs. 7–14 to 7–16. Place a gauze pad behind the head of the pancreas to elevate the duodenum.

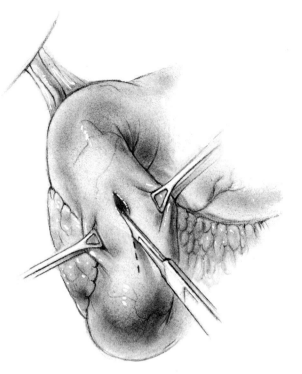

Fig. 56–1

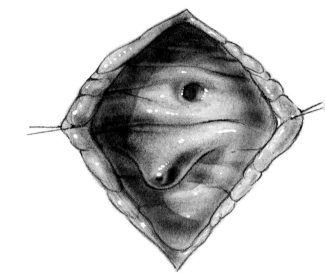

Fig. 56–2

Duodenotomy and Diverticulectomy

Make a 4–5 cm longitudinal incision near the antimesenteric border of the descending duodenum **(Fig. 56–1)**. Identify the ampulla by palpation or visualization **(Fig. 56–2)**. If there is any difficulty in identifying the ampulla in this fashion, do not hesitate to make an incision in the CBD and pass a Coudé catheter down to the ampulla through the CBD incision.

Identify the orifice of the periampullary diverticulum. Insert a forceps into the diverticulum. Grasp the mucosal wall of the diverticulum **(Fig. 56–3)** and gently draw the mucosa into the lumen of the duodenum until the entire diverticulum has been inverted into the lumen of the duodenum **(Figs. 56–4 and 56–5)**. Transect the neck of the diverticulum about 2–3 mm distance away from its junction with the duodenal wall.

Inspect the bed of the diverticulum through the orifice in the duodenum to check for bleeding. Then close the duode-

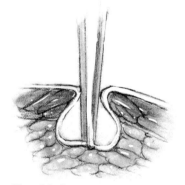

Fig. 56–3

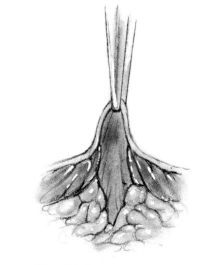

Fig. 56–4

142

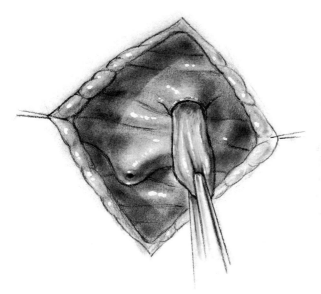

Fig. 56–5

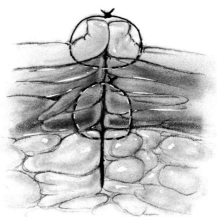

Fig. 56–6

nal wall by suturing the seromuscular layer with interrupted 4–0 Vicryl and invert this layer into the lumen of the duodenum. Close the defect in the mucosa also with inverting sutures of interrupted 5–0 Vicryl **(Fig. 56–6)**.

Close the duodenotomy incision in two layers using interrupted or continuous inverting sutures of 5–0 Vicryl for the mucosal layer and interrupted 4–0 atraumatic cotton Lembert sutures for the seromuscular coat.

Closure and Drainage

Bring a closed-suction drain out from the region of the head of the pancreas through a puncture wound in the right upper quadrant of the abdomen. Close the abdominal wall in routine fashion.

Postoperative Care

Continue nasogastric suction until bowel function has returned.

Give the patient perioperative antibiotics for 24 hours.

Check postoperative levels of serum amylase to detect postoperative pancreatitis.

Postoperative Complications

Acute pancreatitis

Duodenal leakage

References

Eggert A, Teichmann W., Wittmann DH (1982) The pathologic implication of duodenal diverticula. Surg Gynecol Obstet 154:62

Iida F (1979) Transduodenal diverticulectomy for periampullar diverticula. World J Surg 3:103

Landor JH, Fulkerson CC (1966) Duodenal diverticula: relationship to biliary tract disease. Arch Surg 93:182

Manny J, Muga M, Eyal Z (1981) The continuing clinical enigma of duodenal diverticulum. Am J Surg 142:596

Neill SA, Thompson NW (1965) The complications of duodenal diverticula and their management. Surg Gynecol Obstet 120:1251

Pinotti HW, Tacka M, Pontes JF, Battarello A (1971) Juxtaampullar duodenal diverticula as a casue of biliopancreatic disease. Digestion 41:353

Thompson NW (1979) Transduodenal divertculectomy for periampullar diverticula: invited commentary. World J Surg 3:135

Whitcomb JG (1964), Duodenal diverticula. Arch Surg 88:275

57 Operations for Carcinoma of Hepatic Duct Bifurcation

Concept: When to Operate for Carcinoma of the Bile Ducts

Tumors of the Distal Third of the Bile Ducts

For purposes of classification the bile ducts are generally divided into thirds. The proximal third extends from the cystic duct upward. The middle third starts at the cystic duct and includes that portion of the common bile duct (CBD) that is located cephalad to the pancreas. The distal third encompasses the CBD in its course between the pancreas and duodenum, ending at its termination in the ampulla of Vater. Operation for cure in the region of the distal third of the bile duct requires a Whipple pancreatoduodenectomy. Whereas Lees, Zapolanski, Cooperman, and Hermann of the Cleveland Clinic were able to resect only 19% of 32 patients having carcinoma of the distal third of the duct, Tompkins, Thomas, Wile, and Longmire performed the Whipple operation in 12 of their 18 cases with a mortality rate of 8%. Forty-two percent of the cases resected by Tompkins and associates survived for 5 years. There seems little question that pancreatoduodenectomy is the treatment of choice for lesions of the distal CBD.

When the tumor is not resectable, generally a bypass between the hepatic duct and a Roux-Y limb of jejunum (see Chap. 55) offers the best palliation, perhaps supplemented by radiotherapy and chemotherapy.

Tumors of the Middle Third of the Bile Ducts

Although many patients with carcinoma of the hepatic or cystic ducts show early invasion of adjacent structures in the hepatoduodenal ligament (portal vein or hepatic artery), Tompkins and associates were able to resect 16 of the 26 tumors they encountered in this location with no mortality, including three patients who required pancreatoduodenectomy. Thirteen of the patients were treated by duct resection and biliary-enteric anastomosis. Eight underwent palliative long-term intubation of the bile duct. The overall 5-year survival in this group was 12%.

Each of these tumors of the hepatic duct should be evaluated by dissecting out the portal vein and the hepatic artery and tracing these structures to the vicinity of the tumor. If the tumor can be separated from these two vessels, resection is indicated with frozen-section histological examination of the duct margins. Reconstruction should include a hepaticojejunostomy of the Roux-Y type. If the tumor is contiguous with the pancreas, a pancreatoduodenectomy is indicated.

Tumors of the Proximal Third of the Bile Ducts

Resection of Bifurcation Tumors
Some bile duct tumors are located in the proximal portion of the intrahepatic ducts. These are managed by hepatic resection using the same techniques necessary for primary hepatic cell carcinomas of the liver. The majority of primary bile duct cancers seem to arise at or near the bifurca-

144

tion of the common hepatic duct. Long-mire, in discussing the paper by Hart and White, stated that he generally finds it unnecessary to excise liver parenchyma when resecting tumors at the hepatic duct bifurcation because in most patients the junction of the right and left hepatic lobar ducts is situated outside the liver. Tompkins and associates were able to resect 46% of the 47 patients with *proximal* lesions of the bile ducts. They experienced a 23% mortality rate and achieved no 5-year survivals. Cameron, also commenting on Hart and White's paper, stated that he was able to resect only about 20% of the malignant strictures he encountered at the bifurcation of the hepatic duct, while Lees and associates did not resect any of their 36 malignancies at the bifurcation. Tompkins and associates, Adson and Farnell, and Cameron, Gayler, and Zuidema all failed to note any statistically significant increase in survival following resection of ductal cancers in the region of the bifurcation. Since the mortality of resecting these lesions is higher than palliative management by intubating the ducts, it is difficult to advocate a high-risk, difficult resection in the absence of supporting data. In those cases where the tumor is localized, resection is relatively simple; here resection plus a regional lymphadenectomy, as advocated by Adson and Farnell, is indicated. Because of the high recurrence rate after resection, it is advisable to leave indwelling Silastic catheter-stents in the hepatic ducts indefinitely even when resection has been done.

Voyles, Bowley, Allison, Benjamin, and others found that they could identify preoperatively most cases of hilar cholangiocarcinoma, which proved to be unresectable, by performing percutaneous transhepatic cholangiography followed by angiography of the hepatic arteries and the portal vein.

Intubation of Hepatic Ducts

If the patient presents with complete obstruction of the left hepatic duct and partial obstruction of the right duct, it is often not sufficient to drain only one duct, since the bile backed up behind an obstructed duct will often become contaminated with bacteria. The patient will generally develop cholangitis unless adequate drainage of both ducts is accomplished. When ducts are partially obstructed, drainage of both ducts is necessary as intubation of a single duct will cause chronic contamination of those portions of the biliary tree that are in communication with the intubated duct.

When a patient appears to have a large tumor at the bifurcation of the hepatic ducts, as determined by percutaneous transhepatic cholangiography, perform an angiogram to visualize the hepatic arteries and portal vein. If there is encasement of these structures and the percutaneous needle biopsy of the tumor is positive, operation is probably contraindicated. In this case, ask the radiologist to pass a drainage catheter into the partially obstructed right main duct. The catheter can sometimes be passed through the tumor and even into the duodenum; a "pig-tail" will anchor the catheter in place and no external drainage of bile will be necessary. A second catheter will be required in the obstructed left hepatic duct. If the radiologist cannot pass catheters through the tumor, then the patient will be required to wear a plastic bag to collect the bile from each of the catheters that have been inserted into the obstructed hepatic ducts.

When tumors do not appear to be large by cholangiography, laparotomy for possible resection of the tumor, or for the passage of Silastic catheters through the tumor to permit bile drainage, is indicated. It has been our impression that when a Silastic catheter, 4–8 mm in diameter, is inserted into the hepatic duct through the tumor at laparotomy, recurrent postoperative cholangitis occurs less frequently than when a smaller catheter is introduced percutaneously by the radiologist. In either case, the catheters should be changed in the radiology suite at least every 3 months following their insertion. There is insufficient data at this time to determine exactly which patients should be subjected to percutaneous intubation of hepatic ducts by the radiologist or to catheterization of the ducts at laparotomy, as advocated by Terblanche, Saunders, and Louw, and by Cameron, Gayler, and Zuidema.

Indications

Carcinomas of hepatic duct bifurcation

Preoperative Care

Percutaneous transhepatic cholangiography to demonstrate the proximal extent of the tumor

Hepatic angiography, in selected cases

Perioperative antibiotics

Nasogastric tube

Pitfalls and Danger Points

Trauma to liver during transhepatic intubation at laparotomy

Trauma to portal vein or hepatic artery during tumor excision at hilus

Failure to achieve adequate drainage of bile

Operative Strategy

Resection

Cameron, Broe, and Zuidema emphasize that resection of malignant tumors at the bifurcation of the hepatic duct is safe when the surgeon can demonstrate that there is no invasion of the underlying portal vein or liver tissue, and if the proximal extent of the tumor does not reach the secondary divisions of the hepatic ducts. In these cases it is generally not necessary to resect hepatic parenchyma; 37% of Cameron, Broe, and Zuidema's bifurcation malignan-

cies could be resected for cure with no deaths. Patients, who do not meet these criteria of resectability, should undergo transhepatic intubation of the ducts and not resection.

Avoiding hemorrhage during the operation depends on careful dissection of the common hepatic duct and the tumor away from the bifurcation of the portal vein. This is best done by dividing the CBD, mobilizing the gallbladder, and elevating the hepatic duct together with the tumor to expose the portal vein and its bifurcation. In borderline cases, remove the gallbladder and make a preliminary assessment regarding invasion of the portal vein by dissecting beneath the common hepatic duct toward the tumor before dividing the CBD. Cameron and associates (1982) suggest that this dissection may be facilitated if a radiologist has passed percutaneous transhepatic catheters of the Ring type into both the right and left main ducts. Since the bifurcation of the common hepatic duct occurs, in almost all cases, outside the liver, the right and left hepatic ducts can be identified by palpating the transhepatic catheters that have been previously inserted.

Dilating Malignant Strictures of the Hepatic Duct Bifurcation

Most tumors of the hepatic duct involve the bifurcation. If the radiologist has passed percutaneous catheters through the tumor into the common hepatic duct or the common bile duct preoperatively, these catheters, in the right and left hepatic ducts, can be used to facilitate passage of larger, permanent Silastic catheter-stents. The stents should preferably be 6 mm in outer diameter and fairly thick-walled to prevent the tumor from occluding them. Since it is also desirable to catheterize both the right and left hepatic ducts, two such stents are required. Because these two stents rarely fit into the CBD, it is generally necessary to perform a Roux-Y hepaticojejunostomy to permit both stents to enter the jejunum and drain the bile in this fashion. If the occlusion of the left hepatic duct cannot be dilated from below, it is often possible to identify the left hepatic duct above the tumor and to pass a stent through an incision in the hepatic duct above the tumor.

Operative Technique—Resection of Bifurcation Tumors

Incision

In most cases a midline incision from the xiphocostal angle to a point about 5–8 cm below the umbilicus is suitable. It is helpful to apply a chain or an Upper Hand retractor to the right costal margin, to improve the exposure at the hilus of the liver.

Determination of Operability

Perform a cholecystectomy by the usual technique (see Chap. 48). Incise the layer of peritoneum overlying the common he-

patic duct beginning at the level of the cystic duct stump and progressing in a cephalad manner. Also unroof the peritoneum overlying the hepatic artery so that the common hepatic duct and the common hepatic artery have been skeletonized (**Fig. 57–1**). Now dissect along the lateral and posterior walls of the common hepatic duct near the cystic stump and elevate the duct from the underlying portal vein. Try to continue the dissection along the anterior wall of the portal vein towards the tumor in order to make a judgment as to whether the tumor has invaded the portal vein. A more accurate determination will be made later in the dissection after the CBD has been divided and elevated. If there are no signs of gross invasion, then identify the anterior wall of the tumor and try to palpate the Ring catheters, if they have been placed in the right and the left hepatic ducts prior to operation. This will give the

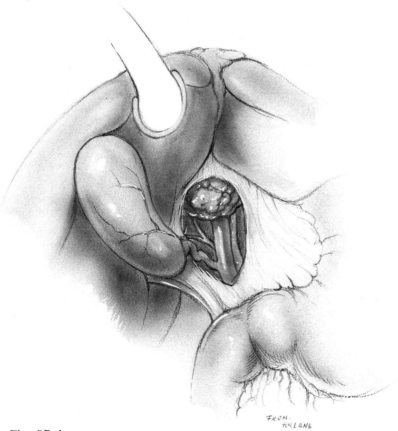

Fig. 57–1.

147

surgeon some idea of the cephalad extent of the tumor. Frequently, this judgment can be made from the preoperative transhepatic cholangiogram. If there is gross invasion by the tumor of hepatic parenchyma, this may be considered a relative contraindication to resection.

For a final determination of the advisability of resecting the tumor, divide the CBD **(Fig. 57–2)** distal to the cystic duct stump. Oversew the distal end of the CBD with continuous 4–0 PG suture material. Dissect the proximal stump of the CBD off the underlying portal vein by going in a cephalad direction **(Fig. 57–3).** Skeletonize the portal vein and sweep any lymphatic tissue towards the specimen. Carefully identify the bifurcation of the portal vein behind the tumor. Perform this portion of the dissection with great caution because lacerating a tumor-invaded portal vein bifurcation will produce hemorrhage that will be difficult to correct if one side of the laceration consists of tumor. During this dissection, pay attention also to the common hepatic and the right hepatic arteries that course behind the tumor. Bifurcation tumors may occasionally invade or adhere to the right hepatic artery.

After demonstrating that the tumor is clear of the underlying portal veins and hepatic arteries, continue the dissection along the posterior wall of the tumor. The right and left hepatic ducts and even secondary branches can often be identified without resecting hepatic parenchyma. It is sometimes difficult by palpation to determine the proximal extent of the tumor. If preoperative catheters have been placed, palpate the right and left duct for the presence of the catheters. After adequate exposure has been obtained, transect the ducts and remove the tumor **(Fig. 57–4).** Perform frozen-section examination of the proximal portions of the right and left ducts in the specimen to determine if the tumor has been completely removed. If the report is positive for tumor, determine whether removing a reasonable additional length of duct is feasible. If this additional duct is resected, it may be necessary to anasto-

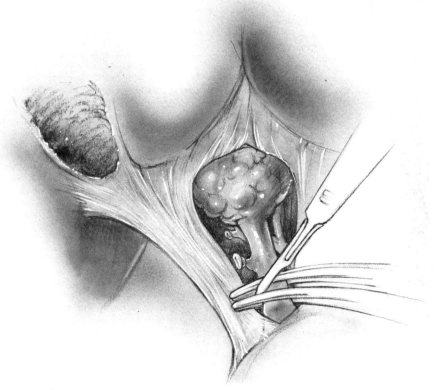

Fig. 57–2

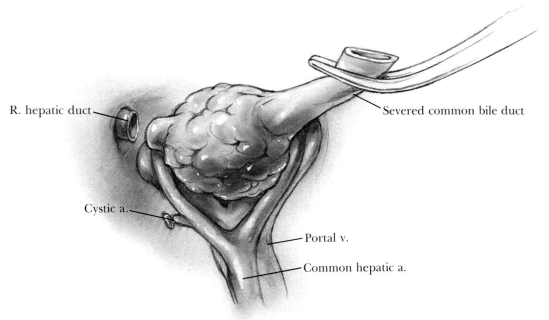

R. hepatic duct

Cystic a.

Severed common bile duct

Portal v.

Common hepatic a.

Fig. 57–3

mose three and four hepatic ducts to the jejunum. Although some adjacent hepatic parenchyma may be left attached to the duct during blunt dissection, it is probably not indicated to perform a major hepatic

resection for tumors at the bifurcation. Then insert Silastic tubes into each severed duct by one of the techniques described below.

Anastomosis

Construct a Roux-Y jejunal limb as described in Chap. 55. Apply a row of 3.5 mm staples with a TA-55 device across the open end of jejunum. Cut the mucosa flush with the stapling device and lightly electrocoagulate the everted mucosa. Bring the closed end of jejunum to the hilus of the liver. Make an incision in the antimesenteric border of the jejunum equal to the diameter of the open left hepatic duct. Anastomose the end of the left hepatic duct to the side of jejunum with interrupted 5–0 Prolene or 5–0 Vicryl sutures in one layer. Perform the same type of anastomosis between the right hepatic duct and a second incision in the jejunum. Pass each Silastic catheter through the anastomosis into the jejunum so that it projects for a distance of 5–6 cm into the jejunum (**Fig.**

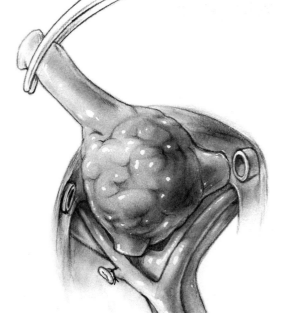

Fig. 57–4

149

57–5). Leave the catheters in place permanently because this tumor has a high rate of recurrence.

In some situations when a tumor excision requires the reattachment of smaller ducts to the jejunum, it may be necessary to remove the jejunal serosa and to suture the jejunal mucosa to the hepatic parenchyma surrounding the divided duct. So long as each duct has been intubated with a Silastic tube and this tube passes through the anastomosis into the jejunum, small deficiencies in the mucosa-to-mucosa approximation will be repaired by the ingrowth of epithelium over a period of months, providing that the Silastic stents remain in place for a period of a year or more.

Drainage and Closure

At the site where the Silastic tube enters the left hepatic duct at the dome of the liver, insert a mattress suture of 3–0 PG into the liver capsule to minimize the possibility of bile draining around the tube at

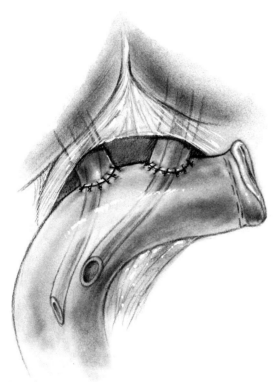

Fig. 57–5

this point. Tie the two tails of this suture around the Silastic tube to anchor it in place. Accomplish the identical maneuver at the point where the second tube enters the anterior surface of the right lobe of the liver. Then make a puncture wound through the abdominal wall in the right upper quadrant. Pass the Silastic tube through this puncture wound. Leave enough slack to compensate for some degree of abdominal distension. Then suture the Silastic tube to the skin securely using 2–0 nylon. Perform the identical maneuver to pass the other Silastic tube that exits from the liver through a puncture wound in the left upper quadrant of the abdominal wall. In addition, place a 2-cm latex Penrose drain near each of the exit wounds in the right and left lobes of the liver and bring them through abdominal stab wounds. A third latex drain should be placed at the hilus of the liver near the hepaticojejunal anastomoses.

Close the abdominal incision in routine fashion.

Operative Technique— Intubation of Hepatic Ducts without Resecting Tumor

Incision

Make a midline incision from the xiphoid to a point 4–5 cm below the umbilicus.

Dilating the Malignant Structure

Identify the common hepatic duct below the tumor. Make a 1.5–2.0 cm incision in the anterior wall of the duct. If the patient has previously undergone percutaneous transhepatic catheterization of the right and left hepatic ducts and if both catheters have passed into the CBD, these catheters may be utilized to draw Silastic tubes into each hepatic duct.

In the absence of intraductal catheters, pass a Bakes dilator into the common hepatic duct and try to establish a channel leading into the right hepatic duct. After the channel has been established, dilate the

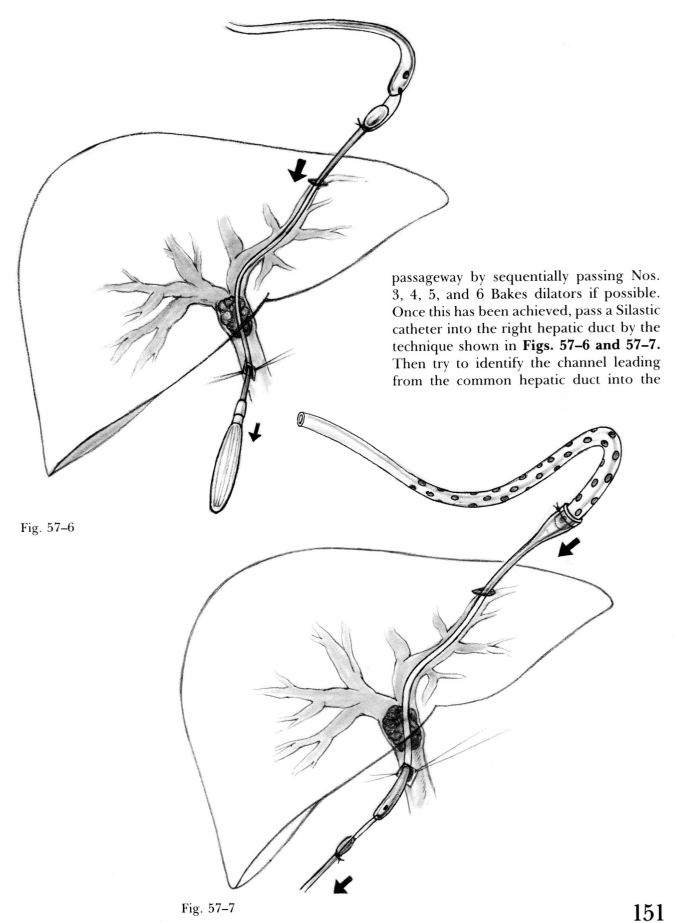

passageway by sequentially passing Nos. 3, 4, 5, and 6 Bakes dilators if possible. Once this has been achieved, pass a Silastic catheter into the right hepatic duct by the technique shown in **Figs. 57–6 and 57–7.** Then try to identify the channel leading from the common hepatic duct into the

Fig. 57–6

Fig. 57–7

151

left hepatic duct with a No. 2 or a No. 3 Bakes dilator. If this channel cannot be established, try to identify the left hepatic duct just above the tumor. Having accomplished this, incise the duct and pass a Silastic tube through the duct and out the parenchyma of the liver on the anterior surface of the left lobe. It will be necessary to anastomose a Roux-Y limb of jejunum to this opening in the left hepatic duct. Pass the Silastic tube through the anastomosis into the jejunum.

Even if the channel can be established through the tumor into both the right and left hepatic ducts, often the CBD will not be sufficiently large to accommodate two Silastic tubes. Consequently, if both the right and the left ducts are intubated, generally a Roux-Y hepaticojejunostomy will be necessary to accommodate the two Silastic tubes. Because of the presence of tu-

mor, it is often not possible to perform mucosa-to-mucosa anastomoses. In this case, simply suture the incised jejunum to the tissues surrounding the point at which the tubes exit from the bile duct. Then pass each tube down into the jejunum for a distance of at least 6 cm **(Fig. 57–8).**

Perform the end-to-side jejunojejunostomy, in completing the Roux-Y anastomosis, at a point 60–70 cm distal to the hepaticojejunostomy, by the method illustrated in Figs. 19–36 to 19–40.

Other Intubation Techniques

There are many techniques aimed at minimizing trauma when passing a tube through the liver into the hepatic ducts. It is helpful to keep the hole in Glisson's capsule as small as possible to minimize the leakage of bile around the tube. If the patient has already undergone a preoperative transhepatic catheterization of the he-

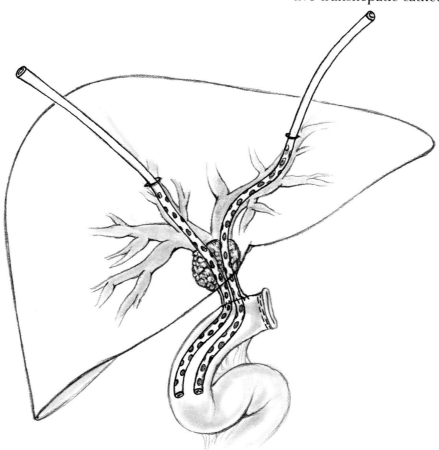

Fig. 57–8

patic duct, and if the point at which this catheter penetrates the liver capsule is in a satisfactory location, one may suture a urological filliform to the end of the intra-ductal catheter. Then by withdrawing the catheter through the liver, the filliform will be brought through the opening in the liver capsule. Urological filliform-followers may then be attached to the end of the filliform so that the path of the catheter can be dilated about 6 mm. Following this step, the Silastic tube can be inserted into the open end of the follower, where it is sutured securely in place. By withdrawing the follower, the Silastic tube catheter can be brought through the liver with minimal trauma and then out through the skin.

In the absence of an intraductal cath-eter, one may utilize the technique of Sparkman (discussion of paper by Cam-eron, Broe, and Zuidema) by passing a Fenger flexible gall duct probe through the cut end of the hepatic duct at the hilus of the liver. This probe is then passed through the hepatic parenchyma to a point on the lower anterior surface of the right lobe. Suture a urethral filliform to the tip of the probe and draw it back to the hilus of the liver. To this filliform, sequentially attach urethral followers to gently dilate the tract. Finally, attach a Silastic catheter to the last follower and draw it through the liver and out through the cut end of the right hepatic duct. Follow a similar se-quence for the left hepatic duct.

Another simple technique is to pass a No. 2 or No. 3 Bakes bile duct dilator through the cut end of the right or left hepatic duct. Pass the dilator through the duct until it reaches a point about 1–1.5 cm from Glisson's capsule in an appropri-ate location on the anterior surface of the liver. Then make a tiny incision in the cap-sule and push the metal dilator through the hepatic parenchyma. Suture the tip of the 10F straight rubber catheter to the Bakes dilator (see Fig. 57–6). This step may be simplified if a small hole has been drilled in the tip of the Bakes dilator to accept the suture (Tatarchuk and White).

After drawing the Bakes dilator downward, the catheter will be led into the hepatic duct at the hilus of the liver. Then insert a Silastic tube, 6 mm in outer diameter, into the flared open end of the French cath-eter and suture it securely in this location (see Fig. 57–7). By drawing the catheter out of the hepatic duct at the hepatic hilus, the Silastic tube will be in the proper loca-tion. Make certain that holes have been punched in the Silastic prior to its inser-tion. These holes should be situated above and below the site of the tumor. One con-venient source of the Silastic tubing is the round Jackson-Pratt drain.

Bring the Silastic catheters out through puncture wounds in the abdomi-nal wall and insert latex drains to the sites from which the plastic catheters exit from the right and left hepatic lobes, and one drain to the hilus of the liver.

Postoperative Care

Attach the Silastic catheters to plastic bags for gravity drainage until there is no drainage of bile along any of the latex drains. Then occlude the Si-lastic catheters. Instruct the patient to irrigate each catheter twice daily with 25 ml of sterile saline. It will be neces-sary to replace the nylon suture fixing the catheter to the skin approximately once every 4–6 weeks.

Instruct the patient to return to the X-ray department every 3 months in order to have the catheters replaced, as sludge tends to occlude many of the openings as time goes by. Replac-ing the catheters is accomplished by passing a sterile guide wire through the Silastic tube; then remove the Si-lastic tube with sterile technique and replace it with another tube of the same type. Remove the wire and per-form a cholangiogram in order to con-firm that the tube has been accurately placed. Then suture the tube to the skin. If the patient develops cholangi-tis, it may be necessary to replace the tube at an earlier time interval than 3 months.

Remove the latex drains when there is no further drainage of bile.

Continue perioperative antibiotics until the latex drains have been removed.

Maintain nasogastric suction until bowel function returns.

Prescribe cimetidine intravenously until the patient has resumed a regular diet to lower the incidence of postoperative gastric "stress" bleeding.

Postoperative Complications

Sepsis, subhepatic or subphrenic

Cholangitis generally will not occur unless there is some element of obstruction to the drainage of bile. If the ducts draining only one lobe of the liver have been intubated, leaving the opposite hepatic duct completely occluded but not drained, cholangitis or even a liver abscess will frequently occur over a period of time. Consequently, in the presence of a tumor at the bifurcation of the hepatic duct which occludes both right and left hepatic ducts, drainage of each duct is necessary. If drainage of both ducts cannot be accomplished in the operating room, then request the radiologist to perform percutaneous transhepatic insertion of a catheter into the undrained duct postoperatively. Routine replacement of the Silastic tubes at intervals of 2–3 months will prevent most cases of postoperative cholangitis.

Leakage of bile around the Silastic tube may occur early if the puncture wound in Glisson's capsule is larger than the diameter of the Silastic tube. If leakage occurs late in the postoperative course, attempt to replace the tube, around which the bile is leaking, with a tube of somewhat larger diameter. If leakage occurs in the immediate postoperative course, check the position of the Silastic tubes by performing cholangiography to ascertain that none of the side holes in the tubes is draining freely into peritoneal cavity.

Upper gastrointestinal hemorrhage late in the postoperative course is reported to occur in as many as 7% of patients with hepaticojejunostomies that divert bile from the duodenum. Patients should be alerted to this possibility and treated promptly with antacid therapy and cimetidine.

References

Adson MA, Farnell MB (1981) Hepatobiliary cancer—surgical consideration. Mayo Clin Proc 56:686

Cameron JL, Broe P, Zuidema GD (1982) Proximal bile duct tumors: surgical management with Silastic transhepatic biliary stents. Ann Surg 196:412

Cameron JL, Gayler BW, Zuidema GD (1978) The use of Silastic transhepatic stents in benign and malignant biliary strictures. Ann Surg 188:552

Hart MJ, White TT (1980) Central hepatic resections and anastomosis for stricture or carcinoma at the hepatic bifurcation. Ann Surg 192:299

Lees CD, Zapolanski A, Cooperman AM, Hermann RE (1980) Carcinoma of the bile ducts. Surg Gynecol Obstet 151:193

Tartarchuk JW, White TT (1979) A new instrument for inserting a U-Tube. Am J Surg 137:425

Terblanche J, Saunders SJ, Louw JH (1972) Prolonged palliation in carcinoma of the main hepatic duct junction. Surgery 71:720

Tompkins RK, Thomas D, Wile A, Longmire WP Jr (1981) Prognostic factors in bile duct carcinoma: analysis of 96 cases. Ann Surg 194:447

Voyles CR, Bowley NJ, Allison DJ, Benjamin IS et al. (1983) Carcinoma of the proximal extrahepatic biliary tree; radiologic assessment and therapeutic alternatives. Ann Surg 197:188

Pancreas

58 Concept: Which Operations for Pancreatic Cancer

Resection versus Bypass

In past decades the mortality rate of pancreatic resection ranged between 20% and 40%. Since the mortality rate far exceeded the incidence of 5-year survival, it could reasonably be argued that the results of bypass procedures were superior to resection. For the period 1953–1973, Aston and Longmire lost 13.8% of 65 patients undergoing a Whipple resection. But those patients undergoing surgery from 1963 to 1973 had a mortality rate of only 5.1%. ReMine experienced a 4.3% mortality in a recent series of total pancreatectomies, while Moosa, Lewis, and Mackie had four deaths in 52 resections (19 Whipple operations and 33 total pancreatectomies). Barton and Copeland reported a 2.3% mortality for 44 Whipple operations for ampullary carcinoma. Representative 5-year survival figures reported by Forrest and Longmire in 1979 ranged from 4% for carcinoma of the pancreas to 24% for ampullary and 25% for distal common bile duct (CBD) cancer. These patients were treated by partial pancreatoduodenectomy. Our hospital mortality is 4.8% in 21 cases.

Since the average mortality rate for a palliative bypass procedure in pancreatic carcinoma is 10%–20% (Brooks, 1983), which exceeds that of pancreatic resection when the latter is performed by an experienced team, we believe that any patient whose tumor can be encompassed by surgical means should undergo resection. We have noted, together with Child, Hinerman, and Kauffman, with Wilson and Block, and with others, that even in patients who are not cured by resection, pancreatectomy provides a considerably greater degree of palliation, especially of pain, than does a bypass operation.

Contraindications to resection include distant metastases, peritoneal seeding, invasion of the root of the mesentery and metastases to distant lymph nodes (e.g., at the celiac axis). A minor degree of invasion of the portal vein or the middle colic vessels does not contraindicate resection.

Which Bypass Operation?

Because patients with inoperable pancreatic cancer are usually in the poor-risk category and can not withstand any serious postoperative complication, the bypass procedure must be selected with care. Operations involving anastomoses to the duodenum are contraindicated because a leak is often fatal in these patients. Using the gallbladder to bypass a malignant obstruction may be short-lived because the tumor may grow up the CBD and occlude the cystic duct. Our preference in this category of patients is an anastomosis between the end of a Roux-Y segment of jejunum and the side of the dilated hepatic duct.

Because the Roux-Y jejunojejunostomy is accomplished by a stapling technique that takes only 1–2 minutes of operating time, the Roux-Y technique can be accomplished expeditiously. It has the additional advantage that leakage of bile from this type of anastomosis is not a serious complication if a drain has been inserted at the time of surgery.

Because 30% of patients with inoperable carcinoma of the head of the pancreas will experience obstruction of the duodenum before they die of cancer, we routinely perform a gastrojejunostomy to the Roux-Y loop in order to prevent this late complication. The gastrojejunostomy, too, is performed by a stapling technique to the greater curvature side of the gastric antrum. The gastrojejunostomy should be located 50–60 cm from the hepaticojejunostomy. Our mortality rate from this procedure has been one death in 52 Roux-Y hepaticojejunostomies.

Total versus Partial Pancreatoduodenectomy (Whipple)

Although the reported 5-year survival rate following resection for ampullary and periampullary cancer has risen in recent years to 25%–30%, the survival following partial pancreatectomy (Whipple) for carcinoma of the pancreas has remained negligible. One reason for this poor survival may be the fact that pancreatic carcinoma is multicentric in origin. Therefore resection of only the head of the pancreas may leave residual carcinoma in the body or the tail. Collins, Craighead, and Brooks noted four cases of tumor extending beyond the line of resection in 11 consecutive Whipple procedures.

There are several reasons why the total pancreatectomy is a safer operation than is the Whipple. Removing the entire pancreas avoids the possibility of postoperative acute pancreatitis as well as the possibility that the patient will develop a leaking pancreaticojejunal anastomosis. The latter complication is responsible for many of the lethal results following pancreatoduodenectomy. In addition to avoiding these complications, total pancreatectomy also permits more complete removal of lymph nodes. Although the total number of cases involved is small, there is suggestive evidence from the data of Brooks and Culebras, of Forrest and Longmire, and of Moosa and associates that the 5-year survival following total pancreatectomy for pancreatic carcinoma is higher than that following partial pancreatectomy.

If the results following total pancreatectomy seem superior to that of the Whipple operation, what are the disadvantages of this procedure? First, the absence of any exocrine secretion from the pancreas requires the supplemental feeding of pancreatic enzymes in order to prevent steatorrhea. Since these enzymes are fairly effective, this does not create a significant disadvantage. A more important drawback of total pancreatectomy is the resulting diabetes.

The diabetes that follows total pancreatectomy tends to be "brittle" and difficult to manage in about 20% of patients. Death from hypoglycemia has been reported as long as 4 years following operation when the patients do not exhibit continued alertness to diabetic control. Although this is true of 20% of patients, the remainder have no more difficulty than do those with diabetes of nonsurgical origin. Consequently we agree with Brooks and Culebras, with ReMine, and with Moosa and associates that total pancreatectomy is now the operation of choice for patients with carcinoma of pancreatic origin.

There are also situations when total pancreatectomy may be indicated even for cancers of ampullary, periampullary, or distal CBD origin. In some of these patients, the pancreas may be very soft and the pancreatic duct may be either small or thin walled, conditions that make the pancreatojejunostomy an insecure anastomosis with increased danger of postoperative leakage. Under these conditions, total pancreatectomy may be a safer operation.

Fortner, Kim, Cubilla, Turnbull, and associates have described a very radical total pancreatectomy that includes the resection and reanastomosis of the superior mesenteric artery and vein. As yet, there are inadequate data to support the use of this procedure.

Distal Pancreatectomy

Distal pancreatectomy is indicated and may be curative in cases of localized cystadenocarcinoma and malignant insulinoma. On the other hand, for duct cell carcinoma of the pancreatic tail, distal pancreatectomy has resulted in no known 5-year survivors. However, in some cases resection may produce excellent palliation.

Is Biopsy Necessary?

When a Whipple pancreatoduodenostomy is inadvertently performed for chronic pancreatitis, the mortality rate is low because the thickened pancreas and pancreatic duct take sutures quite well and thus minimize the incidence of postoperative anastomotic leakage. Also, the postoperative disability is minimal because removing the head of the pancreas does not produce diabetes in patients who do not already suffer from this condition. On the other hand, if total pancreatectomy is done in error, the resulting disability may be a brittle form of diabetes. Therefore, we believe that prior to total pancreatectomy, a serious attempt should be made to confirm the diagnosis of malignancy. In some cases this may be done by performing a biopsy during endoscopic radiographic cholangiopancreatography (ERCP). Alternatively, aspiration of the pancreatic duct during ERCP may produce a positive diagnosis when the specimen is subjected to cytological study. If this is not successful, needle aspiration of the tumor during laparotomy should be carried out. Staining of this aspirate for cytological study is a safe means of obtain-

ing a histological diagnosis. When these procedures fail, a scalpel or Travenol needle biopsy may be successful.

In some cases an experienced pancreatic surgeon may make the diagnosis of carcinoma on the basis of marked enlargement of the pancreatic duct accompanied by a thin-walled dilated CBD and gallbladder. Before doing a total pancreatectomy, we prefer, in most cases, histological confirmation.

Pancreatectomy as a Palliative Procedure

Although pancreatectomy for cancer is generally performed only when there are prospects for cure, this operation does in fact provide better palliation than any other. In agreement with Child and associates, "we are convinced that death from metastatic disease is more humane than death with a painful cancer in place which infiltrates the aorta and regional nerves." A number of patients following pancreatectomy for cancer have survived from 2–5 years without suffering the unrelenting back pain characteristic of this disease. Death generally ensues from liver metastases. Consequently, a surgical team, whose mortality rate is at or below 10%, should be aggressive in performing pancreatectomy whenever the lesion is technically resectable and if there are no distant metastases.

References

Aston SJ, Longmire, WP Jr (1973) Pancreaticoduodenal resection. Arch Surg 106:813

Barton RM, Copeland EM III (1983) Carcinoma of the ampulla of Vater. Surg Gynecol Obstet 156:297

Brooks JR (1983) Surgery of the pancreas. Saunders, Philadelphia

Brooks JR, Culebras JM (1976) Cancer of the pancreas, palliative operation, Whipple procedure, or total pancreatectomy? Am J Surg 131:516

Child III CG, Hinerman DL, Kauffman GL (1978) Pancreatoduodenectomy. Surg Gynecol Obstet 147:529

Collins JJ, Craighead JE, Brooks JR (1966) Rationale for total pancreatectomy for carcinoma of the pancreatic head. N Eng J Med 274:599

Forrest JF, Longmire WP Jr (1979) Carcinoma of the pancreas and periampullary region. Ann Surg 189:129

Fortner JG, Kim DK, Cubilla A, Turnbull A et al. (1977) Regional pancreatectomy: en bloc pancreatic, portal vein and lymph node resection. Ann Surg 186:42

Moosa AR, Lewis MH, Mackie CP (1979) Surgical treatment of pancreatic cancer. Mayo Clin Proc 54:468

ReMine WH (1978) Experience with total pancreatectomy for cancer. Am J Surg 135:186

Wilson SM, Block GE (1974) Periampullary carcinoma. Arch Surg 108:539

59 Partial Pancreatoduodenectomy (Whipple)

Indications

Carcinoma of ampulla

Periampullary and duodenal carcinoma

Periampullary and duodenal carcinoma

Carcinoma of the distal common bile duct (CBD)

Islet cell carcinoma of pancreatic head

Duct cell carcinoma of pancreatic head

Contraindications

Distant metastases (liver)

Distant lymph node metastases (celiac axis)

More than minimal invasion of portal vein, superior mesenteric vessels, or root of small bowel mesentery.

Absence of a surgical team experienced in pancreatoduodenectomy; when a patient suffering from obstructive jaundice has been found to have operable ampullary or pancreatic cancer, perform only a simple cholecystostomy and refer the patient elsewhere.

Preoperative Care

Correct hypoprothrombinemia with vitamin K.

Accomplish nutritional rehabilitation, if necessary.

If the patient's serum bilirubin exceeds 20 mg/dl, the operative mortality rate will be increased. In these cases, preoperative decompression of the biliary tract is advocated by some surgeons. The preferred method of accomplishing this is to have an experienced radiologist insert into the dilated hepatic ductal system a percutaneous drainage catheter (Denning, Ellison, and Carey). This catheter is attached to a drainage bag for a period of 2–3 weeks, during which the bilirubin level will recede. Norlander, Kalin, and Sunblad, after establishing preoperative percutaneous transhepatic drainage in 58 patients with jaundice due to cancer, doubted that this procedure benefited these patients. We are not convinced that preoperative biliary drainage should be performed in all patients whose serum bilirubin exceeds 20 mg/dl.

Perform diagnostic procedures as described below.

Prescribe perioperative antibiotics.

Pass nasogastric tube preoperatively.

Special Diagnostic Procedures in Obstructive Jaundice

After determining the liver chemistry profile in patients suspected of having obstructive jaundice, order a sonogram or CT scan of the pancreas and bile ducts. Sonography will generally reveal whether the bile ducts

161

are dilated, whether there are calculi in the gallbladder, and whether the head of the pancreas is enlarged. In the absence of calculi, if the CBD is enlarged down to its termination and there is no mass seen in the head of the pancreas, an endoscopic radiographic cholangiopancreatogram (ERCP) is indicated. This will often result in successful radiographic visualization of the CBD, and a tumor of the distal bile duct may be suspected by the appearance of this cholangiogram. ERCP will also permit direct observation of the ampulla, which can be biopsied if any abnormality of the ampulla is seen. If there is a periampullary tumor or ulceration, an endoscopic biopsy is the most direct route to a histological diagnosis. It is very helpful preoperatively to have a confirmed diagnosis of a primary carcinoma arising from the ampulla, from the periampullary duodenum, or from the distal CBD, because in these cases total pancreatectomy is not necessary and a Whipple operation can be planned. In tumors that arise from the pancreas, we prefer a total pancreatectomy, as discussed in Chap. 58.

If ERCP is not successful in delineating the cause of the obstructive jaundice, then performing a percutaneous transhepatic cholangiogram will provide an accurate road map of the entire system down to the point of obstruction. This radiographic procedure often differentiates successfully among biliary calculus, ampullary carcinoma, and carcinoma of the head of the pancreas. Occasionally the transhepatic cholangiogram will identify an intrahepatic carcinoma arising at the bifurcation of the left and right main hepatic ducts, or in one or the other hepatic ducts, thereby revealing information that markedly alters the operative plan.

Patients suspected of obstructive jaundice, who do not have enlarged ducts by sonography and in whom percutaneous transhepatic cholangiography is unsuccessful, may benefit from an ERCP, a percutaneous biopsy of the liver, or a CT scan.

Preoperative angiography is often performed prior to pancreatectomy, since it is helpful for the surgeon to know in advance if his patient has an anomalous hepatic artery that originates at the superior mesenteric artery. Lacking this information, the surgeon runs an increased risk of damaging the anomalous artery during the pancreatic dissection. Angiography of the celiac axis may reveal that the splenic artery and vein are completely encased by tumor, in which case it is very likely that the lesion is inoperable. In cases of this type, it may be desirable to biopsy the pancreas under radiographic control with a percutaneous needle. Cytological study of the needle aspirate is often diagnostic of cancer. This may obviate the need for surgery.

Pitfalls and Danger Points

Intraoperative hemorrhage

Trauma to or inadvertent ligation of superior mesenteric artery or vein, an anomalous hepatic artery, or the portal vein

Failure of pancreaticojejunal anastomosis with leakage

Failure of choledochojejunal anastomosis with leakage

Postoperative hemorrhage

Postoperative sepsis

Postoperative acute pancreatitis

Postoperative marginal ulcer with gastric bleeding

Operative Strategy

Avoiding and Managing Intraoperative Hemorrhage

The greatest risk of major intraoperative hemorrhage occurs when the surgeon is dissecting the portal vein away from the neck of the pancreas. This is especially true when an inexperienced pancreatic surgeon has misjudged the resectability of a carcinoma of the pancreas. In this case, while injudiciously trying to separate the portal vein from an invading carcinoma, he can produce a major laceration at a time when he has not yet achieved adequate exposure of the portal vein. Freeing the portal vein is the most dangerous step in this operation. Temporary control of hemorrhage is generally possible in this situation if the surgeon will compress the portal and superior mesenteric veins against the tumor by passing his left hand behind the head of the pancreas.

Next, an experienced assistant will have to divide the neck of the pancreas anterior and just to the left of the portal vein. In some cases, it will be necessary to isolate and temporarily occlude the splenic, the inferior mesenteric, the superior mesenteric, the coronary, and the portal veins in order to achieve proximal and distal control. If tumor has indeed invaded the portal vein, then a patch or a segment of vein may have to be excised, to be replaced by a saphenous vein patch or, in some cases, a vein graft. An end-to-end anastomosis of the portal to the superior mesenteric vein is possible when the segment to be resected is short. To replace longer segments of resected portal vein,

interpose a saphenous or internal jugular vein graft. Ligating the portal vein is often fatal unless the superior mesenteric vein is preserved and is free to drain *into the intact splenic, and then into the short gastric veins.* We know of no 5-year survivals in patients whose tumor has invaded the portal vein.

Avoiding Postoperative Hemorrhage

Braasch and Gray (1977) in a review of 279 Whipple operations noted that postoperative hemorrhage, either from the operative site or the gastrointestinal tract, occurred in 11% of their patients. Among patients who developed postoperative hemorrhage, 58% died. This complication must be regarded as preventable. Postoperative hemorrhage stems from one of the four following causes: (1) stress ulcer; (2) gastrointestinal marginal ulcer; (3) digestion of the retroperitoneal blood vessels by combined leakage of both bile and pancreatic juice; or (4) inadequate ligature of the innumerable blood vessels divided during surgery.

With respect to stress bleeding, it is important to treat the postoperative pancreatectomy patient with cimetidine or antacid therapy or both, so that the intragastric pH will not go below the level of 5.0. Frequent determinations of the gastric pH by aspirating the nasogastric tube will determine the dosage of antacid therapy required in each case. This is identical with the routine followed in an Intensive Care Unit for all surgical patients who are at risk of developing stress bleeding. Antacid therapy is very effective in preventing bleeding from stress ulcers.

To prevent a postoperative marginal ulcer, which follows the Whipple operation in 6% of cases (Grant and Van Heerdon), either perform a vagotomy plus antrectomy or remove at least 65%–75% of the stomach. Of these two methods, Scott, Dean, Parker, and Avant demonstrated the superiority of vagotomy in these cases.

163

Hemorrhage secondary to the digestion of retroperitoneal tissues by activated pancreatic juice is best prevented by observing the operative strategy (outlined below) aimed at preventing leakage from the pancreatic anastomosis.

Hemorrhage that results from a ligature slipping off the gastroduodenal or right gastric artery is a result of careless operative technique. During pancreatectomy, carefully skeletonize each of these two arteries prior to ligating them. Heavy nonabsorbable ligature material should be used and an *adequate stump of vessel must be left distal to the ligature* to prevent slipping. The same principles apply to the branches of the portal and superior mesenteric veins.

Avoiding Leakage from the Pancreaticojejunal Anastomosis

Failure of the pancreaticojejunal anastomosis has in our experience been the most common serious technical complication of pancreatoduodenectomy. As noted by Braasch and Gray (1977), failure of the anastomosis is more common (25%) in patients who have carcinoma of the distal portion of the CBD or of the duodenum because many of these patients do not develop obstruction of the pancreatic duct, which is frequently accompanied by some degree of pancreatitis. Both obstruction and pancreatitis produce thickening of the pancreatic duct and the pancreatic parenchyma. In the absence of this thickening, sewing a small thin-walled duct to the jejunum produces a high failure rate. Some authors (Child, Hinerman, and Kauffman) feel that invagination of the pancreatic stump into the end of jejunum may be superior to the mucosa-to-mucosa anastomosis. However, when the pancreatic parenchyma is soft, suturing it to the open end of jejunum may also be fraught with complications. When a small duct and a soft pancreatic parenchyma are encountered,

the surgeon should consider whether total pancreatectomy might not be the safest alternative, even though it will produce postoperative diabetes.

In cases of ampullary cancer, the pancreatic duct will enlarge and the pancreas itself will become somewhat fibrotic, both of which make an anastomosis more reliable. In addition, inserting a Silastic catheter into the pancreatic duct and bringing it into the jejunum and then out to the skin through a tiny jejunostomy opening will divert the pancreatic secretions to the outside. This will reduce the likelihood of postoperative leakage. Leave the catheter in place for 3 weeks. In performing the anastomosis, insert an outer layer of nonabsorbable sutures to firmly attach the pancreatic parenchyma to the serosa of jejunum. The inner layer consists of very fine sutures that attach the pancreatic duct to the full thickness of the jejunal wall. Although no conclusive data are available, it appears that this technique in cases with dilated pancreatic ducts, gives better results than invaginating the stump of the pancreas into the end of the jejunum.

If a leak of pancreatic juice does occur, it is important to have placed an adequate number of drains in the area of the anastomosis. Leakage of pure pancreatic juice, which has not been activated, will not damage the surrounding tissues, and the pancreatocutaneous fistula will generally close spontaneously without damaging the patient. On the other hand, if leakage from the pancreaticojejunostomy is accompanied by simultaneous seepage of bile into the same region, the pancreatic tryptic ferments become activated and begin to digest the surrounding retroperitoneal tissues. This produces sepsis and hemorrhage, complications that constitute the chief causes of death following pancreatoduodenectomy. Consequently, every attempt should be made to divert the flow of bile from the area of the pancreaticojejunostomy. This may help prevent the bile from refluxing up into the pancreaticojejunal anastomosis.

Treating a Pancreatic Fistula by Removing the Pancreatic Stump

When a patient suffers a pancreatocutaneous fistula that leaks clear pancreatic juice, only expectant therapy is necessary. If after a few days the clear, watery secretion turns green, indicating the admixture of bile with the pancreatic juice, the situation is much more serious. A major leak of bile and pancreatic juice carries with it a high mortality rate. If the patient's condition begins to deteriorate despite adequate drainage, serious consideration should be given to exploring the patient and removing the remnant of pancreas together with the spleen. Although Braasch and Gray (1977) state that such a procedure is extremely hazardous, we performed this procedure successfully on one occasion without much difficulty. Under certain conditions converting the Whipple operation into a total pancreatectomy can constitute a lifesaving operation.

Avoiding Postoperative Marginal Ulcer

As mentioned above, preventing a marginal ulcer following pancreatectomy requires the excision of 65%–75% of the stomach or the combination of vagotomy with antrectomy in order to reduce the gastric acid output. We prefer vagotomy and antrectomy, as do Scott and associates. Alternatively, preserving the antrum and the pylorus as described by Traverso and Longmire does not seem to cause a significant number of postoperative ulcers.

Avoiding Trauma to an Anomalous Hepatic Artery Arising from the Superior Mesenteric Artery

Braasch and Gray (1976) point out that in 20% of 200 cadaveric dissections performed by Michels, the superior mesenteric artery gave rise either to the common hepatic artery or to the right hepatic artery. In most cases, these anomalous hepatic arteries follow a course from the superior mesenteric artery posterior to the pancreas into the hepatoduodenal ligament. Proper anatomical dissection of the superior mesenteric vessels away from the superior uncinate process *with alert palpation of the posterior pancreas* by the surgeon will avoid traumatizing the anomalous hepatic artery. In 1% of the cases in the anatomical study, the common hepatic artery arose from the superior mesenteric and passed *through* the head of the pancreas on its way to the liver. In the 1% of patients in whom this anatomical condition exists, Braasch and Gray (1976) consider pancreatectomy contraindicated. Preoperative angiography to delineate the hepatic arterial supply will help the surgeon avoid injuring these anomalous vessels.

Operative Technique

Incision

Make a midline incision from the xiphoid to a point 10 cm below the umbilicus.

Evaluation of Pathology

If tissue has not been obtained preoperatively by gastroduodenoscopy for the positive histological diagnosis of cancer, then a further attempt should probably be made to biopsy the tumor at operation prior to proceeding with pancreatectomy. Divide the omentum between hemostats to ex-

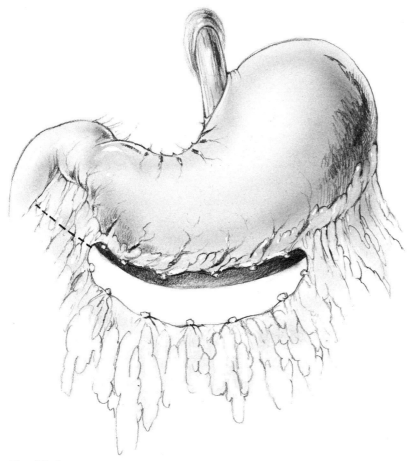

Fig. 59–1

pose the anterior surface of the pancreatic head **(Fig. 59–1)**. If a stony-hard area of tumor is visible either on the anterior or posterior surface of the pancreas, shave the surface of the tumor with a scalpel or remove a wedge of tissue. If the tumor appears to be deep, insert into the tumor a No. 22 needle on a 10 ml syringe containing 4–5 ml of air; aspirate; expel the sample on a sterile slide; spray the slide *promptly* with a fixation solution and submit the slide for immediate cytological study. In most cases we have found cytological examination of smears prepared after thin needle aspiration to be both safe and accurate. If this is not confirmatory for cancer, perform the biopsy with a Travenol Tru-cut needle. If possible, pass a Travenol needle through both walls of the duodenum on its way to the pancreas. This technique helps avoid a postoperative pancreatic fistula. When lesions of the distal common duct are suspected, obtain a tissue sample by passing a small curette through a cholodochotomy incision and scrape the region of the suspected malignancy. Choledochoscopy is an excellent means of obtaining a biopsy of common duct tumors. If a tumor is palpable in the region of the ampulla, make a longitudinal or oblique duodenotomy incision over the mass and excise a sample under direct vision. Close the duodenotomy in an everting fashion by applying Allis clamps and then the TA-55 stapling device. Discard all instruments that have come into contact with the tumor during the biopsy and redrape the field.

If preoperative X-ray visualization of the CBD has not been accomplished by transhepatic cholangiography or ERCP, a cholangiogram or choledochoscopy may

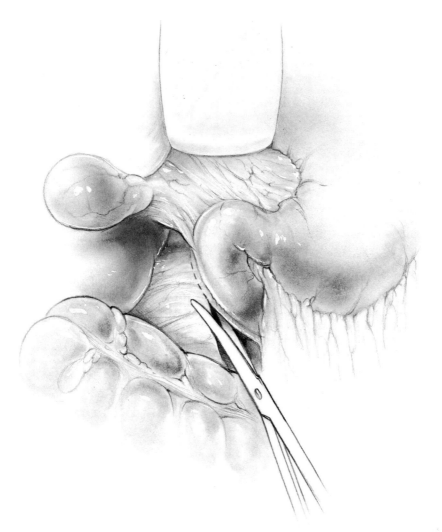

Fig. 59–2

be indicated to rule out an impacted common duct stone as the cause of the patient's jaundice.

Next, evaluate the lesion for operability. Check for metastatic involvement of the liver, of the root of the small bowel mesentery, and of the lymph nodes at the celiac axis. Metastasis to a lymph node along the gastrohepatic or the gastroduodenal artery adjacent to the malignancy does not contraindicate resection.

Invasion of the superior mesenteric or the portal vein is the most common contraindication to resection. Although it is possible to resect a small segment of these veins, and to replace it with a vein patch or a vein graft, the finding that the tumor invades these structures is a contraindication to pancreatectomy.

Determination of Resectability; Dissection of Portal and Superior Mesenteric Veins

Perform an extensive Kocher maneuver by incising the peritoneal attachment **(Fig. 59–2)** along the lateral portion of the descending duodenum. It is not always necessary to liberate the hepatic flexure of the

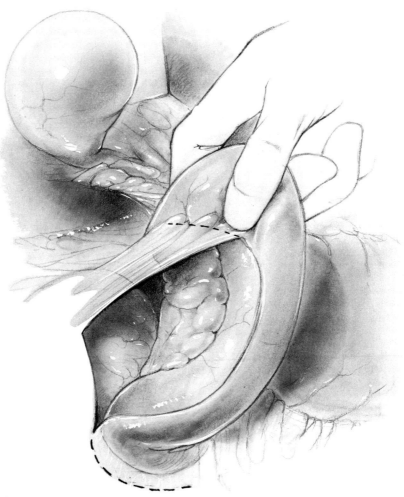

Fig. 59–3

colon to accomplish this maneuver. Insert the left index finger behind a lateral duodenal ligament which attaches the descending duodenum to the fascia of Gerota. Divide this ligament over the index finger and continue this line of dissection toward the third portion of the duodenum as far as the point where the superior mesenteric vein crosses the transverse duodenum **(Fig. 59–3).** Excessive upward traction on the duodenum and pancreas may tear the superior mesenteric vein; so caution is indicated. Continue liberating the duodenum superiorly as far as the foramen of Winslow.

If the head of the pancreas is replaced by a relatively bulky tumor, it would be difficult to expose the superior mesenteric vein. In such cases, after dividing the omentum to expose the anterior surface of the pancreas, identify the middle colic vein and trace it to its junction with the superior mesenteric vein **(Fig. 59–4).** Although this junction may be hidden from view by the neck of the pancreas, one can generally identify the superior mesenteric

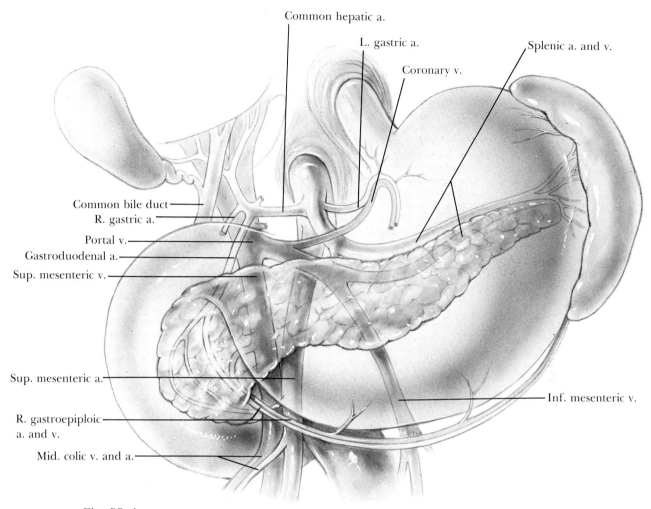

Common hepatic a.

L. gastric a.

Coronary v.

Splenic a. and v.

Common bile duct

R. gastric a.

Portal v.

Gastroduodenal a.

Sup. mesenteric v.

Sup. mesenteric a.

R. gastroepiploic
a. and v.

Mid. colic v. and a.

Inf. mesenteric v.

Fig. 59–4

vein without difficulty by following the middle colic vein. Gentle dissection is important in this area as there are often large fragile branches joining both the middle colic and the superior mesenteric veins with the inferior pancreaticoduodenal vein. If these branches are torn, control of bleeding behind the neck of the pancreas will be difficult.

In the course of this dissection, one can decide whether there is gross invasion of the vena cava or of the superior mesenteric vein, either of which contraindicates resection.

Identify the hepatic artery medial to the lesser curvature of the stomach after incising the filmy avascular portion of the gastrohepatic omentum. Incise the peritoneum overlying the common hepatic artery and sweep the lymph nodes toward the specimen. Continuing this dissection toward the patient's right will reveal the origin of the gastroduodenal artery. Dissect

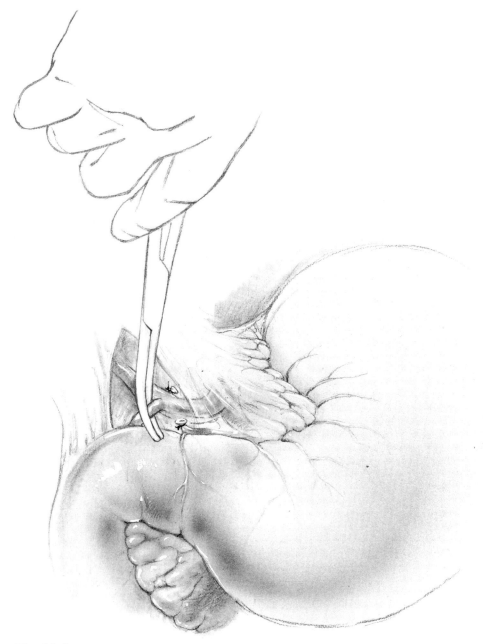

Fig. 59–5

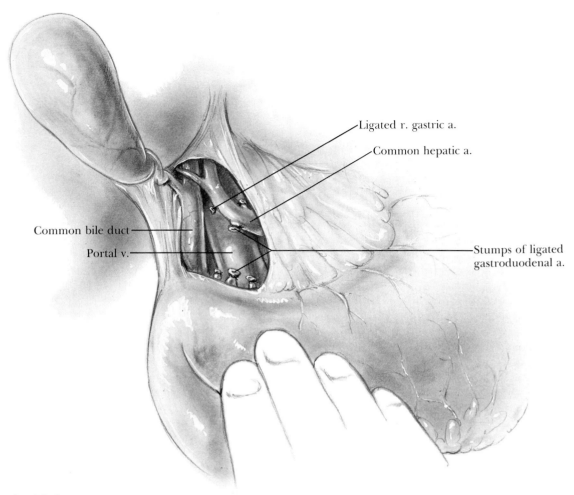

Ligated r. gastric a.

Common hepatic a.

Common bile duct

Portal v.

Stumps of ligated
gastroduodenal a.

Fig. 59–6

this artery free using a Mixter clamp **(Fig. 59–5)** and divide the vessel between two ligatures of 2–0 cotton, leaving about 1 cm beyond the proximal tie to prevent the possibility of the ligature slipping off. Continue the dissection just deep and slightly medial to the divided gastroduodenal artery and identify the anterior aspect of the portal vein **(Fig. 59–6).** In the presence of carcinoma near the head of the pancreas there are often numerous small veins superficial to the portal vein. *Do not use Hemoclips in this area* because they will inadvertently be wiped away during the subsequent dissection and manipulation. Each vessel should be divided and ligated with 3–0 or 4–0 cotton ligatures.

After identifying the shiny surface of the portal vein, gently free this vein from the overlying pancreas, using a peanut sponge dissector. If there is no invasion of the portal vein by tumor, there will be no attachment between the anterior wall of the portal vein and the overlying pancreas; thus a finger can be passed between this vein and the neck of the pancreas **(Fig.**

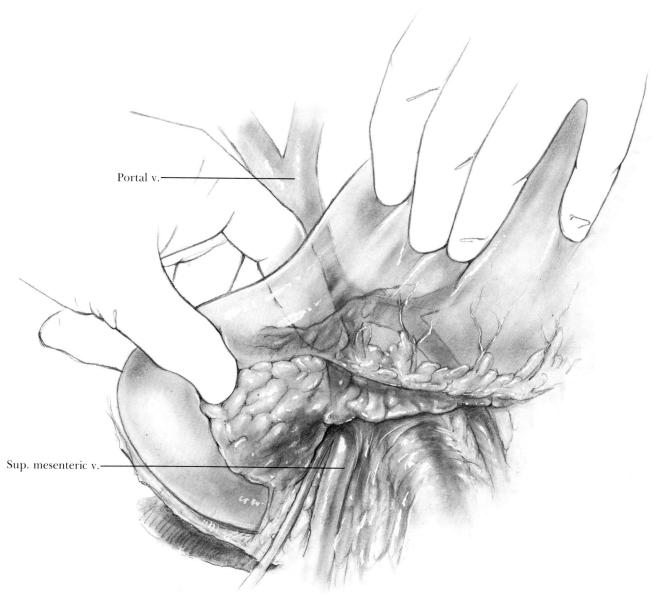

Portal v.—

Sup. mesenteric v.—

Fig. 59–7

59–7). Occasionally, this is easier to accomplish by inserting the finger from below the pancreas, between the superior mesenteric vein and the overlying gland. With one finger inserted between the neck of the pancreas and the superior mesenteric vein, pass the other hand behind the head of the pancreas and try to determine if the tumor has invaded the uncinate process, the posterior side of the portal vein, or the superior mesenteric vessels. If all of the above conditions have been fulfilled, the tumor is probably resectable, and one may proceed now with the pancreatectomy. Execute this dissection carefully since it is the most hazardous in the entire procedure. If the tumor has invaded the portal vein and the finger dissection produces a laceration of the vein, control of the hemorrhage will be extremely difficult. (See discussion above, in the section on Operative Strategy.)

Continue the dissection of the hepatic artery by dividing and ligating the right gastric artery. Incise the peritoneum over the common hepatic artery as far as the porta hepatis. Unroof and expose the CBD and sweep the lymphatic tissue from the porta hepatis down to the specimen, thereby skeletonizing the hepatic artery and CBD.

Cholecystectomy

(See Chap. 48.)

Identify the junction between the cystic and common bile ducts in preparation for a cholecystectomy. Identify, ligate, and divide the cystic artery. Then dissect the gallbladder from its attachment to the liver from above down. When the gallbladder is free and is attached only by the cystic duct, apply a 3–0 suture-ligature to the cystic duct and remove the gallbladder.

Encircle the common hepatic duct just proximal to the point where it is joined by the cystic duct. Apply an occluding temporary ligature or clamp to the hepatic duct and divide it distal to the ligature or clamp, sweeping lymphatic tissue toward the specimen.

Vagotomy and Gastrectomy

(See Chap. 10.)

With the lower portion of the sternum retracted upward and in a cephalad direction by means of either a "chain" or an Upper Hand retractor, expose the anterior surface of the abdominal esophagus. Using a Harrington or Weinberg retractor to elevate the left lobe of the liver, incise the peritoneum overlying the abdominal esophagus transversely. With a peanut sponge dissector separate the esophagus from the crura of the diaphragm. When this has been accomplished, encircle the abdominal esophagus with the index fin-

ger. Resect the anterior and posterior vagal trunks plus any other vagal branches that can be identified.

Palpate the left gastric artery along the lesser curvature of the stomach. Identify a point about halfway between the esophagus and pylorus. Insert a large hemostat between the vascular pedicle and the lesser curvature of the stomach. Doubly ligate the left gastric pedicle by using 2–0 cotton ligatures and divide these vessels, freeing the lesser curvature of the stomach. Now identify the gastroepiploic arcade on the greater curvature at a point approximately opposite the point of division of the left gastric vessels. Ligate and divide this arcade vessel. This will accomplish approximately a 50% gastrectomy. Divide the omentum outside the arcade toward the head of the pancreas.

Now apply the TA-90 stapling device across the body of the stomach and fire the staples (see Fig. 15–45). If the stomach wall is not thickened, use the 3.5 mm staples. Reapply the TA-90 device about 1 cm cephalad to this line of staples and fire again (see Fig. 15–46). Then transect the stomach flush with the stapling device and remove the TA-90. Observe the staple line for bleeding points. These can generally be controlled by electrocoagulation. Apply a sterile rubber glove over the antrum of the stomach in order to avoid contamination from the everted gastric mucosa. Fix the glove in place with an umbilical-tape ligature.

Division of Pancreas

In patients with periampullary or distal CBD tumors there may be no obstruction of the pancreatic duct. In these cases the pancreas may be quite soft in consistency and thus make a duct-to-jejunum anastomosis unsafe. In this case the surgeon may elect to perform a total pancreatectomy by the technique described in Chap. 60. If this option is not selected, place the line of division of the pancreas 3–5 cm to the left of the superior mesenteric vessels. This will leave a remnant of pancreatic tail, which is suitable for implanting into the open end of the jejunum when the pancreatic duct is too small for a good anastomosis. Leaving a small remnant of pancreas will reduce the exocrine secretion and thus reduce the risk of serious leakage; at the same time, there may be sufficient number of islet cells left to prevent diabetes. If this method is elected, carefully free the neck and the body of the pancreas from the underlying splenic vein by working from above and from below. A few small branches from the pancreas to the splenic vein must be divided.

After the neck and body of the pancreas have been elevated, apply a TA-55 stapler across the pancreas **(Fig. 59–8a)**. Use 3.5 mm staples in most cases. Fire the stapling device and divide the pancreas *to the left* of the stapling device **(Fig. 59–8b)**. Identify the pancreatic duct and insert a plastic catheter into the duct to prevent its being occluded by the serial mattress sutures of 4–0 Prolene, which are used to close the pancreatic parenchyma **(Fig. 59–9)**.

In patients, who have an ampullary carcinoma that obstructs the pancreatic duct, the thickened and dilated duct together with the secondary pancreatitis produced by this obstruction makes both the duct and the pancreas suitable for accurate suturing. In these cases, it is not necessary

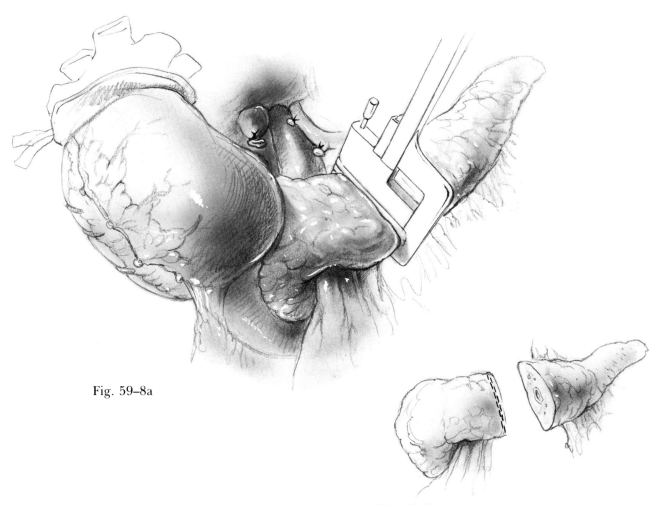

Fig. 59–8a

Fig. 59–8b

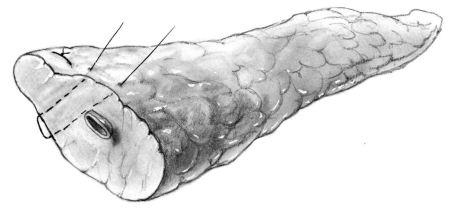

Fig. 59–9

to remove quite so large an amount of pancreas and the line of division may be at any point to the left of the superior mesenteric vein. The same technique of division is used. Generally, a suture-ligature will be necessary for a superior and for an inferior pancreatic artery in the pancreatic stump.

Dissection of Uncinate Process

Now retract the cut, stapled end of pancreas as well as the divided stomach towards the patient's right. This will expose the anterior surface of the superior mesenteric and portal veins **(Fig. 59–10).** Two or three arterial branches of the superior mesenteric artery pass deep to the superior mesenteric vein and into the head of the pancreas. These are generally easy to iden-

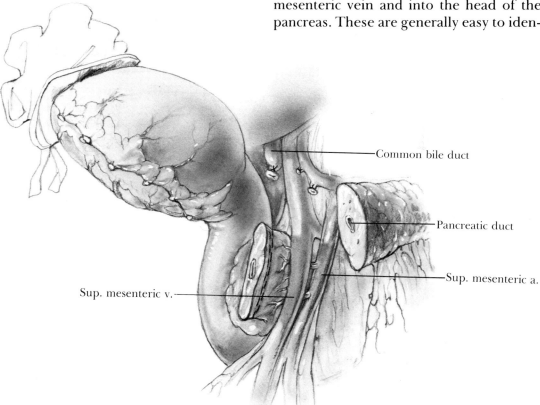

Common bile duct

Pancreatic duct

Sup. mesenteric a.

Sup. mesenteric v.

Fig. 59–10

tify. Divide and ligate each of them with 3–0 cotton. Several branches from the pancreas drain into the superior mesenteric vein from the patient's right. These are also divided and ligated. Thereupon the superior mesenteric vein may be gently retracted to the patient's left, revealing the superior mesenteric artery. The uncinate process may terminate at this point in some fibroareolar tissue, in which case this may be divided under direct vision. More often, a tongue of uncinate process is attached to the posterior surface of the superior mesenteric artery. First pass the left hand behind the uncinate process *to check again that there is no major anomalous hepatic artery* coming from the superior mesenteric. Then, serially apply large Hemoclips to the remnant of the uncinate process along the superior mesenteric artery and divide the uncinate process along the Hemoclips **(Figs. 59–11 and 59–12).** Instead of Hemoclips, one may serially clamp, ligate, and divide the uncinate process. Another convenient method is to apply a TA-55 stapler across the uncinate process prior to dividing it; this will achieve hemostasis if 3.5 mm staples are used. Be certain to avoid injuring the superior mesenteric vein and artery. At the end of this dissection the

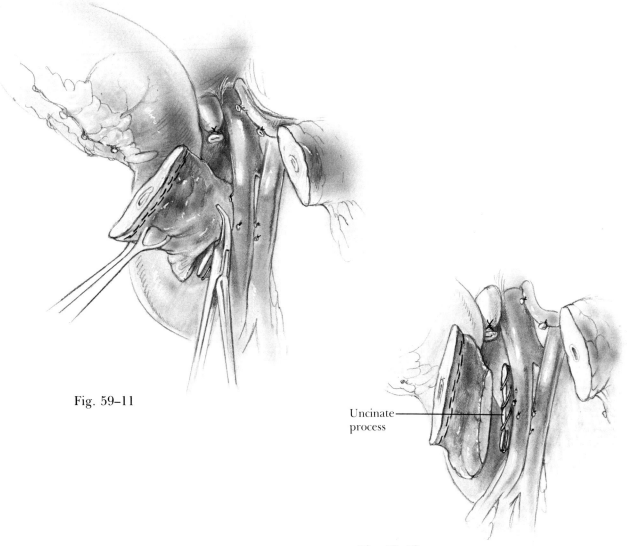

Fig. 59–11

Uncinate process

Fig. 59–12

gastric antrum, the duodenum, and the head of the pancreas will be attached only at the duodenojejunal junction **(Fig. 59–13)**.

It is possible to save 10–12 minutes of operating time by applying a GIA stapler across the fourth portion of duodenum and by dividing the duodenum, thereby releasing the specimen from all of its attachments. This will leave both the proximal and distal segments of divided duodenum closed by means of staples. This method avoids the necessity of dividing the proximal jejunal mesentery and of freeing the duodenojejunal junction from the ligament of Treitz. The stomach, hepatic duct, and pancreas can each then be anastomosed end-to-side to the jejunum. Most surgeons do free the duodenojejunal junction from the ligament of Treitz, divide the mesentery in this region, and divide the jejunum a few centimeters beyond the ligament of Treitz. This procedure is described in the next paragraph.

Dissection and Division of Proximal Jejunum

Expose the ligament of Treitz under the transverse mesocolon and divide it so that the duodenojejunal junction is completely free. Pass the proximal 6–8 cm of jejunum behind the ligament of Treitz into the supramesocolic space. Then serially clamp, divide, and ligate each of the mesenteric branches from the superior mesenteric vessel to the proximal 6–8 cm of the jejunum. This will release the proximal jejunum. Unless it is planned to implant the pancreatic tail into the open end of jejunum, apply a TA-55 stapling device across the proximal jejunum and fire the staples (3.5 mm). Then, using a scalpel, divide the jejunum flush with the stapler. Lightly electrocoagulate the everted mucosa and remove the stapling device. It is not necessary to invert this staple line with a row of sutures. Remove the specimen.

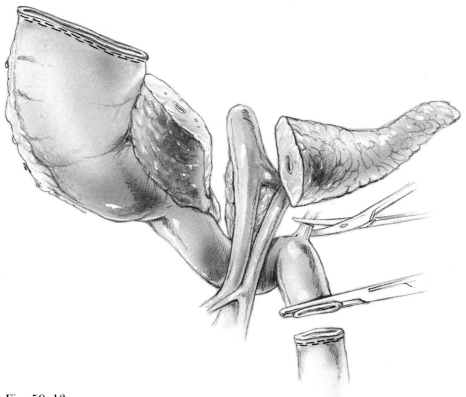

Fig. 59–13

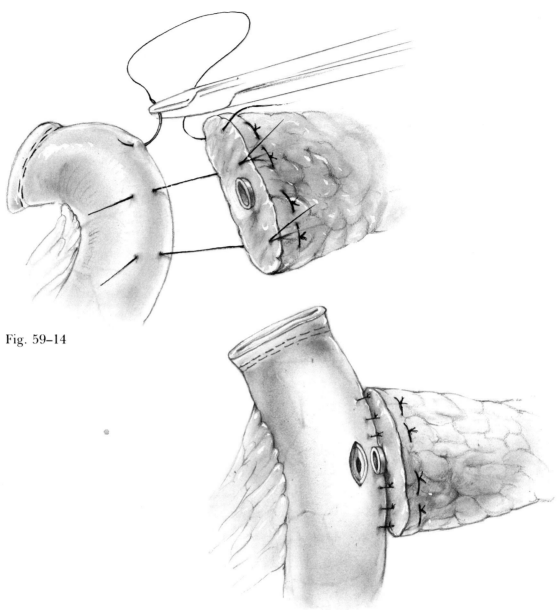

Fig. 59–14

Fig. 59–15

Pancreaticojejunal Anastomosis

Pass 12–15 cm of proximal jejunum through the aperture in the transverse mesocolon. Construct an end-to-side pancreaticojejunostomy along the antimesenteric aspect of the jejunum, beginning at a point about 3 cm from the staple line. Use interrupted 4–0 Prolene to suture the posterior capsule of the pancreas to the seromuscular layer of jejunum (**Fig. 59–14**). Then make a small incision slightly larger than the diameter of the pancreatic duct (**Fig. 59–15**). Approximate the pancreatic duct to the full thickness of the jejunal wall using interrupted 6–0 Prolene sutures (**Fig. 59–16**). Wearing telescopic lenses with a 2½ × magnification is helpful in assuring an accurate anastomosis. After the posterior half of this anastomosis has been completed, insert a Silastic plastic

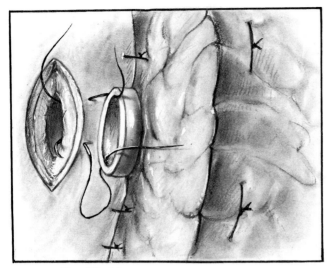

Fig. 59–16

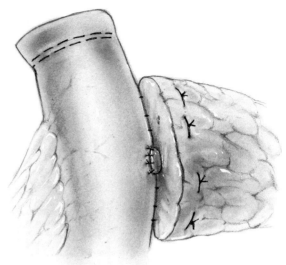

Fig. 59–17

catheter into the pancreatic duct. Cut several side holes near the tip of the catheter. Thread the long end of the catheter into the jejunum. Make no holes in the catheter on the jejunal side of the anastomosis. The catheter will be brought out from the jejunum about 10–15 cm beyond this anastomosis and passed through a stab wound in the abdominal wall for drainage to the outside. Then complete the duct-to-jejunum anastomosis with 6–0 Prolene sutures **(Fig. 59–17)**. Carefully buttress the remainder of the pancreas into the anterior wall of jejunum with additional 4–0 sutures **(Fig. 59–18)**. It is important to suture the Silastic catheter to the pancreas by means of a single 5–0 PG stitch; otherwise it is easily dislodged during subsequent steps of the operation. Also suture the jejunostomy site to the stab wound of the abdominal wall.

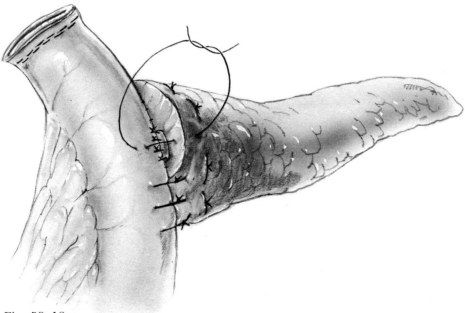

Fig. 59–18

179

An alternative method of anastomosing pancreas to jejunum is to pass 2–3 cm of the pancreatic stump into the lumen. First insert a Silastic catheter into the pancreatic duct as described above. Suture the catheter into the duct with fine Vicryl. Pass 2–3 cm of the pancreatic stump into the open proximal end of the jejunum. Suture it in place with one layer of interrupted 4–0 Prolene Lembert sutures to attach the end of the jejunum to the capsule of the pancreas (**Fig. 59–19).**

Other surgeons prefer to invaginate the jejunum by sewing the pancreas in place with two layers of interrupted sutures (**Fig. 59–20).** Then bring the catheter out through a puncture wound in the jejunum and then out through the abdominal wall.

Hepaticojejunal Anastomosis

Before anastomosing the hepatic duct to jejunum, make a tiny stab wound in the anterior wall of the hepatic duct about 3 cm proximal to its cut end. Insert a Mixter clamp into the hepatic duct through the stab wound. Grasp the *long arm* of a 16F or 18F T-tube (**Fig. 59–21).** and draw it through the stab wound (**Fig. 59–22).** The purpose of this T-tube is to drain bile to the outside until the pancreaticojejunostomy has healed completely.

Then make an incision on the antimesenteric border of the jejunum (**Fig. 59–23).** about 15–20 cm distal to the pancreaticojejunostomy. The jejunal incision should

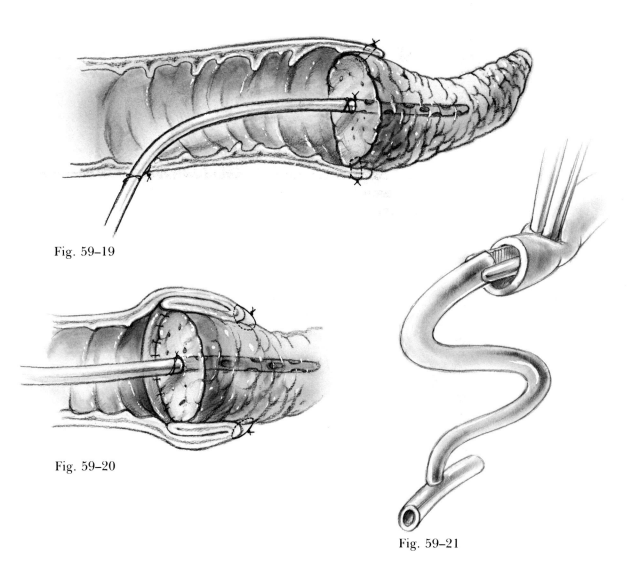

Fig. 59–19

Fig. 59–20

Fig. 59–21

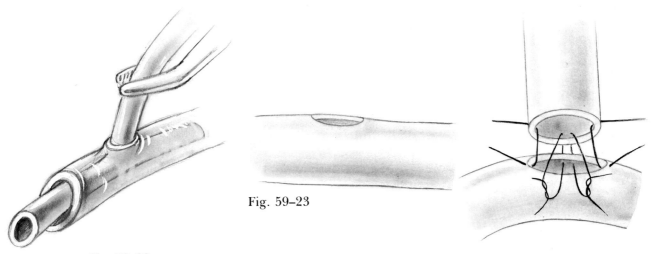

Fig. 59–22

Fig. 59–23

Fig. 59–24

be approximately equal to the diameter of the hepatic duct. Use one layer of interrupted 5–0 Vicryl sutures to approximate the full thickness of hepatic duct to the full thickness of jejunum **(Fig. 59–24).** Tie the knots of the posterior layer of sutures in the lumen. The anterior knots are placed on the serosal surface of the hepaticojejunal anastomosis. On the jejunal side of the anterior layer a "seromucosal" type of stitch (see Vol. I, Fig. B–16) may be used. Leave only 3–4 mm of space between sutures **(Fig. 59–25).** We have not found it

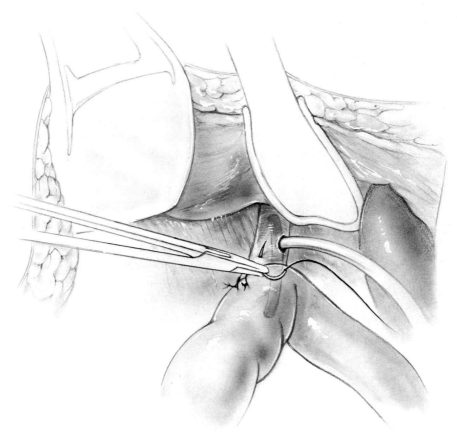

Fig. 59–25

181

necessary to insert two layers of sutures. If the diameter of the hepatic duct is small, enlarge the ductal orifice by making a small Cheatle incision in the anterior wall of the duct.

Gastrojejunostomy

Identify the proximal jejunum, and bring it to the gastric pouch in an antecolonic fashion. Place the antimesenteric border of jejunum in apposition with the posterior wall of the residual gastric pouch for the

gastrojejunal anastomosis. Leave 10–20 cm between the hepaticojejunostomy and the gastric anastomosis. Insert a guy stitch approximating the antimesenteric wall of the jejunum to the greater curvature of the stomach at a point about 3 cm proximal to the previously placed TA-90 staple line. Then, with the electrocautery make small stab wounds in the posterior wall of the

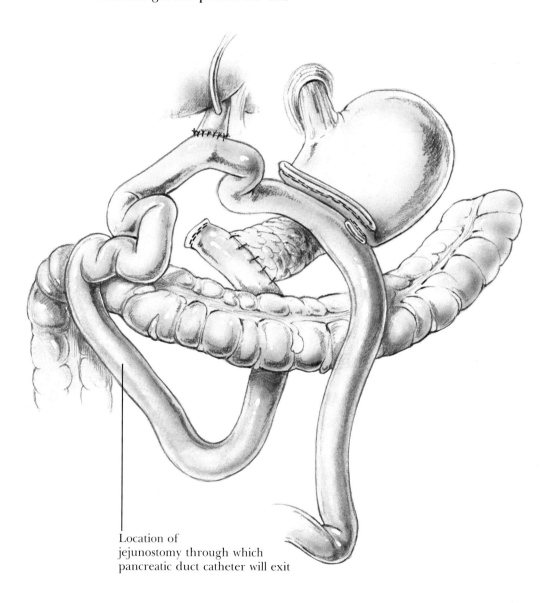

Location of
jejunostomy through which
pancreatic duct catheter will exit

Fig. 59–26

stomach and in the jejunum. Now insert the GIA device, one fork into the gastric lumen and one into the jejunum (see Fig. 15–47). Be certain that there is no extraneous tissue between the walls of the stomach and jejunum. After locking the GIA stapling device, insert a single Lembert stitch to approximate stomach and jejunum at the tip of the GIA. Then, fire the GIA and remove it. Carefully inspect the staple line for bleeding which should be corrected either by cautious electrocoagulation or the insertion of 4–0 PG sutures. Apply Allis clamps to the anterior and posterior terminations of the staple line. Use additional Allis clamps to close the remaining aperture in the gastrojejunal anastomosis.

Apply a TA-55 stapler deep to the line of Allis clamps and fire the staples. (The details of this technique are described in Chap. 15.)

Close the defect in the mesocolon at the region of Treitz's ligament by means of continuous and interrupted sutures of 4–0 PG around the jejunum and its mesentery. Try to isolate the hepaticojejunal anastomosis from the pancreatic anastomosis by suturing the free edge of the omentum to the remaining hepatoduodenal ligament overlying the hepatic duct.

Intermittently during the entire operation, a dilute antibiotic solution is used for irrigating the operative field. **Fig. 59–26** illustrates the completed operation.

Insertion of Drains

Insert a latex drain through a stab wound in the right upper quadrant down to the vicinity of the hepaticojejunostomy. Allow the T-tube to exit through the same stab wound in the right upper quadrant.

Next, bring the pancreatic catheter through a tiny stab wound in the anti-mesenteric wall of the jejunum about 10–15 cm distal to the pancreatic anastomosis. Place a 3–0 cotton purse-string suture around this tiny stab wound. Then make a stab wound in the appropriate portion of the abdominal wall, generally in the right upper quadrant; bring the catheter through this stab wound. Now fix the jejunum to the abdominal wall around the catheter's exit point, using four sutures of interrupted 3–0 PG, one suture to each quadrant. This will prevent intraperitoneal leakage of jejunal content. Connect this catheter to a plastic collecting bag. Alternatively, bring the Silastic catheter through a stab wound in the *proximal* jejunum as depicted in Fig. 59–27.

Through a stab wound in the left upper quadrant, insert a latex and a sump or closed-suction drain to the posterior abdominal cavity in the vicinity of the pancreaticojejunostomy and subhepatic spaces.

Closure

Close the abdominal wall using 1 PDS sutures in the fashion described in Chap. 5.

Operative Technique: Partial Pancreatoduodenectomy with Preservation of Stomach and Pylorus

Concept: When to Preserve the Pylorus

Traverso and Longmire introduced the concept of preserving the pylorus following pancreatoduodenectomy, especially for benign conditions like chronic pancreatitis. We and others (Newman, Braasch, Rossi, and O'Campo-Gonzales) have used this modification of the pancreatoduodenectomy for patients with cancers localized to the ampulla, periampullary duodenum, and the distal CBD. If preservation of the pylorus with its intact vagal innervation is successful, it will avoid the necessity for gastric resection and vagotomy, maintain normal gastric emptying, and eliminate the gamut of postgastrectomy malfunctions.

Following the usual partial or total pancreatoduodenectomy, marginal ulcer may occur unless vagotomy and gastric resection are performed (Scott and associates). It is not yet clear from the data available, whether or not a peptic ulcer will follow partial pancreatoduodenectomy with preservation of the pylorus. By removing the head and neck of the pancreas, a por-

tion of the alkaline pancreatic secretion is eliminated from the intestinal tract. This reduces the buffering capacity of the secretions in the upper intestinal tract and lessens its resistance to peptic ulceration. Reports of early results (Newman et al.) have so far proved favorable but the period of followup observation has been short. Our results in 10 cases have also been favorable.

Whether the survival rate following preservation of the pylorus will be reduced is also an unanswered question. If there is metastatic spread to the subpyloric or the right gastroepiploic lymph nodes, this procedure is contraindicated. It is also contraindicated for carcinoma located in the proximal duodenum. Actually, preserving the proximal 2 cm of duodenum and the left gastroepiploic arcade along the greater curvature of the antrum does not limit resection of the lymph nodes that drain tumors of the ampullary region.

Pitfalls and Danger Points

Same as those mentioned above for the Whipple pancreatoduodenectomy, plus the possibility of inadequate blood supply to the duodenum

Operative Strategy

The important parts of this operation are identical with the Whipple pancreatoduodenectomy except that the pylorus and 2 cm of duodenum as well as all of the vagus nerve branches are preserved. In the hope of reducing the risk of marginal ulceration, we place the duodenojejunal anastomosis closer to the biliary and pancreaticojejunal anastomoses than is the case with the Whipple operation.

Also illustrated in this operative description is a method of bringing the pancreatic catheter to the abdominal wall through a tiny stab wound near the closed proximal end of the jejunal segment (Fig. 59–27). This has the important advantage that the length of the catheter between the pancreatic duct and the abdominal wall is much less than that described under the technique of the Whipple operation (above).

Technique: Modifications for Preserving the Pylorus with Partial Pancreatoduodenectomy

The operative technique used in partial pancreatoduodenectomy with preservation of the pylorus is the same as that described above for the Whipple operation, with the following exceptions:

Do not perform a vagotomy.

Dissect the posterior wall of the duodenum off the head of the pancreas for distance of 2.5 cm after dividing and ligating the gastroduodenal and the right gastric arteries as described above.

Apply the GIA stapling device to the duodenum at a point about 2.5 cm distal to the pylorus. Fire the stapling device. This will transect the duodenum and apply a stapled closure to both the proximal and distal ends of the divided duodenum.

Be careful to avoid injuring the gastroepiploic arcade in the greater omentum along the greater curvature of the stomach, since much of the blood supply to the proximal duodenum will be coming from the intact left gastroepiploic artery down to the pylorus. Beyond this point the duodenum will be fed by the intramural circulation. Additional blood supply comes from the left gastric artery along the lesser curve of the stomach.

Anastomose the end of the duodenum to the antimesenteric side of the jejunum at a point about 20 cm distal to the hepaticojejunal anastomosis. The jejunum should be brought directly from the hepaticojejunostomy to the duodenum for an end-to-side duodenojejunal anastomosis in the supramesocolic space.

The first step in preparing for the anastomosis is to apply several Allis clamps to the line of staples closing the duodenum. Then excise the staple line with a scissors, leaving the duodenum wide open. Observe the cut duodenum for adequacy of bleeding. Although pulsatile flow is not generally seen and the duodenum may be somewhat cyanotic, a fairly brisk ooze of red blood is an indication of satisfactory circulation.

Do not place the anastomosis too close to the pylorus because the close proximity of the suture line to the pylorus will interfere with pyloric function and result in gastric retention. Insert a layer of 4–0 interrupted cotton Lembert sutures to approximate the posterior seromuscular coat of the duodenum to the antimesenteric border of the jejunum. After this has been done, make an incision in the antimesenteric border of the jejunum. Obtain hemostasis with absorbable sutures or electrocoagulation. Then begin the mucosal layer. Use 5–0 atraumatic Vicryl suture material and place the first stitch in the middle of the posterior layer of the anastomosis. Run a continuous locked stitch from this point to the left-hand termination of the posterior layer. Take relatively small bites through the full thickness of duodenum and jejunum. If the bites are small, the continuous suture will not act as a purse string to narrow the anastomosis.

Insert a second 5–0 Vicryl suture adjacent to the first one at the midpoint of the posterior layer. Run this stitch in a continuous locked fashion towards the patient's right. Accomplish closure of the first ante-

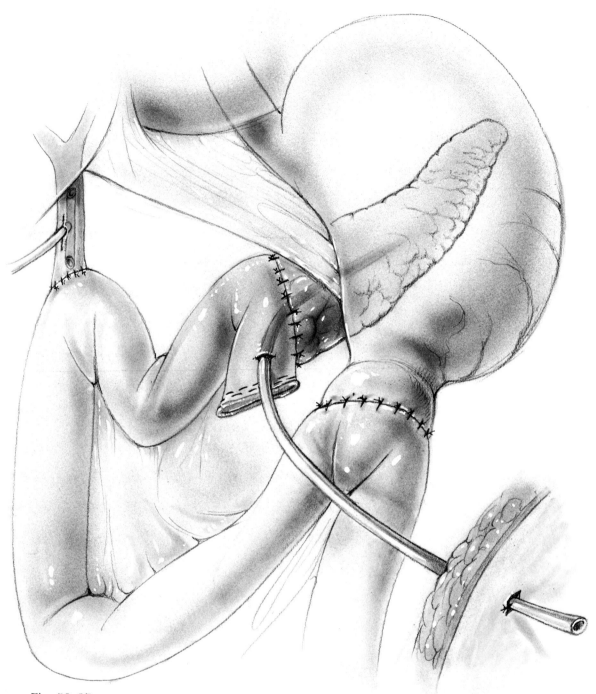

Fig. 59–27

rior layer of the anastomosis by using the same 5–0 Vicryl stitch either as a Connell, a Cushing, or a "seromucosal" stitch. Terminate this layer by tying the ends of the two continuous Vicryl sutures to each other in the middle of the anterior layer. Complete the anterior layer of the anastomosis by inserting interrupted 4–0 cotton Lembert seromuscular sutures.

Fig. 59–27 illustrates the method of draining the pancreatic duct. Insert the Silastic catheter (e.g., the small round Jackson-Pratt catheter) into the pancreatic duct after completing the posterior layers of the pancreaticojejunostomy. Suture the catheter to the pancreas with a 5–0 PG stitch. Then bring it through a puncture wound in the proximal jejunum. Close the jejunal puncture wound around the catheter with a 4–0 cotton suture. Then bring the catheter through a puncture wound of the abdominal wall to the left of the midline incision. Transfix the catheter to the skin with a suture. In most cases it will be possible to suture the jejunum to the parietal peritoneum around the puncture wound through which the catheter exits.

Complications of Pancreatectomy with Stomach and Pylorus Preservation

Delayed Gastric Emptying
This complication will occur if the duodenojejunal suture line abuts the pyloric sphincter muscle and thus interferes with the sphincter's proper functioning.

Pyloroduodenal Ulcer
Superficial ulceration may follow impairment of the duodenal blood supply.

Peptic ulcer of the duodenum or jejunum may occur if the gastric pH following the operation is permitted to fall below 4–5. With the bile diverted into the T-tube and all the pancreatic juice draining to the outside via the pancreatic duct catheter, one of our patients developed a gastric pH of 1 postoperatively while receiving cimetidine 100 mg per hour intravenously. The patient bled from a superficial pyloroduodenal ulcer that healed when the pancreatic secretions were injected into the nasogastric tube together with antacids. In the early postoperative period it is important to administer cimetidine and antacids and to refeed the pancreatic juice.

Postoperative Care

Perioperative antibiotics, which were initiated prior to the operation, are repeated by the intravenous route every 2 or 3 hours during the procedure and then every 6 hours for four doses postoperatively.

Administer cimetidine parenterally. Test the intragastric pH on the sample of gastric juice aspirated through the nasogastric tube every 2 hours. Administer additional dosages of antacid, if necessary, in doses sufficient to keep the pH at or above the level of 5.0.

Intravenous fluids should be administered in sufficient quantities to assure normal urine output. In older patients, it is extremely helpful to have the guidance of pulmonary artery wedge pressures and sometimes of cardiac output determinations. Some of our patients have required 8 or more liters of isotonic fluid on the day of operation to maintain cardiovascular homeostasis even in the absence of significant blood loss. Since this is an extensive operation, one can expect considerable sequestration of fluids into the "third space." By the 3rd postoperative day there is frequently a brisk diuresis, at which time intravenous fluids should be limited in volume.

Oral feeding should be interdicted for 7 days in order to give the biliary and pancreatic anastomoses time to heal. Patients who have lost as much as 10–15 pounds in weight prior to operation, should have total parenteral nutrition.

Both the T-tube and the pancreatic catheter are left in place for 21 days. If there has been no drainage of pancreatic juice or bile by the 7th or 8th day, the latex drains may be mobilized and gradually removed. Remove the sump drain on day 8–10 unless significant amounts of fluid are being aspirated.

If a clear, watery secretion drains from the operative site, this represents a pancreatocutaneous fistula, which will probably heal with the passage of time. If this leak of pancreatic

187

juice becomes complicated by the admixture of bile and pus, the tryptic enzymes become activated and start digesting the tissues in the vicinity of the anastomosis. This complication can be serious and even fatal. Initially, attempt conservative therapy by continuous irrigation of the anastomotic site through the sump catheter using sterile saline containing appropriate dilute antibiotics. A dosage of 1–2 liters per day seems appropriate. If, despite this management, the patient's-condition continues to deteriorate, relaparotomy for removal of the remaining tail of pancreas together with the spleen may prove lifesaving.

Postoperative Complications

Leakage from pancreatic anastomosis

Leakage from biliary anastomosis

Postoperative sepsis

Postoperative hemorrhage. In our experience both sepsis and hemorrhage are most often the result of leakage from the pancreaticojejunal anastomosis. In some cases this may be due to the development of acute pancreatitis in the pancreatic tail. As discussed above, the only solution to this vicious cycle, in some cases is surgical removal of the residual pancreas.

Postoperative gastric bleeding. If the gastric pH is kept elevated by antacid therapy, bleeding from stress ulceration is extremely rare.

Thrombosis of the superior mesenteric artery or vein. Although we have never encountered this complication, thrombosis can occur. It can be prevented by dissecting these two vital structures with care and precision.

Hepatic failure

Gastric bezoar. We have had two patients who developed gastric phytobezoars following pancreatoduodenectomy with vagotomy. Both were treated with gastric lavage and with medication, which included papain and cellulase, with satisfactory results.

References

Braasch JW, Gray BN (1976) Technique of radical pancreatoduodenectomy. Surg Clin N Amer 56:631

Braasch JW, Gray BN (1977) Considerations that lower pancreatoduodenectomy mortality. Am J Surg 133:480

Child CG III, Hinerman DL, Kauffman GL (1978) Pancreatoduodenectomy. Surg Gynecol Obstet 147:529

Denning D, Ellison C, Carey L (1981) Postoperative percutaneous transhepatic biliary decompression lowers operative morbidity in patients with obstructive jaundice. Am J Surg 141:61

Grant CS, Van Heerdon JA (1979) Anastomotic ulceration following subtotal and total pancreatectomy. Ann Surg 190:1

Newman KD, Braasch JW, Rossi RL, O'Campo-Gonzales (1983) Pyloric and gastric preservation with pancreatoduodenectomy. Am J Surg 145:152

Norlander A, Kalin B, Sunblad R (1982) Effect of percutaneous transhepatic drainage upon liver function and postoperative mortality. Surg Gynecol Obstet 155:161

Scott HW Jr, Dean RH, Parker T, Avant G (1980) The role of vagotomy in pancreaticoduodenectomy. Ann Surg 191:688

Traverso LW, Longmire WP Jr (1980) Preservation of the pylorus in pancreaticoduodenectomy: a follow-up evaluation. Ann Surg 192:306

60 Total Pancreatoduodenectomy

Indications

Duct cell carcinoma of pancreas

Contraindications

Distant metastases

Absence of an experienced surgical team

Patient who lacks alertness and intelligence to manage diabetes

Invasion of portal or superior mesenteric vein

Preoperative Care

(See Chap. 59.)

Pitfalls and Danger Points

Operative or postoperative hemorrhage

Trauma to superior mesenteric artery and vein, or to anomalous right hepatic artery

Devascularization of omentum and possibly stomach

Operative Strategy

In addition to the points discussed concerning the operative strategy of the Whipple operation (Chap. 59), remember that division of both the gastroduodenal and the splenic arteries results in complete devascularization of the omentum unless special effort is exerted to preserve the left gastroepoploic artery. Complete omentectomy is generally performed as part of a total pancreatectomy.

Also remember that division of the splenic artery, the short gastric, the right gastric, and the gastroduodenal arteries leaves the gastric pouch dependent on the left gastric artery for its blood supply. For this reason, do not divide the left gastric artery at its point of origin from the celiac axis. Rather, it should be divided along the lesser curvature distal to the point where the branches to the proximal stomach and esophagus arise.

Operative Technique

Incision

Except for very stocky patients, we use a long midline incision from the xiphoid to a point 10 cm below the umbilicus, as described in Chap. 5.

Evaluation of Pathology; Kocher Maneuver

The technique followed here is identical with that shown in Figs. 59–2 and 59–3.

Determination of Resectability; Dissection of Portal and Superior Mesenteric Veins

This technique is identical with that described in Figs. 59–4 to 59–7, except that

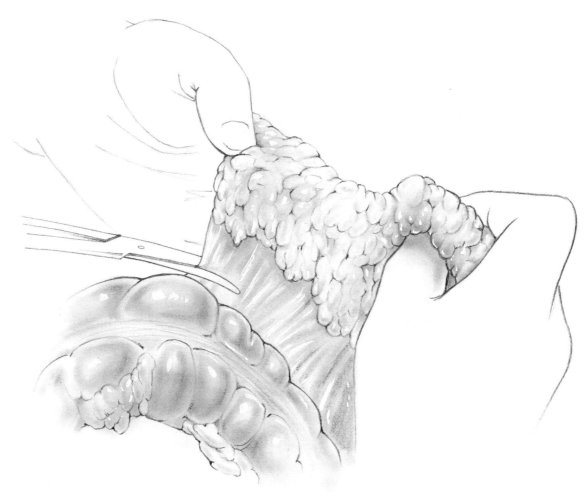

Fig. 60–1

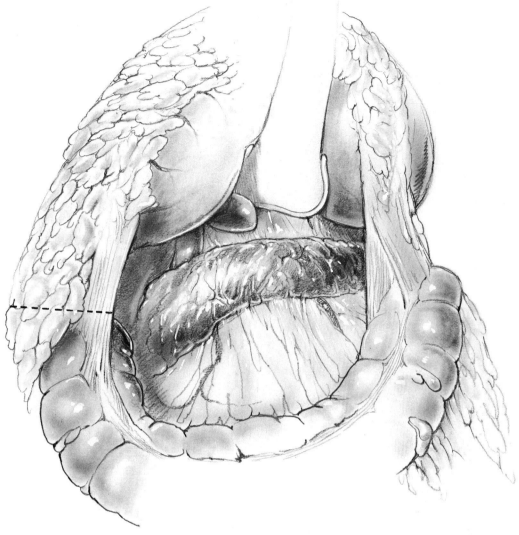

Fig. 60–2

instead of dividing the omentum between clamps, detach the omentum from the transverse colon so that it may be removed with the specimen **(Figs. 60–1 and 60–2).**

Splenectomy and Truncal Vagotomy

With the stomach and omentum retracted in a cephalad direction, identify the splenic artery along the superior surface of the

pancreas. Open the peritoneum over the splenic artery at a point 1–2 cm distal to its origin at the celiac axis. With a right-angled Mixter clamp, free the posterior surface of the artery and apply a 2–0 cotton

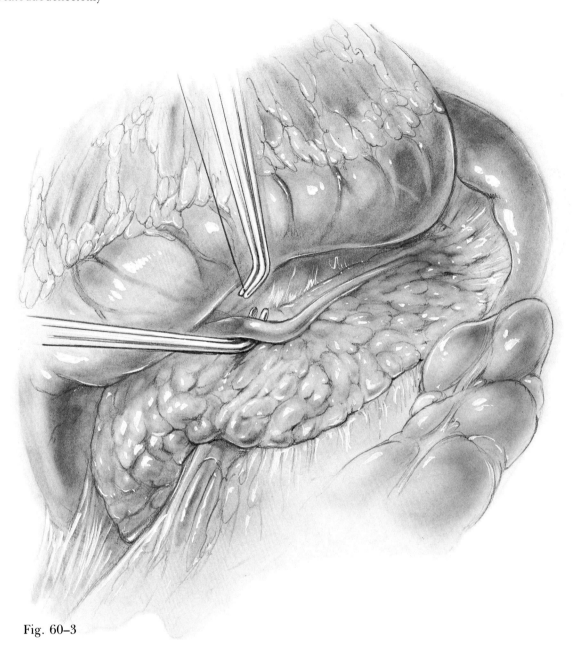

Fig. 60–3

ligature **(Fig. 60–3).** Ligate the vessel but do not divide it at this point in the operation.

Then apply a chain retractor to the left costal margin in order to improve the exposure of the spleen. Make an incision in the avascular lienophrenic fold of the peritoneum **(Figs. 60–4a and 60–4b).** Electrocoagulate any bleeding vessels. Elevate the tail of the pancreas together with the spleen. Divide the attachments between the lower pole of the spleen and the colon. Expose the posterior surface of the spleen and identify the splenic artery and veins at this point. If there is any bleeding, ligate these vessels.

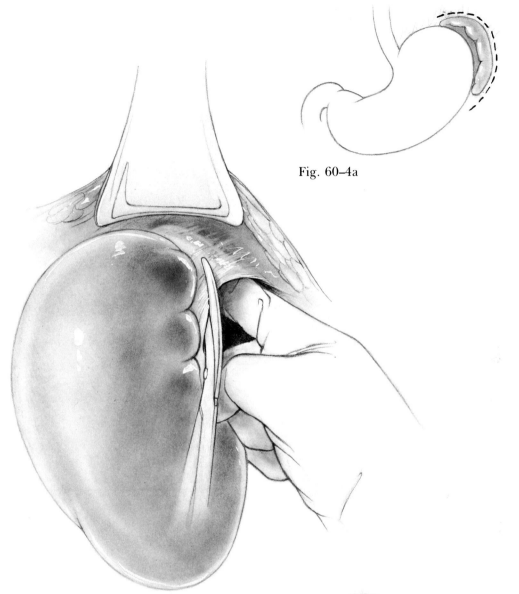

Fig. 60–4a

Fig. 60–4b

Insert moist gauze pads into the bed of the elevated spleen.

At this time remove the chain retractor from the left costal margin and place it in the region of the sternum. Apply traction with the chain in a cephalad and anterior direction, exposing the abdominal esophagus. Incise the peritoneum over the abdominal esophagus. Use a peanut-gauze dissector to separate the crus of the diaphragm from the esophagus (**Fig. 60–5**) and perform a truncal vagotomy as described in Vol. I, Chap. 10.

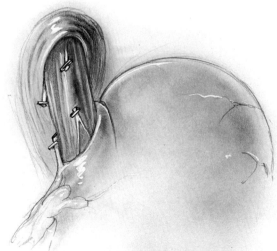

Fig. 60–5

193

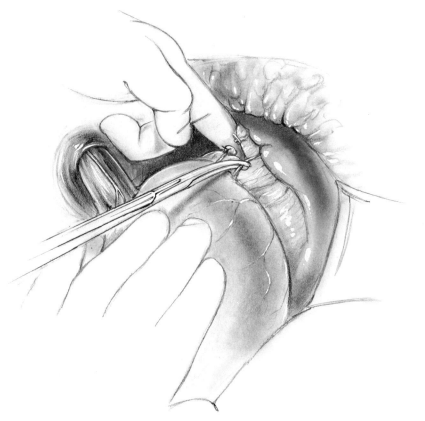

Fig. 60–6

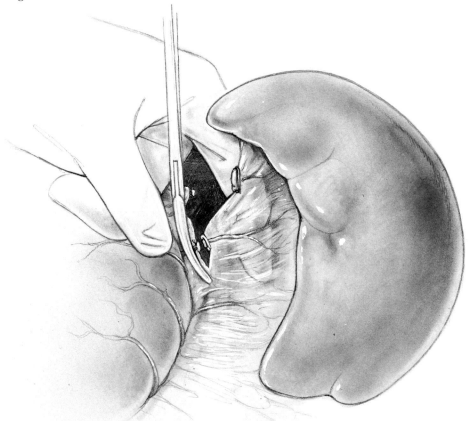

Fig. 60–7

Mobilizing the Distal Pancreas

Now identify the proximal short gastric vessel. Insert the left index finger beneath the gastrophrenic ligament. Apply a Hemoclip to the distal portion of the vessel. Ligate the gastric side of the vessel with 2–0 or 3–0 cotton and divide it **(Fig. 60–6)**. Continue the dissection in this manner until all of the short gastric vessels have been divided **(Fig. 60–7)**.

Now redirect attention to the tail and body of the pancreas. It will be seen that this organ is covered by a layer of posterior parietal peritoneum. This is avascular and should be incised first along the superior border of the pancreas and then again along the inferior border of the pancreas after elevating the tissue with the index finger **(Fig. 60–8)**. As the pancreas is elevated from the posterior abdominal wall, follow the posterior surface of the splenic vein to the point where the inferior mesen-

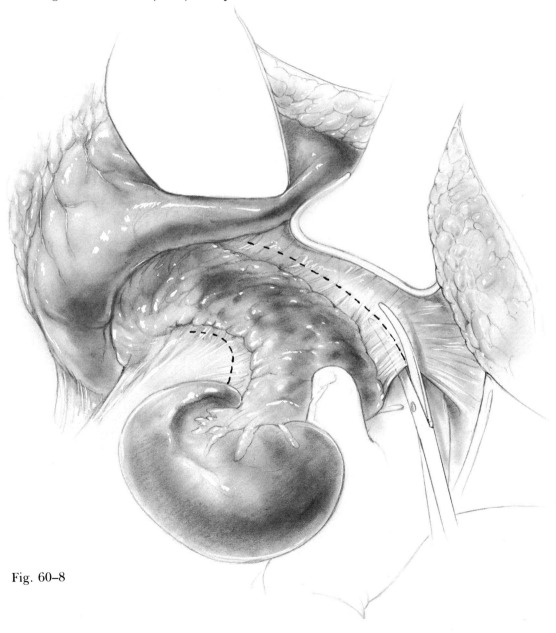

Fig. 60–8

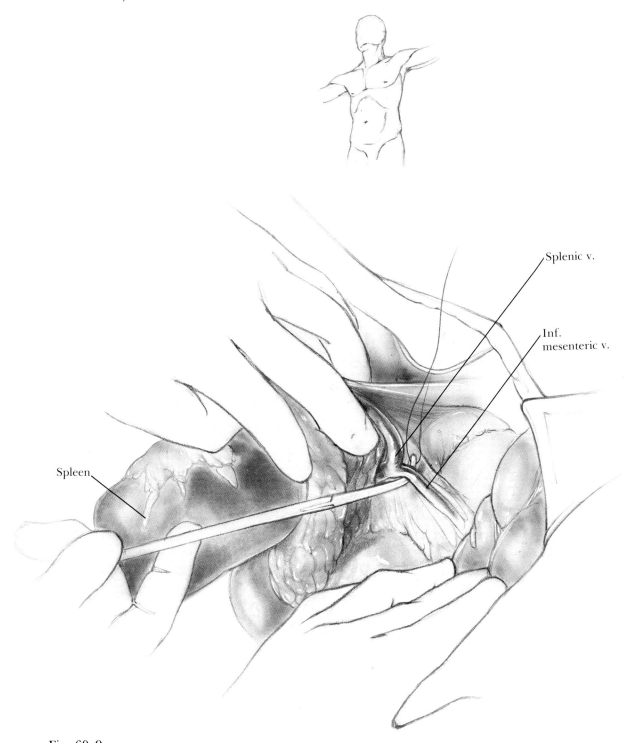

Fig. 60–9

teric vein enters. Then divide this vessel between 2–0 cotton ligatures **(Fig. 60–9).** Follow the splenic artery to its point of origin where the previous ligature will be seen. Doubly ligate the proximal stump of the splenic artery and apply a similar ligature to the distal portion of the splenic artery. Divide between these ties. Then carefully dissect the junction of the splenic and portal veins away from the posterior wall

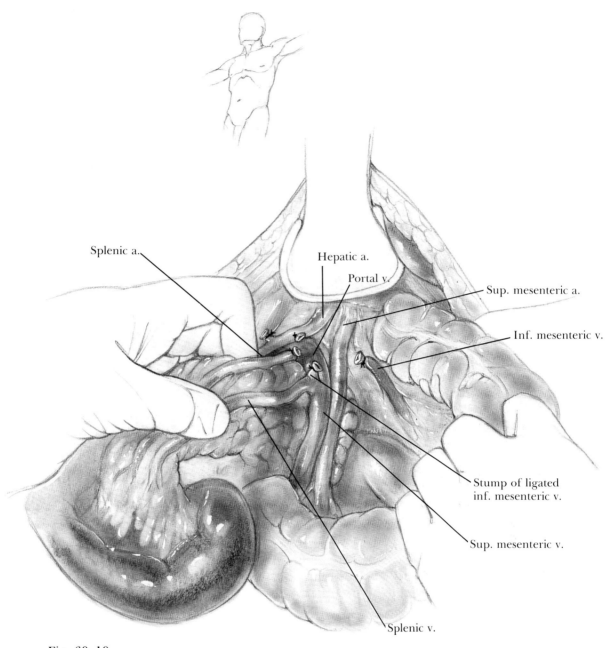

Splenic a.

Hepatic a.

Portal v.

Sup. mesenteric a.

Inf. mesenteric v.

Stump of ligated
inf. mesenteric v.

Sup. mesenteric v.

Splenic v.

Fig. 60–10

of the pancreas. After 2 cm of the terminal portion of the splenic vein has been cleared **(Fig. 60–10),** divide the splenic vein between 2–0 cotton ligatures.

Hemigastrectomy

Select a point on the lesser curvature of the stomach about half way between the pylorus and the esophagogastric junction. Divide and ligate the left gastric vessels at this point. Clear the omentum from the greater curvature of the stomach so that a hemigastrectomy can be accomplished. Then divide the stomach between two applications of the TA-90 stapling device

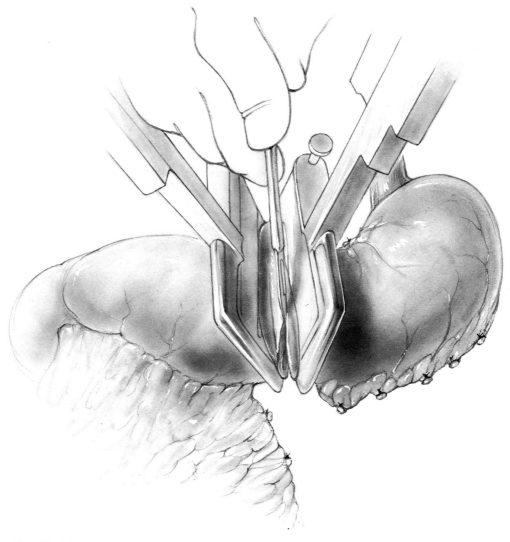

Fig. 60–11

(Fig. 60–11). Lightly coagulate the everted mucosa of the gastric stump. Apply a sterile rubber glove to the specimen side of the divided stomach and fix it in place with an umbilical tape ligature.

Cholecystectomy and Division of the Hepatic Duct

The hepatic duct, portal vein, and hepatic artery have already been stripped of overlying peritoneum and lymph nodes. At this time, divide and ligate the cystic artery. Remove the gallbladder by dissecting it out of the liver bed from above down **(Fig. 60–12).** Obtain complete hemostasis in the liver bed with electrocautery. Ligate the cystic duct. Divide it and remove the gallbladder.

Dissect the hepatic duct free from the portal vein at a point just above its junction

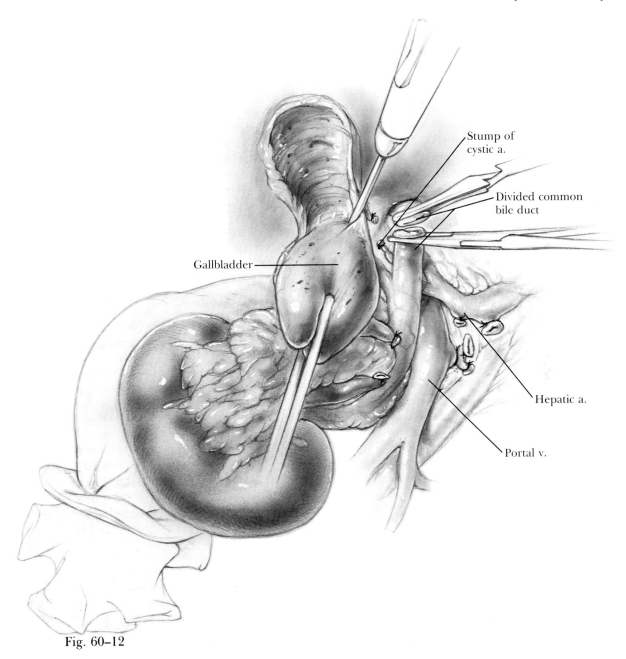

Stump of
cystic a.

Divided common
bile duct

Gallbladder

Hepatic a.

Portal v.

Fig. 60–12

with the cystic duct. Free about 1.5 cm of
hepatic duct. Apply a ligature to the distal
end and an atraumatic bulldog clamp to
the proximal end and divide the duct.

Freeing the Uncinate Process

Retract the spleen, pancreas, and duodenum to the patient's right. Gentle dissection will disclose 3–4 venous branches
between the posterior surface of the pancreatic head and the portal-superior mes-

199

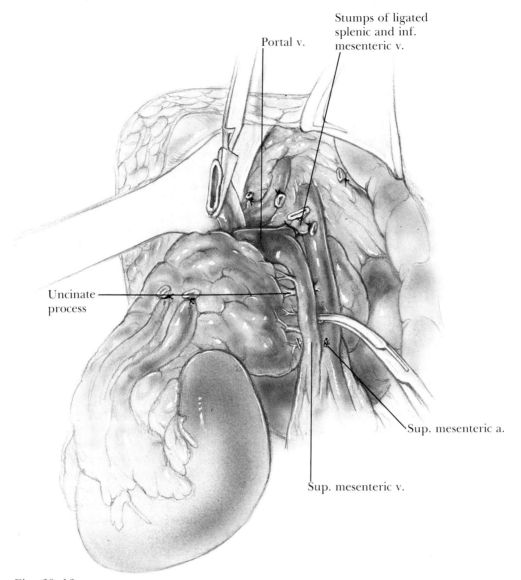

Portal v.

Stumps of ligated
splenic and inf.
mesenteric v.

Uncinate
process

Sup. mesenteric a.

Sup. mesenteric v.

Fig. 60–13

enteric veins **(Fig. 60–13).** Ligate each of these vessels with 3–0 cotton and divide them. Then it will be possible gently to retract the portal vein to the right. At this point the superior mesenteric artery can generally be clearly identified. In some cases it is easy to identify several arterial branches that can be dissected free, divided, and individually ligated **(Fig. 60–14).** More commonly, a fibrotic segment

of uncinate process goes posterior to the superior mesenteric artery. This is difficult to dissect free. In these cases, the uncinate process may either be divided between straight Crile hemostats, or large Hemoclips may be applied and the uncinate process serially divided between the Hemoclips, always keeping the superior mesenteric artery in view (see Figs. 59–11 and

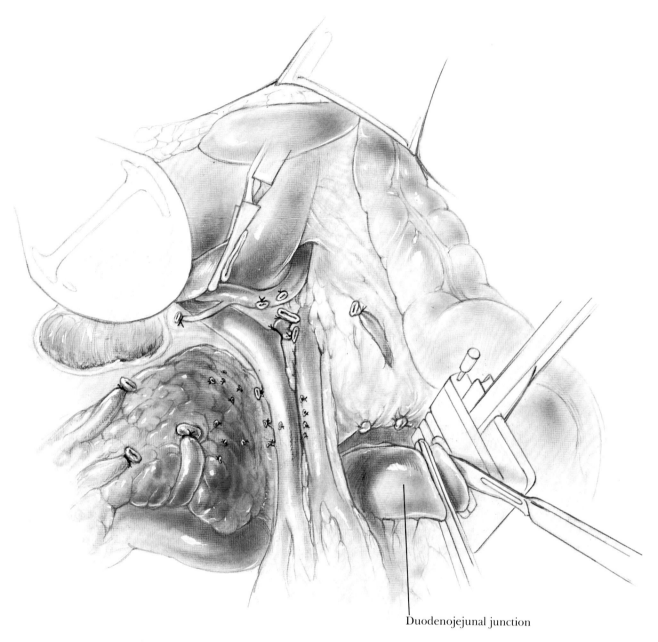

Duodenojejunal junction

Fig. 60–14

59–12). Alternatively apply a TA-55 stapler to the uncinate process and divide the process flush with the stapling device. Before dividing the uncinate process, always remember to palpate along its posterior surface to be sure that an anomalous hepatic artery does not arise from the superior mesenteric artery and pass through this uncinate process, thus making it vulnerable to injury at this point in the operation.

Mobilizing the Duodenojejunal Junction

Expose the ligament of Treitz by elevating the transverse colon. Divide all of the attachments between the terminal duodenum and the ligament of Treitz by sharp dissection. Next divide the first 3–4 blood vessels to the jejunum after drawing the jejunum behind the superior mesenteric vessels to the patient's right. After this segment of mesentery has been freed, apply

201

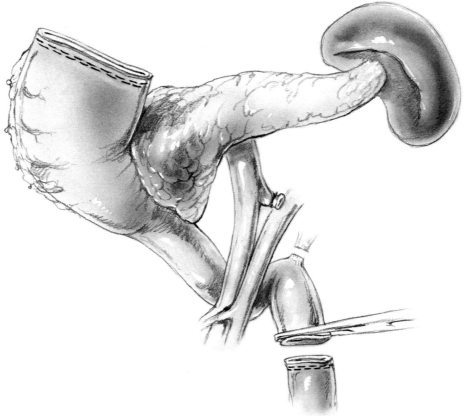

Fig. 60–15

a TA-55 stapling device with 3.5 mm staples across the jejunum. Fire the staples. Apply an Allen clamp to the specimen side of the jejunum. Divide the specimen with a scalpel, flush with the stapler (Fig. 60–14). After removing the stapling device, lightly electrocoagulate the everted mucosa and remove the specimen **(Fig. 60–15).**

Hepaticojejunostomy

If the diameter of the hepatic duct is small, enlarge it by making a small Cheatle incision along its anterior aspect.

In order to insert a T-tube across the anastomosis, make a 3 mm incision on the anterior wall of the hepatic duct at a point about 2–3 cm proximal to its cut end. Then insert a right-angled hemostat through this incision into the lumen of the hepatic duct. Grasp the long limb of a No. 16 T-tube

and draw it through the lumen and out through the small puncture wound (see Figs. 59–21 and 59–22).

Bring the proximal jejunum in an antecolonic fashion up to the hepatic duct. Make an incision along the antimesenteric border of the jejunum about equal to the diameter of the hepatic duct. Excise any redundant jejunal mucosa by electrocautery. We use one layer of either 4-0 or 5-0 Vicryl sutures for this anastomosis. Since this material is absorbable, it does not matter whether the knots are tied inside or outside the lumen of the anastomosis.

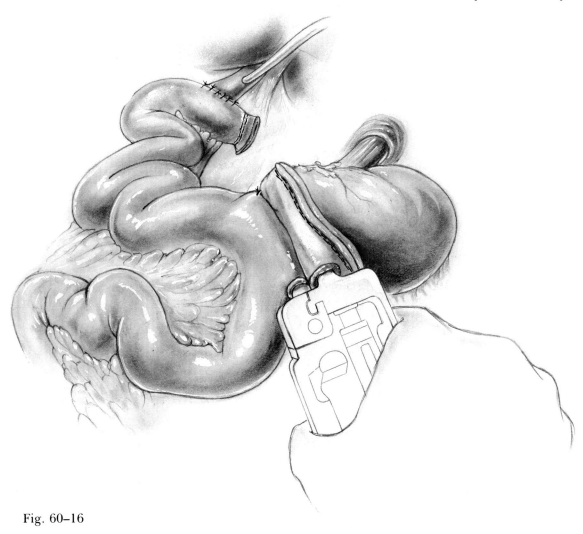

Fig. 60–16

Insert the first suture through the full thickness of the jejunum and then through the hepatic duct at the left lateral border of the anastomosis. Insert the second suture in the same fashion at the right lateral margin of the anastomosis. Before tying these sutures bisect the posterior anastomosis by placing the next suture at the midpoint between the first two and tie it (see Fig. 59–24). Insert the remaining sutures of the posterior layer so as to invert the jejunal mucosa.

Now complete the anterior layer of the anastomosis with a single row of interrupted through-and-through sutures of 5–0 Vicryl. If there is any difficulty about inverting the jejunal mucosa, use a Lembert or a seromucosal suture on the jejunal side and a full-thickness stitch on the hepatic duct side.

Gastrojejunostomy

At a point about 50 cm downstream from the hepaticojejunal anastomosis, construct a stapled gastrojejunostomy (**Figs. 60–16** and 60–17) by the technique described in Chap. 15 (Figs. 15–47 to 15–50). Bring the T-tube out through a stab wound in the right upper quadrant. Irrigate the entire operative field with a dilute antibiotic solution. Be certain that hemostasis is complete. Insert a large Jackson-Pratt suction-drainage catheter in the right upper quadrant of the operative field and bring it out through a stab wound in the abdominal wall.

Close the midline incision in routine fashion. Close the skin with interrupted nylon sutures or staples.

Postoperative Care

Those principles of postoperative care described in Chap. 59 apply to total pancreatectomy except that there is no possibility of a pancreatic fistula. The suction-drainage catheters are removed sometime after the 4th postoperative day unless a significant amount of drainage persists. The T-tube is left in place for 12–14 days.

The most important element of post-operative care following total pancreatectomy is the regulation of the resulting diabetes. The greatest danger is the hypoglycemia that develops from administering too much insulin. Perform blood sugar determi-

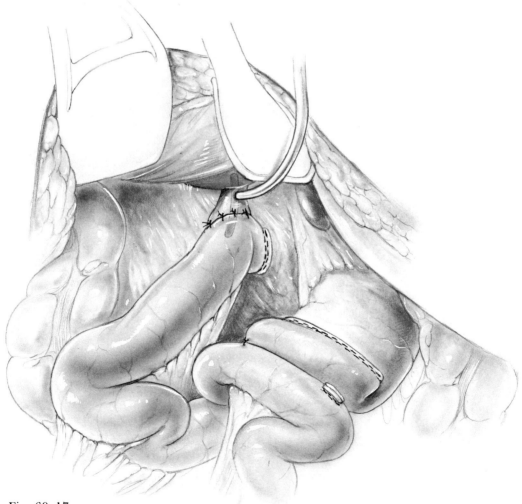

Fig. 60–17

nations every 3–4 hours for the first few days. Do not try to keep the blood sugar level below 200 mg/dl. Especially during the early postoperative period, the diabetes is quite brittle and an overdose of only a few units of insulin may produce hypoglycemic shock. There is much more danger from hypoglycemia than from diabetic acidosis. Administer regular insulin in doses of 2–5 units every few hours as necessary. Frequently no more than 10–20 units are required per day.

After the patient begins to eat, he may be switched to one of the longer-acting insulin products. The patients and his relatives should be carefully instructed in the symptoms of hypoglycemia.

Repeated measurements of the gastric pH are vital to prevent postoperative gastric hemorrhage. Use both intravenous cimetidine and oral antacids to keep the gastric pH at 5 or above.

A sufficient dose of pancreatic enzymes must be given to prevent steatorrhea. This may require as little as three or as many as 8–9 tablets of Viokase before each meal. The newer products, like Pancrease, are more concentrated and smaller doses will suffice.

Postoperative Complications

Insulin shock

Postoperative gastric bleeding due to stress ulceration or marginal ulcer

Postoperative hemorrhage

Postoperative sepsis

Leakage from biliary anastomosis

Mesenteric venous thrombosis

Hepatic failure

61 Distal Pancreatectomy

Indications

Malignant tumors of body or tail: cyst-adenocarcinoma; malignant insulinoma or gastrinoma; duct cell carcinoma (rarely resectable)

Benign tumors that cannot be locally excised (e.g., insulinoma)

Pseudocysts of tail (selected)

Chronic pancreatitis localized to body and tail

Preoperative Care

Angiography occasionally localizes a tumor (e.g., insulinoma).

Operations for insulinoma require careful monitoring of the blood sugar at frequent intervals prior to and during operation.

Patients suspected of having a gastrinoma should have this diagnosis confirmed by serial serum gastrin levels before and after administration of intravenous secretin.

Pitfalls and Danger Points

Lacerating splenic or portal vein

Operative Strategy

Avoiding Damage to Blood Vessels

Once the decision has been made that the lesion in the pancreas should be resected, locate the splenic artery at a point a few centimeters beyond its origin at the celiac axis. Ligate the vessel in continuity to reduce the size of the spleen and to reduce the volume of blood loss if the splenic capsule is ruptured during the dissection.

The greatest danger in resecting the body and tail of the pancreas arises when a malignancy in the body obscures the junction between the splenic and portal veins. Invasion, by tumor, of the portal vein is an indication of inoperability. If elevation of the tail and body of the pancreas together with the tumor should result in a tear at the junction of the splenic and portal veins, and this accident occurs before the tumor has been completely liberated, it may be extremely difficult to repair the lacerated portal vein. If an accident of this type should occur, it may be necessary to find the plane between the neck of the pancreas and the portal vein, and then to divide the pancreas across its neck while manually occluding the lacerated vein. With the portal and superior mesenteric veins exposed after the neck of the pancreas has been divided, occluding vascular clamps may be applied and the laceration repaired. This complication can generally be avoided by careful inspection of the tumor after elevating the tail of the pancreas and by observing the area where the splenic vein joins the portal. If the tumor extends beyond this junction, it is probably inoperable.

Avoiding Pancreatic Fistula

We have used the TA-55 stapling device for 7–8 years to accomplish closure of the cut end of the remaining pancreas after resecting the body and tail of this organ (Pachter, Pennington, Chassin, and Spencer). When the stapler is used across the neck of a pancreas of average thickness, the staples seem to occlude the cut end of the pancreatic duct successfully; no supplementary sutures are needed to prevent a fistula.

If the stapler is not used, be certain to occlude the cut pancreatic duct by inserting a nonabsorbable mattress suture.

Operative Technique

Incision and Exposure

In the average patient a long midline incision from the xiphoid to a point about 6–10 cm beyond the umbilicus provides adequate exposure for mobilizing the spleen and the tail of the pancreas. In an obese or a very muscular individual with a wide costal angle, a long transverse or left subcostal incision is a suitable alternative.

Exploration; Liberating the Omentum

After exploring the abdomen for possible metastatic deposits, expose the body and tail of the pancreas by liberating the omentum from its attachments to the transverse colon. An alternative method is to divide the omentum between hemostats. This will expose the anterior surface of the pancreas. In order to palpate the posterior surface, it will be necessary to incise the layer of peritoneum that covers the pancreas and then continues down to the transverse colon forming one leaflet of the transverse mesocolon. Incise this layer along the infe-

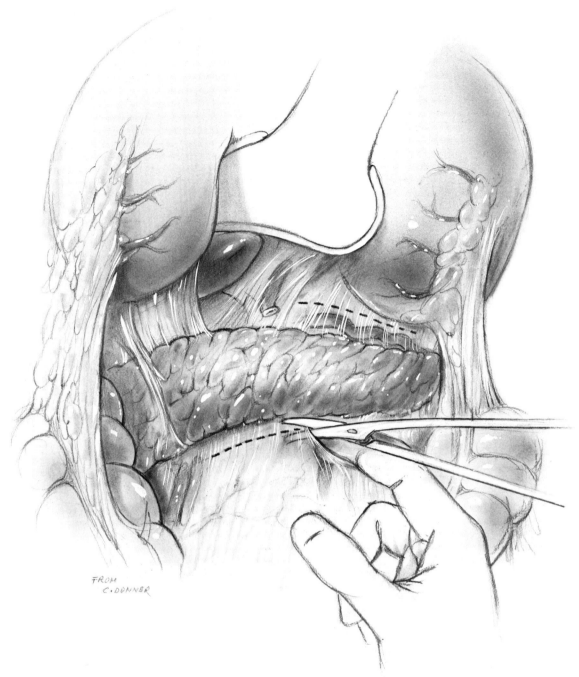

Fig. 61–1.

rior border of the tail of the pancreas (**Fig. 61–1).** The only major blood vessel deep to this layer of peritoneum is the inferior mesenteric vein that travels from the transverse mesocolon to join the inferior border of the splenic vein just before the splenic vein joins the portal. After completing this incision, insert the index finger behind the pancreas and use the fingertip to elevate the peritoneum along the superior margin of the pancreas (**Fig. 61–2).** Then incise this layer of peritoneum with a scissors, avoiding the sometimes convoluted splenic artery that runs along the superior border of the pancreas deep to the layer of peritoneum. After these two peritoneal incisions have been made, palpate the tail and body

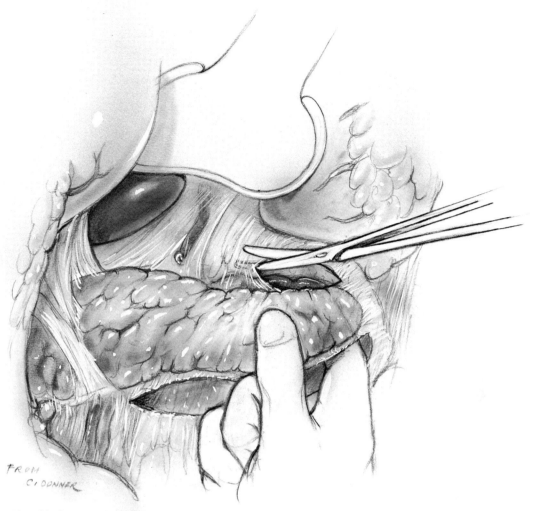

Fig. 61–2.

of the pancreas between the thumb and forefinger to evaluate the pathology.

If the surgeon is searching for a gastrinoma, he should also perform a Kocher maneuver and palpate the descending duodenum and the head of the pancreas. Some non-beta cell tumors of the pancreas can be palpated as small projections from the pancreas into the posterior wall of the descending duodenum. Many of the benign tumors can be excised locally or may be shelled out by gentle dissection.

Identifying Splenic Artery

Palpate the splenic artery along the upper border of the neck of the pancreas at a point a few centimeters from its origin. If there is some confusion as to the identity of the artery, occlude it with the fingertip and palpate the hepatoduodenal ligament to determine whether it is the hepatic artery that has been occluded. If the hepatic artery pulsation is normal, then open the peritoneum overlying the splenic artery. Encircle it with a right-angle clamp and ligate it in continuity with 2–0 cotton (see Fig. 64–2).

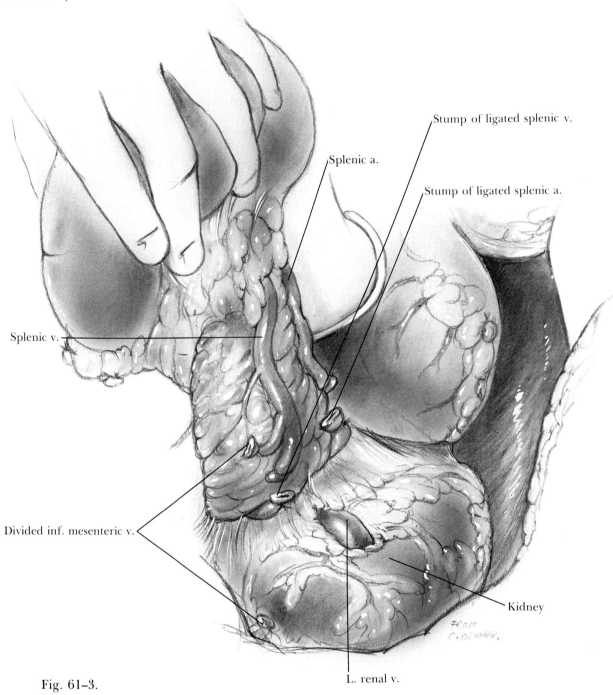

Splenic a.

Stump of ligated splenic v.

Stump of ligated splenic a.

Splenic v.

Divided inf. mesenteric v.

Kidney

L. renal v.

FROM
C. DENNER.

Fig. 61–3.

Mobilizing Spleen and Pancreas

Retract the spleen to the patient's right, placing the splenorenal ligament on stretch. Incise this ligament (see Fig. 65–1) with a Metzenbaum scissors or electrocoagulator. Continue this incision up to the diaphragm and down to include the splenocolic ligament. Now elevate the spleen and the tail of the pancreas by fingertip dissection from the renal capsule. The greater omentum may be attached to the lower portion of the spleen. Dissect this away from the spleen. It should now be possible to elevate the spleen and the tail and body of the pancreas up into the incision leaving the kidney and adrenal gland behind. Cover these structures with a large moist gauze pad.

The spleen remains attached to the greater curvature of the stomach by means of the intact left gastroepiploic and short gastric vessels. Divide each of these structures individually between hemostats and then ligate each with 2–0 cotton (see Figures 64–2 and 64–4). Inspection of the posterior surface of the pancreas will reveal the splenic vein. Dissecting along the inferior border of the pancreas will unroof the inferior mesenteric vein on its way to join the splenic vein. Identify, encircle, and divide the inferior mesenteric vein between 2–0 cotton ligatures.

Dividing the Splenic Artery and Vein

Gently elevate the splenic vein by sweeping the areolar tissue away from this vessel with a peanut dissector until the junction between the splenic and portal veins is identified. At this point encircle the splenic vein with a right-angle clamp at a point about 2 cm proximal to its junction with the portal vein. Pass two ligatures of 2–0 cotton around the splenic vein and tie these two ligatures about 1.5 cm apart. Divide the vein between the two ligatures (**Fig. 61–3**).

Then identify the previously ligated splenic artery. Tie a second ligature around this artery and divide the vessel distal to the two ligatures. This will leave the specimen attached only by the neck of the pancreas in the region of the portal vein.

Dividing the Pancreas

If the pancreas is average in thickness, it is a simple matter to apply a TA-55 stapler across the neck of the pancreas. Use 3.5 mm staples in most cases. Fire the staples and divide the pancreas flush with the stapler using a scalpel. Remove the specimen.

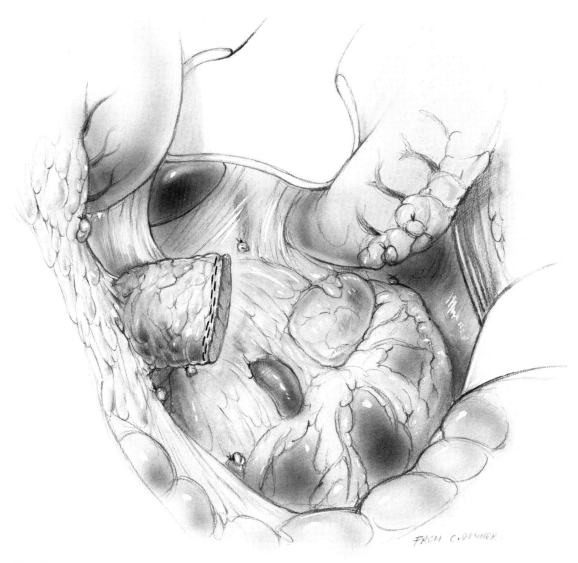

Fig. 61–4.

Then remove the stapling device and inspect the cut edge of the pancreas carefully for bleeding points **(Fig. 61–4)**. It is frequently necessary to suture-ligate a superior pancreatic artery near the upper border of the remaining pancreas. We have not found it necessary to identify or to suture the pancreatic duct when using a stapled closure of the transected pancreas.

Alternatively, one may occlude the transected pancreas with interlocking interrupted mattress sutures of 3–0 nonabsorbable suture material. If the pancreatic duct is identified, occlude this duct with a separate mattress suture.

Closure and Drainage

Place a flat Jackson-Pratt multiperforated closed-suction drainage catheter down to the site of the divided pancreas and bring the catheter out through a puncture wound in the abdominal wall.

Close the incision in routine fashion after ascertaining that complete hemostasis in the pancreatic and splenic beds has been achieved.

212

Postoperative Care

Attach the drainage catheter to a closed-suction system. Leave the drain in place 4–6 days. If a pancreatic duct fistula is suspected, leave the drain in place for a longer period of time.

Perform frequent checks of the serum amylase and the blood sugar to detect postoperative pancreatitis and diabetes.

Postoperative Complications

Pancreatic fistula. If this complication develops, it will generally recede spontaneously in 1–4 weeks. If it does not recede in that period of time, perform an X-ray sinogram with an aqueous contrast medium.

Acute pancreatitis in the residual pancreas is a possible but uncommon complication.

Diabetes mellitus of mild degree sometimes occurs after an extensive distal pancreatectomy.

Reference

Pachter HL, Pennington R, Chassin JL, Spencer FC (1979) Simplified distal pancreatectomy with the autosuture stapler; preliminary clinical observations. Surgery 85:166

62 Operations for Pancreatic Cyst

Concept: When to Operate and Which Operation to Do

Cystadenoma versus Pseudocyst

The proper operation for cystadenoma, a neoplasm that has the potential of containing malignancy, is a resection. On the other hand, most pseudocysts may be cured by drainage. Therefore it is important to make an accurate diagnosis before selecting the operation for a pancreatic cyst. A pseudocyst, which is often preceded by one or more attacks of acute pancreatitis, frequently produces upper abdominal pain, occasionally nausea and vomiting, mild leukocytosis, and an elevated serum amylase. The cystadenoma, on the other hand, produces few symptoms. In any case, during the course of performing a drainage operation on a suspected pseudocyst, always excise a segment of the cyst wall for immediate frozen-section histopathology to rule out cystadenoma or cystadenocarcinoma. This is particularly important because resecting a cystadenocarcinoma results in a highly satisfactory 5-year survival rate (over 50%). If the cyst is lined by epithelium, it is *not* a pseudocyst and should be resected, not drained.

Timing of Operation

In the case of *cystadenoma,* perform a resection as soon as the patient is properly prepared.

The pancreatic *pseudocyst* begins its existence as nothing more than an accumulation of secretion and exudate surrounding the pancreas in the lesser sac after an epi-sode of acute pancreatitis. These cysts may be detected sometimes by no other means than sonography or computerized tomography.

After a period of time the wall of the pseudocyst develops a fibrotic lining, which makes a cystogastric or cystojejunal anastomosis feasible. Prior to the development of this fibrotic wall, suturing the cyst to a portion of the gastrointestinal tract may be dangerous. Consequently, operation is not indicated during the first 6 weeks following the initial formation of the pseudocyst unless serial sonography shows rapid growth or unless some complication occurs. Abscess, rupture of the cyst with peritonitis, and hemorrhage have been reported during this initial 6-week period of observation by Bradley, Clements, and Gonzales. Immediate operation is, of course, indicated for these complications. On the other hand, these authors found that at least 40% of their patients showed complete resolution of the pseudocyst *during* this 6-week period. *After* the passage of 6 weeks, they noted only one case of spontaneous resolution in 33 patients studied in contrast with 17 serious complications, which included intraperitoneal rupture (with two deaths), cystenteric fistula, common bile duct obstruction, and hemorrhage.

Frey emphasized that hemorrhage in patients with pancreatic pseudocysts is most often due to rupture of a pseudoaneurysm. This type of aneurysm occurred most frequently in the splenic artery and

214

ruptured into the pseudocyst, but pseudo-aneurysms were also found in the gastro-duodenal and the inferior pancreatico-duodenal arteries. In patients who have formed cystenteric fistulas, rupture of a pseudoaneurysm produces hemorrhage into the gastrointestinal tract and occasionally hemobilia.

Because of the high incidence of serious complications occurring in patients with conservatively managed pseudocysts, all such cysts require operation unless they resolve themselves in 6 weeks, or unless the cyst is less than 5 cm in diameter as measured on the sonogram (Bradley et al.; Frey; Martin et al.; Shatney and Lillehei). Whether it is safe to persist in the nonoperative management of a small (5 cm) pseudocyst for an indefinite period of time is a point concerning which there is inadequate data for a definitive opinion at this time.

Choice of Operation

External Drainage by Laparotomy or Percutaneous Catheter

External drainage is the operation of choice in all pseudocysts that have not yet developed a wall fibrotic enough to withstand suturing and in the unusual case of the pseudocyst that is in fact a large abscess cavity containing frank pus. We rarely encounter a patient who is "too sick" to withstand a cystojejunostomy or a cystogastrostomy, although Martin, Catalano, Cooperman, Hecht et al. feel that external drainage is not such a poor second choice. In their series, the longest period of continuous drainage from the cystocutaneous fistula was 4 months, although most fistulas stopped draining within 6 weeks. Other authors report a high incidence of persistent fistulas, recurrent cysts, and other complications following external drainage (Frey; Sandy, Taylor, Christensen, Scudamore et al.).

Marsupialization, or suturing the wall of the cyst to the skin, is rarely indicated. If the cyst wall is thick enough to suture to the skin, it is thick enough to undergo a cystenteric anastomosis.

Another method of instituting external drainage is to pass a needle and then a catheter into the pseudocyst by a transcutaneous route under the control of computed tomography (Karlson, Martin, Frankuchen, Mattern, and associates). This technique of draining a pancreatic pseudocyst must be judged an experimental procedure until more data becomes available concerning its merits and its complications.

Cystogastrostomy

This operation is indicated only when the anterior wall of the cyst is firmly attached to the posterior wall of the stomach. Under these conditions it is an excellent operation. Otherwise, suturing the free wall of a cyst to the free wall of the stomach assumes the risk of a postoperative gastric fistula, which is indeed a disastrous complication. Because the wall of a pseudocyst is primarily fibrous and contains no discrete blood supply, there is always some risk that an anastomosis to this structure will fail. And because most large pseudocysts are indeed firmly attached to the posterior wall of the stomach, cystogastrostomy is probably the most commonly performed operation for pancreatic pseudocyst.

Cystoduodenostomy

The warning stated above applies with even greater force to cystoduodenostomy. If the cyst wall is not densely attached to the wall of the duodenum, do not perform cystoduodenostomy because a duodenal leak in this situation will often be fatal, as it was in the case of two patients reported by Frey.

Roux-Y Cystojejunostomy

This operation is indicated whenever an anastomosis must be performed to the an-

215

terior wall of a cyst that is not firmly attached to either stomach or duodenum. If a defunctionalized limb is used, one that is over 50 cm long, the dehiscence of a cystojejunal anastomosis will not be a life-threatening complication because the fluid leaking from this type of anastomosis will not contain the powerful digestive ferments that flow from leaking gastric or duodenal anastomoses.

Distal Pancreatectomy
When a patient with a pancreatic pseudocyst suffers also from a pseudoaneurysm in the back wall of the cyst, simply performing a drainage procedure, whether internal or external, will not prevent postoperative hemorrhage (Frey). While the older literature concerning postoperative hemorrhage following cystogastrostomy attributed the bleeding to some technical error in the anastomosis (Huston, Zeppa, and Warren), it is highly likely that the bleeding resulted from the rupture into a cyst of a pseudoaneurysm. Frey noted that 10.8% of his operative cases were found to have pseudoaneurysms on preoperative angiography. "Since hemorrhage . . . was a significant factor in the majority of deaths of patients with pseudocysts," Frey states that "all pseudocysts having an associated pseudoaneurysm should, whenever possible, be treated by excision." Three patients in Frey's series, none of whom had bled preoperatively or had any evidence of blood in the cysts at operation, underwent a simple drainage procedure, and all three exsanguinated postoperatively. A pseudoaneurysm in the wall of the cyst was the source of the hemorrhage in each case.

When a pseudoaneurysm is actively bleeding, local control by ligating the artery in the wall of a chronically inflamed cyst may not be effective since the suture will often cut through the artery postoperatively, with consequent rebleeding. Resection of the cyst together with adjacent pancreas and division of the artery in an uninflamed area proximal to the pseudoaneurysm will eliminate the threat of hemorrhage.

When an arteriogram does not demonstrate a pseudoaneurysm, it is probably not necessary to excise a pseudocyst, even if it contains blood at the time of operation (Frey; Grace and Jordan).

The only other indication for resecting a pancreatic pseudocyst occurs when a patient suffers such severe pain from irreversible chronic pancreatitis that distal pancreatectomy is indicated for this purpose alone.

Whipple Pancreatoduodenectomy
When arteriography demonstrates a pseudoaneurysm of the pancreaticoduodenal artery in the head of the pancreas, Frey believes that a Whipple pancreatoduodenectomy is indicated to remove the serious threat of exsanguinating hemorrhage. Otherwise, most pseudocysts in the head of the pancreas or in the uncinate process can be treated by internal drainage. Even though the mortality rate of pancreatoduodenectomy for pancreatitis is lower than that after cancer, this radical procedure is not often indicated for pancreatic pseudocysts except in patients who have a pseudoaneurysm in the head of the pancreas.

Indications

Any pseudocyst that measures over 5 cm in diameter by sonography or CT scan requires operation if it persists for more than 6 weeks.

Preoperative Care

Visualize the cyst by sonogram or CT scan.

Complete an upper GI X-ray series.

Rule out the presence of gallstones or bile duct obstruction by sonography, oral cholecystography, or endoscopic radiographic cholangiopancreatography (ERCP).

Perform angiography of the splenic artery and pancreas in all cases.

Administer perioperative antibiotics.

Insert a nasogastric tube preoperatively.

Pitfalls and Danger Points

Anastomotic leak

Postoperative hemorrhage

Mistaken diagnosis (abdominal aortic aneurysm, cystedenocarcinoma)

Overlooking a pseudoaneurysm in the wall of a cyst

Operative Strategy

Avoiding Anastomotic Leakage

As discussed above, do not perform either a cystogastronomy or a cystoduodenostomy unless the wall of the cyst is firmly attached to the wall of the stomach or duodenum. In the latter case make the anastomosis through the area of attachment. Otherwise, perform a Roux-Y cystojejunostomy because leakage from this anastomosis is far less dangerous to the patient than is leakage from either stomach or duodenum.

Also, be certain that the wall of the pseudocyst is thick enough to make the anastomosis safe. Although this degree of thickening is generally presumed to require the passage of 6 weeks, a thick wall may occasionally be noted as soon as 3 weeks after the onset of the cyst (Grace and Jordan). If there is doubt about the adequacy of the cyst wall, perform an external drainage operation.

Avoiding Diagnostic Errors

Although preoperative angiography is helpful in ruling out the presence of an abdominal aortic aneurysm that may resemble a pancreatic pseudocyst, always inspect the pancreatic cyst carefully with the tentative hypothesis that it may, in fact, be an aortic aneurysm. Also, insert a needle into the suspected cyst and aspirate to see if it contains blood. When the cyst is pulsatile, proceed with great caution, as the cyst may contain a free rupture of a pseudoaneurysm of the splenic artery.

Also, perform a biopsy of the cyst wall to rule out cystadenocarcinoma.

Pseudoaneurysm

When arteriography has demonstrated a leaking pseudoaneurysm of the splenic artery in a large pseudocyst, it is wise to ask the angiographer to pass a balloon catheter into the proximal splenic artery in order to occlude the artery preoperatively. Sometimes the area of inflammation extends close to the origin of the splenic artery, making proximal control in the operating room, under emergency conditions, quite difficult.

It is preferable to resect a cyst containing a pseudoaneurysm to prevent postoperative rupture and hemorrhage, rather than to drain it.

The Jaundiced Patient

While jaundice in the presence of a pseudocyst may well be the result of extrinsic pressure by the cyst against the distal common bile duct, it is also important to rule out the presence of calculi or periductal pancreatic fibrosis as the cause of bile duct obstruction. Preoperative ERCP is helpful, but performing an operative cholangiogram after the cyst has been drained will determine whether further surgery of the bile duct is necessary. If the jaundice is due to chronic fibrosis in the head of the pancreas, a bypass operation will be required. It may be necessary to perform a side-to-side choledochojejunostomy to the defunctionalized limb of the Roux-Y distal to the cystojejunostomy.

Operative Technique

External Drainage

Make a long midline incision. Explore the abdomen. Identify the pseudocyst. After making an incision in the greater omentum to expose the anterior wall of the cyst, insert a needle into the cyst to rule out the presence of fresh blood. Then incise the cyst wall and evacuate all of the cyst contents. Take a sample for bacteriological analysis. If the cyst wall is too thin for anastomosis, insert soft sump suction and latex drains and bring them out through an adequate stab wound in the left upper quadrant.

If the cyst wall is thick enough to permit suturing to the skin for marsupialization, the wall is adequate for cystojejunostomy.

If the cyst wall is thick enough to permit suturing, but the contents of the cyst appear to consist of pus and to resemble a large abscess, make a Gram stain. Sometimes what appears to be pus is only grumous detritus. If the Gram stain does not show a large number of bacteria, it is possible to perform an internal drainage operation. Otherwise, marsupialize a 4–5 cm window in the anterior cyst wall by suturing it to the anterior fascia of a large 5-cm stab wound in the abdominal wall.

Close the abdominal incision in the usual fashion after lavaging the abdominal cavity with a dilute antibiotic solution.

Cystogastrostomy

Make a midline incision from the xiphoid to the umbilicus. Explore the abdomen. If the gallbladder contains stones, perform a cholecystectomy and a cholangiogram. Explore the lesser sac by exposing the posterior wall of the stomach from its lesser curvature aspect. If the cyst is densely adherent to the posterior wall of the stomach, a cystogastrostomy is the operation of choice. If the retrogastric mass is pulsatile, consider seriously whether the mass represents an aortic aneurysm. Expose the aorta at the hiatus of the diaphragm and prepare a suitable large vascular clamp for emergency occlusion of this vessel, should this be necessary. If the surgeon has had no previous experience with this maneuver,

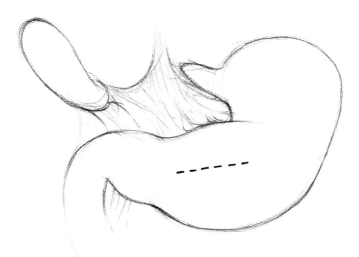

Fig. 62–1

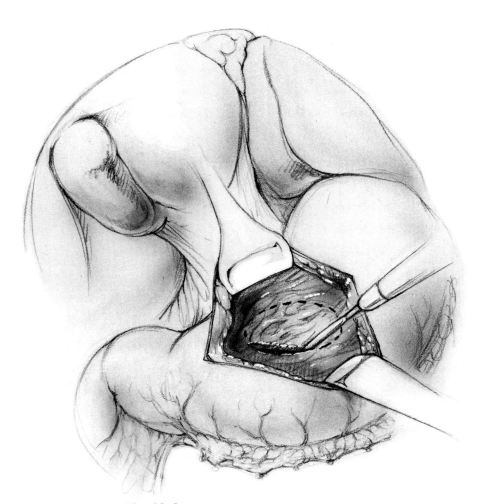

Fig. 62–2

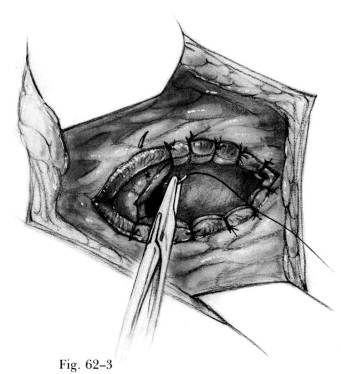

Fig. 62–3

he should request the presence of a vascular surgeon.

Make a 6–8 cm incision in the anterior wall of the stomach **(Fig. 62–1)** opposite the most prominent portion of the retrogastric cyst. Obtain hemostasis with an electrocautery or ligatures. Then insert an 18-gauge needle through the back wall of the stomach into the cyst and aspirate. If no blood is obtained, make an incision about 5–6 cm in length through the posterior wall of the stomach and carry it through the anterior wall of the cyst. Excise an adequate ellipse of tissue from the anterior wall of the cyst for frozen-section histopathology to rule out the presence of a cystadenoma or cystadenocarcinoma **(Fig. 62–2).**

Then approximate the cut edges of the stomach and cyst by means of continuous or interrupted 3–0 PG sutures **(Fig. 62–3).** Close the defect in the anterior wall

219

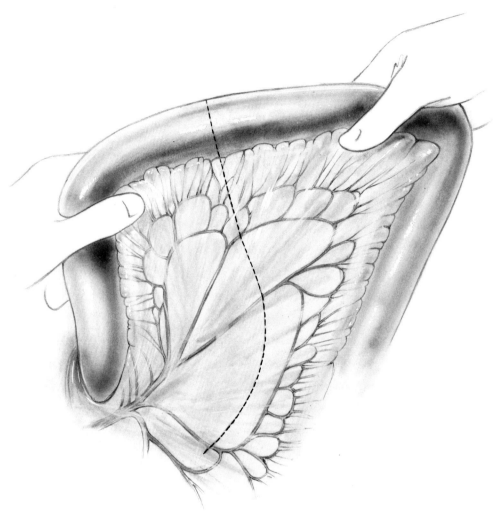

Fig. 62–4

of the stomach by applying 4–5 Allis clamps and then perform a stapled closure by using the TA-90 stapler. If the gastric wall is not thickened, use the 3.5 mm staples. Lightly electrocoagulate the everted gastric mucosa. Suture-ligate any arterial bleeders with 4–0 PG.

Roux-Y Cystojejunostomy

Make a long midline incision. Explore the abdomen. Check the gallbladder for stones. Expose the anterior wall of the cyst by dividing the omentum overlying it. Pre-

pare a segment of jejunum at a point about 15 cm beyond the ligament of Treitz. Divide the jejunal mesentery as illustrated in **Fig. 62–4.** Then divide the jejunum between two Allen clamps. Liberate enough of the mesentery of the distal jejunal segment to permit the jejunum to reach the cyst without any tension.

Make a small window in an avascular portion of the transverse mesocolon and deliver the distal jejunal segment into the supramesocolic space. Excise a window of anterior cyst wall, about 3–4 cm in diameter. Send it for frozen-section histopathological examination. Perform a one-layer anastomosis between the open end of jejunum and the window in the anterior wall. Insert interrupted Lembert 3–0 or 4–0 Vicryl sutures. Then use 4–0 Vicryl sutures to attach the mesocolon to the jejunum at the point where it passes through the mesocolon.

Anastomose the divided proximal end of the jejunum to the antimesenteric border of the descending limb of the jejunum at a point 50–60 cm beyond the cystojejunal anastomosis. Align the open proximal end of jejunum so that its opening points in a cephalad direction make a 1.5 cm incision in the antimesenteric border of the descending jejunum using electrocautery (see Fig. 19–36). Insert the forks of the GIA stapling device into both limbs of jejunum so that the GIA will grasp the antimesenteric borders. Then fire the GIA device making a side-to-side anastomosis (Fig. 19–37).

Apply an Allis clamp to the anterior termination of the GIA staple line and another Allis clamp to the posterior termination of the GIA staple line and draw these two points apart. Then insert a guy suture to approximate the midpoints of the cephalad and caudal lips of jejunum (see Fig. 19–38). Complete the anastomosis by tri-angulation. Apply Allis clamps to the tissue between the guy suture and the anterior termination of the GIA staple line. Apply a TA-55 device with 3.5 staples deep to the guy suture and the Allis clamps. Close the TA-55 and fire, creating an everting closure (see Fig. 19–39). Excise the redundant mucosa with a heavy scissors, but be careful not to detach the guy suture. Lightly electrocoagulate the mucosa. Then apply Allis clamps to approximate the jejunum between the guy suture and the posterior termination of the GIA staple line. Apply a TA-55 device just deep to the guy suture and the Allis clamps. Fire the TA-55. Excise the redundant tissue and lightly electrocoagulate the everted mucosa. Remove the TA-55 (see Fig. 19–40). Be sure that the ends of the GIA staple line have been included in each of the two applications of the TA-55. This method will create a large end-to-end anastomosis, completing the Roux-Y procedure.

Use 4–0 PG sutures to close the defect in the jejunal mesentery.

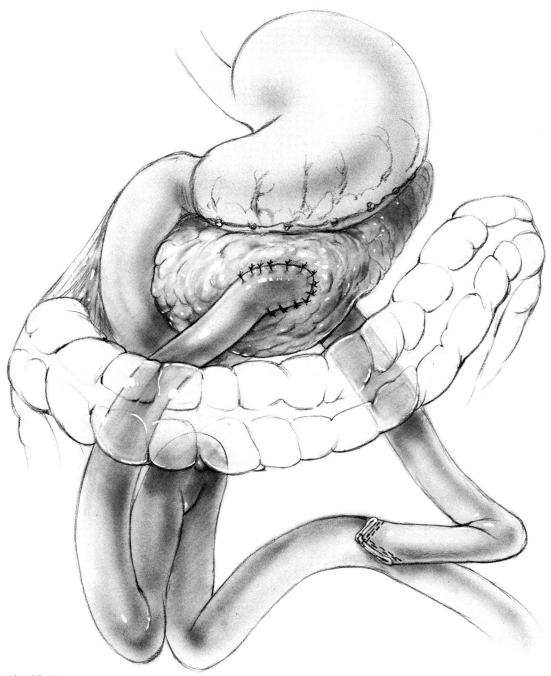

Fig 62–5

The completed cystojejunostomy is illustrated in **Fig. 62–5.**

If the cyst wall is of adequate quality, no drains need be used. Close the incision in the usual fashion.

Distal Pancreatectomy

The technique of distal pancreatectomy has been described in Chap. 61.

Whipple Pancreatoduodenectomy

The technique for the pancreatoduodenectomy is described in Chap. 59.

Postoperative Care

Nasogastric suction until the patient passes flatus

Perioperative antibiotics are indicated. If the culture report of the cyst contents comes back positive, administer the appropriate antibiotics for 7 days.

In cases of external drainage, administer antibiotics depending on the culture reports. Leave at least one drain in place until the amount of fluid obtained is minimal and also a radiographic study with aqueous contrast material shows that the cyst has contracted down to the size of the drain. It may be helpful to instill a dilute antibiotic solution at 8–12 hour intervals into the sump drain.

Postoperative Complications

Acute pancreatitis

Persistent fistula following external drainage

Abscess

Postoperative bleeding into gastrointestinal tract (rare if pseudoaneurysms have been excised).

References

Bradley II EL, Clements Jr JL, Gonzalez AC (1979) The natural history of pancreatic pseudocysts: a unified concept of management. Am J Surg 137:135

Frey CF (1978) Pancreatic pseudocyst-operative strategy. Ann Surg 188:652

Grace RR, Jordan Jr PH (1976) Unresolved problems of pancreatic pseudocysts. Ann Surg 184:16

Huston DG, Zeppa R. Warren DW (1976) Postoperative hemorrhage after pancreatic cystogastrostomy. Ann Surg 177:689

Karlson KB, Martin EC, Fankuchen EI, Mattern RF et al. (1982) Percutaneous drainage of pancreatic pseudocysts and abscesses. Radiology 142:619

Martin Jr EW, Catalano P, Cooperman M, Hecht C et al. (1979) Surgical decision-making in the treatment of pancreatic pseudocysts: internal versus external drainage. Am J Surg 138:821

Sandy JT, Taylor RH, Christensen RM, Scudamore C et al. (1981) Pancreatic pseudocyst: changing concepts in management. Am J Surg 141:574

Shatney CH, Lillehei RC (1979) Surgical treatment of pancreatic pseudocysts: analysis of 119 cases. Ann Surg 189:386

63 Pancreaticojejunostomy (Puestow) for Chronic Pancreatitis

Concept: Which Therapy for Chronic Pancreatitis

Pathogenesis

Chronic pancreatitis of the type severe enough to require surgery generally follows chronic alcohol abuse. It is rare after an attack of biliary pancreatitis if the biliary calculi are removed. Occasionally trauma to the pancreas or congenital abnormalities of the pancreatic ducts may produce chronic pancreatitis.

Objectives of Surgery

It is unlikely that any type of operation will significantly preserve pancreatic function. The only objective that surgery can be expected to accomplish is relief of pain. This can be achieved in some patients by an extensive pancreaticojejunostomy, an operation that presumably relieves the patient's pain by decompressing the partially obstructed pancreatic ducts. Another method of alleviating intractable pain in chronic pancreatitis is resection of part or all of the diseased pancreas. The drawback to resection operations is that they may produce diabetes, which can be very difficult for the alcoholic patient to manage. A number of alcoholic patients, following extensive pancreatic resection, will die late in the postoperative course due to a complication of diabetes control.

Although another objective of pancreatic surgery is to preserve the exocrine function of the pancreas, there is no convincing data that pancreaticojejunostomy accomplishes this aim.

Choice of Operation

Sphincteroplasty

Even when sphincteroplasty is accompanied by a septotomy that enlarges the orifice of Wirsung's duct, it is not an effective operation for the usual type of chronic pancreatitis seen in the alcoholic patient. Theoretically, if there is a localized obstruction at the orifice of Wirsung's duct, sphincteroplasty combined with ductopalsty is a logical procedure to relieve this obstruction. Because an isolated obstruction of this type is quite rare, however, there is, in our opinion, scant indication for this operation in chronic pancreatitis.

Pancreaticojejunostomy, Roux-Y

Pancreaticojejunostomy is the operation of choice in patients with intractable pain from chronic pancreatitis only if the pancreatic duct is dilated to a diameter over 5 mm. Since there are multiple points of ductal obstruction in most patients with this disease, the pancreatic ductogram in the typical case will resemble a "chain of lakes." When the indications for pancreaticojejunostomy are restricted to patients who have large ducts, 80% will experience satisfactory relief of pain following this operation according to Prinz and Greenlee. When the pancreatic duct is not enlarged, pancreaticojejunostomy is contraindicated. The diameter of the pancreatic duct can generally be determined preoperatively by endoscopic radiographic cholangiopancreatography (ERCP). Otherwise, it will be necessary to obtain a pancreatic ductogram in the operating room prior to performing a pancreaticojejunostomy.

Pancreatic Resection
(See Chaps. 59–61.)

Whipple Pancreatoduodenectomy
When the chronic pancreatitis appears to be located primarily in the head of the pancreas or the uncinate process, or when these areas are the site of a pseudoaneurysm, a resection of the head of the pancreas may be necessary. In this case the usual Whipple operation is modified by preserving the stomach and pylorus, as illustrated in Chap. 59. In performing this operation for chronic pancreatitis, it may be somewhat more difficult to free the portal vein from the pancreas than when one does a Whipple operation for ampullary carcinoma. However, anastomosing the cut end of the pancreatic duct to the jejunum will be more secure because the duct in chronic pancreatitis is fibrotic and holds sutures quite well with a low rate of postoperative pancreatic fistula. The mortality rate following pancreatoduodenectomy for chronic pancreatitis is probably no more than 3%, a figure lower than that which follows the same operation in patients with carcinoma. When the tail and body of the pancreas are preserved, the incidence of postoperative diabetes will be low.

Distal Pancreatectomy
When the primary location of the chronic pancreatitis appears to be localized in the body and tail of the pancreas, and when the pancreatic duct is too small for a successful side-to-side pancreaticojejunostomy, then resecting the distal portion of the pancreas may be indicated if the patient suffers intractable pain. If it is possible to dissect the fibrotic pancreas away from the splenic vein, it may occasionally be possible to perform a distal pancreatectomy with preservation of the spleen. Otherwise, this operation is done by the technique described in Chap. 61. Distal pancreatectomy for pancreatitis in the alcoholic patient is not generally effective in relieving pain according to White and Hart.

Subtotal and Total Pancreatectomy
Frey and Child performed an 80%–95% pancreatectomy with preservation of the duodenum. A 2-cm remnant of the pancreatic head was left on the duodenum and the pancreatoduodenal blood vessels were preserved to guarantee adequacy of the duodenal blood supply. Special attention must be devoted to avoiding trauma to the distal common bile duct. If the uncinate process is diseased, it must be resected or the patient's pain may not be relieved. Although the technical details can be mastered, this has not proved to be a very satisfactory operation for a chronic alcoholic because of the difficulty that the alcoholic patient will experience in controlling the resulting diabetes. The same objection applies to a total pancreatoduodenectomy for intractable chronic pancreatitis in the alcoholic patient.

Nonsurgical Treatment

Some internists believe that if they persist in conservative management of patients with intractable pain from chronic pancreatitis, the disease will "burn out" and pain will eventually be relieved. There is no evidence that this concept is valid. On the other hand, long-term survival of the alcoholic patient with chronic pancreatitis is not likely, whether or not he has undergone a successful operation for the pancreatitis. This is because most of the patients do not discontinue their consumption of alcohol, and the cause of death is generally some complication of alcoholism. Aside from encouraging the patient to change his drinking habits, medical management requires medication for pain and enzyme replacement therapy for malabsorption secondary to exocrine insufficiency.

A positive indication for continuing nonsurgical management of chronic pancreatitis is the presence of severe hepatic cirrhosis, especially with portal hypertension.

Indications

Chronic pancreatitis producing *intractable* pain not responsive to medical treatment. If the pancreatic duct is dilated (diameter of 5–7 mm), perform pancreaticojejunostomy. Otherwise, pancreatic resection of some type may be required.

Preoperative Care

Evaluate hepatic function.

Rule out portal hypertension.

Establish nutritional rehabilitation if necessary.

Order ERCP.

Complete an upper GI X-ray series to rule out duodenal obstruction.

Rule out biliary calculi by X-ray or sonography.

Pitfalls and Danger Points

Failure to rule out portal hypertension

Overlooking pancreatic carcinoma (In any large series of operations for chronic pancreatitis, there will be a few cases of pancreatic carcinoma. It is possible that chronic pancreatitis does indeed predispose the patient to pancreatic cancer. Before deciding on an operative procedure, biopsy suspicious areas. Aspiration cytology in the operating room may be helpful in this situation.)

Operative Strategy

Since the dilated pancreatic ducts are thick walled and fibrotic the pancreaticojejunal anastomosis is a safe procedure in these cases. One layer of sutures generally suffices.

Operative Technique

Exposure

Make a midline incision from the xiphoid to a point 4–5 cm below the umbilicus. Separate the greater omentum from the middle of the transverse colon for a sufficient distance to expose the pancreas. Divide the peritoneal attachments between the pancreas and the posterior wall of the stomach.

Incising the Pancreatic Duct

The main pancreatic duct is generally located about one-third of the distance from the cephalad to the caudal margin of the pancreas. If the duct cannot be palpated, inserting a 22-gauge needle and attempting to aspirate pancreatic juice may serve to locate the pancreatic duct. If the duct has not been successfully visualized by a preoperative ERCP, perform a ductogram in the operating room by aspirating 2 ml of pancreatic juice with a 22-gauge needle; inject an equal amount of dilute Hypaque into the duct. If there is suspicion that the common duct is obstructed by the chronic pancreatitis, perform a cholangiogram in the operating room.

Once the pancreatic duct has been identified, it should be opened by making an incision along its anterior wall. The incision should open the entire duct from the head to the tail of the pancreas. This may be done with a Potts scissors or with a scalpel (**Fig. 63–1**). Continue the duct incision further into the head of the pancreas than is shown in the illustrations. Secure hemostasis with an electrocautery. Occasional bleeding points may require a fine PG suture-ligature. If a stricture of the pancreatic duct is encountered, insert a probe through the strictured area and incise the anterior wall of the duct with a scalpel over the probe. Remove any calculi or debris that may have collected in the ductal system.

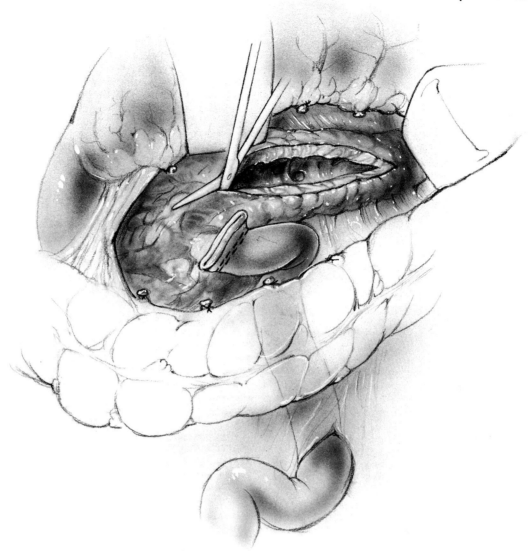

Fig. 63–1

Constructing the Roux-Y Jejunostomy

Prepare the proximal jejunum for a Roux-Y as illustrated in Fig. 55–1. Select a suitable point about 12–15 cm beyond the ligament of Treitz. After a sufficient amount of mesentery has been divided, apply the TA-55 stapling device to the jejunum and fire the 3.5 mm staples. Apply an Allen clamp just proximal to the stapling device. Divide the jejunum flush with the cephalad side of the stapler with a scalpel. Lightly electrocoagulate the everted mucosa and remove the stapler.

Make a 3-cm incision in an avascular area of the transverse mesocolon. Pass the limb of jejunum through this incision and position it side-to-side to the open pancreatic duct. The stapled cut end of the jejunum should be approximated to the tail of the pancreas and the distal jejunum to the head. Now incise the antimesenteric border of jejunum over a length approximately equal to the incision in the pancreatic duct using a scalpel or electrocautery. Since the fibrotic pancreas accepts sutures nicely, one layer of sutures is sufficient. For the posterior layer of the anastomosis, approximate the full thickness of the jejunum to the incision in the pancreatic

227

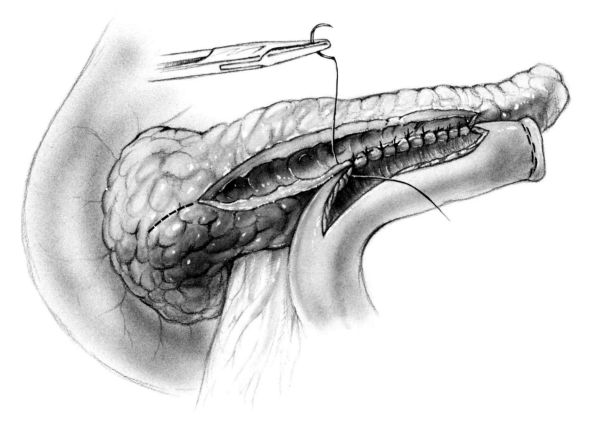

Fig. 63–2

duct. Use 4–0 Vicryl interrupted sutures. Insert the needle through both the mucosal and seromuscular portions of the jejunal wall. Then pass the needle through the fibrotic parenchyma of pancreas and through the pancreatic duct. Tie the suture with the knot inside the lumen of the pancreatic duct **(Fig. 63–2).** For the anterior layer of the anastomosis use a seromucosal or Lembert stitch on the jejunum. Then pass the needle through the full thickness of the duct including some of the pancreatic parenchyma **(Figs. 63–3** and **63–4a** and **63–4b).**

Close the defect in the mesocolon by inserting fine interrupted sutures between the mesocolon and the serosa of the jejunum.

At a point at least 50 cm distal to the pancreaticojejunostomy, construct an end-to-side jejunojejunostomy to complete the Roux-Y anastomosis. We generally accomplish this amastomosis by stapling as described in Figs. 19–36 to 19–40.

If desired, make a puncture wound in the left upper quadrant and insert a Jackson-Pratt closed-suction silicone drainage catheter down to the region of the pancreaticojejunal anastomosis. Close the abdomen in routine fashion.

Postoperative Care

Discontinue nasogastric suction as soon as bowel function has resumed. At this time, also initiate oral feeding. Administer perioperative antibiotics for 24 hours.

Postoperative Complications

Pancreatic fistula

Abdominal or wound infection

228

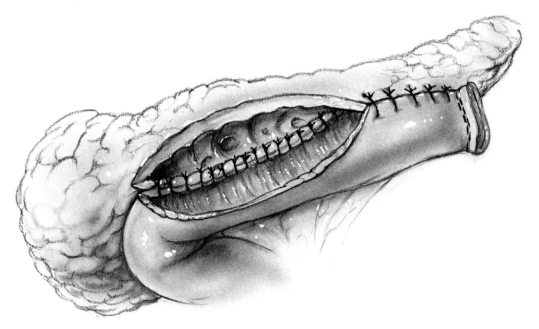

Fig. 63–3

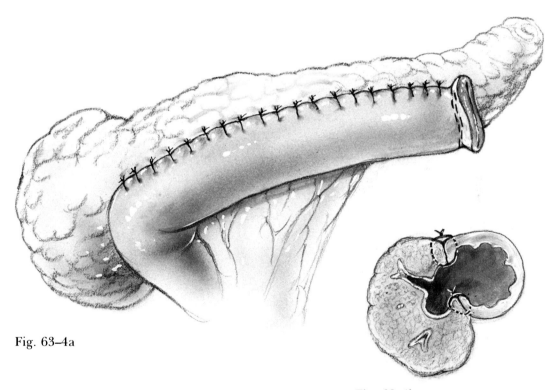

Fig. 63–4a

Fig. 63–4b

References

Frey CF, Child CG III (1976) Pancreatectomy for chronic pancreatitis. Ann Surg 184: 403

Prinz RA, Greenlee HB (1981) Pancreatic duct drainage in 100 patients with chronic pancreatitis. Ann Surg 194:313

White TT, Hart HJ (1979) Pancreaticojejunostomy versus resection in the treatment of chronic pancreatitis. Am J Surg 138:129

229

Spleen

64 Splenectomy for Disease

Indications

Since the specific therapy for the group of diseases that require splenectomy is often in a state of flux and since some of the conditions are complicated by problems of coagulation, it is important that the indications and timing for surgery be worked out in close cooperation with an experienced hematologist. Splenectomy is generally indicated for patients with hereditary anemias (spherocytosis, elliptocytosis, nonspherocytic hemolytic anemia), primary hypersplenism, and chronic idiopathic thrombocytopenic purpura. Patients with autoimmune hemolytic anemia, secondary hypersplenism, thalassemia, myelofibrosis, chronic lymphatic leukemia, and lymphoma also may benefit from splenectomy in selected situations. Until recently splenectomy was a routine part of the staging procedure for patients with Hodgkin's disease, but this is no longer universally accepted.

Primary splenic tumor

Splenic abscess

Splenic cysts, parasitic and nonparasitic

Under unusual circumstances, a large number of other diseases may be benefited by splenectomy, such as Gaucher's disease, sarcoidosis, Felty's syndrome, Neimann-Pick's disease, and Fanconi's syndrome.

Preoperative Care

Consult with an experienced hematologist concerning blood coagulation factors in the patient and the careful cross-matching of an adequate quantity of blood. For patients with thrombocytopenia, preparations should be made to have platelets and other coagulation factors on reserve. Do not administer the platelets prior to ligating the splenic artery in patients with thrombocytopenia as the platelets will be promptly destroyed.

Insert nasogastric tube prior to operation.

Administer perioperative antibiotics.

Remember that in patients with giant splenomegaly, portal hypertension, and pancytopenia (as may occur in myelofibrosis), preoperative occlusion of the splenic artery by transcatheter infarction of the spleen may be accomplished in the angiography suite (Levy, Wasserman, and Pitha). Splenectomy should be performed promptly after completion of the splenic artery occlusion, as necrosis of the spleen and sepsis are otherwise likely to occur.

Pitfalls and Danger Points

Intraoperative hemorrhage

Postoperative hemorrhage

Injuring the greater curvature of the stomach

233

Injuring the pancreas

Postoperative sepsis, especially in immunologically impaired patients

Failure to remove accessory spleen

Operative Strategy

Avoiding Intraoperative Hemorrhage

Perhaps the single most important method of avoiding serious intraoperative bleeding is to be sure that the exposure is adequate for each step of the operation. For the large spleen, this requires a long incision, although it is rarely necessary to perform a thoracic extension. Frequently, the use of a chain retractor to elevate the left costal margin will greatly improve exposure.

A second important method of avoiding the laceration of a major vein is the meticulous dissection and individual ligation of each of the important vessels. When performing splenectomy for hematological disorders, we prefer to isolate the splenic artery as the first step in the splenectomy. The splenic artery may be approached from the lesser curvature portion of the stomach by entering the lesser sac at this point. An alternative approach is to divide the gastrocolic omentum, thereby exposing the upper border of the pancreas. When the splenic artery is ligated before manipulating the spleen, it will be noted that a large spleen frequently diminishes considerably in size and thus makes the dissection safer.

Patients with portal hypertension, as in myelofibrosis, also require clamping and ligating of the splenophrenic and splenorenal ligaments.

Preventing Postoperative Hemorrhage

At the conclusion of the splenectomy, it is important to achieve complete hemostasis in the bed of the spleen, especially along the tail of the pancreas, the left adrenal gland, and the posterior abdominal wall. Some of the bleeding points can be con-

trolled by electrocoagulation; others require clamping. Bleeding from the tail of the pancreas almost always necessitates the insertion of fine suture-ligatures on atraumatic needles because the blood vessels tend to retract into the pancreatic tissue. If there is diffuse oozing due to inadequate platelets or other coagulation deficiencies, it may be necessary after the spleen is removed to administer platelets, fresh frozen plasma, and other coagulation factors. After administering these substances and testing the blood for various coagulation deficiencies, continue to observe the operative site until the bleeding stops. Do not simply insert a few drains and close the abdomen. The latter course will often lead to the development of a large hematoma in the left upper quadrant. Some of these hematomas may become infected and cause a subphrenic abscess.

Avoiding Pancreatic Injury

The greatest risk of injuring the tail of the pancreas occurs when the splenic blood supply is being ligated and divided at the hilus of the spleen. When carrying out this step, it is important clearly to identify the tail of the pancreas and to divide the blood vessels without injuring the pancreas. If each clamp contains only a blood vessel and not other tissue, then the pancreas will not be crushed by a large hemostat. Nor will it be transected inadvertently.

Avoiding Trauma to the Stomach

During the course of clamping and dividing the short gastric vessels it is easy—especially when a large spleen is being removed—to include the wall of the gastric greater curvature within a hemostat aimed at a short gastric vessel. In other situations, the serosa of the stomach may be denuded during the process of dissecting out these

234

blood vessels. In either case, the injury may result in a gastric fistula, a serious and life-threatening complication. Consequently, take care to identify clearly each of the vessels and to achieve hemostasis and division of the short gastric vessels without damaging the stomach.

In addition, a postoperative gastric fistula may be avoided if the greater curvature is inverted with a continuous or interrupted layer of seromuscular Lembert sutures. In this way the ligated stumps of the short gastric vessels and any possibly traumatized gastric wall are inverted together. In cases where division of the short gastric vessels has been accomplished with great ease and under conditions of good visibility, one may be able to guarantee that the greater curvature has not been traumatized. In these cases, it may not be necessary to invert this region of the stomach.

Preventing Postoperative Sepsis

In the immunologically deficient patient, subphrenic sepsis in the bed of the excised spleen may occur, especially in those patients who have sustained a postoperative hematoma. Therefore, the first step in preventing this complication is to ascertain that good hemostasis has been achieved. Secondly, we believe that the use of prophylactic antibiotics administered intravenously at the induction of anesthesia and repeated at intervals for the next 24 hours, is an important means of helping to prevent this complication. This is especially true if there is any danger that the stomach or colon may be entered during a difficult dissection. Whether irrigating the field and the abdominal wound with a dilute antibiotic solution provides any *additional* protection is not statistically validated at this time; however, we choose to carry out this type of lavage during splenectomy.

We agree with Traetow, Fabri, and Carey that inserting a drain to the splenic bed appears to increase the incidence of postoperative subphrenic sepsis. This is especially true for the latex type of drain that permits the entrance of bacteria from the skin down the drain tract. If the pancreas has been injured, or if the hemostasis cannot be completely controlled despite intensive effort, then a drain is necessary. However, it is important to use a closed-suction type of drain, either one or two, passed through snug puncture wounds and sutured to the skin. By applying iodophor ointment to these puncture wounds around the suction catheter daily and covering with sterile gauze, the incidence of drain tract infection and subphrenic abscesses will probably be less than if a latex drain is used (see Vol. I, Chap. 3). Also, removing the drain within 5 days appears to lower the risk of infection.

Accessory Spleen

Occasionally, the presence of a residual accessory spleen will impair the therapeutic effect of a splenectomy. In some reported cases, performing a second laparotomy and removing an accessory spleen has resulted in considerable improvement. Consequently, it is important in patients splenectomized for hematological diseases to identify and remove accessory spleens. The most common locations of accessory spleens are in the hilus of the spleen as well as in the gastrosplenic, the splenocolic, and the splenorenal ligaments. Also search the perirenal area, the tail of the pancreas, the small bowel mesentery, and the presacral region for accessory spleens, although these locations are less commonly the site of an accessory spleen than is the area around the splenic hilus.

Operative Technique

Incision

In the patient who has a small spleen, as is often the case with idiopathic thrombocytopenic purpura, a long left subcostal incision reaching at least to the anterior axillary line, provides excellent exposure. In some cases the subcostal incision may be improved by a Kehr extension up the middle to the xiphocostal junction, as illustrated **Fig. 64–1.** In patients with marked splenomegaly, a long midline incision may be preferable, especially if the patient has a narrow costal arch. Use an electrocoagulator to incise the abdominal wall. In order to provide adequate exposure, a midline incision must extend a considerable distance below the umbilicus. Then, apply a chain retractor to elevate the left costal margin and to draw it in a cephalad and lateral direction.

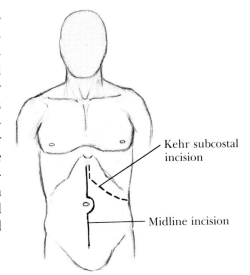

Kehr subcostal incision

Midline incision

Fig. 64–1

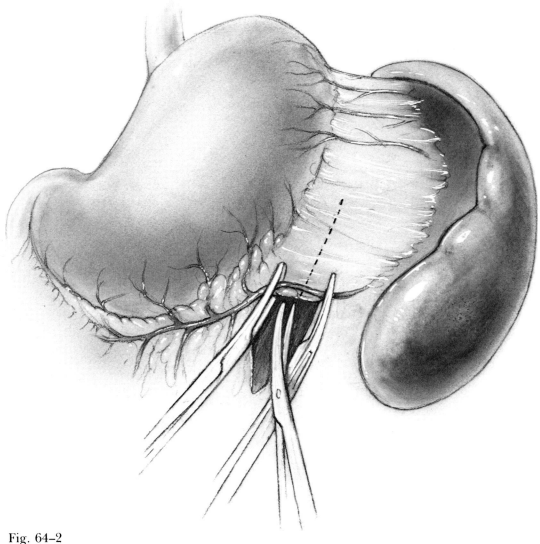

Fig. 64–2

Ligating the Splenic Artery

Incise the avascular portion of the gastrohepatic ligament along the middle of the lesser curvature portion of the stomach and elevate the stomach to expose the upper border of the pancreas. Palpate the splenic artery as it courses along the upper border of the pancreas towards the spleen. If it appears that ligating the splenic artery near the pancreatic tail will be difficult, then identify the pancreas behind the lesser curvature of the stomach and incise the peritoneum over the splenic artery above the body of the pancreas. Carefully pass a blunt-tipped right-angle Mixter clamp around the splenic artery. Temporarily, occlude this artery either with a vas-

cular clamp or by doubly encircling it with a Vesseloop or a narrow umbilical tape fixed in place with a small hemostat.

In most cases, approach the splenic artery by opening the gastrocolic omentum outside the gastroepiploic arcade, applying clamps, dividing and ligating serially with 2–0 cotton. Also divide and ligate the left gastroepiploic vessel **(Fig. 64–2).** After a window in the omentum has been achieved, identify the splenic artery by palpating along the superior border of the pancreatic body or tail. Open the peritoneum over the artery and encircle the artery with a 2–0 cotton ligature **(Fig. 64–3).** Then tie this ligature.

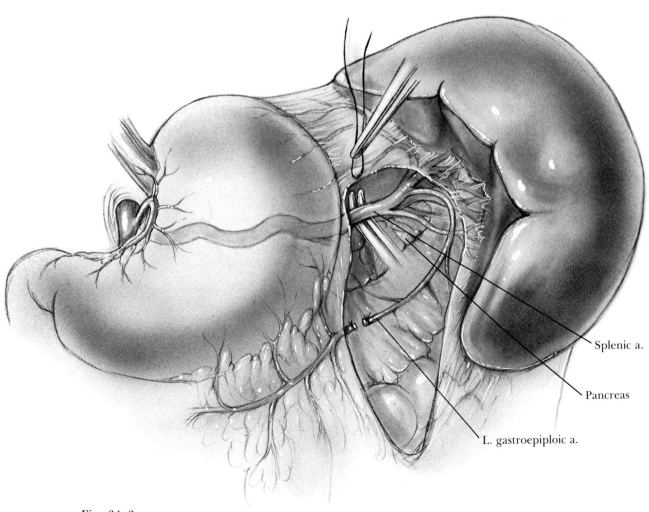

Splenic a.

Pancreas

L. gastroepiploic a.

Fig. 64–3

Sometimes, accomplishing the identification of the splenic artery requires division of the lower short gastric vessels. If this step has not already been accomplished, then identify, clamp, divide, and ligate these structures with 2–0 cotton **(Fig. 64–4).** Continue the division of the short gastric vessels in a cephalad direction as long as the exposure is satisfactory. If the upper short gastric vessel is not long enough to be divided easily at this time, delay this until the spleen has been completely mobilized.

Mobilizing the Spleen

With the left hand, retract the spleen in a medial direction to expose the splenophrenic and splenorenal ligaments. These are generally avascular. Divide the ligaments with a Metzenbaum scissors or an electrocautery. Only in the presence of portal hypertension will it be necessary to ligate a number of bleeding vessels in these ligaments. Insert the left index finger behind the incised splenorenal ligament and continue the incision both by sharp and blunt dissection until the spleen has been freed from the capsule of Gerota and the diaphragm **(Figs. 64–5** and **64–6).**

In the same plane, slide the hand behind the posterior surface of the pancreas and elevate both the tail of the pancreas and the attached spleen into the abdominal incision. Tearing the splenic capsule by rough maneuvering during this step, will produce unnecessary bleeding and possible postoperative peritoneal splenosis. Apply a number of moist gauze pads to the bed of the spleen in the posterior abdominal wall.

Slide the index finger behind the splenocolic ligament and divide this ligament, releasing the colon and its attached omentum from the lower pole of the spleen. This dissection will leave the spleen attached only by the splenic artery and vein and perhaps one or two remaining short gastric vessels.

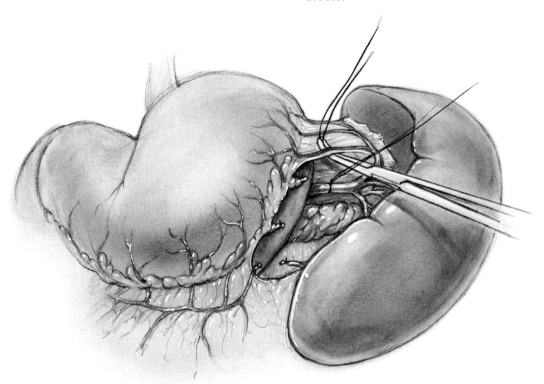

Fig. 64–4

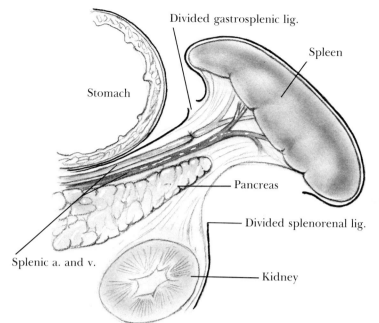

Stomach

Divided gastrosplenic lig.

Spleen

Pancreas

Divided splenorenal lig.

Splenic a. and v.

Kidney

Fig. 64–5

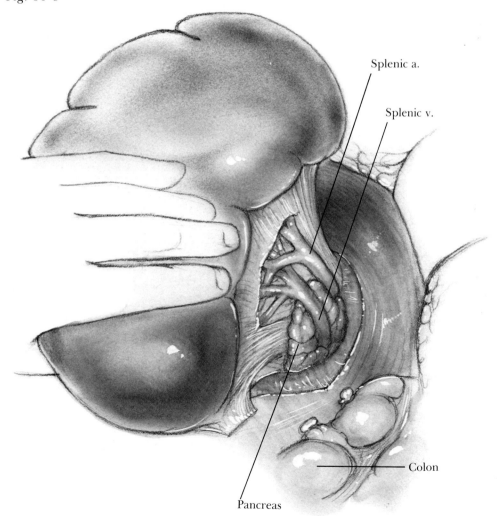

Splenic a.

Splenic v.

Colon

Pancreas

Fig. 64–6

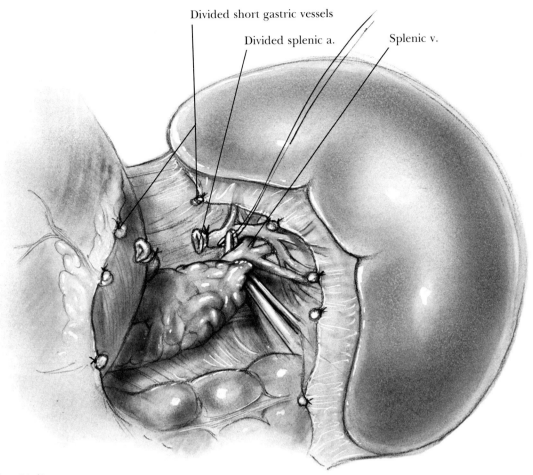

Divided short gastric vessels

Divided splenic a.

Splenic v.

Fig. 64–7

Ligating the Splenic Vessels

With the spleen elevated out of the abdominal cavity, search the posterior aspect of the splenic hilus for the tail of the pancreas. Gently separate the tail of the pancreas from the posterior wall of the splenic artery and vein. Carefully divide and ligate small branches of the splenic vessels entering the tail of the pancreas. Identify the previously ligated splenic artery. Ligate the artery again near the hilus. Leave sufficient stump of splenic artery (1 cm). Then divide the splenic artery. Further dissection will reveal the splenic vein. This may be a large structure, or it may have divided into several branches by the time it reaches the splenic hilus. Carefully encircle either the main splenic vein or each of its branches with 2–0 cotton ligatures **(Fig. 64–7).** Tie the ligatures and divide the veins between ligatures. Remove the spleen.

Search the area of the pancreatic tail, the kidney, the gastrosplenic ligament, the

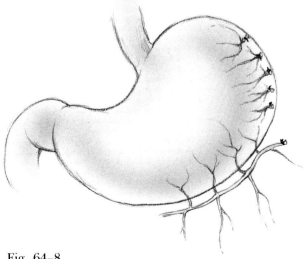

Fig. 64–8

omentum, the small and large bowel mesentery, and the pelvis for accessory spleens. Remove the gauze pads from the splenic bed and accomplish complete hemostasis utilizing an electrocoagulator and

Inverting the Greater Curvature of Stomach

Carefully inspect the greater curvature of the stomach. If there is the slightest suspicion of any damage to the tissue in this area, turn in the greater curvature together with the ligated stumps of the short gastric vessels. Use continuous or interrupted Lembert sutures of 4–0 atraumatic PG suture material to accomplish this step, which will avoid a possible gastric fistula (**Figs. 64–8** to **64–11**).

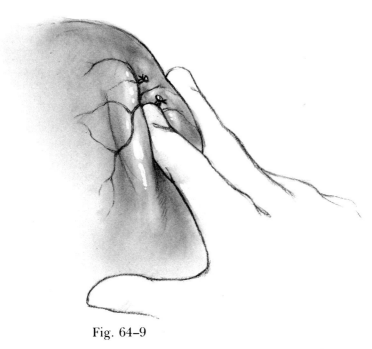

Fig. 64–9

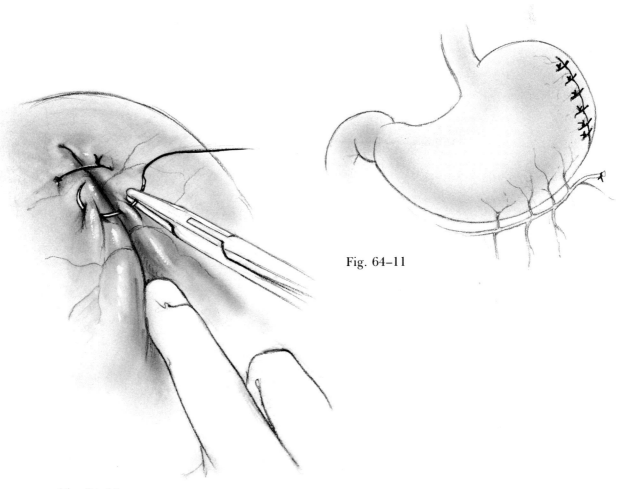

Fig. 64–11

Fig. 64–10

Abdominal Closure

Irrigate the upper abdomen with a dilute antibiotic solution. After aspirating this solution with a suction device, close the abdomen in routine fashion. Do not insert any drains unless there has been an injury to the pancreas or unless complete hemostasis has not been possible to achieve. In either of these cases, insert one or two medium-sized plastic closed-suction drains of the Hemovac or Jackson-Pratt types, through one or two puncture wounds in the area of the splenic bed and apply suction.

Postoperative Care

Continue nasogastric suction until bowel function has resumed.

Continue perioperative antibiotics for 24 hours.

Continue steroid medication in those patients who were on this therapy prior to and during operation.

Monitor the patient's blood coagulation status and check for postoperative bleeding. Frequently, the platelet count will rise postoperatively. This does not generally require any treatment except in patients with myelofibrosis. Patients with this disease have been reported to suffer postoperative portal vein thrombosis. They should probably receive prophylactic treatment with aspirin and low-dose heparin (Gordon, Schaffner, Bennett, and Schwartz).

The leucocyte count may also rise markedly following splenectomy. This does not necessarily indicate sepsis.

If a patient has undergone a total splenectomy, be certain that the patient and his family are aware of the risks of overwhelming postsplenectomy sepsis. The patient should wear a Medic-Alert bracelet recording the fact that he has undergone splenectomy. Administer Pneumovax vaccine. This will protect against a majority of the types of pneumococcal infections. Young children should probably receive prophylactic treatment with penicillin throughout childhood. It is not clear that prophylactic antibiotics are indicated in adult life.

Postoperative Complications

Bleeding
Subphrenic abscess
Acute pancreatitis
Gastric fistula
Venous thrombosis

References

Gordon DH, Schaffner D, Bennett JM, Schwartz SI (1978) Postsplenectomy thrombocytosis: its association with mesenteric, portal, and/or renal thrombosis in patients with myeloproliferative disorders. Arch Surg 113:713

Levy J, Wasserman P, Pitha N (1979) Presplenectomy transcatheter occlusion of the splenic artery. Arch Surg 114:198

Traetow WD, Fabri PJ, Carey LC (1980) Changing indications for splenectomy. Arch Surg 115:447

65 Operation for Splenic Trauma

Concept: Splenectomy or Splenorrhaphy

Following splenectomy for trauma, children experience fatal sepsis at a rate 58 to 65 times greater than that experienced by the nonsplenectomized child. Sudden in onset, the sepsis is often fatal within 24 hours despite good medical treatment. It is generally caused by the encapsulated *Pneumococcus, Meningococcus, Hemophilus,* or sometimes *Eschericia coli.* Although the cases of fatal sepsis appear to be somewhat more common when a splenectomy is performed in a child under the age of 5 years, and although the fatal sepsis is likely to occur within 2 years of the splenectomy, there are many reports of fatal sepsis due to meningitis, pneumonia, and other causes, sometimes occurring many years after splenectomy. While it is difficult to determine exactly how much increase there is in the risk of fatal sepsis following splenectomy for trauma in the adult, there is general agreement that there is indeed some increase in this risk (Leonard, Giebink, Baesl, and Krivit; Schwartz, Sterioff, Mucha, Melton, and Offord; Singer).

For all of the above reasons, it is imperative not to remove the traumatized spleen in children unless conservative management is not safe. In adults also the spleen should be salvaged unless it has been pulverized, separated from its blood supply, or unless the patient is unstable and preservation of the spleen would increase the risk of operative or postoperative fatality.

Children who have evidence of isolated trauma to the spleen can, in most cases, be successfully managed by nonoperative means (Ein, Shandling, Simpson, and Stephens) unless they have lost more than 25%–30% of their blood volume. These children should be observed in an intensive care unit with frequent monitoring of vital signs for 2–3 days. After an additional 4–5 days of observation, including serial liver-spleen scanning, the child may be sent home. After an additional week of bed rest at home, and 3–4 weeks of restricted activity, the child may return to his normal way of life. Delayed splenic rupture during or after nonoperative management has been quite uncommon.

Whether conservative management is also indicated in the good-risk adult patient is a question that has not yet been answered. In the adult, where the injury is more likely to be an automobile accident rather than an athletic injury, there is a greater risk of overlooking serious injuries unrelated to the spleen if nonoperative management is pursued in a large number of cases. Nonoperative therapy is not at this time recommended for the usual splenic injury to the adult. The remainder of this chapter concerns itself with the management of splenic trauma in the adult patient, although the child in whom nonoperative management has failed, can be managed by the same surgical principles.

Indications

Splenectomy is indicated for the traumatized spleen if the patient's condition is unstable, if he has suffered multiple injuries, if there is gross fecal contamination, if the spleen is fragmented beyond repair, or if the spleen has been separated from its blood supply. Do not risk the patient's life at any time in order to preserve an injured spleen, especially in patients over age 50.

Splenorrhaphy or partial splenectomy is indicated in good-risk patients who do not have the above indications for splenectomy.

Preoperative Care

Resuscitate the patient by means of adequate fluid and blood replacement.

Insert a nasogastric tube.

If the diagnosis is in doubt, perform a liver-spleen or CT scan.

Pitfalls and Danger Points

Failure to control bleeding

Traumatizing the pancreas

Operative Strategy

Splenectomy

Unlike the technique described for the removal of the diseased spleen in Chap. 64, in removing the injured spleen initiate the dissection for removing the injured spleen by dividing the splenorenal and splenocolic ligaments as the first step in the operation. This will permit delivery of the spleen and the tail of the pancreas into the incision. Then hemostasis can be maintained by compressing the splenic artery between the thumb and index finger during the rest of the dissection. In the rare case where a giant spleen has been traumatized, it may be advantageous to identify the splenic artery (see Fig. 64–1) and to ligate it before delivering the enlarged spleen.

Iatrogenic Injuries

In past years, 20%–40% of all splenectomies have been performed as a result of iatrogenic injuries with an average mortality rate of 15% (Morgenstern, 1977). Most cases of iatrogenic splenic injuries result from avulsing a patch of the splenic capsule when the stomach or the transverse colon is retracted away from the spleen. Since the splenic pulp has not been damaged in most of these injuries, it is a simple matter to control the bleeding by applying a hemostatic agent, such as Surgicel or Avitene, and then by tamponading the area with a large gauze pad. Prior to closing the abdomen, remove the gauze pad carefully and inspect the area for bleeding. This technique is not effective if the injury occurs at the hilus of the spleen.

Splenic Fracture

The splenic artery and vein divide into 2–4 trunks prior to entering the spleen. The intrasplenic branches generally travel in a horizontal direction. Since most splenic fractures also travel in a transverse direction, often only one or two small blood vessels have been torn. To achieve hemostasis may require only that a hemostatic agent, Hemoclips, or suture-ligatures be applied; or that the laceration be sutured; or that a partial splenectomy be performed. Partial splenectomy is indicated if a portion of the spleen has been separated from its blood supply. This is suggested by a cyanotic discoloration of the devascularized segment compared to the remainder of the spleen.

Principles basic to all splenic suturing are adequate exposure combined with a *complete mobilization of the spleen* into the abdominal incision. This step is followed by temporary occlusion of the splenic artery by means of a Vesseloop and debridement of the devitalized tissue. Only by dividing the splenorenal and splenocolic ligaments and delivering the spleen together with the tail of the pancreas into the incision, can adequate repair of a ruptured spleen be undertaken. The best suture material appears to be 2–0 chromic catgut on an atraumatic straight or curved needle.

After replacing the repaired spleen into its natural bed, always wait 10–15 minutes and reinspect the spleen to be sure that the bleeding has indeed been completely controlled.

In some cases, a narrow pedicle of viable omentum may be placed into a fracture and sutured into place with continuous chromic catgut.

After removing a portion of the spleen, it is not necessary to apply sutures to close the cut end of the spleen if good hemostasis can be achieved by means of Hemoclips and suture-ligatures in the splenic pulp. When sutures are inserted, they should penetrate the capsule and then be returned as a mattress stitch. In tying the sutures, take care not to tie them so tightly that they rupture the capsule. If the proper tension is applied to the knot, bolsters of teflon, omentum, or Surgicel will not often be necessary.

Further discussions of surgical techniques for preserving the spleen can be found in papers by Morgenstern and Shapiro and by Buntain and Lynn.

Operative Technique

Incision

In the unstable patient, make a midline incision from the xiphoid to a point well below the umbilicus. In the stable patient, a midline incision is suitable for the patient with a narrow costal arch. For the wide-bodied patient, make a long left subcostal incision, dividing the muscular layers with the electrocoagulator to accelerate the operation. A Kehr extension, which extends up the midline from the medial tip of the subcostal incision and divides the linea alba to the xiphocostal junction, provides excellent exposure. In both the midline and the subcostal incisions, exposure is further enhanced by retracting the left costal margin anterolaterally and in a cephalad direction by means of the "chain" retractor.

Splenectomy

When the spleen is shattered, or when the hilus has sustained sufficient damage to separate the spleen from its blood supply, or when the patient's condition is unstable, emergency splenectomy is the operation of choice. In performing splenectomy for trauma, it is not necessary to isolate and ligate the splenic artery as a first step in the operation (as described in Chap. 64) unless the traumatized spleen is greatly enlarged due to a preexisting disease.

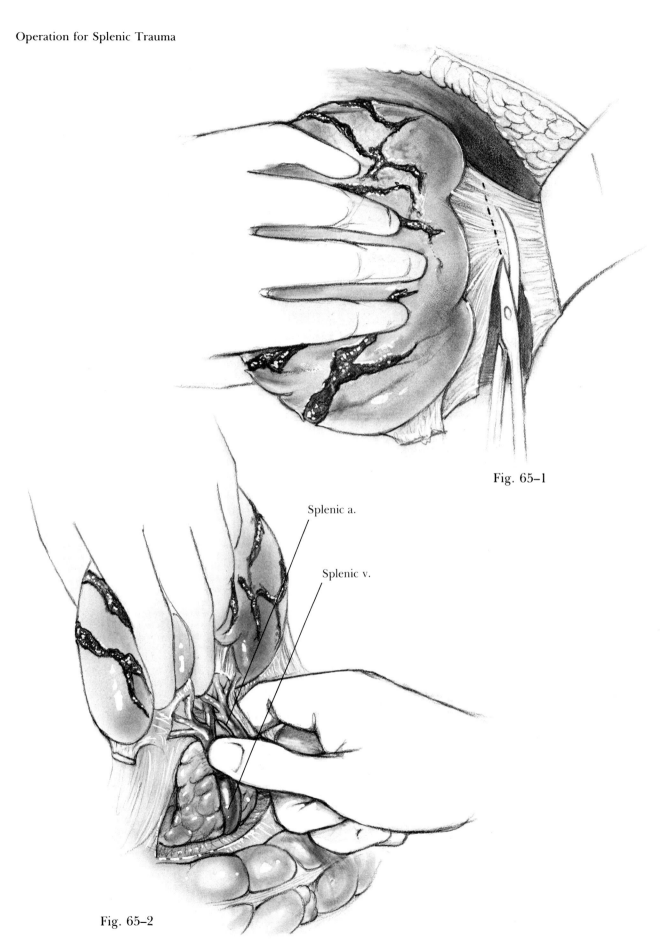

Fig. 65–1

Splenic a.

Splenic v.

Fig. 65–2

Take a position on the patient's right and retract the spleen in a medial direction with the left hand. Then divide the splenorenal, the splenophrenic, and the splenocolic ligaments **(Fig. 65–1)**. In an emergency situation the experienced surgeon can often perform much of this dissection bluntly with his fingers. After the ligaments have been divided, slide the right hand behind the tail of the pancreas and elevate the tail of the pancreas together with the damaged spleen into the incision. Hemostasis can be achieved promptly by compressing the splenic artery between the thumb and index finger in the space be-

tween the tip of the pancreas and the hilus of the spleen **(Fig. 65–2)**. Pack the posterior abdominal wall with moist gauze pads. Expose the posterior aspect of the splenic hilus and identify the splenic artery and vein. It is generally simple to divide these structures between hemostats or ligatures **(Fig. 65–3)**. This will control most of the bleeding. Now, deliberately dissect out each of the short gastric vessels. Next, divide each vessel between Adson hemostats and remove the spleen and then ligate each of the hemostats with 2–0 or 3–0 cotton. Be sure to apply a second ligature to the splenic artery for added security and to control the minor bleeding points around the tail of the pancreas with fine suture-ligatures. Finally, remove the gauze pads

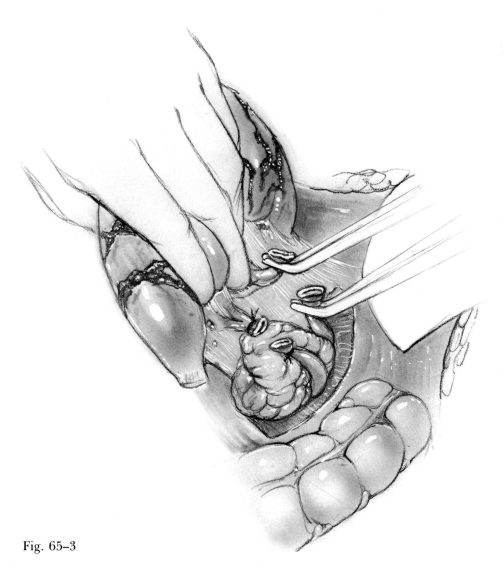

Fig. 65–3

from the splenic bed and achieve complete hemostasis with ligatures and electro-coagulation.

With this technique there need not be any haste to obtain hemostasis, because early in the operation the surgeon can control most of the bleeding by compressing the vessels at the hilus of the spleen with his fingers. Otherwise, hasty dissection may traumatize the tail of the pancreas.

Carefully inspect the greater curvature of the stomach. If there is any suspicion that the stomach wall has been injured during the dissection or the ligation of the short gastric vessels, insert Lembert sutures to invert this area of stomach as shown in Figs. 64–8 to 64–11.

Selecting the Optimal Technique for Splenic Preservation

Avulsion of Capsule; Superficial Injuries
Iatrogenic injury to the spleen, occurring during the course of vagotomy, hiatus hernia repair, or colon resection has constituted in many institutions the most common single indication for splenectomy in past years. Most of these injuries have involved the avulsion of a relatively small patch of splenic capsule. Superficial inju-

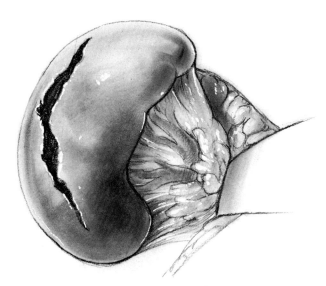

ries of this type are best treated by the application of topical hemostatic agents (see below) rather than splenectomy. A large subcapsular hematoma, on the other hand, is best treated by incising the capsule, by exposing the bleeding points, and then by applying topical hemostatic agents.

Partial Transverse Fracture
The transverse fracture that does not penetrate through the entire thickness of the spleen is a common injury because of the transverse distribution of the splenic blood supply. It is eminently suitable for repair by suturing after hemostasis has been obtained. A description of this technique is given in the section on splenorrhaphy below.

Complete Transverse Fracture
When a transverse fracture of the spleen has divided the organ into two or more segments, it is necessary to determine the viability of each segment. This is easily done because the nonviable spleen develops a purple discoloration. Remove the nonviable segments and retain the viable portion of the spleen after achieving hemostasis. Preserving from one-third to one-half of the normal spleen is very likely to prevent a significant diminution of the patient's immune response to infection. The technique for hemisplenectomy is given below. Be sure to identify and ligate the hilar artery that supplied the amputated segment of spleen.

Longitudinal Fracture
Severe blunt injuries may produce a longitudinal fracture in the long axis of the spleen (Fig. 65–4). Because this type of fracture may lacerate a large number of the transverse branches of the splenic artery and vein, hemostasis is more difficult than is the case with transverse injuries. After controlling the arterial bleeders with Hemoclips and suture-ligatures, the residual oozing can generally be managed by inserting a narrow pedicle of viable omentum and fixing it in place by means of a series of capsular sutures (Fig. 65–5).

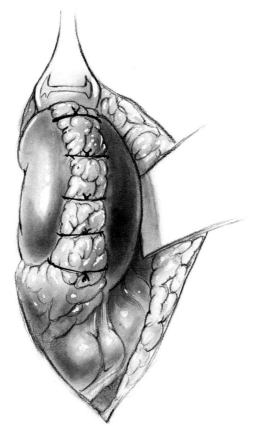

Fig. 65–5

Stellate Fracture

After exploring the depths of the fracture and removing clotted blood, treat the superficial fractures by suturing the capsule. Closing the capsule in this fashion will generally control bleeding from superficial fractures. Alternatively, applying Avitene to the stellate fracture may successfully control all but the arterial bleeders. The efficiency of this topical agent may be enhanced by also inserting capsular sutures.

Any splenic fracture, that significantly involves the hilus of the spleen, generally requires a partial splenectomy to control hilar bleeding, rather than capsular sutures.

Applying Topical Hemostatic Agents

Most of the topical hemostatic agents (Gelfoam, Oxycel, Surgicel, and Avitene) provide a framework for the deposition of platelets, which accelerates the formation of a blood clot. None of these agents will control rapid bleeding. Consequently, it is necessary to slow down the bleeding from the surface of a damaged spleen by local pressure for a few minutes. If the oozing surface is fairly smooth, apply a double sheet of Surgicel gauze. Cover this with a dry gauze pad. Apply even pressure with the gauze pad for 10 minutes. Then gently remove the gauze pad while taking care not to dislodge the sheet of Surgicel, which should now be adherent to the raw surface.

If the bleeding surface is irregular in nature, Avitene is a much better choice than Surgicel. It is very effective for oozing surfaces from traumatized capillaries and sinusoids. In applying Avitene, make certain to use only absolutely dry instruments. Use a forceps to apply enough Avitene to cover the entire bleeding surface for a thickness of 3–4 mm. Apply the Avitene quickly and cover it with a dry gauze pad. Apply constant pressure for at least 5 minutes. If bleeding breaks through one portion of the Avitene, apply an additional layer of dry Avitene. If bleeding continues to break through, remove the Avitene and pursue further efforts to reduce the rate of bleeding by applying Hemoclips or suture-ligatures. Rapid bleeding makes the Avitene gel prematurely, thus making it useless as a hemostatic agent.

Splenorrhaphy

Mobilizing the Spleen

Do not try to repair the spleen without completely mobilizing the spleen and the tail of the pancreas by the same technique described above (see Fig. 65–1). Be sure to free any attachments between the spleen and the omentum. Adequate exposure may also require the division of the lower short gastric vessels. Be very careful not to cause further injury to the spleen when dividing the splenic ligaments. Evacuate liquid and clotted blood from the area. Place a large gauze pad against the posterior abdominal wall in the area of the dissection and ele-

249

vate the spleen and tail of the pancreas into the incision. If any of these maneuvers initiates brisk bleeding, compress the splenic artery and vein between the thumb and index finger at the hilus (see Fig. 65–2). Ligate any of the small vessels at the hilus that may have been lacerated by the trauma.

Suturing the Splenic Capsule

In the case of fractures that have not penetrated the full thickness of the spleen, remove devitalized tissue and blood clot from the traumatized areas. Use a narrow-tipped suction device to provide exposure and occlude bleeding arteries by accurately applying small or medium-sized Hemoclips. In the case of bleeding veins, or arteries that have retracted, use 4–0 or 5–0 vascular sutures. Residual oozing of blood from the sinusoids can be controlled by closing the capsule with interrupted sutures of 2–0 chromic catgut on a medium-sized gastrointestinal atraumatic needle, as illustrated in **Fig. 65–6.** If necessary, these sutures may be inserted in such fashion that they interlock. In other cases, a continuous suture of the same material may prove to be effective. In tying these sutures, take great care not to apply force sufficient to tear the delicate splenic cap-

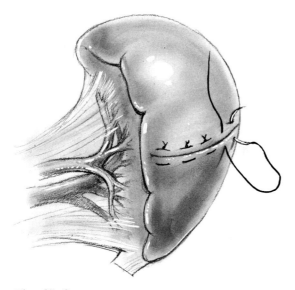

Fig. 65–6

sule. Tie the sutures just tight enough to achieve hemostasis without tearing the spleen. If necessary, use strips or pledgets of teflon felt or even Surgicel gauze; insert the sutures through these pledgets to protect the splenic capsule when the suture is being tied.

Partial Splenectomy

Dividing the Spleen

With a Vesseloop doubly looped around the splenic artery, occlude the splenic artery by applying tension to the Vesseloop with a small hemostat. Then, aspirate all blood clots from the area of injury, especially at the splenic hilus. Ligate the traumatized vessels at the hilus, preserving the blood supply to that portion of the spleen which will be retained. Use a narrow-tipped suction device to expose the bleeding points in the line of the fracture. Use the suction tip to develop a transverse division of the spleen. Apply small Hemoclips to bleeding vessels and continue the dissection until the traumatized section of the spleen has been entirely severed. Remove the specimen. Then release the Vesseloop encircling the splenic artery and observe the cut edge of the splenic remnant for hemostasis. Generally, some oozing will persist requiring suturing of the cut end of the spleen. Use 2–0 chromic catgut on a straight atraumatic needle **(Fig. 65–7).** Although their use should not often be necessary, it is possible to protect the delicate splenic capsule by applying a strip of teflon felt on the anterior surface of the spleen and a second on the posterior surface. Then insert the sutures through the teflon felt as shown on **Fig. 65–8.** Tie each of these mattress sutures. This will achieve satisfactory hemostasis along the cut edge of the spleen.

Replace the splenic remnant in its natural position after making certain that hemostasis is complete in the posterior abdominal wall and in the splenic bed. Use electrocoagulation along the posterior abdominal wall, but if there are bleeding points in the tail of the pancreas, occlude

Postoperative Care

Administer perioperative antibiotics for 12–24 hours.

Observe the patient in an intensive care unit or in another area where vital signs can be carefully observed for 2–3 days. Order hemoglobin and hematocrit determinations every 8 hours for the first 48 hours and then daily for the next 3–4 days.

If there is no significant bleeding or drainage, remove the drain by the 2nd postoperative day.

Keep the patient at bed rest for the first day or two. Thereafter cautiously resume ambulation. Patients, who have had a splenorrhaphy or partial splenectomy, should avoid vigorous athletics for a period of 4–6 weeks.

If a patient has undergone a total splenectomy, be certain that the patient and his family are aware of the risks of overwhelming postsplenectomy sepsis. The patient should wear a Medic-Alert bracelet recording the fact that he has undergone splenectomy. Administer Pneumovax vaccine. This will protect against a majority of the types of pneumococcal infections. Young children should probably receive prophylactic treatment with penicillin throughout childhood. It is not clear that prophylactic antibiotics are indicated in adult life.

Postoperative Complications

Postoperative bleeding. If proper hemostasis has been attained during the operation, this complication is rare.

Infarction of the splenic remnant.

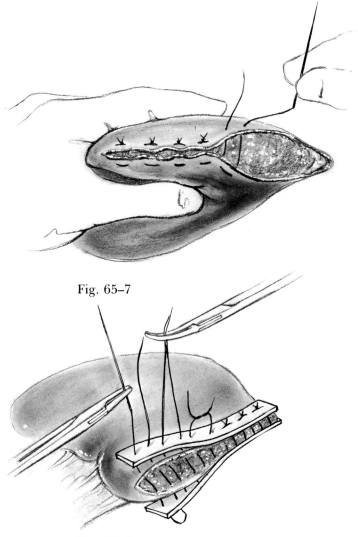

Fig. 65–7

Fig. 65–8

these bleeding points by means of 4–0 or 5–0 suture-ligatures.

Do not close the abdominal incision for at least 10–15 minutes in order to inspect the splenic remnant after it has been replaced into the abdomen. If there is any bleeding, again deliver the remnant of spleen into the abdominal incision and control the bleeding.

Abdominal Closure and Drainage

Close the abdominal incision in the usual fashion after inserting a flat Silastic Jackson-Pratt closed-suction drainage tube through a puncture wound in the left upper quadrant down to the vicinity of the splenic bed.

References

Buntain WL, Lynn H (1979) Splenorrhaphy: changing concepts for the traumatized spleen. Surgery 86:748

Ein SH, Shandling B, Simpson JS, Stephens CA (1978) Nonoperative management of traumatized spleen in children: how and why. Surgery 13:117

Leonard AS, Giebink GS, Baesl TJ, Krivit W (1980) The overwhelming post-splenectomy sepsis problem. World J Surg 4:423

Morgenstern L (1977) The avoidable complications of splenectomy. Surg Gynecol Obstet 145:525

Morgenstern L and Shapiro SJ (1979) Techniques of splenic conservation. Arch Surg 114:449

Pachter HL, Hoffstetter SR, Spencer FC (1981) Evolving concepts in splenic surgery. Ann Surg 194:262

Schwartz PL, Sterioff S, Mucha P, Melton LJ, Offord KP (1982) Postsplenectomy sepsis and mortality in adults. JAMA 248:2279

Singer DB (1973) Postsplenectomy sepsis. In: Rosenberg HS, Bolande RP, (eds) Perspectives in pediatric pathology, Year Book Publishers, Chicago, 1:285

Esophagus

66 Concept: Operations for Reflux Esophagitis, Stricture, Short Esophagus, and Paraesophageal Hernia

Parahiatal and Paraesophageal Hernia

Parahiatal Hernia

Most acquired diaphragmatic hernias enter the chest through the esophageal hiatus. In the typical case, this constitutes a sliding hernia of the esophagogastric junction up into the mediastinum, dragging a fold of peritoneum along with it, just as is the case with a sliding hernia of the cecum. When the abdominal esophagus remains properly attached to the preaortic fascia by means of the phrenoesophageal ligaments, a herniation of the fundus or body of the stomach through the diaphragmatic hiatus into the chest is termed a "paraesophageal" hernia.

MacDougall, Abbott, and Goodhand described five cases where the stomach entered the chest through a congenital defect in the diaphragm, which was situated a few centimeters to the right of the esophageal hiatus, a true *parahiatal* hernia. These authors attributed the defect in the diaphragm to the persistence of a right pneumatoenteric recess. Other authors (Hill and Tobias) state that they have never encountered a true parahiatal hernia that penetrated the diaphragm via any other pathway than the esophageal hiatus itself. In our own experience, we have encountered only one case where the hernia penetrated the left side of the diaphragmatic crus through a defect about 1.5 cm to the left of the normal hiatus. It seems clear that a true parahiatal hernia is extremely rare. A paraesophageal hernia, with a normally situated esophagogastric junction and a normal low esophageal sphincter, is also uncommon, constituting perhaps less than 2% of all acquired diaphragmatic hernias.

Differentiating Paraesophageal from Sliding Hiatus Hernia

By definition, the paraesophageal hernia requires that the esophagogastric junction be fixed to the area of the preaortic fascia and median arcuate ligament. These patients do not suffer from reflux esophagitis. If the paraesophageal hernia is freely reducible, the patients may experience no symptoms. Occasionally, they will suffer from a chronic anemia when a large portion of the stomach is herniated into the chest. This is probably secondary to chronic venous hypertension caused by the diaphragm constricting the stomach, resulting in chronic oozing of blood into the gastric lumen. In some cases gastric ulcer in a herniated stomach may occur because of partial obstruction and stasis.

Paraesophageal Hiatus Hernia with Gastric Volvulus, Obstruction, or Strangulation

The patient with a paraesophageal hernia may have a large portion of the stomach in the chest. Since both the esophagogastric junction and the duodenum are fixed in position, the result is a volvulus of the stomach. This may cause complete obstruction. Since one point of obstruction is at the esophagogastric junction, the patient may be unable to vomit. Generally, an incarcerated paraesophageal hernia produces severe substernal pain. In advanced cases, the blood supply to the herniated stomach is impaired, resulting in necrosis, perforation, empyema, septic shock, and death.

An X ray of the chest, demonstrating a mass in the posterior mediastinum with an air–fluid level, will confirm the diagnosis of a diaphragmatic hernia. Because of the danger that a paraesophageal hernia may strangulate, surgery is indicated in any good-risk patient even if he has no symptoms. All symptomatic patients require surgical repair as this disease results from a mechanical problem for which there is no medical therapy.

Some patients, who appear to suffer from a typical paraesophageal hernia, actually do have a sliding component. It is important to identify these patients because they may have an incompetent lower esophageal sphincter and will develop reflux esophagitis unless an antireflux procedure is combined with a repair aimed at correcting the paraesophageal hernia. In these cases the esophagogastric junction is not firmly attached to the area of the median arcuate ligament, a point that generally can be confirmed by X ray studies.

Surgical Repair

If the neck of a *parahiatal* hernia is indeed surrounded by diaphragmatic muscle of good quality, the repair is simple. Remove the sac and close the defect in the diaphragm with several sutures of 0 or 2–0 Tevdek. Paraesophageal hernias can also generally be repaired through the abdominal approach. An attempt should be made gently to insert a nasogastric tube into the herniated portion of stomach prior to op-

eration. After surgical exposure has been obtained, reduce the herniated stomach and omentum. Generally it is not difficult to tease the large hernial sac down from the mediastinum into the abdomen. Then excise the sac, making no attempt to close the remaining peritoneal defect. Narrow the enlarged hiatal opening by inserting interrupted 0 Tevdek sutures to approximate the crura behind the esophagus as described in the repair of a sliding hiatus hernia. With an 18F nasogastric tube in the esophagus, it should be possible for the surgeon to insert his index finger between the esophagus and the newly repaired hiatal orifice.

Now, if there is any suggestion that the esophagogastric junction is not firmly fixed to the median arcuate ligament, or that the patient may be susceptible to reflux esophagitis, perform a posterior gastropexy by the technique of Hill (see Chap. 68) or some modification of that operation.

Sometimes the herniated gastric pouch is the site of a chronic gastric ulcer due to compression by the muscle of the diaphragm. It is not necessary to resect the ulcer or any part of the stomach as simple repair of the hernia will result in satisfactory healing of the ulcer, unless there is some abnormality of gastric function in addition to the paraesophageal hernia.

Sliding Hiatus Hernia

When to Operate

Occasionally a patient may have a normal high pressure zone at the esophagogastric junction even though he has a sliding hernia with this junction high in the mediastinum. This patient will be free of symptoms and does not require surgery. Surgery is indicated for symptomatic reflux esophagitis and its complications when they cannot be successfully controlled by medical management. Patients, who do not have any hiatus hernia, also require an antireflux operation if the lower esophageal sphincter is incompetent and they suffer from reflux esophagitis that cannot be controlled. Among the serious complications of gastroesophageal reflux are ulceration, bleeding, stricture, and aspiration pneumonitis. Most physicians believe it is the acid that damages the esophagus, producing pain and other complications. However, bile, when it refluxes into the esophagus, also causes pain and stricture formation. Bile may be even more potent in this respect than the gastric acid.

It is generally agreed that medical management is the treatment of choice for mild reflux esophagitis. However, once a stricture has formed, surgery is necessary for long-term relief. Dilating the stricture, without performing an antireflux operation, results in prompt recurrence of the stricture.

Operations for Preventing Reflux

Belsey Mark IV Procedure

Belsey's operation, described by Baue and Belsey and by Skinner and Belsey, was a great step forward in the surgery of hiatus hernia because it was aimed at preventing reflux as well as repairing the hernia. A long-term followup study has been reported by Orringer, Skinner, and Belsey indicating a recurrence rate of 14.7% after 10 years. The Belsey operation can be done only by the thoracic approach. This procedure is likely to fail if the esophagus is not long enough to descend into the abdominal cavity *without tension.* The tension will cause the sutures, which create the partial fundoplication, to pull out of the esophagus with collapse of the repair.

Hill Posterior Gastropexy

In this operation the surgeon narrows the lumen of the esophagogastric junction by turning in the tissues on the lesser curvature side with sutures. These same sutures

are fixed to the median arcuate ligament. If this maneuver is successful, it guarantees that 4–7 cm of esophagus will be within the abdominal cavity. Also, the resting pressure at the esophagogastric junction is restored to the normal value.

The posterior gastropexy, described by Hill (1967 and 1977), is done transabdominally. Postoperative complications, such as the "gas bloat" syndrome, are rare. Hill's postoperative studies, including manometric and acid reflux measurement, have demonstrated excellent long-term results.

Although we have experienced good results with this operation, there are a few disadvantages. The operation is difficult to reproduce or to teach with precision because the pillars of adipose tissue and phrenoesophageal ligaments, which are sutured on the lesser curvature of the stomach, vary from patient to patient. Therefore, the amount of tissue inverted into the esophagogastric junction may vary also. Hill has attempted to rectify this drawback by measuring the intraesophageal pressure during the operation so that he can calibrate the degree of inversion according to the pressure being recorded. On the other hand, Orringer, Schneider, Williams, and Sloan reported that intraoperative pressure measurements were unreliable and not reproducible. Inexperienced surgeons find it difficult to identify and dissect out the median arcuate ligament, which is an essential step in this operation. There is also the possibility that the surgeon, not expert in Hill's technique, will injure the celiac artery while dissecting the median arcuate ligament.

Nissen Fundoplication

Nissen's operation involves a complete wrap of the lower esophagus by a segment of gastric fundus. This operation can be performed equally well in the abdomen or in the chest. Studies by DeMeester, Johnson, and Kent, by Dilling, Peyton, Cannon, and Kanaly, and by Skinner and DeMeester have suggested that the Nissen operation is superior to those of Belsey and of Hill when it comes to preventing gastroesophageal reflux. Woodward, Rayl, and Clarke reported a significant incidence of gastric bloating following the Nissen fundoplication as well as the inability to belch or even to vomit. However, Donahue and Bombeck demonstrated that using a loose wrap in making the fundoplication will avoid this complication in almost every case. This has also been our experience.

On the negative side, many complications have been reported to follow defective suturing in this operation. The gastric wrap may slip down so that it surrounds and obstructs the body of the stomach. If the hiatal opening is too large, the fundoplication may herniate into the chest and produce stasis in the herniated gastric pouch with gastric ulcer and bleeding, or even perforation. The Nissen operation may be impossible to perform if the patient has already undergone a high subtotal gastrectomy.

Personal Viewpoint

When the thoracic approach is used, we prefer Nissen's repair to Belsey's because it is simpler to perform and appears to be more effective in preventing reflux. Transabdominally, the Nissen and Hill repairs both are effective operations; the choice between them depends on the preference of the surgeon.

Operations for Esophageal Stricture Secondary to Reflux

Dilatation of Stricture with Transthoracic Nissen Repair

When the transthoracic approach is used, the anesthesiologist can pass Maloney bougies through the patient's mouth and dilate the stricture while the surgeon guides the bougie through the lumen. After this has been successfully completed, it is necessary to perform an operation to prevent further reflux. The Nissen operation is then performed. After completing this step, reduce the fundoplication into the abdomen and close the crura behind the esophagus.

Long-standing fibrotic strictures can cause foreshortening of the esophagus. In these cases, even dissection of the esophagus up to the arch of the aorta will not achieve significant lengthening and it is not possible to replace the esophagogastric junction into the abdominal cavity *without tension.* If tension is present and the repair is forced into the abdominal cavity, recurrence of both the hernia and the reflux will be common. Some surgeons (Woodward, Pennell) prefer to handle this problem by leaving the esophagogastric junction in the thoracic cavity after performing a Nissen fundoplication. In this case it is necessary to enlarge the hiatal opening to permit the body of the stomach to pass through without constriction. It is also necessary to carefully suture the gastric wall to the muscular ring of the hiatus or else bowel will herniate into the chest between the stomach and the hiatus. Many complications have been reported by Richardson, Larsen, and Polk and by Mansour, Burton, Miller, and Hatcher following an intrathoracic fundoplication. Some of these complications are gastric ulceration and perforation in the intrathoracic stomach, esophagopleurocutaneous and gastropleurocutaneous fistulas, and perigastric herniation of bowel into the chest.

Because of these complications, we restrict the use of the transthoracic Nissen fundoplication *only* to those patients whose esophagus is pliable and is *long enough to pass into the abdomen without tension.* Otherwise, we perform a Collis gastroplasty to lengthen the esophagus before creating an antireflux valve.

Dilatation of Stricture with Collis Gastroplasty and Antireflux Procedure

Whenever there is any question at all concerning the ease with which 5–7 cm of esophagus can be passed into the abdomen, we agree with Pearson and Henderson and with Urschel, Razzuk, Wood, and Galbraith that the esophagus should be lengthened by a Collis gastroplasty. Even if the esophagus is not short in length, when the distal end is rigid with fibrosis, trying to create a valve to prevent reflux will be ineffective because the rigid esophageal wall cannot be compressed. Rigidity of the distal esophagus is, therefore, a second indication for a Collis gastroplasty. The Collis operation is not difficult to perform in the chest, especially with the help of the GIA stapling device. When a fibrotic esophagus is baked into the mediastinum, sharp dissection is required to release it. Dissect the esophagus as far as the inferior pulmonary vein in these cases; further cephalad dissection does not achieve significant lengthening. Then the Collis gastroplasty will add another 5–9 cm to the length of the esophagus.

Following this lengthening procedure, Pearson and Henderson and Urschel and colleagues added a Belsey 270° fundoplication to prevent reflux. Orringer and Sloan (1977) and Henderson (1977) were unable to duplicate the successful antireflux effect of the Collis–Belsey operation reported by Pearson and by Urschel. They prefer to perform a modified Nissen fundoplication following the Collis gastroplasty. Although there has not been any randomized study comparing the Collis–Belsey and the Collis–Nissen operations, at this time we prefer the Collis–Nissen as described by Henderson (1979) and by Orringer and Sloan (1979) because it is simpler and appears to be more effective (Henderson 1977, Orringer and Sloan 1977, and Orringer and Orringer 1982).

Esophageal Resection with Colon or Jejunal Interposition

On rare occasions, the esophageal fibrosis is so advanced that attempting to dilate the stricture will result in rupture of the esophagus. An esophageal laceration can sometimes be converted into an esophagoplasty with a Thal gastric patch (Woodward et al.). However, most of the time the traumatized lower esophagus will have to be resected. Irreversible damage to the lower esophagus may also occur during an operation for severe esophagitis in a patient who has had several previous operations in this area.

In repairing the defect that remains following resection of the lower esophagus, several requirements should be satisfied. First, the operation should be safe. Second, the reconstruction should prevent future reflux. Third, the repair should permit free passage of food from the mouth to the stomach. Two procedures seem to fulfill these requirements. In 1965 Belsey reported 92 cases in which the distal esophagus was replaced by a segment of colon whose blood supply was based on the left colic artery. The mortality rate was 4.3% when this procedure was performed for benign disease. Successful long-term results with the colon interposition operation were also reported by Glasgow, Cannon, and Elkins and by Wilkins. Merendino and Dillard suggested the interposition of an isoperistaltic segment of proximal jejunum between the distal esophagus and stomach. Polk found that the jejunal interposition operation was effective in preventing reflux. His mortality rate was 4%. Both the jejunum and the colon interposition operations need to be performed only under highly unusual circumstances. For this reason, there is not enough data to determine whether one is better than the other. If the esophagus must be resected above the level of the inferior pulmonary vein, the jejunal interposition is contraindicated (Polk), but the colon procedure is feasible.

Another procedure to replace the esophagus that has recently achieved attention is the cervical esophagogastrostomy as described by Akiyama. Although this operation requires only one anastomosis, we prefer the colon interposition. We reduce the operating time by performing the colocolic and the cologastric anastomoses with stapling devices (see Figs. 28–33 to 28–36 and 70–2 to 70–6).

Esophagoplasty and Thal Patch

Thal described a method of repairing a lower esophageal stricture by making a longitudinal incision through the constricted area. He then sutured the fundus of the stomach into the defect created in the esophagus by this incision. Later modifications (Woodward et al.) included applying a split-thickness skin graft to the gastric wall to replace the defect in the esophageal mucosa, as well as creating a Nissen fundoplication around the repair. The repaired esophagus and the fundoplication are left in the thoracic cavity, a situation that is followed by many complications as discussed above. This procedure is possible only in strictures of the lower esophagus where adjacent gastric fundus is available for the repair. Although the operation appears to be straightforward, it has not gained widespread popularity. Woodward reported satisfactory results with the Thal operation, but we have not had any experience with this procedure. In most esophageal strictures, even when they are severe, gradual dilatation leads to a surprisingly high percentage of good results without requiring either an incision of the stricture or a resection of the esophagus. In each case dilatation of the stricture should be followed by an antireflux operation or the stricture will recur.

Operation for Barrett's Esophagus

In Barrett's esophagus, chronic reflux has produced metaplasia of the squamous epithelium of the esophagus distal to the stricture, so that the epithelium becomes columnar in nature. Some strictures in patients suffering from the Barrett esophagus may occur as high as the aortic arch. These patients can be treated by dilatation of the stricture followed by an antireflux operation. In the absence of further gastroesophageal reflux, the successfully dilated stricture will generally not recur.

It should be recognized that the incidence of malignancy (adenocarcinoma) in the Barrett esophagus seems to be higher than when the esophagus is lined with squamous epithelium. For this reason, these patients should be followed by semi-annual esophagoscopy.

Management of Patients with Failed Operations for Reflux Esophagitis

Recurrent Reflux Esophagitis after Transabdominal Operation

Some patients with a failed Nissen fundoplication or Hill posterior gastropexy operation can be successfully explored and repaired by a second abdominal procedure. However, Henderson and Marryatt (1981) warn that in *most* operations for recurrence the upper stomach will be densely adherent to both the liver and the spleen. They advocate the routine use of a thoracoabdominal incision for these cases and almost always employ a Collis–Nissen repair. After an average followup period of 2.5 years in 97% of 121 patients, they achieved excellent results in 94% of their operations for recurrent esophagitis; their advice is well worth following.

Roux-Y Bile Diversion for Recurrent Reflux Esophagitis Following Repeated Failed Operations

When a patient has undergone two or three failed surgical attempts to correct gastroesophageal reflux, Payne and also Royston, Dowling, and Spencer recommend a procedure that does not necessitate reexploring the esophagogastric junction. The procedure consists of vagotomy and antrectomy combined with a Roux-Y gastrojejunostomy (see Chap. 71). This operation is particularly appropriate in patients who have already had a vagotomy and antrectomy during one of their previous operations. It is especially suitable in poor-risk patients who may not be candidates for a thoracotomy and extensive reconstruction of the esophagogastric junction. The combination of vagotomy, antrectomy, and Roux-Y diversion prevents the reflux of either acid or bile into the esophagus, with relief of symptoms. In the good-risk patient with many failed operations for reflux, one might prefer to perform a colonic or jejunal interposition operation, rather than the biliary diversion procedure, because there is more data to support these operations than there is for the Roux-Y. In several critical situations, however, we have had successful results with Payne's operation.

Reflux Esophagitis Following Esophagogastrectomy

After esophagogastrectomy for lesions of the distal esophagus or proximal stomach, an *end-to-side* esophagogastric anastomosis will generally prevent gastroesophageal reflux. When the surgeon has erroneously performed this anastomosis in an end-to-end fashion, he should anticipate a high incidence of serious reflux esophagitis. When this esophagitis will not respond to conservative management, a biliary diversion may be of benefit (Smith and Payne). In these cases, vagotomy has invariably been performed during the esophagogastrectomy. Generally, a significant portion of the acid-secreting gastric mucosa has been resected, so that it is the bile rather than the acid which is causing damage to the esophagus. In this situation, dividing the duodenum 2–3 cm beyond the pylorus and anastomosing it to jejunum by the Roux-Y technique (see Chap. 71) will eliminate the reflux of bile. Before electing to perform the Roux-Y procedure, one should ascertain that it is indeed bile that is refluxing into the esophagus by performing an esophagoscopy or a radionuclide scan.

Whenever more than 50%–60% of the stomach has to be removed for a proximal gastric tumor, it is preferable to perform a total gastrectomy with an esophagojejunal anastomosis by the Roux-Y technique than to do an end-to-end esophagogastrostomy. If this policy is followed, postoperative reflux esophagitis will not be a problem.

Operation for Schatzki's Ring

Schatzki's ring is a thin diaphragmlike membrane across the lower esophagus. This generally occurs in patients with hiatus hernia and an incompetent sphincter. The lumen of the Schatzki ring is rarely less than 1 cm in diameter so that it does not produce obstructive symptoms very often, although a large piece of meat can occasionally occlude its lumen.

When a patient who has a tight Schatzki ring is undergoing surgery for reflux esophagitis, the Schatzki ring may be dilated from above by the anesthesiologist with Maloney bougies or by the surgeon via a small gastrotomy incision with Hegar's dilators from below. It is not generally necessary to perform surgery for the Schatzki ring in the absence of reflux esophagitis.

Thoracic, Abdominal, or Thoracoabdominal Incision?

In patients who have had no previous operations in the area of the esophagogastric junction, the abdominal incision is preferred. With the help of a "chain" or Upper

Hand retractor, the exposure for an antireflux operation is generally quite good. Additionally, other diseases, such as cholelithiasis and duodenal ulcer can be treated surgically at the same time that the hiatus hernia is being repaired. The abdominal approach is *contraindicated* if there is evidence that the esophagus is short. In many patients the esophagus appears to be foreshortened because of the sliding nature of the hiatus hernia. However, in the absence of significant esophageal fibrosis the esophagogastric junction can be brought back into the abdominal cavity without tension. On the other hand, during esophagoscopy it may be evident that there is a thick fibrotic stricture or that the lower esophagus appears to be fixed in the mediastinum. Under these conditions a transthoracic approach is preferable. Attempts at transabdominal dissection of the lower esophagus are fraught with the danger of traumatizing both the esophagus and the vagus nerves. Also, many of these patients will require a Collis gastroplasty to lengthen the esophagus. This operation is much easier to perform through the chest than through the abdomen.

When a patient is undergoing the second or third operation for recurrent gastroesophageal reflux, he should always be positioned on the operating table so that the initial approach can be extended by making a left thoracoabdominal incision (see Vol. I, Figs. 8–3 to 8–7). Although some surgeons prefer to achieve additional exposure by making separate laparotomy and thoracic incisions, thus avoiding division of the costal margin, we have never hesitated to combine the thoracic and the abdominal incisions because division of the costal margin creates no disability if the cartilage is repaired with one or two nonabsorbable sutures. The exposure provided by the thoracoabdominal incision surpasses that of any other combination of incisions. In performing the thoracoabdominal incision for recurrent hiatus hernia, do not make a radial incision from the esophageal hiatus to the costal margin be-

cause this will disrupt the function of the diaphragm by cutting the phrenic nerve. A 12–15 cm incision in the periphery of the diaphragm offers excellent exposure without cutting any branches of the phrenic nerve.

Secondary operations for esophageal reflux are difficult procedures that carry a significant mortality rate. Zucker, Peskin, and Saik reported that 3 of 17 patients (17.6%) undergoing such operations died and 46% developed a complication. All of the fatal cases had been performed by an exclusively transabdominal approach.

References

Akiyama H (1980) Surgery for carcinoma of the esophagus. Curr Probl Surg 17:56

Baue AE, Belsey R (1967) The treatment of sliding hiatus hernia and reflux esophagitis by the Mark IV technique. Surgery 62:396

Belsey R (1965) Reconstruction of the esophagus with left colon. J Thorac Cardiovasc Surg 49:33

DeMeester TR, Johnson LF, Kent AH (1974) Evaluation of current operations for the prevention of gastroesophageal reflux. Ann Surg 180:511

Dilling EW, Peyton MD, Cannon JP, Kanaly PJ et al. (1977) Comparison of Nissen fundoplication and Belsey Mark IV in the management of gastroesophageal reflux. Am J Surg 134:730

Donahue PC, Bombeck CT (1977) The modified Nissen fundoplication-reflux prevention without gas bloat. Chir Gastroenterol 11:15

Glasgow JC, Cannon JP, Elkins RC (1979) Colon interposition for benign esophageal disease. Am J Surg 137:175

Henderson RD (1977) Reflux control following gastroplasty. Ann Thorac Surg 24:206

Henderson RD (1979) Nissen hiatal hernia repair: problems of recurrence and continued symptoms. Ann Thorac Surg 28:587

Henderson RD, Marryatt G (1981) Recurrent hiatal hernia: management by thoracoabdominal total fundoplication gastroplasty. Can J Surg 24:151

Hill LD (1967) An effective operation for hiatal hernia: an eight year appraisal. Ann Surg 166:681

Hill LD (1977) Progress in the surgical management of hiatal hernia. World J Surg 1:425

MacDougall JI, Abbott AC, Goodhand TK (1963) Herniation through congenital diaphragmatic defects in adults. Can J Surg 6:301

Mansour KA, Burton HG, Miller JI Jr, Hatcher CR Jr (1981) Complications of intrathoracic Nissen fundoplication. Ann Thorac Surg 32:173

Merendino KA, Dillard DH (1955) The concept of sphincter substitution by an interposed jejunal segment for anatomic and physiological abnormalities at the esophagogastric junction. Ann Surg 142:486

Orringer MB, Orringer JS (1982) The combined Collis–Nissen operation: early assessment of reflux control. Ann Thorac Surg 33:543

Orringer MB, Schneider R, Williams GW, Sloan H (1980) Intraoperative esophageal manometry: is it valid? Ann Thorac Surg 30:13

Orringer MB, Skinner DB, Belsey RHR (1972) Long-term results of the Mark IV operation for hiatal hernia and analyses of recurrences and their treatment. J Thorac Cardiovasc Surg 63:25

Orringer MB, Sloan H (1977) Complications and failings of the combined Collis–Belsey operation. J Thorac Cardiovasc Surg 74:726

Orringer MB, Sloan H (1978) Combined Collis–Nissen reconstruction of the esophagogastric junction. Ann Thorac Surg 25:16

Payne WS (1970) Surgical treatment of reflux esophagitis and stricture associated with permanent incompetence of the cardia. Mayo Clin Proc 45:553

Pearson FG, Henderson RD (1973) Experimental and clinical studies of gastroplasty in the management of acquired short esophagus. Surg Gynecol Obstet 136:737

Pennell TC (1981) Supradiaphragmatic correction of esophageal reflux structures. Ann Surg 193:655

Polk HC Jr (1980) Jejunal interposition for reflux esophagitis and esophageal stricture unresponsive to valvuloplasty. World J Surg 4:731

Richardson JD, Larson GM, Polk HC Jr (1982) Intrathoracic fundoplication for shortened esophagus. Am J Surg 143:29

Royston CMS, Dowling BL, Spencer J (1975) Antrectomy with Roux-en-Y anastomosis in the treatment of peptic esophagitis with stricture. Br J Surg 62:605

Skinner DB, Belsey R (1967) Surgical management of esophageal reflux and hiatus hernia. J Thorac Cardiovasc Surg 53:33

Skinner DB, DeMeester TR (1976) Gastroesophageal reflux. Curr Probl Surg 13:1

Smith J, Payne WS (1975) Surgical technique for management of reflux esophagitis after esophagogastrectomy for malignancy; further application of the Roux-en-Y principle. Mayo Clin Proc 50:588

Urschel HC, Razzuk MA, Wood RE, Galbraith NF, et al. (1973) An improved surgical technique for the complicated hiatal hernia with gastroesophageal reflux. Ann Thorac Surg 15:443

Wilkins EW Jr (1980) Long-segment colon substitution for the esophagus. Ann Surg 192:722

Woodward ER, Rayl JE, Clarke JM (1970) Esophageal hiatus hernia. Curr Probl Surg 7:1

Zucker K, Peskin GW, Saik RP (1982) Recurrent hiatal hernia repair; a potential surgical dilemma. Arch Surg 117:413

67 Transabdominal Fundoplication (Nissen)

Indications

Reflux esophagitis without good response to medical therapy, whether or not an anatomical hiatus hernia is present. If a previous operation has been performed at the esophagogastric junction for reflux, a transthoracic or thoracoabdominal approach is preferred. (For a discussion of alternative operations for reflux esophagitis, see Chap. 66.)

Preoperative Care

Preoperative esophagoscopy to confirm the presence of reflux esophagitis

Barium esophagram and gastrointestinal X-ray series; check for disordered gastric emptying

Perioperative antibiotics

Manometric studies of esophageal motility in cases where diffuse esophageal spasm, scleroderma, or achalasia is suspected

A 24-hour continuous recording of lower esophageal pH is useful in deciding whether a patient's pain is indeed coincident with reflux of gastric juice into the esophagus.

Pass a nasogastric tube prior to operation.

Pitfalls and Danger Points

Inadequate mobilization of gastric fundus and abdominal esophagus

Injury to spleen or to vagus nerves

Fundoplication wrap too tight or too wide

Inadequate fundoplication suturing

Undiagnosed esophageal motility disorders, such as achalasia, diffuse spasm, aperistalsis, or scleroderma

Hiatal closure too tight, causing obstruction of esophagus

Hiatal closure too loose, permitting postoperative paraesophageal herniation

Injury to left hepatic vein or vena cava when incising triangular ligament to liberate left lobe of liver

Operative Strategy

Mobilizing the Gastric Fundus

In order to perform a hiatus hernia repair efficiently, it is essential that the lower 5–7 cm of esophagus and the entire gastric fundus from the gastroesophageal junction down to the upper short gastric vessel be completely mobilized from all attachments to the diaphragm and the posterior abdominal wall. To accomplish this, use the "chain" or Upper Hand retractor to elevate the sternum. Identify the gastrophrenic ligament by passing the left hand behind the stomach so that the fingertips will identify this avascular ligament, which attaches the greater curvature to the diaphragm. The ligament extends from the gastroesophageal junction down to the first short gastric vessel. It is simple to divide once it has been stretched by the surgeon's left hand behind the stomach. Although in a few cases no short gastric vessels need to be divided, there should be no hesitation to divide 1–3 proximal short gastric vessels so that the fundoplication wrap can be applied loosely.

On the lesser curvature aspect of the gastroesophageal junction, it is necessary to divide the proximal portion of the gastrohepatic ligament. This ligament generally contains an accessory left hepatic artery arising from the left gastric artery and going to the left lobe of the liver as well as the hepatic branch of the left vagus nerve. Division of the accessory left hepatic artery has, in our experience, not proved harmful. Do not divide the left gastric artery itself. Preserving the left gastric artery helps to prevent the fundoplication from slipping in a caudal direction (Polk). The lower esophagus is freed by incising the overlying peritoneum and phrenoesophageal ligaments; continue this incision in a semicircular fashion so that the muscular margins of the diaphragmatic crura are exposed down to the median arcuate ligament. During all of this mobilization, look for the major branches of the anterior and posterior vagus nerves and preserve them.

If the esophagus is foreshortened by esophagitis and fibrosis, a simple fundoplication is an inadequate operation. Unless 5–7 cm of esophagus can be brought without tension into the abdomen, do not perform fundoplication without also creating a Collis gastroplasty (see Chap. 69).

Preventing Injury to Spleen

Splenic trauma is reported to be a common complication of the Nissen operation. Rogers, Herrington, and Morton noted that 26% of their series of fundoplication operations underwent splenectomy because of operative trauma. Injury to the spleen is generally a preventable complication. With the use of the "chain" or Upper Hand retractor there is no reason for any retractor to come into contact with the spleen. Most often the mechanism of splenic injury is traction upon the body of the stomach toward the patient's right. This maneuver avulses a portion of the splenic capsule where it is attached to the omentum or to the gastrosplenic ligament. Early in the operation, make it a point to look at the anterior surface of the spleen. Note where the omentum may be adherent to the splenic capsule. If necessary, divide these attachments under direct vision. Otherwise, simply apply a moist gauze pad over the spleen and avoid lateral traction upon the stomach. Traction on the gastroesophageal junction in a caudal direction does not generally cause any injury to the spleen.

If a portion of the splenic capsule has been avulsed, this can almost always be managed by applying a sheet of Surgicel or powdered Avitene followed by 10 minutes of pressure. Other splenic injuries can be repaired by suturing with 2–0 chromic catgut (see Chap. 65). Extensive disruption of the spleen at its hilus is an indication for splenectomy.

How Tight Should the Fundoplication Be?

The Nissen operation produces a high pressure zone in the lower esophagus but not because the seromuscular sutures themselves reduce the lumen of the esophagus. Rather, the gastric air bubble rises to the area of the plication and transmits sufficient pressure to keep the esophagus partially occluded. This pressure is not sufficient to prevent the passage of food, however. For this reason, it is not necessary that the fundoplication be tight enough actually to constrict the esophagus. A loose wrap seems to accomplish an effective antireflux effect without causing the inability to vomit or belch and without giving the patient the "gas bloat" syndrome. Most surgeons perform the plication with a 40F bougie in place to avoid too tight a wrap. Whether or not the indwelling bougie is used, it is possible to judge the tightness of the wrap by applying Babcock clamps to each side of the gastric fundus and tentatively bringing them together in front of the esophagus. This will mimic the effect of the sutures. The surgeon should be able to pass one or two fingers between the wrap and the esophagus without difficulty with an 18F nasogastric tube in place. Otherwise readjust the fundoplication so that it is loose enough for this maneuver to be accomplished.

Even though the fundoplication wrap seems somewhat loose, the postoperative barium esophagram will show a narrow tapering of the distal esophagus.

How Wide Should the Fundoplication Be?

One cause of postoperative dysphagia is making the fundoplication wrap too wide. In the usual Nissen operation, do not wrap more than 3–4 cm of esophagus. Recent reports advocate wraps of lesser length.

When they perform a fundoplication to prevent reflux simultaneously with an extensive esophageal myotomy for diffuse esophageal spasm, Henderson and Ryder utilize a one-stitch wrap, 0.5 cm wide. These authors also use a 0.5 cm wrap when they perform the Collis–Nissen operation in patients with scleroderma who have severe reflux esophagitis.

Henderson and Marryatt (1983) employ a Nissen fundoplication wrap only 1.0 cm in width (three stitches) together with a Collis gastroplasty in patients with severe reflux esophagitis who do not suffer any disorder of esophageal motility.

Avoiding Fundoplication Suture Line Disruption

Polk and other authors have noted that an important cause of failure after Nissen fundoplication has been disruption of the plication because the sutures broke. For this reason, use 2–0 sutures. Generally the sutures that were found to have broken were silk. We have used 2–0 Tevdek because it retains its tensile strength for many years while silk gradually degenerates in the tissues. It is also important not to pass the suture into the lumen of the stomach or esophagus. If this error is committed, tying the suture too tight will cause strangulation and possible leakage. Some insurance against the latter complication may be obtained if the major fundoplication sutures are turned in with a layer of continuous 4–0 Prolene seromuscular Lembert sutures as recommended by Orringer and Sloan.

Avoiding Postoperative Dysphagia

Transient mild dysphagia during the first 2–3 weeks following operation is common and probably is secondary to local edema. However, some patients have difficulty in swallowing for many months after a hiatus hernia operation. There are several possible causes for this dysphagia. (1) It is possible to make the fundoplication wrap so tight or so wide that permanent dysphagia may ensue. (2) The defect in the hiatus may be sutured so tightly that the hiatus impinges on the lumen of the esophagus and prevents the passage of food. With an 18F nasogastric tube in place, after the crural sutures have been tied to repair the defect in the hiatus, the surgeon should still be able to insert his index finger without difficulty between the esophagus and the margins of the hiatus. There is no virtue in closing the hiatus snugly around the esophagus. (3) A final cause of dysphagia in patients who have experienced this symptom as one of their preoperative complaints is the presence of an esophageal motility disorder like achalasia or aperistalsis. Patients who present to the surgeon with reflux esophagitis and who also complain of dysphagia should have preoperative esophageal manometry to rule out motility disorders that may require surgery either in addition to the antireflux procedure or instead of this operation.

Failure to Bring the Esophagogastric Junction into the Abdomen

If the surgeon cannot mobilize the esophagogastric junction from the mediastinum and bring it into the abdomen while performing a transabdominal repair of a hiatus hernia, he can infer that fibrosis has been sufficient in the esophagus to have foreshortened it. This can generally be suspected prior to operation by the fact that the lower esophagus is strictured. In our opinion, these patients require a transthoracic Collis–Nissen operation. Although it is possible to perform the Collis–Nissen procedure in the abdomen, this is quite difficult. If it cannot be accomplished transabdominally, it will be necessary to open the chest either through a separate incision or through a throacoabdominal extension and to perform the Collis–Nissen operation, which appears to be the best long-term insurance against recurrent reflux esophagitis in these patients (see Chap. 69).

Unsettled Questions of Technique

Combining Nissen Operation with Posterior Gastropexy

Cordiano, Rovere, Agugiaro, and Mazzilli and Kaminski, Codd, and Sigmund have advocated that the Nissen fundoplication be sutured to the median arcuate ligament in order to prevent any possibility of the fundoplication herniating through the hiatus into the chest postoperatively. They accomplish this by passing the two lowermost fundoplication sutures through the median arcuate ligament before tying them. Although this may appear to be a rational extension of the Nissen operation, there are as yet no followup studies to validate the efficacy of this modification. Also, there is the danger that attaching the Nissen sutures to the median arcuate ligament may cause the wrap to slip downward on the stomach.

Dividing Short Gastric Vessels

Although Polk states that he rarely has to divide the short gastric vessels, we find that dividing several of the proximal short gastric arteries and veins does facilitate mobilizing enough of the fundus to permit a loose fundoplication wrap without tension. Since it is easy to pass the fundus behind the esophagus in a tentative fashion, one can estimate in each case whether there will be sufficient mobility of the fundus without dividing the short gastric vessels or whether further dissection is necessary. It is essential to achieve adequate mobility of the fundus.

Dividing Triangular Ligament of Liver

In many descriptions of the technique for transabdominal repair of a hiatus hernia, division of the triangular ligament is routinely performed to free the left lobe of the liver and to help to expose the hiatus. In most cases of hiatus herniorrhaphy, excellent exposure of the hiatus can be obtained by placing a deep Harrington or Weinberg retractor on the left lobe of the liver and elevating it. If the lobe does have to be mobilized and the triangular ligament divided, remember that this ligament leads directly to the junction of the left hepatic vein and the vena cava. If the avascular triangular ligament is divided without paying close attention, the incision can easily continue into the vena cava. An injury at the junction of the left hepatic vein and the inferior vena cava can be serious because these two large veins are surrounded by liver at this point. Consequently, the control of a venous laceration here is extremely difficult.

Keeping the Fundoplication from Slipping by Inserting Additional Esophagogastric Sutures

Various methods have been advocated to keep the fundoplication from sliding in a caudal direction, where it will constrict the middle of the stomach instead of the esophagus and produce an "hour-glass" stomach with partial obstruction. The most important means of preventing this caudal displacement of the wrap is to include the wall of the esophagus in each of the fundoplication sutures. Also, catch the wall of the stomach *just* below the gastroesophageal junction within the lowermost suture. This suture will anchor the lower portion of the wrap (see Fig. 67–10). Leonardi, Crozier, and Ellis advocate an additional suture line between the upper margin of the gastric wrap and the adjacent esophagus.

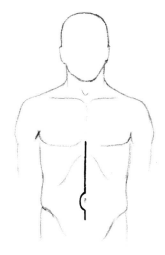

Fig. 67–1

Operative Technique

Incision

Elevate the head of the operating table 10°–15°. Make a midline incision beginning at the xiphoid and continue about 2–3 cm beyond the umbilicus **(Fig. 67–1)**. Explore the abdomen. Insert a "chain" or Upper Hand retractor to elevate the lower portion of the sternum. Reduce the hiatus hernia by traction along the anterior wall of the stomach. Look at the anterior surface of the spleen to determine whether there are omental adhesions to the capsule that may result in avulsing the capsule later in the operation. Place a moist gauze pad over the spleen. In most cases it is not necessary to free the left lobe of the liver; simply elevate the left lobe with a Harrington or Weinberg retractor in order to expose the diaphragmatic hiatus.

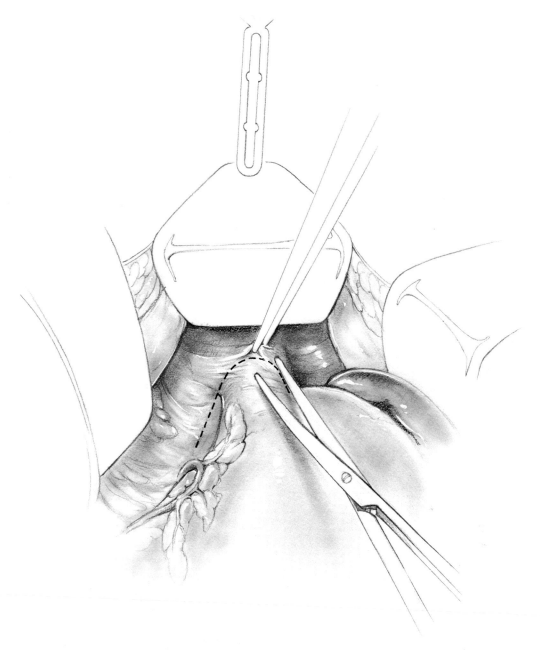

Fig. 67–2

Mobilizing Esophagus and Gastric Fundus

Make a transverse incision in the peritoneum overlying the abdominal esophagus **(Fig. 67–2)** and continue this incision into the peritoneum overlying the right margin of the crus. Then divide the peritoneum overlying the left margin of the diaphragmatic hiatus. Separate the hiatal musculature from the esophagus using a peanut dissector until most of the circumference of the esophagus has been exposed. Then pass the index finger *gently* behind the esophagus and encircle it with a latex drain

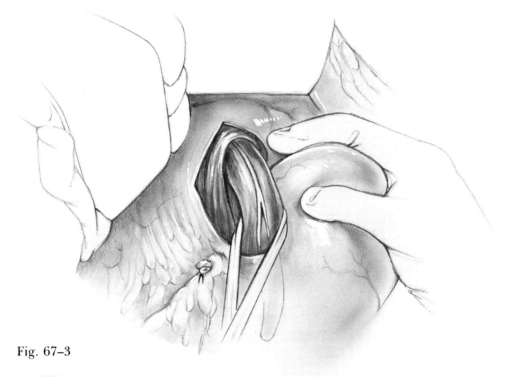

Fig. 67–3

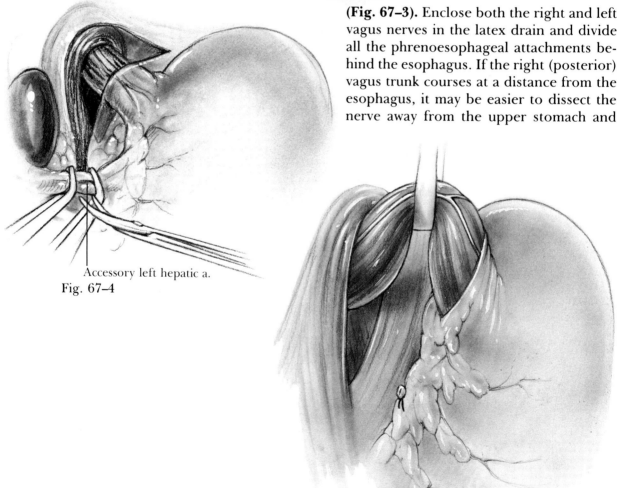

(Fig. 67–3). Enclose both the right and left vagus nerves in the latex drain and divide all the phrenoesophageal attachments behind the esophagus. If the right (posterior) vagus trunk courses at a distance from the esophagus, it may be easier to dissect the nerve away from the upper stomach and

Accessory left hepatic a.

Fig. 67–4

Fig. 67–5

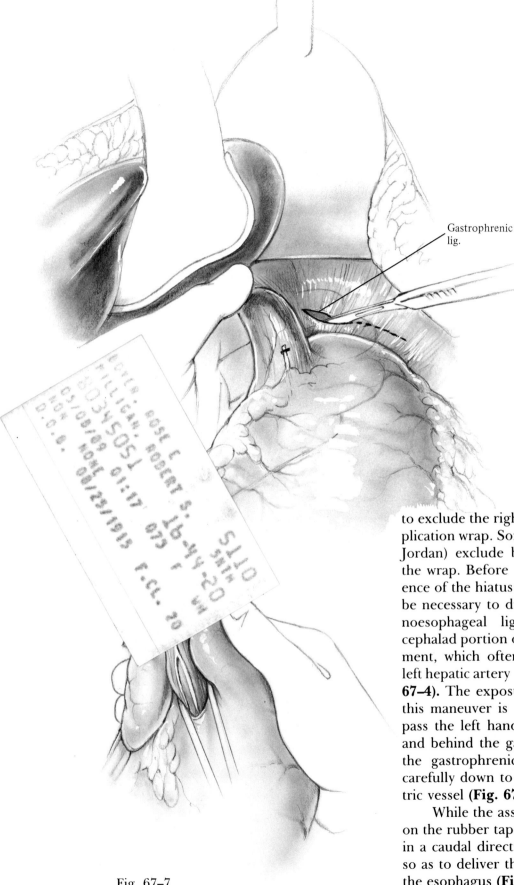

Gastrophrenic
lig.

Fig. 67–7

to exclude the right vagus from the fundo-plication wrap. Some authors (Herrington; Jordan) exclude both vagus trunks from the wrap. Before the complete circumference of the hiatus can be visualized, it will be necessary to divide not only the phrenoesophageal ligaments but also the cephalad portion of the gastrohepatic ligament, which often contains an accessory left hepatic artery that may be divided (**Fig. 67–4**). The exposure at the conclusion of this maneuver is seen in **Fig. 67–5.** Now pass the left hand behind the esophagus and behind the gastric fundus to identify the gastrophrenic ligament. Divide this carefully down to the proximal short gastric vessel **(Fig. 67–6).**

While the assistant is placing traction on the rubber tape to draw the esophagus in a caudal direction, pass the right hand so as to deliver the gastric fundus behind the esophagus **(Fig. 67–7).** Apply Babcock

271

clamps to the two points on the stomach where the first fundoplication suture will be inserted and bring these two Babcock clamps together tentatively to assess whether the fundus has been mobilized sufficiently to accomplish the fundoplication without tension. **Fig. 67–8,** a cross-section view, demonstrates how the gastric fundus surrounds the lower esophagus and the vagus nerves.

Generally there will be inadequate mobility of the gastric fundus unless one divides the proximal 1–3 short gastric vessels. Ligate each with 2–0 cotton.

Repairing the Hiatal Defect

Using 0 Tevdek sutures on a large atraumatic needle, start at the posterior margin of the hiatal defect and take a bite, 1.5–

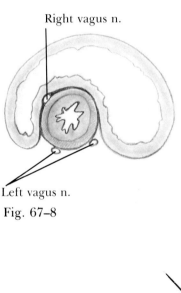

Right vagus n.

Left vagus n.

Fig. 67–8

2.0 cm in width, of the crus and its overlying peritoneum on each side of the hiatus. Insert the next suture about 1.0–1.2 cm cephalad and continue this process until the index finger can just be inserted *comfortably* between the esophagus and the margin of the hiatus **(Fig. 67–9).**

Suturing the Fundoplication

Ask the anesthesiologist to pass a 40F Maloney dilator into the stomach. Insert the first fundoplication suture by taking a bite of the fundus on the patient's left using 2–0 atraumatic Tevdek. Pass the needle through the seromuscular surface of the gastric lesser curve just distal to the esophagogastric junction and then take a final bite of the fundus on the patient's right. Attach a hemostat to tag this stitch but do not tie it. Each bite should contain 5–6 mm of tissue including submucosa, but it should not penetrate the lumen. Do not pierce any of the vagus nerves with a stitch. In order to perform a fundoplication without tension, it is necessary to insert the gastric sutures a sufficient distance lateral to the esophagogastric junction. Place additional sutures, as illustrated in **Fig. 67–10,** at intervals of about 1 cm. Each suture should contain one bite of fundus, then

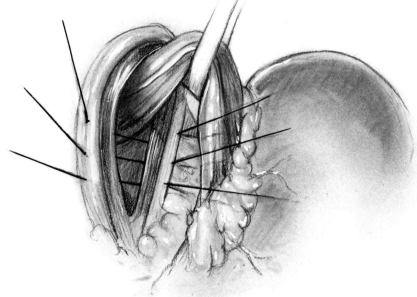

Fig. 67–9

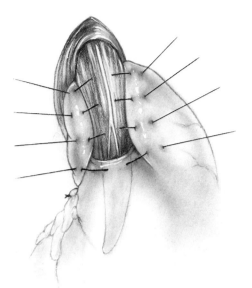
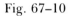

Fig. 67–10

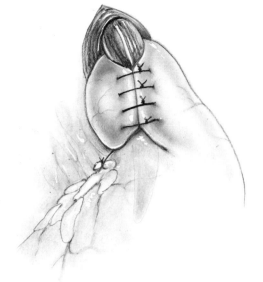

Fig. 67–11

esophagus, and then the opposite side of the fundus. No more than 3 cm of esophagus should be encircled by the fundoplication. Now tie all of these sutures (**Fig. 67–11).** Remove the Maloney dilator from the esophagus and insert an 18F nasogastric tube. It should be possible to insert one or two fingers between the esophagus and the Nissen wrap (**Fig. 67–12).**

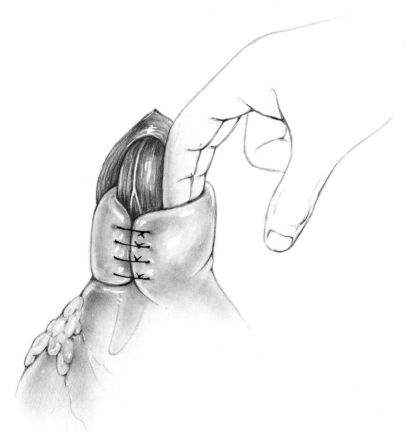

Fig. 67–12

273

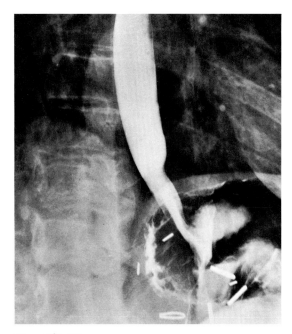

Fig. 67–13.

Optionally, at this point one may invert the layer of fundoplication sutures by inserting a continuous seromuscular layer of 4–0 Prolene Lembert sutures. (This layer is not illustrated.)

Testing Antireflux Valve

Ask the anesthesiologist to inject 300–400 ml saline solution into the nasogastric tube. Then have him withdraw the tube into the esophagus. Now try to expel the saline by compressing the stomach. If the saline cannot be forced into the esophagus by moderate manual compression of the stomach, the fundoplication has been demonstrated to comprise a competent antireflux valve.

Abdominal Closure

Irrigate the abdomen and the subcutaneous tissues with a dilute antibiotic solution. Then close the abdomen without drainage in routine fashion.

Postoperative Care

Continue nasogastric suction until gastrointestional function resumes. Then initiate oral feeding.

Order a barium esophagram before the patient is discharged. If a satisfactory repair has been accomplished, a 3–4 cm length of distal esophagus will become progressively more narrow, tapering to a point at the gastroesophageal junction. If this tapering effect is not noted, it suggests that the wrap may be too loose. Successful antireflux procedures, whether by the Nissen, the Hill, the Belsey, or the Collis–Nissen technique, all show a similar narrowing of the distal esophagus on the postoperative esophagram. A typical postoperative barium esophagram is shown in **Fig. 67–13.**

Postoperative Complications

Dysphagia, usually transient

"Gas bloat" (rare)

Disruption of fundoplication

Slipping downward of fundoplication with obstruction

Postoperative paraesophageal hernia (Leonardi et al.) if hiatal defect was not properly closed

Herniation of fundoplication into thorax

Esophageal or gastric perforation by deep necrosing sutures

Persistent gastroesophageal reflux

References

Cordiano C, Rovere GQD, Agugiaro S, Mazzilli G (1976) Technical modification of the Nissen fundoplication procedure. Surg Gynecol Obstet 143:977

Henderson RD, Marryatt G (1983) Total fundoplication gastroplasty; long-term follow-up in 500 patients. J Thorac Cardiovasc Surg 85:81

Henderson RD, Ryder DE (1982) Reflux control following myotomy in diffuse esophageal spasm. Ann Thorac Surg 34:230

Herrington JR Jr (1983) Treatment of combined sliding and paraesophageal hiatal hernia; emphasis on protection of the vagus nerves. Contemp Surg 22:19

Jordan PH Jr (1978) Parietal cell vagotomy facilitates fundoplication in the treatment of reflux esophagitis. Surg Gynecol Obstet 147:593

Kaminski DL, Codd JE, Sigmund CJ (1977) Evaluation of the use of the median arcuate ligament in fundoplication for reflux esophagitis. Am J Surg 134:724

Leonardi HK, Crozier RE, Ellis FH (1981) Reoperation for complications of the Nissen fundoplication. J Thorac Cardiovasc Surg 81:50

Orringer MB, Sloan H (1978) Combined Collis–Nissen reconstruction of the esophagogastric junction. Ann Thorac Surg 25:16

Polk HC Jr (1976) Fundoplication for reflux esophagitis: misadventures with the operation of choice. Ann Surg 183:645

Rogers DM, Herrington JL, Morton C (1980) Incidental splenectomy associated with Nissen fundoplication. Ann Surg 191:153

68 Posterior Gastropexy (Hill)

Indications
(See Chap. 66.)

Hiatus hernia with reflux esophagitis resistant to conservative management is a clear indication. Successful execution of this operation requires that the esophagus be long enough to suture the esophagogastric junction to the level of the median arcuate ligament without tension (5–7 cm of intra-abdominal esophagus).

Preoperative Care

Esophagoscopy

X rays of the esophagus and upper gastrointestinal tract

Esophageal manometry, if there is any suspicion of diffuse esophageal spasm, achalasia, or scleroderma

Passage of 18F nasogastric tube the morning of the operation

Twenty-four-hour esophageal pH monitoring in selected patients

Pitfalls and Danger Points

Hemorrhage from laceration of celiac or inferior phrenic artery

Injury to spleen

Improper calibration of lumen of lower esophageal sphincter

Excessive narrowing of diaphragmatic hiatus

Failure to identify the median arcuate ligament

Injury to left hepatic vein or vena cava when incising triangular ligament to liberate left lobe of liver

Operative Strategy

Dissecting the Median Arcuate Ligament

The median arcuate ligament constitutes the anterior portion of the aortic hiatus, the aperture in the diaphragm through which the aorta passes. This ligament, a condensation of preaortic fascia, arches over the anterior surface of the aorta just cephalad to the origin of the celiac artery and joins the right crus of the diaphragm at its insertion onto the vertebral column. This band of fibrous tissue covers about 3 cm of the aorta above the celiac axis and is in turn covered by crural muscle fibers. It can be identified by exposing the celiac artery and pushing this vessel posteriorly with the finger at the inferior rim of the median arcuate ligament. In Hill's operation, the surgeon dissects the celiac artery and the celiac ganglion away from the overlying median arcuate ligament in the midline, avoiding the two inferior phrenic arteries that arise from the aorta just to the right and just to the left of the midline. Nerve fibers from the celiac ganglion must be cut to liberate the median arcuate ligament.

An alternative method of identifying the median arcuate ligament is to visualize the anterior surface of the aorta above the aortic hiatus. A few fibers of preaortic fascia may have to be incised. Then with the left index fingernail pushing the anterior wall of the aorta posteriorly, pass the fingertip in a caudal direction. The fingertip will pass behind a strong layer of preaortic fascia and median arcuate ligament. Blocking further passage of the fingertip, at a point about 2–3 cm caudal to the upper margin of the preaortic fascia, is the attachment of the inferior border of the median arcuate ligament to the aorta at the origin of the celiac artery. The pulsation of the celiac artery is easily palpated by the fingertip, which is lodged between the aorta and the overlying ligament. Vansant, Baker, and Ross believe that the foregoing maneuver constitutes sufficient mobilization of the median arcuate ligament and that the ligament need not be dissected free from the celiac artery and ganglion to perform a posterior gastropexy. We believe that a surgeon, who has not had considerable experience in liberating the median arcuate ligament from the celiac artery, may find Vansant's modification to be safer than Hill's approach. If one succeeds in catching a good bite of the preaortic fascia and median arcuate ligament by Vansant's technique, the end result should be satisfactory. Hill himself has recommended that the inexperienced surgeon adopt Vansant's modification (see Herrington, Skinner, Sawyers, Hill et al., 1978, p. 52). If, in the course of performing the Hill operation, the celiac artery or aorta is lacerated, do not hesitate to divide the median arcuate ligament and preaortic fascia in the midline since this step may be necessary to expose the full length of the laceration.

Calibrating the Esophagocardiac Orifice

In addition to fixing the esophagocardiac junction to the median arcuate ligament, the Hill operation serves to narrow the entrance of the lower esophagus into the stomach by partially turning in the lesser curvature aspect of the esophagogastric junction. Calibration of this turn-in is important if reflux is to be prevented without, at the same time, causing chronic obstruction. Hill (1977) now uses intraoperative manometry to measure the pressure at the esophagocardiac junction before and after completing the gastropexy. He believes that a pressure of 50–55 mm Hg will assure that the calibration is proper. Orringer, Schneider, Williams, and Sloan reported that intraoperative pressures did not correlate at all with pressures obtained at postoperative manometry, perhaps because of the variable influence of preoperative medication and anesthetic agents.

If intraoperative manometry is not used, then the adequacy of the repair should be tested by invaginating the anterior wall of the stomach along the indwelling nasogastric tube upward into the esophagogastric junction. Prior to the repair, the index finger will pass freely into the esophagus because of the incompetent lower esophageal sphincter. After the sutures have been placed and drawn together, but not tied, the tip of the index finger should be able to palpate the esophageal orifice but should not quite be able to enter the esophagus alongside the 18F nasogastric tube. This method of calibration has been successful in our hands.

Liberating Left Lobe of Liver

Although most authors, who describe transabdominal repair of a hiatus hernia, advocate dividing the triangular ligament in order to liberate the left lobe of the liver and improve exposure of the hiatus, we have often not found this step to be necessary, just as we have not found it necessary in performing truncal or proximal gastric vagotomy. By elevating the left lobe of the liver with a deep Harrington or Weinberg retractor, the anterior margin of the hiatus is generally easy to expose, making the division of the triangular ligament a superfluous maneuver.

Operative Technique

Incision and Exposure

With the patient in the supine position, elevate the head of the table about 10°–15° from the horizontal. Make a midline incision from the xiphoid to a point about 4 cm below the umbilicus **(Fig. 68–1).** Insert a "chain" or Upper Hand retractor to elevate the lower portion of the sternum and draw it forcefully in a cephalad direc-

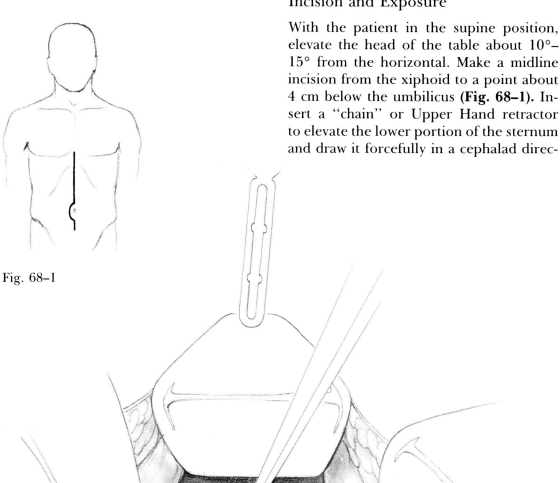

Fig. 68–1

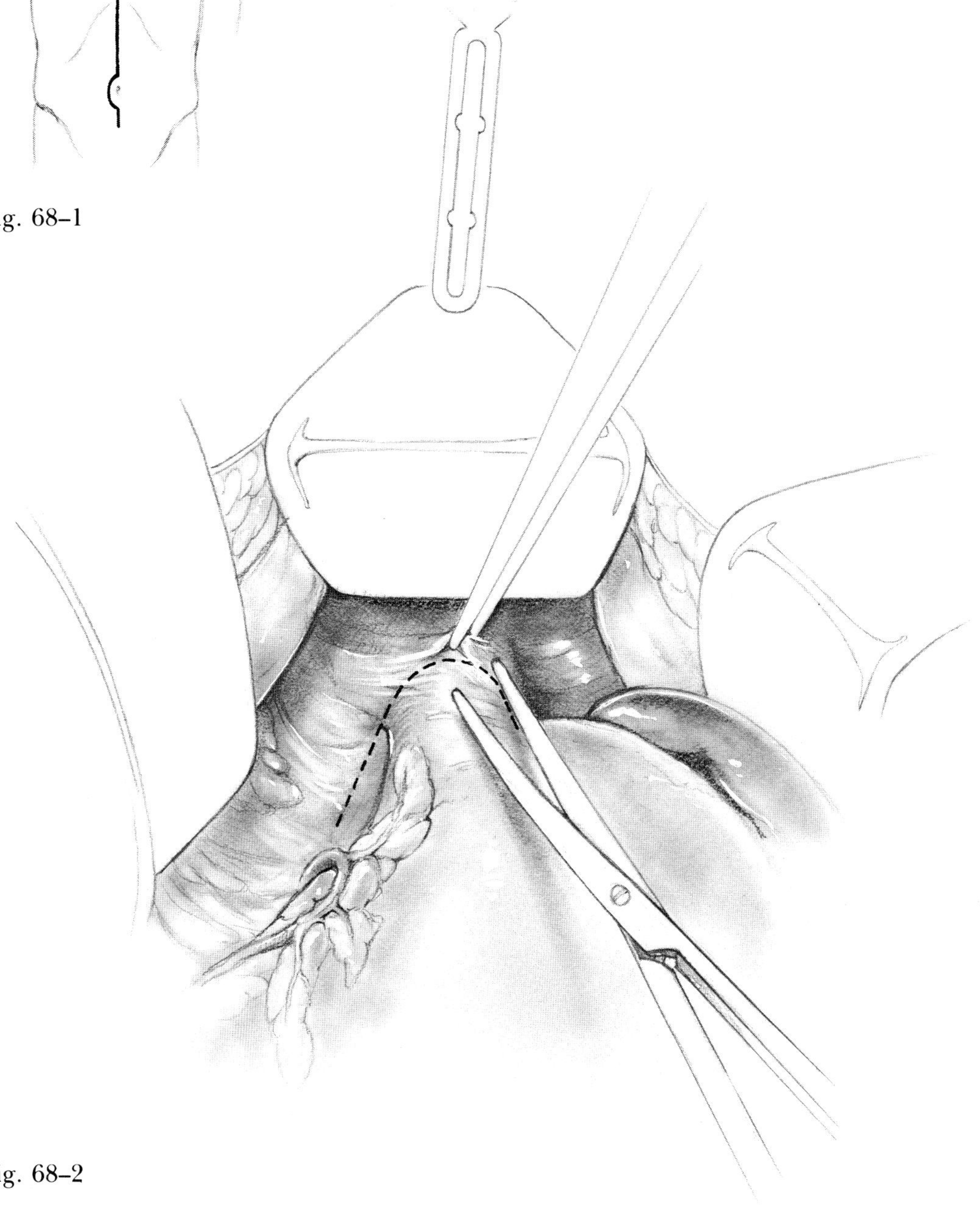

Fig. 68–2

tion. Explore the abdomen for incidental pathology such as duodenal ulcer, cholelithiasis, chronic pancreatitis, or colon disease.

Mobilizing the Esophagogastric Junction

Identify the peritoneum overlying the abdominal esophagus by palpating the indwelling nasogastric tube. Divide this peritoneum with a Metzenbaum scissors and continue the incision over the right and left branches of the crus **(Fig. 68–2)**. After exposing the crus, elevate this muscle by inserting a peanut sponge dissector between the crus and the esophagus, first on the right and then on the left. Then insert the left index finger to encircle the esophagus by gentle dissection. If the esophagus is inflamed owing to inadequately treated esophagitis, it will be easy to perforate it by rough finger dissection. Identify and protect both the right and left vagus nerves. Then encircle the esophagus with a latex drain and free it from posterior attachments by dividing the phrenoesophageal ligaments **(Fig. 68–3)**.

Make an incision in the avascular portion of the gastrohepatic ligament. Continue this incision in a cephalad direction toward the right side of the hiatus. In the course of dividing the gastrohepatic ligament, it is often necessary to divide an accessory left hepatic branch of the left gastric artery **(Fig. 68–4)**. At the conclusion of this step, the muscular portion of the crura surrounding the hiatus should be clearly visible throughout the circumference of the hiatus.

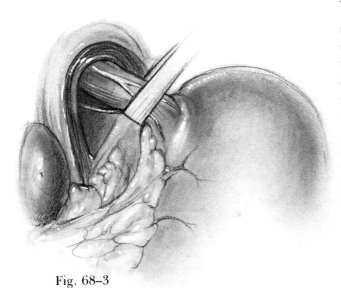

Fig. 68–3

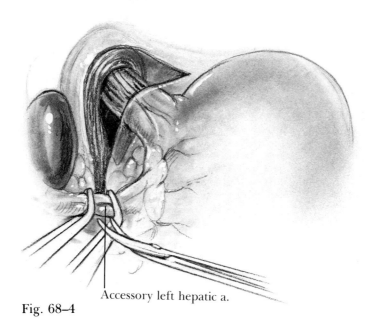

Accessory left hepatic a.

Fig. 68–4

279

The only structure binding the gastric fundus to the posterior abdominal wall now is the gastrophrenic ligament. The best way to divide this ligament is to insert the left hand behind the esophagogastric junction; then bring the left index finger between the esophagogastric junction and the diaphragm. This will place the ligament on stretch. Divide this avascular ligament **(Fig. 68–5)** from the esophagogastric junction along the greater curvature down to the first short gastric artery. It is often necessary to divide the first two short gastric vessels to achieve proper mobilization. This may be done by applying a Hemoclip to the splenic side and a 2–0 cotton ligature to the gastric side of the short gastric vessel.

Avoid injuring the spleen by carefully inspecting the anterior surface of this organ prior to dissecting in this region. Divide any attachments between the omentum and the splenic capsule since traction on the omentum would otherwise cause avulsion of the capsule and bleeding.

Inserting the Crural Sutures

Ask the first assistant to retract the esophagus toward the patient's left. Then narrow the aperture of the hiatus by approximating the crural bundles behind the esophagus. Use 0 Tevdek atraumatic sutures on a substantial needle. Take a bite of 1.5–2.0 cm of crus on the left and then a similar bite on the right. Include the overlying peritoneum together with the crural muscle **(Fig. 68–6)**. Do not tie these sutures at this time but tag each with a small hemostat. It is sometimes helpful to grasp the left side of the crus with a long Babcock or Allis clamp. Do not apply excessive traction with these clamps or with the sutures as the crural musculature will tend to split along the line of the muscle fibers. Insert 3–4 sutures of this type as necessary. Then tentatively draw the sutures together and insert the index finger into the remaining hiatal aperture. It should be possible to

insert a fingertip into the remaining aperture alongside the esophagus with its indwelling nasogastric tube. Narrowing the hiatal aperture more than this may cause permanent dysphagia and will not help reduce reflux. Do not tie the crural sutures at this point.

Identifying the Median Arcuate Ligament

Hill's Method

After the lower esophagus and proximal stomach have been completely freed, identify the celiac artery and use the left index finger to press it posteriorly into the aorta. If the index finger slides in a cephalad direction, its tip will meet the lower border of the median arcuate ligament. Between the aorta and median arcuate ligament there are branches of the celiac ganglion as well as the right and left inferior phrenic arteries, which arise from the aorta in this vicinity. It is necessary to divide some of the nerve fibers, but once the inferior margin of the ligament is freed from the aorta in the midline, it is possible to pass an instrument in a cephalad direction without encountering any further resistance. Hill passes a Goodell cervical dilator between the median arcuate ligament and the aorta to protect the aorta while sutures are being inserted into the lower border of the ligament. He states that if a small diaphragmatic branch of the aorta is disrupted, the bleeding will often subside with pressure. However, it is possible for the inexperienced surgeon to induce major hemorrhage by traumatizing the arteries in this vicinity. Caution is indicated.

Vansant's Method

Vansant, Baker, and Ross described another technique of identifying and liberating the median arcuate ligament by approaching it from its superior margin. In order to do this, identify the anterior surface of the aorta in the hiatal aperture between the right and left branches of the crus. Occasionally, it will be necessary to

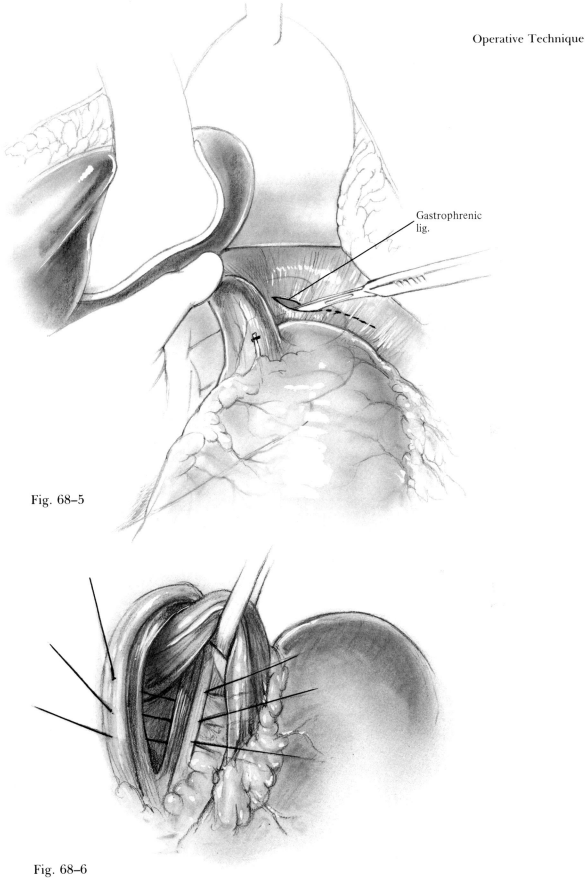

Gastrophrenic
lig.

Fig. 68–5

Fig. 68–6

dissect away some areolar tissue. With the left index fingernail pressing posteriorly against the aorta about 4 cm cephalad to the diaphragm, slide the index finger in a caudal direction. Deep behind the confluence of the diaphragmatic crura, the tip of the index finger will pass behind a dense band of preaortic fascia that crosses over the aorta as the aorta passes through the aortic hiatus in the posterior diaphragm. The width of this band is variable but averages perhaps 3 cm. At the lower margin of this band the fingertip will encounter the pulsation of the celiac artery, which arises from the anterior wall of the aorta at the inferior margin of the median arcuate ligament. The median arcuate ligament lies between the fingertip and a thin layer of muscle fibers representing the caudal confluence of the diaphragmatic crura. With the index finger in place, Vansant and associates insert three interrupted atraumatic sutures of No. 1 braided silk into the median arcuate ligament. Tag each suture with a hemostat, leaving each needle attached for later use in suturing the posterior gastropexy.

Suturing Posterior Gastropexy

Hill's Method
Rotate the esophagogastric junction so that the lesser curvature surface faces anteriorly and the posterior phrenoesophageal fascial bundle and the gastric wall adjacent to it are visible to the surgeon. Demonstrate the anterior and posterior vagal trunks to avoid piercing them by a suture. Apply Babcock clamps, one to the posterior and one to the anterior phrenoesophageal bundle. Hill then places one anchoring suture to fix the posterior phrenoesophageal bundle to the left border of the median arcuate ligament. Tie this suture. Then insert 4–5 gastropexy sutures taking first a bite of the anterior phrenoesophageal bundle, then the posterior phrenoesophageal bundle and, finally, the inferior border of the median arcuate ligament. The cephalad gastropexy suture

is the key suture with respect to calibrating the diameter of the esophageal lumen at the lower esophageal sphincter. Hill tentatively ties the upper suture and then measures the intraluminal pressure with an indwelling intraesophageal manometer catheter. He aims at an intraluminal pressure of 50–55 mm Hg. If the pressure is significantly below 50 mm Hg he takes additional sutures until the pressure has been raised to the proper level. A reading of 60 mm Hg or more indicates that the sphincter will be too tight. After tying all of the gastropexy sutures, take a final measurement of the intraluminal pressure.

Vansant's Method
Vansant and colleagues identify the median ligament by the technique described above. With an index finger in place between the preaortic fascia and the aorta, they insert three interrupted atraumatic sutures of No. 1 braided silk and tag each suture with a hemostat, leaving each needle attached. Then they close the hiatus with several interrupted sutures and insert the requisite sutures, approximating the anterior and posterior phrenoesophageal bundles. The phrenoesophageal sutures are tied. Then, they use the three preplaced #1 braided silk sutures to fix the phrenoesophageal bundles to the median arcuate ligament by passing each of these sutures through the phrenoesophageal bundles.

Author's Technique
Rotate the esophagogastric junction so that the lesser curvature aspect of the stomach faces anteriorly. Then place a large Babcock clamp on the anterior and another clamp on the posterior phrenoesophageal bundle. Between these two bundles, the longitudinal muscle fibers of the esophagus can be seen as they join the lesser curvature of the stomach. Where to place the proximal suture is an important consideration. Placing it too high will cause

excessive narrowing of the esophageal lumen; placing it too low will not adequately increase the intraluminal pressure in the lower esophageal sphincter area. We use 2–0 atraumatic Tevdek and include a few millimeters of adjacent gastric wall together with the phrenoesophageal bundle in order to insure that the submucosa has been included in the suture. After placing the first suture, cross the two ends or insert the first throw of a tie. Then estimate the lumen of the esophagastric junction by invaginating the stomach with the index finger along the indwelling nasogastric tube. If this maneuver is attempted before tying down the suture, the finger will pass easily into the lumen of the esophagus in patients who have an incompetent lower esophageal sphincter. After the first suture is tentatively closed, only the very tip of the index finger should be able to enter the esophagus. In the absence of intraoperative esophageal manometry, this is the best

method of calibrating the proper placement of the gastropexy sutures.

If the first suture has been judged to be properly placed, tag it with a hemostat and insert 3 additional sutures of atraumatic 2–0 Tevdek into the phrenoesophageal bundles at intervals of about 1 cm, caudal to the first suture. Place a hemostat on each suture as a tag. After all the sutures have been placed, tighten them all and again use the index finger to calibrate the lumen of the esophagogastric junction once more. If this is satisfactory, expose the anterior wall of the aorta in the hiatal aperture behind the esophagus. With the index fingernail closely applied to the anterior wall of the aorta, pass the fingertip in a caudal direction beneath the preaortic fascia and median arcuate ligament down to the point where the fingertip palpates the pulsation of the celiac artery. Then, remove the index finger and replace it with a narrow right-angled retractor such as the Army-Navy retractor **(Fig. 68–7).** Be certain that the retractor is indeed deep to

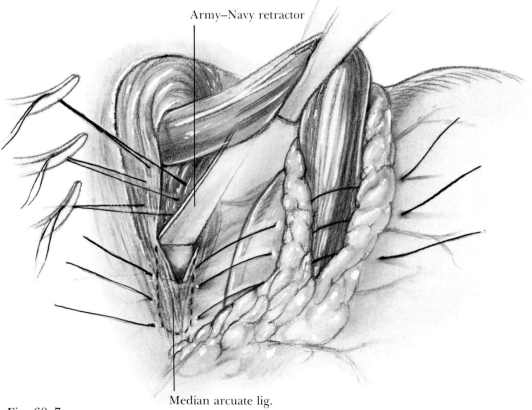

Army–Navy retractor

Median arcuate lig.

Fig. 68–7

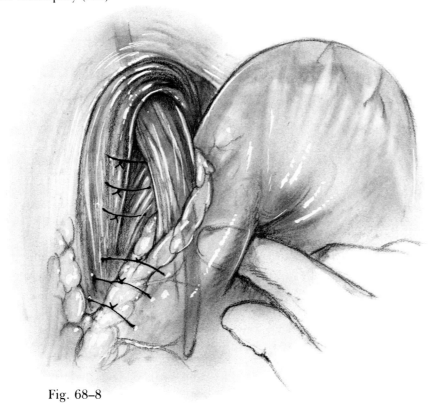

Fig. 68–8

the median arcuate ligament. This retractor will serve to protect the aorta while the gastropexy sutures are being inserted through the preaortic fascia.

Now identify the proximal suture that has already been placed in the phrenoesophageal bundles. Pass this suture through the preaortic fascia. Be sure to take a substantial bite of the tissue anterior to the Army-Navy retractor. Pass the needle deep enough so that it makes contact with the metal retractor. Otherwise, only some overlying crural muscle fibers may be included in the stitch. This will not be strong enough to assure a long-term successful result. After the first stitch has been passed through the preaortic fascia, tag it with a hemostat and pass each of the remaining phrenoesophageal sutures through the preaortic fascia by the same technique and tag each with a hemostat (see Fig. 68–7).

Another good method of expediting the suturing of the median arcuate ligament is to use a large right-angle bronchus clamp. Insert the tip of the clamp behind the median arcuate ligament instead of the Army-Navy retractor. Use the clamp to vigorously draw the median arcuate ligament anteriorly. Pass the needle with the suture through the median arcuate ligament just deep to the clamp. This assures that a large bite of ligament is included in each stitch. Be certain not to injure the underlying aorta with the needle.

At this point, check the entire area for hemostasis. Then tie the previously placed crural sutures (Fig. 68–6), thus narrowing the aperture of the hiatus. After these sutures have been tied, the index finger should pass freely into the hiatal aperture with an indwelling 18F nasogastric tube in the esophagus. If this is not the case, replace the proximal crural suture as necessary.

Now tie each of the previously placed *gastropexy* sutures and cut all of the ends **(Fig. 68–8).**

Testing the Antireflux Valve

A simple method of testing the efficacy of the antireflux valve is to have the anesthesiologist inject about 500 ml of saline into the nasogastric tube. Then ask him to withdraw the tube to a point above the esophagogastric junction. In the presence of a competent antireflux valve, compressing the saline-filled stomach will fail to force the saline into the esophagus.

Abdominal Closure

Irrigate the abdomen and the subcutaneous tissues with saline or a dilute antibiotic solution. Close the abdomen without drainage in routine fashion.

Postoperative Care

Continue nasogastric suction until gastrointestinal function resumes.

X ray the esophagogastric junction with a barium swallow before the patient is discharged from the hospital.

Postoperative Complications

Dysphagia (usually transient)

Persistence or recurrence of gastroesophageal reflux. This, as well as other complications following the Hill operation, are uncommon.

References

Herrington JL, Skinner D, Sawyers J, Hill LD et al. (1978) Surgical management of reflux esophagitis. Contemp Surg 12:42

Hill LD (1967) An effective operation for hiatal hernia; an eight year appraisal. Ann Surg 166:681

Hill LD (1977) Progress in the surgical management of hiatal hernia. World J Surg 1:425

Orringer MB, Schneider R, Williams GW, Sloan H (1980) Intraoperative esophageal manometry: is it valid? Ann Thorac Surg 30:13

Vansant JH, Baker JW, Ross DG (1976) Modification of the Hill technique for repair of hiatal hernia. Surg Gynecol Obstet 143:637

69 Transthoracic Gastroplasty (Collis) and Nissen Fundoplication

Indications

As discussed in the previous chapters (see esp. Chap. 66), this operation is indicated in patients with reflux esophagitis that has caused a significant degree of fibrosis, constriction, and *shortening of the esophagus*. In some patients without much esophageal shortening, advanced fibrosis itself will interfere with the antireflux efficiency of a fundoplication because the rigid esophageal walls will not be compressed by the fundoplication. For this reason, Pearson and Henderson; Urschel, Razzuk, Wood, Galbraith et al.; and Orringer and colleagues (see Chap. 66) believe that almost every esophageal stricture caused by reflux should be treated by a Collis gastroplasty and an antireflux procedure. A previous high subtotal gastrectomy generally contraindicates a Collis gastroplasty. Most patients with recurrent reflux esophagitis after a previous operation will require a thoracoabdominal Collis–Nissen operation. This operation is indicated whenever the esophagogastric junction cannot *without tension* be brought down to the level of the median arcuate ligament.

Preoperative Care

Esophagram and upper gastrointestinal X-ray series

Esophagoscopy with biopsy of stricture

Attempt to dilate the esophageal stricture up to size 40F. This can generally be done with Maloney dilators.

Insert a nasogastric tube down to the stricture on the morning of the operation.

If the patient has severe fibrosis and an advanced stricture, he may be one of the rare cases whose stricture cannot be dilated and thus requires resection and possible colon interposition. In such a case, perform a preoperative barium colon enema and routine bowel preparation. Among those patients who should receive preoperative bowel preparation are those whose strictures could not be dilated to the size of a 40F bougie. An angiogram of the colonic blood supply may also be helpful.

When esophagoscopy reveals severe acute ulcerative esophagitis with inflammation and bleeding, a 2–3 week period of preoperative treatment with cimetidine and/or a continuous intra-esophageal antacid drip will reduce the inflammation and lessen the risk of intraoperative perforation of the esophagus.

Pitfalls and Danger Points

Esophageal perforation

Hemorrhage resulting from traumatizing or avulsing the accessory left hepatic artery, the inferior phrenic artery, the ascending branch of the left gastric artery, a short gastric vessel, or the inferior pulmonary vein

Laceration of spleen

Inadvertent vagotomy

Inadequate suturing, permitting the fundoplication to slip postoperatively

Operative Strategy

Performing an Adequate Gastroplasty

The object of performing a gastroplasty is to lengthen a shortened esophagus for an extent sufficient to prevent any tension whatever from being exerted on the antireflux operation and hernia repair. This newly constructed esophagus ("neoesophagus") consists of a tube made from the lesser curvature of the stomach. The anesthesiologist passes a 50F Maloney dilator into the stomach and the tube is constructed by applying a GIA stapling device precisely at the esophagogastric junction parallel to and snug up alongside the Maloney dilator. When the GIA device is fired, the esophageal tube will be lengthened by approximately 5 cm. If the GIA has been placed snug against the esophagogastric junction, there will be no irregularities or outpouching at this point. In patients with advanced strictures, it is often necessary to apply the GIA a second time to construct a neoesophagus about 7 cm in length if tension is to be avoided.

If the gastric walls being approximated in the stapling device are of average thickness or less, it is probably not necessary to oversew the staple line, assuming that the surgeon is experienced in using staples for gastrointestinal anastomoses. He will check to see that the staples have been shaped into the form of a proper "B."

Also, he must be certain to check that the point, where the second application of the GIA meets the first row of staples, is securely closed. In the absence of all these conditions, we agree with Orringer that the precaution of oversewing the GIA staple line on the stomach is indicated. This is especially true if the gastric walls are somewhat thick or if the surgeon is inexperienced in using stapling techniques.

Mobilizing Esophagus and Stomach

Not only is it important to completely mobilize the distal esophagus, at least as far up as the inferior pulmonary vein, but the proximal stomach must be entirely free of attachments, just as is the case when a Nissen fundoplication is being performed through an abdominal approach. Only with full mobilization can this operation be accomplished without tension. This requires dividing the phrenoesophageal and the gastrophrenic ligaments, freeing the hiatus throughout its complete circumference from any attachments to the stomach or lower esophagus, as well as dividing an accessory left hepatic artery, which courses from the left gastric artery across the proximal gastrohepatic ligament to help supply the left lobe of the liver. After mobilization has been accomplished, the remaining maneuvers in the Collis–Nissen operation are not difficult.

If the esophagus is inadvertently perforated during the dissection, it will require careful judgment by the surgeon in deciding whether it is safe to suture the esophageal laceration or whether a resection and colon or jejunum interposition is necessary. If it is elected to suture the laceration, try to cover the suture line with a flap of parietal pleura (see Figs. 74–1 to 74–3).

Avoiding Hemorrhage

Avoiding unnecessary bleeding in any operation requires careful dissection and a knowledge of vascular anatomy. This is especially important when mobilizing the stomach through a thoracic approach, because losing control of the accessory left hepatic, a short gastric, or an inferior phrenic artery causes the proximal bleeding arterial stump to retract deep into the abdomen. Controlling these retracted vessels will be difficult and may require a laparotomy, or at least a peripheral incision in the diaphragm. Preventing this complication is not difficult if the dissection is orderly and the surgeon is aware of the anatomical location of these vessels.

Similarly, careful dissection and avoidance of traction along the greater curvature of the stomach will help prevent damaging the spleen.

Avoiding Esophageal Perforation

When the distal esophagus is baked into a fibrotic mediastinum, sharp scalpel dissection is safer than blunt dissection if injury to the esophagus and the vagus nerves are to be avoided. Sometimes the fibrosis terminates 8–9 cm above the diaphragm. If so, the esophagus and the vagus nerves can easily be encircled at this point. This will provide a plane for the subsequent dissection of the distal esophagus.

Operative Technique

Incision

With the patient in the lateral position with the left side up, make a skin incision in the sixth intercostal space from the costal margin to the tip of the scapula **(Fig. 69–1)**. Then identify the latissimus dorsi muscle and insert the index finger beneath it. Transect this muscle with the electrocoagulating device. Then divide the underlying anterior serratus muscle in similar fashion **(Fig. 69–2)**. In both cases it is preferable to divide these muscles somewhat caudal to the skin incision. This will help to preserve muscle function.

Then use the electrocautery to divide the intercostal muscles along the upper border of the seventh rib **(Fig. 69–3)** and open the pleura. Complete this opening from the costal margin to the region of the lateral spinal muscles. Separate the periosteum and surrounding tissues from a 1-cm segment of the posterior portion of the seventh rib lateral to the spinal muscles. Excise a 1-cm segment of this rib **(Fig. 69–4)**. Then divide the intercostal neuro-

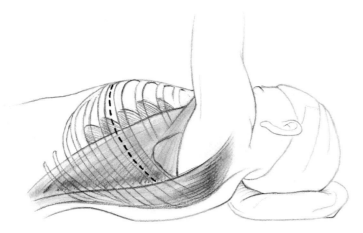

Fig. 69–1

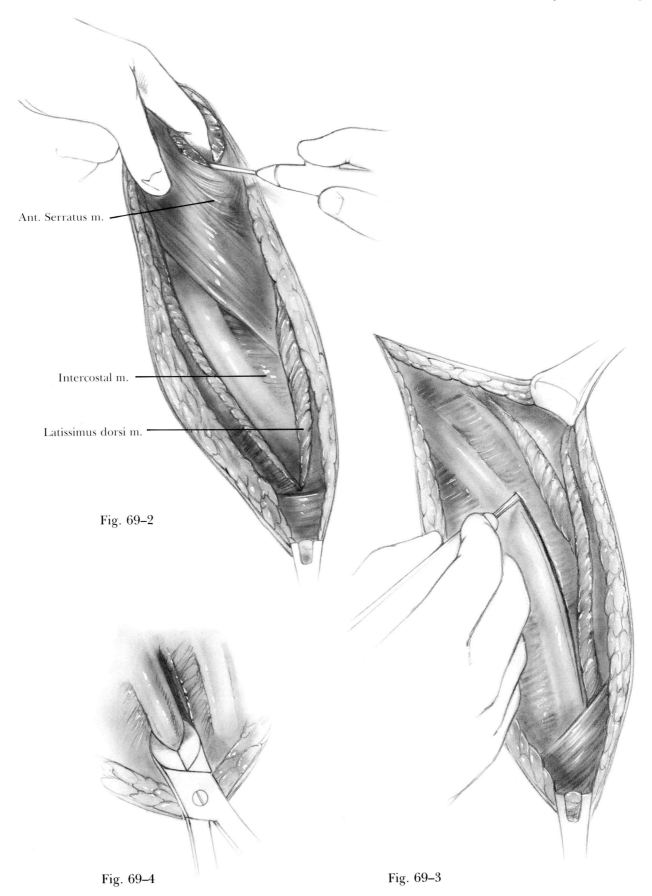

Ant. Serratus m.

Intercostal m.

Latissimus dorsi m.

Fig. 69–2

Fig. 69–4

Fig. 69–3

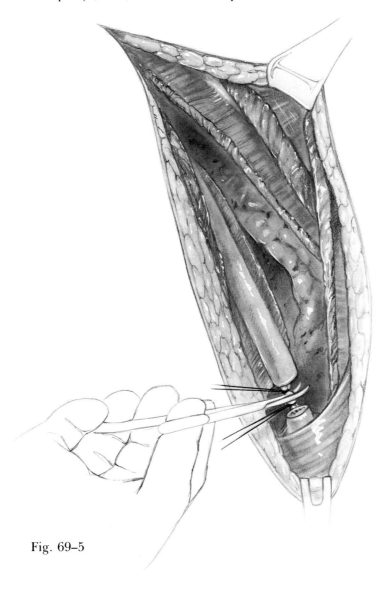

Fig. 69–5

vascular bundle that runs along the inferior border of this rib **(Fig. 69–5).**

Insert a Finochietto retractor into the incision and gradually increase the distance between the blades of the retractor over a 10-minute period to avoid causing rib fractures.

In patients who have undergone previous surgery of the distal esophagus or proximal stomach, do not hesitate to continue this incision across the costal margin, converting it into a thoracoabdominal incision to facilitate dissection on the abdominal aspect of the diaphragmatic hiatus (see Vol. I, Figs. 8–5 to 8–7).

Liberating the Esophagus

Incise the inferior pulmonary ligament with the electrocoagulator and then compress the lung and retract it in both an anterior and cephalad direction by using moist gauze pads and Harrington retractors. Incise the mediastinal pleura just medial to the aorta **(Figs. 69–6 and 69–7).** Encircle the esophagus with the index finger using the indwelling nasogastric tube as a guide. If this cannot easily be done, it may be necessary to initiate sharp dissection at a somewhat higher level where the fibrosis may be less advanced. Encircle the esophagus and the vagus nerves with a 2-cm latex drain. Continue the dissection of

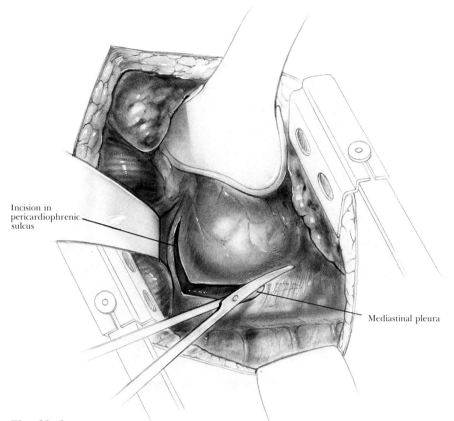

Incision in pericardiophrenic sulcus

Mediastinal pleura

Fig. 69–6

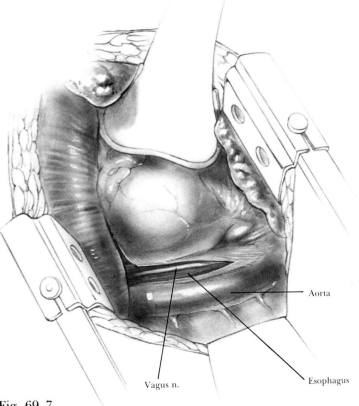

Aorta

Vagus n.

Esophagus

Fig. 69–7

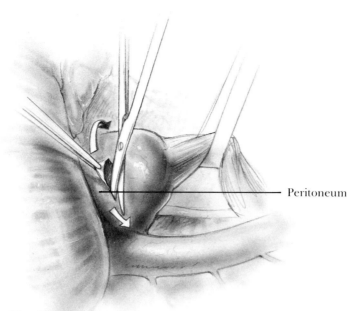

Fig. 69–8

the esophagus from the inferior pulmonary vein down to the diaphragmatic hiatus. After the mediastinal pleura has been incised down to the hiatus, continue the incision anteriorly and divide the pleura of the peri-cardiophrenic sulcus (see Fig. 69–6). Otherwise, the medial aspect of the hiatal ring will not be visible.

If the right pleural cavity has been inadvertently entered, simply place a moist gauze pad over the rent in the pleura to prevent excessive seepage of blood into the right chest and continue the dissection.

Excising the Hernial Sac

Identify the point where the left branch of the crus of the diaphragm meets the hernial sac. By applying traction to the diaphragm, some attenuated fibers of the phrenoesophageal ligament and preperitoneal fat will be encountered. Incise these tissues as well as the underlying peritoneum **(Fig. 69–8)**. Continue the incision in the peritoneum in a circumferential fashion, opening the lateral and anterior aspects of the hernial sac; expose the greater curvature of the stomach. Insert the left

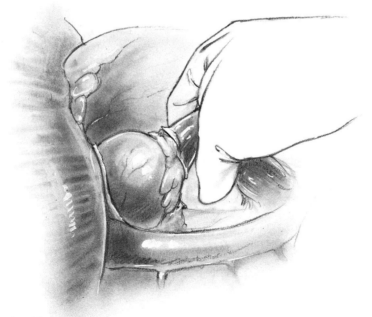

Fig. 69–9

index finger into the sac and continue the incision along the medial (deep) margin of the hiatus using the finger as a guide **(Fig. 69–9).** A branch of the inferior phrenic artery may be noted posteriolaterally near the left vagus nerve. This is divided, and ligated with 2–0 cotton. In attempting to circumnavigate the proximal stomach, the index finger in the hernial sac will encounter an obstruction on the lesser curvature side of the esophagogastric junction. This represents the proximal margin of the gastrohepatic ligament, which often contains a 2–4 mm accessory left hepatic artery coming off the ascending left gastric artery. By hugging the lesser curvature side of the cardia with the index finger, this finger can be passed between the stomach and the gastrohepatic ligament, thus delivering the ligament into the chest, deep to the stomach. Identify the artery and ligate it proximally and distally with 2–0 cotton. Divide it between the two ligatures **(Fig. 69–10).** After this step, it should be possible to pass the index finger around the entire circumference of the proximal stomach and encounter no attachments between the stomach and the hiatus. Throughout these maneuvers, repeatedly check on the location of the vagus nerves and preserve them.

Excise the peritoneum that constituted the hernial sac.

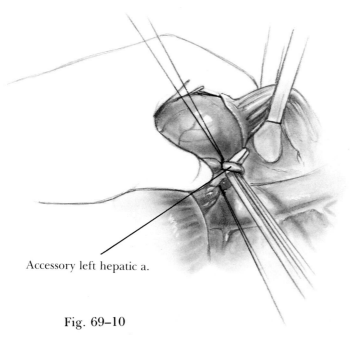

Accessory left hepatic a.

Fig. 69–10

Dilating an Esophageal Stricture

Ascertain that the esophagus is lying in a straight line in the mediastinum. Ask the anesthesiologist or a surgical assistant to pass Maloney dilators into the esophagus through the mouth after removing the indwelling nasogastric tube. As the dilator is passed down the esophagus, guide it manually into the lumen of the stricture. Successively larger bougies are passed up to size 50–60F. This can be successfully accomplished in probably 95% of cases. Occasionally forceful dilatation of this type may cause the lower esophagus to burst in the presence of unyielding transmural fibrosis. In this case, resect the damaged esophagus and perform a colonic or jejunal interposition between the healthy esophagus and the stomach.

Dividing the Short Gastric Vessels

Continue the dissection along the greater curvature of the stomach in an inferior direction until the first short gastric vessel is encountered. Use a long right-angled Mixter clamp to encircle this vessel with two 2–0 cotton ligatures. Tie each ligature leaving at least 1 cm between them. Divide between ligatures. Continue this process until about five proximal short gastric vessels have been divided and about 12–15 cm of greater curvature has been mobilized.

Gastroplasty

Check that the esophagogastric junction has indeed been completely mobilized. Identify the point at which the greater curvature of the stomach meets the esophagus. Overlying this area is a thin fat pad perhaps 3 cm in diameter. Carefully dissect this fat pad away from the serosa of the

293

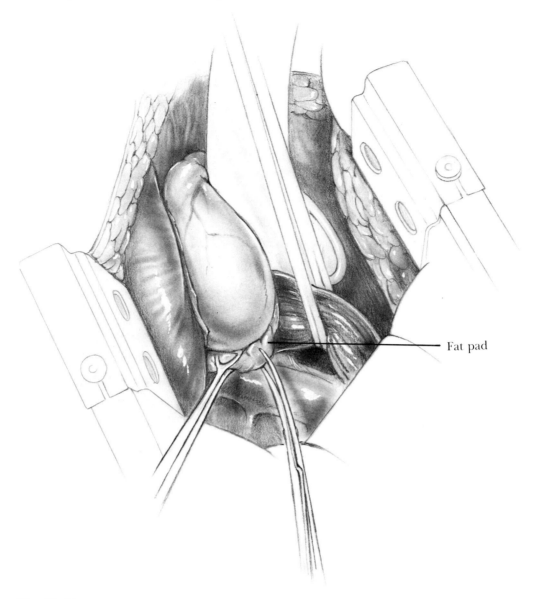

Fat pad

Fig. 69–11

stomach and the longitudinal muscle of the esophagus **(Fig. 69–11)**. Avoid damaging the anterior vagus nerve.

Pass a 56–60F Maloney dilator into the stomach and position it along the lesser curvature. Then apply the GIA stapler par-

allel to and closely adjacent to the Maloney dilator while a Babcock clamp retracts the greater curvature of the stomach in a lateral direction **(Fig. 69–12)**. Fire the stapler and remove it. Check to see that the staples have been shaped into an adequate "B" formation and that there are no leaks. Lightly electrocoagulate the everted mucosa. This maneuver will have lengthened the esophagus by approximately 4–5 cm **(Fig. 69–13)**. In most cases an additional length of neoesophagus will be necessary. Reload the GIA with a new cartridge. Then

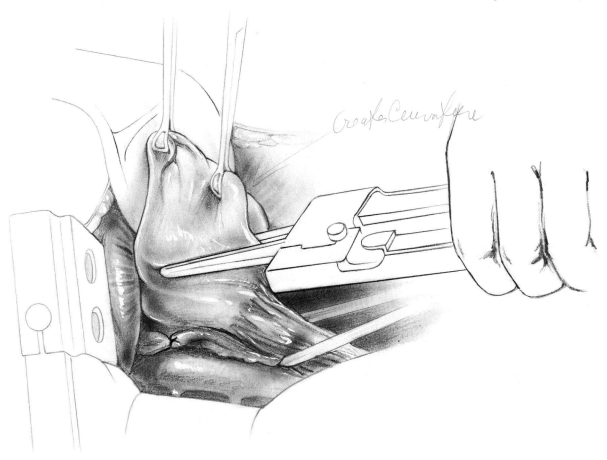

Fig. 69–12

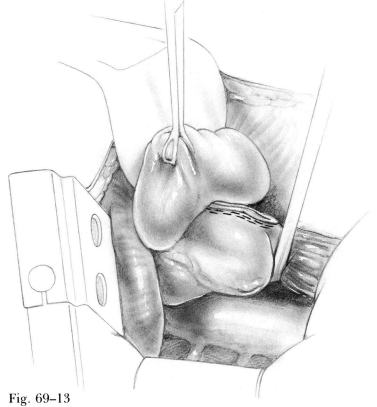

Fig. 69–13

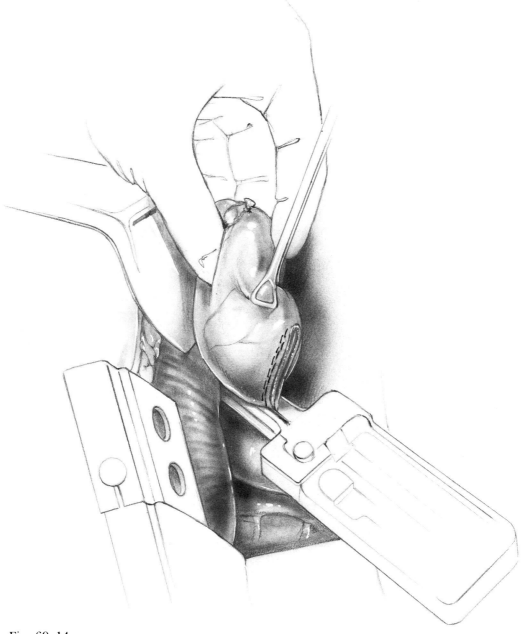

Fig. 69–14

reapply it again parallel to and snug up against the dilator in the lesser curvature of the stomach **(Fig. 69–14).** Apply the GIA to the 3-cm mark. Lock the device and fire it, thereby adding an additional 3 cm to the length of the neoesophagus **(Fig. 69–15).** Again check the integrity of the staple line. Although this step is not shown in the illustrations, it is probably wise as a precautionary measure to oversew the staple lines with two continuous Lembert sutures of either 4–0 Prolene or PG suture

material, one continuous suture to invert the staple line along the neoesophagus and the second continuous suture to invert the staple line along the gastric fundus. A continuous suture of the Lembert type is suitable, taking care not to turn in an excessive amount of tissue, as this will narrow the neoesophagus unnecessarily. If the gastric walls are of average or less than average thickness, and if the staples have been

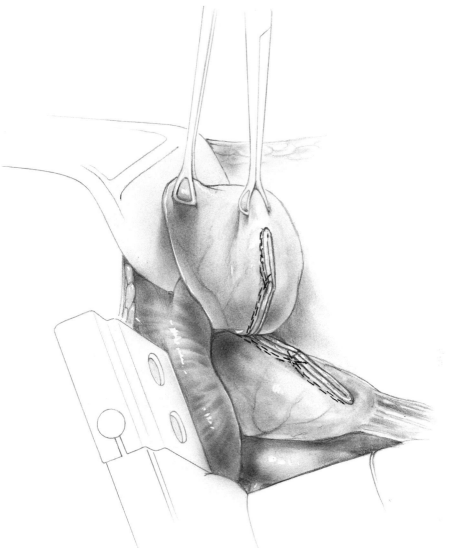

Fig. 69–15

properly placed, this suture line is probably not essential.

Performing a Modified Nissen Fundoplication

Since the neoesophagus has utilized a portion of the gastric fundus, there may not be sufficient remaining stomach to perform the Nissen fundoplication in the classical manner. Instead, as seen in **Fig. 69–16,** the apex of the gastric fundus is wrapped around the neoesophagus in a counterclockwise fashion.

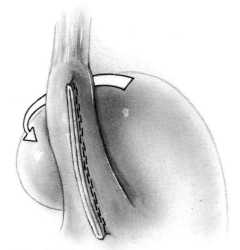

Fig. 69–16

297

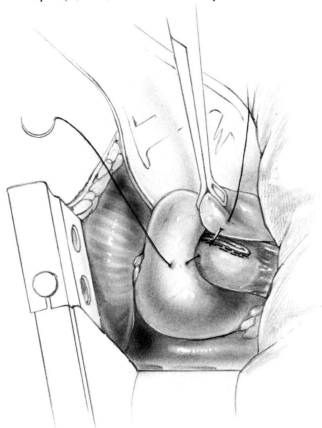

Fig. 69–17

Before inserting any sutures, remove the indwelling large Maloney dilator and replace it with one sized 46F. Place a large Hemoclip at the site of the new esophagogastric junction (i.e., the junction of the neoesophagus with the stomach) as a radiographic marker. The fundoplication should encircle the neoesophagus and the immediately adjacent stomach for a length of 3–4 cm **(Fig. 69–17).** About 3 cm of the neoesophagus and 1 cm of adjacent stomach are included in the fundoplication sutures.

Fig. 69–17 illustrates the insertion of the first Nissen fundoplication stitch including a 5–6 mm bite of gastric wall, then a bite of the neoesophagus, and finally a bite of the opposite wall of the gastric fundus. These bites should be deep to submu-

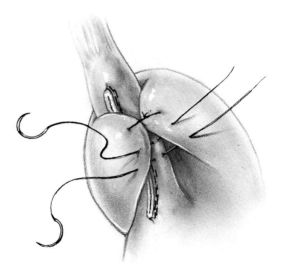

Fig. 69–18

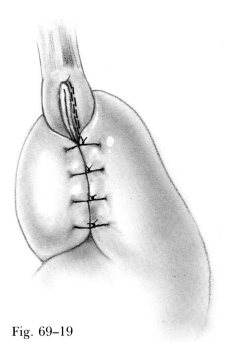

Fig. 69–19

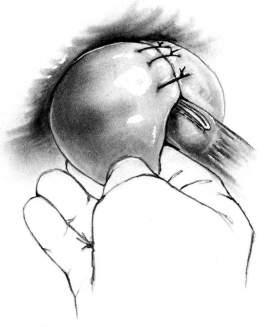

Fig. 69–20

cosa but not into the lumen of the stomach. Although Orringer uses 2–0 silk for this step, we prefer 2–0 Tevdek. A total of 4 fundoplication sutures are used at about 1-cm intervals **(Figs. 69–18 and 69–19).** Now remove the Maloney dilator from the esophagus and replace it with a nasogastric tube. **Fig. 69–20** illustrates that the fundoplication wrap around the neoesophagus is loose enough to admit the fingertip. Orringer then inverts the layer of fundoplication sutures by oversewing it with a continuous Lembert seromuscular suture of 4–0 Prolene. This step is not illustrated.

299

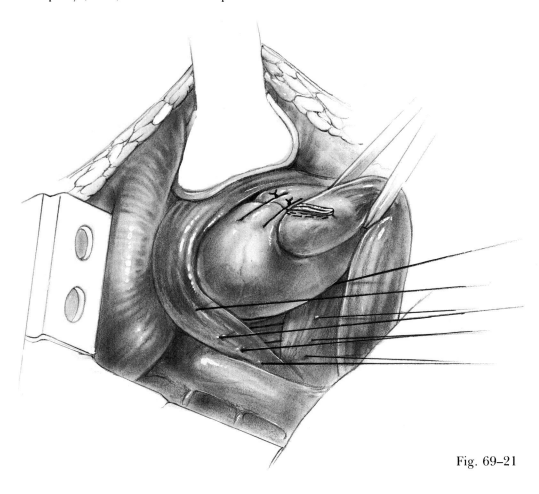

Fig. 69–21

Closing the Hiatal Defect

Close the defect in the posterior portion of the hiatus by inserting 0 Tevdek interrupted sutures through the right and left margins of the hiatus. Take a bite 1.5–2.0 cm in width and include overlying parietal pleura. After checking for hemostasis, reduce the fundoplication into the abdomen. This should slide down with ease. Then tie each of the sutures leaving space for the surgeon's fingertip alongside the esophagus or neosophagus, with a naso-gastric tube in place (**Figs. 69–21 and 69–22**). Place a Hemoclip at the edge of the hiatus as a marker. It is not necessary to resuture the incision in the mediastinal pleura.

Irrigate the mediastinum and thoracic cavity with warm saline and check for complete hemostasis. Insert a No. 36F plastic multiperforated intercostal drainage tube through a puncture wound below the level of the incision and bring the tube up the posterior gutter above the hilus of the lung. Insert 3–5 interrupted No. 2 PG pericostal sutures and tie them to approximate the ribs. Close the overlying serratus and latissimus muscles in two layers with 2–0 PG continuous sutures. Close the skin with continuous or interrupted fine nylon sutures.

Postoperative Care

Continue nasogastric suction until gastrointestinal function has resumed.

Continue perioperative antibiotics for 24–48 hours.

Order a barium esophagram X ray on the 7th postoperative day.

Remove the chest drainage tube on the 3rd day unless drainage is excessive.

Postoperative Complications

Obstruction. Not rarely there will be a partial obstruction at the area of the fundoplication due to edema during the first 2 weeks following surgery. If the wrap is too tight, this obstruction may persist.

Recurrent gastroesophagel reflux. This is uncommon after the Collis–Nissen procedure unless the fundoplication suture line disrupts.

Leakage from the gastroplasty or fundoplication sutures. This complication is rare. If the fundoplication sutures are inserted into the lumen of the stomach and then the suture is tied with

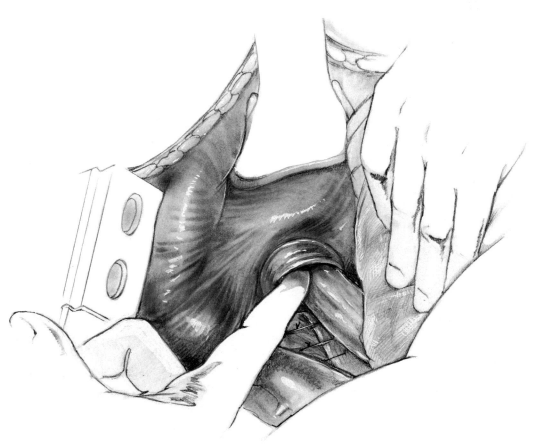

Fig. 69–22

strangulating force, a leak is possible. The risk of this occurring may be reduced by oversewing the fundoplication sutures line with a continuous Lembert seromuscular suture.

Necrosis of the gastroplasty tube. This complication was reported by Orringer and Orringer in an operation for recurrent hiatus hernia. They warn that traumatizing the lesser curve of the stomach may doom a gastroplasty tube.

References

Orringer MB, Orringer JS (1982) The combined Collis–Nissen operation: early assessment of reflux control. Ann Thorac Surg 33:534

Orringer MB, Sloan H (1978) Combined Collis–Nissen reconstruction of the esophago-gastric junction. Ann Thorac Surg 25:16

Pearson FG, Henderson RD (1973) Experimental and clinical studies of gastroplasty in the management of acquired short esophagus. Surg Gynecol Obstet 136:737

Urschel HC, Razzuk MA, Wood RE, Galbraith NF, et al. (1973) An improved surgical technique for the complicated hiatal hernia with gastroesophageal reflux. Ann Thorac Surg 15:443

70 Operations to Replace or Bypass the Esophagus: Colon or Jejunum Interposition; Gastric Pull-Up

Concept: To Replace or to Bypass the Esophagus

Colon Interposition or Bypass

Using the colon (or jejunum) to replace resected segments of the esophagus permits the surgeon to preserve intact a functioning stomach. Performing the cologastric anastomosis 8–9 cm down from the gastric cardia will generally minimize gastrocolic reflux. Achieving a sufficient length of viable colon is, with rare exceptions, a relatively simple task. One drawback to using the colon as a substitute esophagus is the risk of impairing the venous blood flow either by injuring the veins in the colon mesentery or impairing venous return by leaving an inadequate aperture in the diaphragm or at the apex of the thorax for the colon and its mesentery. Under these conditions venous infarction can occur. Following careful surgery, this complication should be quite rare. Belsey experienced one colon infarct in 92 left colon interposition operations. This complication appears to be more common when the right colon is used as opposed to the left colon (Wilkins). When performed for benign disease, the left colon interposition is a safe operation. Belsey reported a 4.3% mortality, but no anastomotic leaks. Skinner, in discussing a paper by Mansour, Hansen, Hersh, Miller, and others, stated that they had had no hospital deaths in 40 consecutive operations for colon interposition after the resection of nondilatable benign strictures of the esophagus. Also, Skinner's long-term functional results following the use of the left colon interposition have been good. Belsey, after following his patients for 1–6 years, reported 81% good and 17% satisfactory results. Wilkins followed a group of 21 patients for 5–24 years and reported excellent functional results. Glasgow, Cannon, and Elkins also reported good or excellent results and no operative deaths following 17 left and 1 right colon interposition operations for benign esophageal disease. These patients had been followed for 1–6.5 years. Good results following colon interposition in children were reported by Kelly, Shackelford, and Roper.

Gastrocolic regurgitation has rarely been symptomatic, although some patients have noted a slow transit time for a bolus of food to pass from the colon into the stomach.

The major objection to using the colon as an esophageal substitute has been the fact that more time is required to perform three anastomoses, as compared to the single esophagogastric anastomosis, which is required following a gastric pull-up in the neck. With modern stapling techniques, the colocolonic and the cologastric anastomosis can each be accomplished in a matter of a very few minutes, and the colon can be mobilized rapidly by an experienced colon surgeon. We do not feel that there is a significant difference in the time or the complexity of surgery when one compares the colon with the gastric esophageal substitute, provided that the surgeon is equally experienced and skilled in both areas.

303

Jejunum Interposition

For patients requiring the replacement of a relatively short segment of the esophagus, interposing a segment of jejunum is extremely effective in preventing further reflux. Polk noted no evidence nor any symptoms of reflux following 28 such operations in patients who had previously undergone many failed surgical procedures for the complications of reflux esophagitis. Polk's mortality was 4%. Moylan, Bell, Cantrell, and Merendino also reported very good functional results in 16 of 17 patients followed 10–17 years. Since peristalsis in the jejunum is considerably more vigorous than in the colon, it may well be that for patients, who have had many failed operations for reflux esophagitis, interposing the jejunum may be more effective for a short segment replacement than the colon. However, mobilizing a 15–20 cm segment of jejunum with preservation of both venous and arterial circulation can be difficult and time consuming. The jejunum interposition is contraindicated if the segment of jejunum must reach above the level of the inferior pulmonary vein.

Gastric Pull-Up

It has long been recognized that resection of a peptic stricture of the lower esophagus followed by esophagogastrostomy is often followed by disastrous consequences (Belsey). This is true because even when the esophagogastric anastomosis is made end-to-side, postoperative gastroesophageal reflux may occur. In patients, who undergo esophagogastrectomy for carcinoma of the esophagus, this may not be a prominent symptom because of their limited life expectancy. On the other hand, Orringer and Orringer (1982) have recommended total thoracic esophagectomy with esophagogastric anastomosis in the neck for patients with benign esophageal diseases such as neuromotor disorders or strictures that have failed to respond to multiple previous operations. When the stomach is stretched to reach the neck, it becomes a tubular or-

gan and the incidence of reflux esophagitis is said to be insignificant. Orringer claims that, following the gastric pull-up operation, the functional results are good. Nevertheless we have noted that regurgitation can be a significant problem both in the immediate postoperative period and at a later date. The patients must be instructed to sleep with the head of the bed elevated in most cases if aspiration is to be prevented. In 1977 Orringer, Kirsh, and Sloan stated:

> We believe that colonic interposition with isoperistaltic left colon based on the ascending branch of the left colic artery as described by Belsey, is currently the best method of esophageal reconstruction for benign disease in relatively healthy patients in the first four to five decades of life. The relative size, length, constancy of blood supply, and ease of mobilization of the left colon and transverse colon through a left thoracoabdominal incision make this segment of bowel ideal for either one stage esophagectomy and reconstruction or for substernal bypass.

Skinner; Wilkins; Glasgow, Cannon, and Elkins; and Belsey—as well as this author—agree with the above statement. However, Orringer and Orringer (1983) later changed this opinion so that they now believe "that transhiatal esophagectomy without thoracotomy is the preferred approach in virtually all patients requiring esophageal resection." Follow the esophagectomy with a gastric pull-up, these authors advise.

Reversed Gastric Tube

First reported in 1955 by Heimlich and also by Gavriliu, the reversed gastric tube has achieved a certain degree of acceptance as a substitute for the esophagus in adults as well as in children. Heimlich (1975) reported performing this operation in 67 patients with a 4.2% operative mortality and with good functional results. Nine of these patients had previously undergone colon or jejunum interposition operations that had failed. This operation requires the construction of a tube 30 cm by 2.5 cm in size from the greater curvature of the stomach, with its blood supply based on the left gastroepiploic artery and vein. This tube is generally anastomosed to the cervical esophagus. It can be brought to the neck by way of the bed of the resected thoracic esophagus, by the substernal route, or by the subcutaneous route, all with equally good results according to Heimlich. Anderson and Randolph noted satisfactory results with the gastric tube interposition in children.

Since we have no experience with this operation, and since there are few reports documenting its risks and end results, a description of the operative technique is not included in this volume.

Concept: To Preserve the Esophagus with a Bile Diversion Operation

Reflux Esophagitis Following Esophagogastrectomy

When a proximal gastrectomy has been performed with removal of more than half the stomach, it may not be possible to perform an end-to-side esophagogastric anastomosis because the remaining pouch of antrum is too small. In these patients reflux esophagitis is likely to occur. When a proximal gastrectomy is performed for cancer, truncal vagotomy combined with hemigastrectomy will generally eliminate any significant amount of acid secretion; reflux esophagitis nevertheless occurs because bile often backs up into the esophagus through an incompetent pyloric sphincter. The reflux of bile produces more damage to the esophagus than is provoked by the reflux of acid. This situation may be remedied by performing a total gastrectomy with an esophagojejunostomy by the Roux-Y technique. However, this may be difficult as a secondary operation, requiring a thoracoabdominal incision. In an elderly poor-risk patient, an alternative is to transect the duodenum about 2 cm beyond the pylorus. Close the duodenal stump. Then anastomose the proximal cut end of the duodenum to a Roux-Y segment, 60 cm in length. Since there is no significant amount of acid being secreted by the residual gastric pouch, and since bile reflux is eliminated by the Roux-Y operation, reflux esophagitis will subside. In performing this operation, be sure to *preserve the right gastric and right gastroepiploic blood supply* to the gastric remnant because these two vessels constitute its only blood supply.

When the patient has undergone an esophagogastrectomy for benign disease, and there is some doubt whether a complete vagotomy was performed, preoperative acid studies of the gastric pouch may be beneficial. Anastomosing a Roux-Y segment of jejunum to a gastric pouch that produces a significant amount of acid may produce a marginal ulcer. In this case the bile diversion operation is probably contraindicated unless a simultaneous vagotomy can be accomplished. Smith and Payne have reported success in relieving reflux esophagitis after esophagogastrectomy by the use of Roux-Y bile diversion.

Reflux Esophagitis Following Multiple Failed Antireflux Operations

Patients, who have had multiple failed operations aimed at eliminating gastroesophageal reflux, may be helped by a Collis–Nissen operation (see Chap. 69). If they have a nondilatable stricture, a resection and jejunum or colon interposition will be necessary. However, approaching the esophagogastric junction after several previous operations can be a formidable as

305

well as hazardous undertaking in some patients. In such cases, one can consider performing a distal gastrectomy followed by closure of the duodenal stump and anastomosis of the gastric pouch to a Roux-Y limb of jejunum. Payne advocated performing truncal vagotomy in all of these patients. He reported a series of 15 cases, 6 of whom also suffered from strictures. Seven of the patients had acquired a short esophagus secondary to chronic esophagitis. Two of the patients suffered from scleroderma of the esophagus with esophagitis and stenosis. Both had previous failed surgery. Another three patients had severe esophagitis and strictures following treatment of achalasia. All of the patients achieved relief of their esophagitis and the strictures responded nicely to dilatations following distal gastrectomy and Roux-Y gastrojejunostomy. Payne pointed out that this operation did not relieve the problem of gastroesophageal regurgitation. Consequently, some of the patients suffered from regurgitation of a bland liquid into the mouth when stooping or recumbent. This regurgitation did not produce any irritation. For this reason bile diversion is not an ideal solution to the problem of recurrent esophageal reflux, but the operation, in some patients, will be much safer than a repeated attack upon the esophagogastric junction.

It is interesting that Royston, Dowling, and Spencer performed the same operation in eight patients with severe esophagitis and strictures of long duration, but they did not include vagotomy. All of their patients had excellent results over a followup period of 11–20 months. In fact, some of the patients with strictures showed spontaneous resolution and did not require dilatation. Apparently, performing an adequate distal gastrectomy may reduce the gastric acidity sufficiently for the patient to tolerate a Roux-Y anastomosis to the gastric pouch without producing a marginal ulcer. If a marginal ulcer does occur, a transthoracic vagotomy may be necessary.

Indications

Short-Segment Interposition

Reflux esophagitis with nondilatable stricture

Repeated failed operations for reflux esophagitis

Total Replacement or Bypass of Thoracic Esophagus

Caustic burns of esophagus with permanent stricture

Failed operations for neuromotor disorders of the esophagus with reflux and permanent stricture

Resection of esophagus for postemetic perforation or intrathoracic anastomotic leaks

Bypass of inoperable obstructing esophagogastric carcinoma

(See also Table 70–1)

Preoperative Care

Nutritional rehabilitation whenever indicated

Perioperative antibiotics

If colon interposition is contemplated, preoperative barium colon X ray and arteriography of the superior and inferior mesenteric vessels to delineate colon circulation

Routine bowel preparation if colon is to be employed

Operative Technique—Colon Interposition, Long Segment

Incision—Resection of Esophagus

In patients who have experienced irreversible strictures following a caustic burn of the esophagus, there is no quantitative data to determine whether removing the de-

TABLE 70–1. Indications for Various Types of Esophageal Substitution

	Colon Inter-position or Bypass	Jejunum Interposition	Gastric Pull-Up	Reverse Gastric Tube
Benign Disease				
Short lesion	Yes	Yes	No	No
Long lesion—adult	Yes	No	No	Yes
Malignant Disease[a]				
Inoperable Esophageal CA	Yes	No	Yes	Yes
Inoperable Esophagogastric CA	Yes	No	Yes	No
CA Thoracic Esophagus–				
Subtotal Esophagectomy	?	No	Yes	No
CA Cervical Esophagus–				
Pharyngolaryngectomy	?	No	Yes	No

[a] CA = carcinoma, carcinoma of

stroyed esophagus carries with it a greater risk than the risk of the patient developing esophageal carcinoma if the organ is left behind. In the young patient we would tend to remove the esophagus and replace it with a long segment of left colon using a 6th interspace left thoracoabdominal incision (see Vol. I, Figs. 8–3 to 8–8). Patients, who have irreversible peptic esophagitis, will require resection of the esophagus. Otherwise, continued gastroesophageal reflux has been shown frequently to produce ulcerations and hemorrhage in the remaining esophagus. For this condition, transthoracic esophagectomy is generally performed. It is also performed on patients who have undergone failed operations for neuromotor esophageal disorders or who have had diversion–exclusion operations (see Chap. 74) for esophageal perforations or for anastomotic leakage. On the other hand, Orringer and Orringer (1983) do not open the chest in most of these patients; instead, they perform a transhiatal esophagectomy from the abdominal and cervical approaches.

We prefer a 6th interspace left thoracoabdominal incision for most of these esophagectomies. Close the gastroesophageal junction in an area relatively free of disease using the TA-55 or TA-90 stapler on the stomach side. Also close the esophageal end with another application of the stapling device. Dissect the esophagus out of the mediastinum. If the esophagus is markedly fibrotic, this dissection may require a scalpel. After the esophagus has been freed to the arch of the aorta, dissect the esophagus out from beneath the arch of the aorta as illustrated in Vol I, Fig. 8–27. Temporarily leave the esophagus in its bed until the colon has been liberated.

Colon Dissection

The initial step in preparing a long colon segment is to liberate the hepatic flexure as well as the entire transverse and descending colon. If necessary, extend the thoracoabdominal incision below the umbilicus. Also dissect the omentum away from the transverse colon and its mesentery, as illustrated in Figs. 19–5 and 19–6 and in Figs. 28–1 to 28–6.

With this accomplished, inspect the blood supply of the left and transverse colon. Preserving the left colic artery will in almost every case permit transection of the middle colic vessels close to the point of origin and will yield a segment of colon that could include a good portion of the descending colon as well as the right colon,

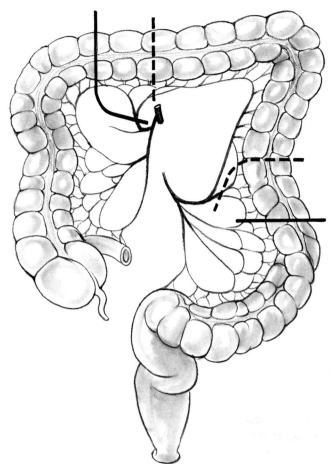

Fig. 70–1.   Solid lines indicate points of division for creating a long-segment colonic interposition; dotted lines, for a short-segment interposition

if that should be necessary. We have not encountered any cases where the "marginal artery" did not continue unimpeded from the left colon around to the right portion of the transverse colon. However, this should be checked by careful palpation of the marginal artery as well as transillumination of the mesentery. If there is any doubt concerning the adequacy of the blood supply, apply bulldog vascular clamps along the marginal artery at the points selected for division and check the adequacy of the pulse in the vessels being retained to supply the transplanted segment. Use an umbilical tape to measure the distance between the upper neck and midstomach. Lay this tape along the marginal artery of the colon to achieve a rough estimate of the amount of colon necessary for the interposition operation. Always add an additional 5–7 cm to this estimate. Divide the mesentery in roughly the locations identified in **Fig. 70–1.** Also divide the inferior mesenteric vein at the lower border of the pancreas.

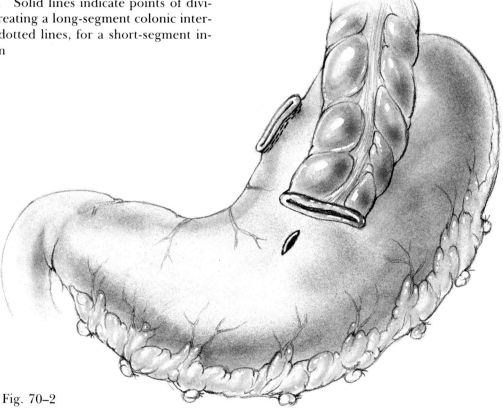

Fig. 70–2

Transect the colon at the proximal and distal margins of the segment selected for transplantation. Restore continuity to the colon by performing a stapled anastomosis as illustrated in Figs. 28–33 to 28–36. Close the proximal (right) margin of the colon transplant (temporarily) with a TA-55 stapler and leave the distal end of the colon segment open.

Cologastrostomy

Elevate the stomach with its attached omentum away from the pancreas. Divide the avascular attachments between the peritoneum overlying the pancreas and the back wall of the stomach. Also incise the avascular portion of the gastrohepatic omentum. Then draw the colon transplant with its mesentery in an isoperistaltic direction through the retrogastric plane and through the opening in the gastrohepatic omentum. Be certain not to twist the mesentery.

Now prepare to anastomose the open end of the distal colon to a point on the stomach approximately one-third of the distance down from the fundus to the pylorus. The anastomosis may be made on the anterior or the posterior side of the stomach. As illustrated in **Fig. 70–2,** make a 1.5 cm vertical incision in the stomach about one-third of the way down from the fundus. Then insert the GIA stapler, one fork in the stab wound of the stomach and one in the open lumen of the colon. Insert the GIA to a depth of 3 cm and lock the instrument **(Fig. 70–3).** Then fire the stapling device and remove it. Inspect the staple line for bleeding. Then apply one Allis clamp to the left extremity of the GIA staple line and another Allis clamp to the right termination of the GIA staples. Insert a guy suture through the midpoint of the stab wound of the stomach as illustrated

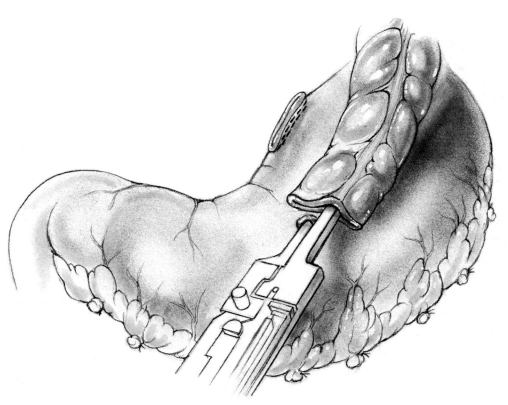

Fig. 70–3

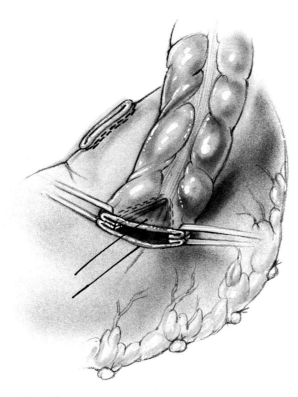

Fig. 70–4

in **Fig. 70–4.** Close the remaining defect by two applications of the TA-55 stapler. First, apply the stapler just deep to the Allis

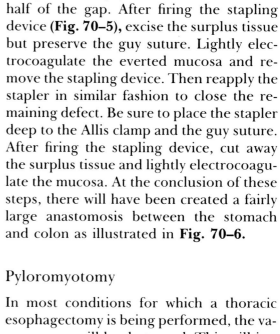

clamp and the guy suture to close the left half of the gap. After firing the stapling device **(Fig. 70–5),** excise the surplus tissue but preserve the guy suture. Lightly electrocoagulate the everted mucosa and remove the stapling device. Then reapply the stapler in similar fashion to close the remaining defect. Be sure to place the stapler deep to the Allis clamp and the guy suture. After firing the stapling device, cut away the surplus tissue and lightly electrocoagulate the mucosa. At the conclusion of these steps, there will have been created a fairly large anastomosis between the stomach and colon as illustrated in **Fig. 70–6.**

Pyloromyotomy

In most conditions for which a thoracic esophagectomy is being performed, the vagus nerves will be destroyed. This will impair gastric emptying to a fairly severe degree in about 20% of cases. In order to prevent this complication, a pyloromyotomy may be performed by the technique illustrated in Figs. 7–17 to 7–19.

Advancing the Colon Segment to the Neck

Be certain to enlarge the diaphragmatic hiatus (see Fig. 7–20) sufficiently so that the veins in the colon mesentery will not be compressed by the muscles of the hiatus. The most direct route to the neck is along the course of the original esophageal bed in the posterior mediastinum. This may be accomplished by placing several sutures between the proximal end of the colon transplant and the distal end of the esophagus; then draw the colon up into the neck by withdrawing the esophagus into the neck. This will bring the colon into the posterior mediastinum behind the arch of the aorta and into the neck posterior to the trachea. If there is no constriction in the chest along this route, the sternum and clavicle at the root of the neck are also not likely to compress the colon. On the other hand, if a substernal tunnel is selected for passing the colon up to the

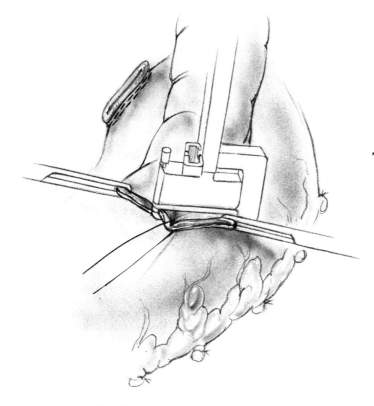

Fig. 70–5

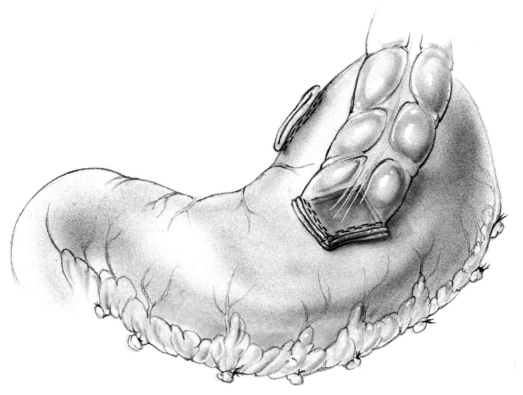

Fig. 70–6

neck, it is generally necessary to resect the head of one clavicle and a 1–2-cm width of adjacent sternal manubrium in order to be certain that there will not be any venous obstruction at that point.

Check to see that the tube of colon from the neck to the abdominal cavity lies in a straight line and that there is no surplus of colon in the chest. Leaving redundant colon in the thorax may produce a functional obstruction to the passage of food. After this item has been checked, suture the colon to the muscle of the diaphragmatic hiatus with interrupted sutures of atraumatic 4–0 Tevdek at intervals of about 2 cm around the circumference of the colon. This will help maintain a direct passageway from the neck into the abdomen and will also avoid the complication of small intestine herniating into the chest between the colon and the margins of the hiatus. Be sure not to pass the needle deep to the submucosa of the colon as colonic leaks have been reported from this error.

Dissecting the Cervical Esophagus

Change the position of the patient's left hand, which is now suspended from the ether screen. Bring the left hand laterally and place it along the left side of the patient. Turn the head slightly to the right and make an incision along the anterior border of the left sternomastoid muscle and continue the dissection as described in Figs. 7–27 to 7–30. Be careful not to damage either the left or the right recurrent laryngeal nerve. After dissecting the esophagus free down into the superior mediastinum, extract the thoracic esophagus by applying gentle traction in the neck. In this way the thoracic esophagus and the attached colon interposition segment may be drawn gently into the neck. At the same time, feed the colon into the diaphragmatic hiatus in the abdomen. Divide the distal cervical esophagus and remove the thoracic esophagus. Inspect the end of the colon. This should not be cyanotic as this indicates venous obstruction. Also, there should be a good pulse in the marginal artery. Draw the closed stapled end of the colon transplant to a point about 6–7 cm above the cut end of the esophagus and, taking care not to penetrate the lumen of the colon, suture the colon to the prevertebral fascia with several interrupted 4–0 sutures.

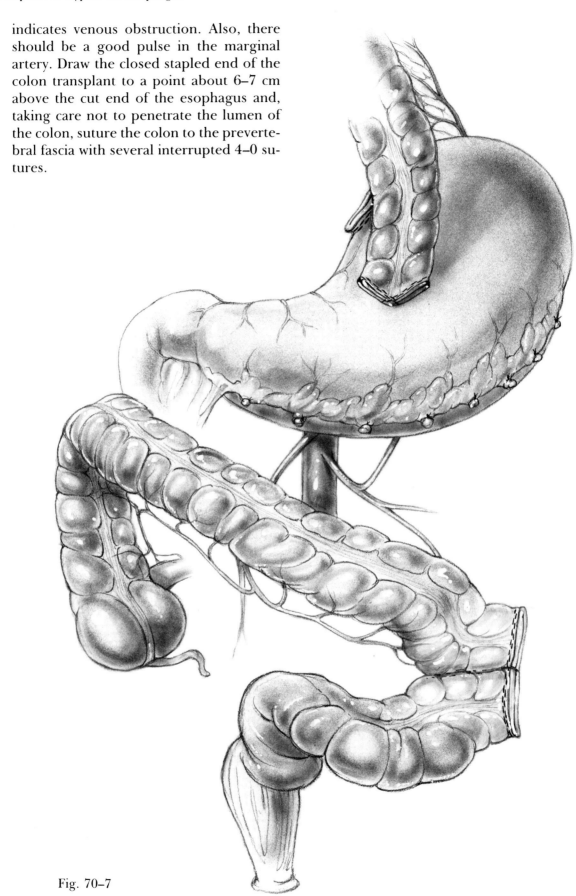

Fig. 70–7

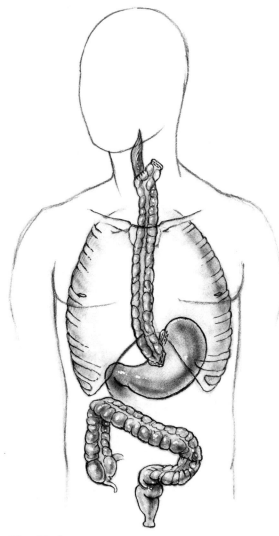

Fig. 70–8

Esophagocolonic Anastomosis

Perform an end-to-side esophagocolonic anastomosis at a point about 4 cm below the proximal end of the colon by using a technique similar to that described in Figs. 7–22 to 7–26 and by using interrupted 4–0 Prolene Cushing sutures for the outer layer and 5–0 Vicryl to the mucosal layer. Before closing the anterior portion of the anastomosis, ask the anesthesiologist to pass a nasogastric tube into the esophagus and guide this tube through the anastomosis into the colon.

During the course of this operation, whenever a hollow viscus is opened, irrigate the operative field with a dilute antibiotic solution.

Retrosternal Passage of Colon Transplant

When the posterior mediastinum is not a suitable pathway for the colon, or if the esophagus has not been removed, make a retrosternal tunnel to pass the colon up to the neck. If the left lobe of the liver is large, or if it appears to be exerting pressure on the posterior aspect of the colon transplant, liberate the left lobe by dividing the triangular ligament. This will permit the left lobe to fall in a posterior direction and thereby relieve this pressure. If the xiphoid process curves posteriorly and impinges on the colon, resect the xiphoid.

Enter the plane just deep to the periosteum of the sternum. Start the dissection with Metzenbaum scissors. Then insert one or two fingers of the right hand; finally pass the entire hand just deep to the sternum up to the suprasternal notch. This is generally an avascular plane. Orient the colon segment so that the mesentery enters from the patient's left side. Resect the medial 3–4 cm of clavicle. Then rongeur away about 1–2 cm of adjacent sternal manubrium in order to be certain that the aperture at the root of the neck is sufficiently large to avoid any venous obstruction in the mesentery. Pass a long sponge-holder into the retrosternal tunnel from the neck down into the abdomen, and suture the proximal end of the colon segment to the tip of the sponge-holder. Gently pass the colon into the substernal tunnel while simultaneously drawing the sutures in a cephalad direction.

Orringer, Kirsh, and Sloan point out that there will be fewer symptoms from resection of the clavicular head if it is performed on the side opposite the dominant hand. Once it has been ascertained that the circulation to the colon segment is good, perform the esophagocolonic anastomosis as above. The final appearance of the colon interposition is depicted in a diagrammatic fashion in **Figs. 70–7 and 70–8.**

313

Closure

Close the cervical incision in layers with interrupted 4–0 PG sutures. Insert one or two latex drains to the general vicinity of the anastomosis and leave these in place for 7–10 days. Close the skin in the usual fashion.

Close the thoracoabdominal incision as illustrated in Figs. 8–36 to 8–42.

Operative Technique—Colon Interposition, Short Segment

In rare cases with benign peptic strictures of the lower esophagus, it will not be possible to dilate the stricture, even in the operating room, without rupturing the esophagus. If there is no significant amount of disease above the level of the inferior pulmonary ligament, resect the diseased esophagus down to the esophagogastric junction and replace the missing esophagus with a short isoperistaltic segment of colon to extend from the divided esophagus to a point about one-third of the distance between the fundus and pylorus of the stomach. For a short-segment operation it is not necessary to divide the middle colic artery, and only the left half of the transverse colon and the splenic flexure need be employed. Otherwise, the operation is very much the same as described above. The cologastric anastomosis is identical. The esophagocolonic anastomosis may be sutured either in an end-to-end fashion, in an end-to-side fashion, or even by a stapling technique. The latter involves inserting a proper EEA cartridge (generally EEA-28 or EEA-25) into the open proximal end of the colon segment. The anastomosis is made between the end of the esophagus and the side of the colon by the EEA technique. Then, after disengaging the instrument, explore the anastomosis visually, and with a finger through the open end of the colon. If the exploration appears to be satisfactory, then close the opening in the colon about 1 cm away

from the EEA anastomosis by using a TA-55 stapler. Excise the redundant tissue and remove the stapler.

Operative Technique—Jejunum Interposition

Incision and Mobilization

Although Polk advocates performing mobilization of the esophagogastric junction through an upper midline abdominal incision, we much prefer the left 6th interspace thoracoabdominal incision with a vertical midline abdominal component. This is true because the jejunal interposition operation is performed primarily in patients who have had multiple failed previous operations for reflux esophagitis. The Collis–Nissen gastroplasty combined with dilatation of the esophageal stricture will suffice in most patients. This leaves a few of the most advanced cases that require either a colon (short-segment) or jejunum interposition. In order to make the esophagogastric dissection as safe as possible, the combined thoracoabdominal incision is much to be preferred over an abdominal approach or even using both a laparotomy and a separate thoracotomy incision. It should also be emphasized that creating a jejunal segment is much more difficult than the short-segment colon interposition. In performing the thoracoabdominal incision, incise the diaphragm with the electrocautery in a circumferential fashion as depicted in Fig. 8–8.

Now dissect the left lobe of the liver carefully away from the anterior wall of the stomach; in doing so, approach the dissection from the lesser curvature aspect of the stomach. At the same time, incise the gastrohepatic omentum by going up towards the hiatus. This may require division of the accessory left hepatic artery, provided this has not been done at a previous operation (see Fig. 68–4). It may also be difficult to free the upper stomach from its posterior attachments to the pancreas. Careful dissection with good exposure from the thoracoabdominal incision should make it possible to preserve the spleen from irreparable injury. At the conclusion of this dissection, the upper portion of the stomach and lower esophagus should be free. Freeing the esophagus in the upper abdomen may be expedited by first dissecting the esophagus out of its bed in the lower mediastinum.

Resection of Diseased Esophagus

After the esophagus has been freed from its fibrotic attachments in the mediastinum and upper stomach, select a point near the esophagogastric junction for resection. If the upper stomach has been perforated during this dissection and it can be included in the specimen, do so. If the upper stomach is not excessively thickened, apply a TA-55 or TA-90 stapling device with 4.8 mm staples and fire the stapling device. Transect the esophagogastric junction just above the stapling device. Lightly electrocoagulate the everted mucosa and remove the stapler. Deliver the transected esophagus into the chest and select the point of transection on the esophagus above the stricture. A mild degree of mucosal inflammation in the esophagus is acceptable at the point of transection. Remove the specimen.

If the point of division of the esophagus is not higher than the inferior pulmonary vein, a jejunal interposition is a good method of establishing continuity (Polk). If the esophagus must be transected at a higher level, use either a short segment of colon for the interposition, or remove the remainder of the thoracic esophagus and reestablish continuity either by means of a long-segment colon interposition from the neck to the stomach or by bringing the stomach up into the neck for this purpose as described below.

Mobilizing the Jejunum Graft

Because the vascular anatomy of the proximal jejunum varies somewhat from patient to patient, it is necessary to individualize the dissection according to the conditions encountered. First, try to stretch the proximal jejunum in a cephalad direction in order to determine where the greatest mobility is located. Be certain to leave intact at least the first major jejunal artery to the proximal jejunum. The average length of jejunal segment to be transplanted varies between 12 and 20 cm, and the pedicle should consist of at least one major arcade vessel with careful preservation of the veins. Most jejunal grafts fail not because of poor arterial circulation but because the veins have been injured or compressed at some point in their course. Follow the principles illustrated in Fig. 19–11, and try to preserve a vascular pedicle containing two arcade vessels with their veins intact. Occasionally the method illustrated in Fig. 19–12, of resecting a segment of jejunum but leaving its entire mesentery, will help to provide a vigorous blood supply to the transplanted jejunal segment. In dividing an arcade vessel, be sure to place the point of transection sufficiently proximal to a bifurcation so that the continuity of the "marginal" artery and vein will not be interrupted. Divide the jejunum proximally and distally; preserve a segment measuring 15–20 cm for interposition. Close both proximal and distal segments of jejunum temporarily by applying a TA-55 stapler.

Now make an incision of the transverse mesocolon through its avascular portion just to the left of the middle colic vessels. Carefully pass the jejunal graft together with its vascular pedicle through this incision into the previously dissected lesser sac behind the stomach. Be absolutely certain that the incision in the mesentery does not constrict the veins of the vascular pedicle. Also be careful not to twist the pedicle. Pass the proximal portion of the jejunal segment through the hiatus into the chest. Be certain that the hiatus is large enough so that it does not compress the veins in the vascular pedicle.

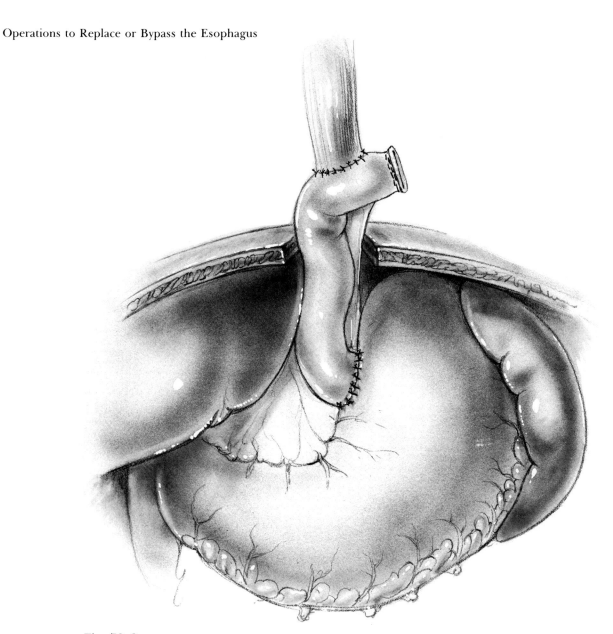

Fig. 70–9

Esophagojejunostomy

Establish an end-to-side esophagojejunal anastomosis on the antimesenteric border of the jejunum beginning about 1 cm distal to the staple line on the proximal closed end of the jejunal segment. A technique similar to that described in Figs. 19–13 to 19–23 using 4–0 atraumatic interrupted cotton Cushing or Lembert sutures for the outer layer and interrupted or continuous 5–0 Vicryl for the mucosal layer may be employed. Pass the nasogastric tube through this anastomosis down to the lower end of the jejunal graft.

Jejunogastrostomy

Place the jejunogastric anastomosis at a point 5–7 cm below the proximal margin of the stomach in an area of stomach that is relatively free of fibrosis and that permits the vascular pedicle to be free of tension. This may be done by the same suture technique as mentioned above (see Figs. 19–13 to 19–23), but if there is sufficient length of jejunum, it may also be performed by a stapled anastomosis similar to that described in Figs. 70–2 to 70–6. The appearance of the completed anastomosis is shown in **Fig. 70–9.**

Jejunojejunostomy

Reestablish the continuity of the jejunum by creating a functional end-to-end anastomosis using the stapling technique described in Figs. 21–12 to 21–16. Then carefully resuture the defect in the jejunal mesentery without compressing the vascular pedicle jejunal graft.

Use interrupted 4–0 Tevdek sutures to approximate the diaphragmatic hiatus to the seromuscular wall of the jejunum to avoid herniation of bowel through the hiatus. Be certain not to compress the vascular pedicle.

Gastrostomy; Pyloromyotomy

Although the nasogastric tube has been passed through the jejunal graft into the stomach in order to maintain the position of the graft, there is a risk that the nasogastric tube may be inadvertently removed before the patient's gastrointestinal tract has resumed function. For this reason, perform a Stamm gastrostomy as described in Figs. 17–1 to 17–5 and remove the nasogastric tube.

Most surgeons advocate performing a pyloromyotomy or pyloroplasty in this type of operation because it is assumed that the vagus nerves have been interrupted during the course of dissecting a heavily scarred esophagus out of the mediastinum. Polk stated that this step may not be necessary.

Closure

Repair the diaphragm and close the thoracoabdominal incision as illustrated in Figs. 8–36 to 8–42 after inserting a large catheter into the thorax. No abdominal drains are utilized. Intermittently during the operation, whenever a hollow viscus has been opened, irrigate the operative field with a dilute antibiotic solution.

Operative Technique— Transhiatal Esophagectomy without Thoracotomy; Gastric Pull-Up

Abdominal Incision

Removing the esophagus by dissecting through the diaphragmatic hiatus from below, and through the neck from above, is especially suitable for patients who have a reasonably normal esophagus. For instance, after pharyngolaryngectomy, removing the esophagus without a thoracotomy, followed by drawing the stomach into the neck for a pharyngogastrostomy can offer an expeditious method of replacing the esophagus. Orringer and Sloan (1978) warned that "if there is even the slightest amount of tension between the stomach and pharynx, we believe that colonic interposition should be performed, for . . . a pharyngogastric anastomotic disruption may ultimately result in a fatal carotid or innominate artery erosion." Orringer and Orringer (1983) have extended the indications of the transhiatal esophagectomy to include all patients with carcinoma of the thoracic or cervical esophagus on the assumption that all operations for esophageal carcinoma are only palliative and do not require a wide field excision. Although we still believe that early carcinoma of the esophagus may benefit by transthoracic wide excision, those patients with midthoracic carcinoma, who have positive nodes in the abdomen or a metastasis to the liver, would benefit from the esophagectomy without thoracotomy especially if they have limited pulmonary reserve.

With the patient in the supine position, prepare the neck, the anterior chest and the entire abdomen. Make a midline incision from the xiphoid to a point 5 cm below the umbilicus. Insert an Upper Hand retractor and elevate the sternum strongly in a cephalad direction. Incise the peritoneum over the abdominal esophagus and encircle the esophagus with a latex drain.

317

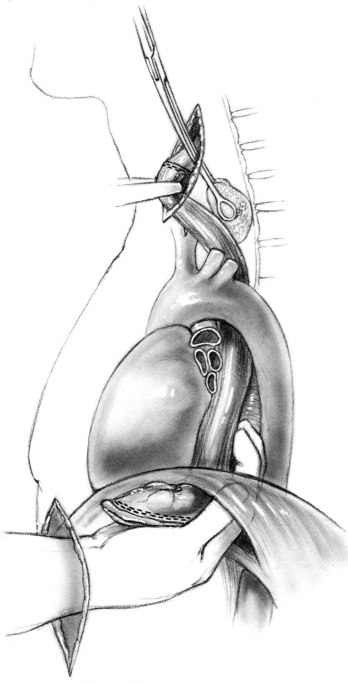

Fig. 70–10

Identify the margins of the diaphragmatic hiatus. If the hiatus is small, enlarge it by making an incision in an anterior direction using the electrocautery. Divide and ligate the transverse phrenic vein that crosses over this incision.

Esophageal Dissection in the Mediastinum

In dissecting the esophagus away from its attachments in the mediastinum, we differ from Orringer and Sloan in that we believe most of this dissection should be done accurately under direct vision. Exposure can be improved by inserting a narrow Harrington or Deaver retractor into the anterior margin of the hiatus. The surgeon would benefit from wearing a headlight to illuminate the mediastinum. Using a blunt Metzenbaum scissors and finger dissection it is possible to identify the blood vessels surrounding the esophagus and to occlude them with Hemoclips prior to transection. Divide the major vagal trunks while dissecting the esophagus from the pleura and the pericardium. This type of dissection can be pursued without difficulty in most patients up to the level of the carina. Do not attempt to include any surrounding soft tissue or lymph nodes in the specimen; rather, keep the dissection close to the wall of the esophagus. If tumor is encountered that cannot be easily separated from other mediastinal structures, abandon this dissection and perform a thoracotomy.

Cervical Dissection

Make an incision along the anterior border of the left sternomastoid muscle down to and across the sternal notch. Develop this dissection as illustrated in Figs. 7–28 to 7–30. Be careful not to apply traction to the recurrent laryngeal nerve; dissect it away from the esophagus. Gently encircle the cervical esophagus and use blunt dissection to free the esophagus from its attachments in the upper mediastinum. Be especially careful in dissecting the esophagus away from the membranous portion of the trachea. During this step in the dissection it is wise to ask the anesthesiologist to decompress the balloon of the endotracheal tube for a minute or two when the dissection is being conducted along the upper posterior trachea. Keep the fingers closely applied to the wall of the esophagus so that the dissection does not extend any distance away from the esophageal wall, especially in the region of the membranous trachea and carina. Surround the upper esophagus with a latex drain and apply mild traction. A small sponge grasped in a sponge-holder may be used to dissect the esophagus away from the tissues of the superior mediastinum (Fig. 70–10). There is a small area of dissection in the vicinity of the carina which is difficult to visualize, either from below or from above. Pass the right hand into the mediastinum from below and left hand from above. With this type of bimanual dissection, it should be possible to free the remaining attachments of the esophagus bluntly.

Apply a TA-55 stapling device across the esophagus very low in the neck and transect the esophagus above the stapling device. Then, remove the esophagus into the abdomen. Place several large moist gauze pads into the mediastinum while the gastric dissection is being conducted.

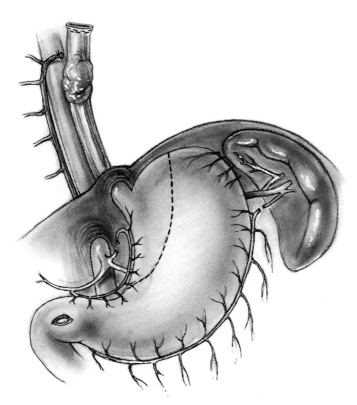

Fig. 70–11

Mobilizing the Stomach

Complete the liberation of the upper stomach and divide the omentum as described in Figs. 7–10 to 7–12. Be certain not to damage any portion of the right gastroepiploic arcade as this constitutes the major remaining blood supply to the stomach. If necessary, leave 5–10 cm of omentum lateral to the gastroepiploic arcade attached to the greater curvature. Elevate the stomach and identify and divide the coronary vein and left gastric artery (see Fig. 7–13). Perform an extensive Kocher maneuver as illustrated in Figs. 7–14 to 7–16. Then perform a pyloromyotomy (see Figs. 7–17 to 7–19). The stomach should now be free of all attachments. The Kocher maneuver should permit the pylorus to come close to the diaphragmatic hiatus without tension.

According to Akiyama, the most important step in preparing the stomach for an anastomosis in the neck is to apply traction to the highest point on the gastric fundus as determined by the stretchability of the remaining stomach. He then advocates removing the lesser curvature, for two reasons: (1) the vascularity of the lesser curvature portion of the stomach following division of the left gastric artery is reduced; (2) with the upper 50%–60% of lesser curvature removed, the fundus can be stretched further into the neck without excessive tension. Although the illustration in Fig. 70–11 relates to a patient with esophageal carcinoma, even patients with benign disease would benefit from removing almost the same amount of stomach along the lesser curvature. This also tends to convert the stomach into a tubular structure rather than a reservoir. If staples are used along the lesser curvature, as recommended by Akiyama, be certain to fire the staples only while considerable cephalad traction is being applied to the gastric fundus at its highest point **(Fig. 70–12)**. We use the TA-90 stapler with 4.8 mm staples if the stomach is even slightly thickened, or 3.5 mm staples for the perfectly normal stomach. Apply a TA-90 roughly along the line demonstrated in Fig. 70–12. Slightly more gastric fundus may be preserved if desired. One application of the TA-90 will generally not suffice to cover the entire dis-

tance. In this case, after applying the TA-90 to the stomach, drive the alignment screw through both walls of the stomach and rotate the wingnut until the screw is in its bed. Then tighten the TA-90 and fire. Apply Allen clamps or another TA-90 cartridge to the specimen side and divide the stomach flush with the TA-90 stapler. Remove the stapler. During the second application of the TA-90 device run the staple line across the portion of the stomach that has been perforated by the alignment screw and excise it with the specimen. Close the TA-90 device and fire the staples. Two applications of the TA-90 will suffice. Lightly electrocoagulate the everted mucosa and remove the specimen. When the TA-90 stapling device has been used, we do not find it necessary to oversew these staple lines. If the GIA device is used, we generally do oversew the staple lines because the GIA device does not permit the surgeon to use a large enough staple to guarantee viability of the tissue distal to the staples.

Advancing the Stomach to the Neck

Akiyama prefers to use the substernal route for the stomach's course to the neck if the patient has carcinoma of the thoracic esophagus because he fears that recurrent carcinoma in the mediastinum may invade and occlude the gastric tube. Akiyama states that in most cases he can deliver the gastric tube into the neck without very often resecting the clavicle or manubrium, provided that the sternal origins of the left sternohyoid and sternothyroid muscles have been transected. Orringer and Orringer (1983) advocate passing the stomach through the original esophageal bed in the posterior mediastinum behind the arch of the aorta because this is the most direct route and does not require any dissection at the root of the neck nor resection of the clavicle.

Remove the gauze packing from the mediastinum. Pass the right hand through

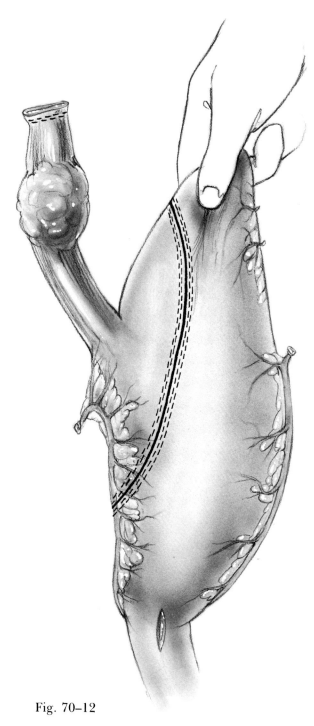

Fig. 70–12

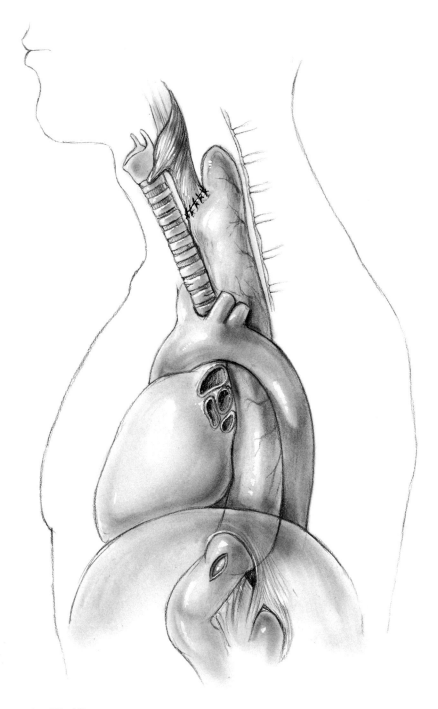

Fig. 70–13

the hiatus up into the neck to confirm that there is free passage. Then gently direct the gastric tube along this route and bring it out in the neck. It should reach the hypopharynx without tension. Check to see that the hiatus is large enough so that it does not exert pressure on the epiploic veins. Suture the upper portion of the gastric fundus to the prevertebral fascia as high as possible in the neck. Use interrupted 4–0 Tevdek sutures. Then anastomose the esophagus to the anterior wall of the gastric tube at a point about 5–6 cm beyond its apex. A one-layer anastomosis between the end of the esophagus and the side of the gastric tube sutured with interrupted 4–0 Prolene may be used, as advocated by Orringer and Sloan (1978) **(Fig. 70–13).**

321

An alternative two-layer method is depicted in Figs. 7–31, 7–32, and 7–24 to 7–26. Pass the nasogastric tube across the anastomosis into the thoracic portion of the gastric tube.

Closure

Close the cervical incision in layers with interrupted 4–0 PG, after inserting a 1.5 cm latex drain down to a point near the anastomosis. Close the abdominal cavity without drainage by using the modified Smead-Jones closure described in Chap. 5 and No. 1 PDS sutures. Close the skin with interrupted fine nylon, a subcuticular continuous 4–0 PG, or staples.

Intermittently during the operation, when a hollow viscus had been opened, irrigate the operative field with a dilute antibiotic solution.

Because there is potential for blood loss during the phase of the thoracic dissection that is performed bluntly, these patients should have a pressure monitor in the radial artery and in the poor-risk patient, another monitor to measure pulmonary artery wedge pressure.

Postoperative Care

If the patient develops signs of postoperative sepsis, keep a high index of suspicion that the colon bypass may have become infarcted. Because this is a fatal complication, do not hesitate to explore the neck (long-segment bypass) or the chest (short-segment bypass) whenever a serious suspicion exists that colon infarction has occurred.

Continue nasogastric suction until bowel function resumes.

Maintain the chest catheter on some type of underwater drainage for 4–5 days, or until the volume of drainage becomes insignificant.

In patients with anastomoses of the cervical esophagus, leave the drain in place for 7–10 days.

Postoperative Complications

Venous infarction of colon or jejunum

Anastomotic leak, especially in cases of anastomoses involving the cervical esophagus

Stricture of the cervical anastomosis, especially after leaks

Intestinal obstruction due to adhesions

Trauma to recurrent laryngeal nerve during dissection of cervical esophagus

Pneumothorax and intraoperative or postoperative hemorrhage, which may occur with transhiatal esophagectomy

References

Akiyama H (1980) Surgery for carcinoma for the esophagus. Curr Probl Surg 17:56

Anderson KD, Randolph JG (1978) Gastric tube interposition: a satisfactory alternative to the colon for esophageal replacement in children. Ann Thorac Surg 25:521

Belsey R (1965) Reconstruction of the esophagus with the left colon. J Thorac Cardiovasc Surg 49:33

Glasgow JC, Cannon JP, Elkins RC (1979) Colon interposition for benign esophageal disease. Am J Surg 137:175

Heimlich HJ (1975) Reversed gastric tube (RGT) esophagoplasty for failure of colon, jejunum and prosthetic interpositions. Ann Surg 182:154

Kelly JP, Shackelford GD, Roper CL (1983) Esophageal replacement in children: functional results and long-term growth. Ann Thorac Surg 36:634

Mansour KA, Hansen HA II, Hersh T, Miller JI Jr et al. (1981) Colon interposition for advanced nonmalignant esophageal stricture: experience with 40 patients. Ann Thorac Surg 32:584

Moylan JP Jr, Bell JW, Cantrell JR, Merendino KA (1970) The jejunal interposition operation: a follow-up on seventeen patients followed 10–17 years. Ann Surg 172:205

Orringer MB, Kirsh MM, Sloan H (1977) Esophageal reconstruction for benign disease: technical considerations. J Thorac Cardiovasc Surg 73:807

Orringer MB, Orringer JS (1982) Esophagectomy. Definitive treatment for esophageal neuromotor dysfunction. Ann Thorac Surg 34:237

Orringer MB, Orringer JS (1983) Esophagectomy without thoracotomy: a dangerous operation? J Thorac Cardiovasc Surg 85:72

Orringer MB, Sloan H (1978) Esophagectomy without thoracotomy. J Thorac Cardiovasc Surg 76:643

Payne WS (1970) Surgical treatment of reflux esophagitis and stricture associated with permanent incompetence of the cardia. Mayo Clin Proc 45:553

Polk HC Jr (1980) Jejunal interposition for reflux esophagitis and esophageal stricture unresponsive to valvuloplasty. World J Surg 4:741

Royston CMS, Dowling BL, Spencer J (1975) Antrectomy with Roux-en-Y anastomosis in the treatment of peptic oesophagitis with stricture. Br J Surg 62:605

Smith J, Payne WS (1975) Surgical technique for management of reflux esophagitis after esophagogastrectomy for malignancy. Further application of Roux-en-Y principle. Mayo Clin Proc 50:588

Wilkins EW Jr (1980) Long-segment colon substitute for the esophagus. Ann Surg 192:722

71 Bile Diverting Operations in the Management of Reflux Esophagitis

Concept and Indications

Esophagitis Following Repeated Failed Operations for Gastroesophageal Reflux

After several failed procedures for gastroesophageal reflux, one may elect to attack the esophagogastric junction another time by performing either a Collis–Nissen operation or a jejunal interposition procedure. If the patient is a poor-risk candidate for a formidable repeat dissection in the region of the esophagogastric junction, or if the technical difficulties are overwhelming, a possible alternative is a distal gastrectomy combined with a Roux-Y gastrojejunostomy. In 1970 Payne reported 15 patients who were suffering from "permanent incompetence of the cardia" and who were treated by vagotomy, hemigastrectomy, and Roux-Y gastrojejunostomy. All had severe esophagitis and six of the patients had serious strictures. Three patients suffered from achalasia and two from scleroderma of the esophagus. All of the patients had satisfactory results, although long-term followup has not been reported. Similar results were reported by Royston, Dowling, and Spencer in a series of eight patients, six of whom had undergone multiple previous operations at the esophagogastric junction. These authors stated that "none of the patients had any heartburn from the day of operation onwards." These good results persisted during a followup period of 11–20 months.

Because this operation is not supported by extended data and followup study, its use should probably be limited to those patients who are not suitable candidates for an operation aimed directly at eliminating gastroesophageal reflux.

Reflux Esophagitis Following Esophagogastrectomy

When the lower esophagus is resected, especially for a benign disease, and an anastomosis is made between the esophagus and the stomach in the lower chest, reflux esophagagitis is a common complication. This is especially true if the anastomosis is made in an end-to-end fashion. The same complication does not occur as often after resection for cancer. However, since survival of patients with esophagogastric carcinoma is limited, the complications following gastroesophageal reflux in this group of patients has not received much attention.

One method of treating esophagitis following esophagogastrectomy is to reexplore the chest to interpose an intrathoracic short segment of isoperistaltic jejunum between the esophagus and the gastric pouch. Another option is to perform a total gastrectomy with a Roux-Y esophagojejunostomy. A third method of treating esophagitis following esophagogastrectomy is to transect the anastomosis, to reposition the gastric pouch into the abdomen and to replace the esophagus by a long-segment interposition of colon from the neck to the gastric pouch. All of the above operations are formidable undertakings, not without significant risk. A safer

324

operation, suggested by Smith and Payne is based on the presumption that the original esophagogastrectomy has almost invariably included a truncal vagotomy as well as the excision of a significant portion of the acid-secreting cells of the stomach. For this reason, in most of these patients the esophagitis is due to the reflux of bile. Smith and Payne recommend division of the proximal duodenum. This is followed by closing the duodenal stump and anastomosing the proximal end of the duodenum to a Roux-Y segment of jejunum, a procedure that will avoid any reflux of bile if the length of the Roux-Y segment is 50–60 cm. Although a large data base in support of this operation does not exist, we have had two excellent results using it, and the procedure is relatively simple and safe.

Preoperative Care

In case of doubt whether a previous vagotomy has been done, perform appropriate studies of gastric acidity.

Perform esophagoscopy to evaluate the esophagus and to detect the presence of bile.

If bile reflux has not been demonstrated on esophagoscopy, obtain radionuclide studies for bile reflux.

Insert a nasogastric tube prior to operation.

Pitfalls and Danger Points

Incomplete vagotomy
Traumatizing liver, pancreas, or stomach

Operative Strategy

If transabdominal vagotomy does not appear to be feasible due to excessive scar tissue around the abdominal esophagus, one may make a transthoracic incision and perform a truncal vagotomy in the chest.

Operative Technique— Vagotomy and Antrectomy with Bile Diversion

Incision and Exposure

Ordinarily a long midline incision from the xiphoid to a point about 5 cm below the umbilicus will be adequate for this operation. Divide the many adhesions and expose the stomach. Evaluate the difficulties of performing a hemigastrectomy, as opposed to the other available operations aimed at correcting the gastroesophageal reflux anatomically. Insert an Upper Hand or chain retractor and determine whether a transabdominal vagotomy is feasible.

Vagotomy

If it is feasible to perform an abdominal truncal vagotomy, follow the procedure described in Chap. 10. If dissecting the area of the esophagogastric junction appears to be too formidable a task, then it will be necessary to turn the patient to the lateral position and perform a left thoracotomy for a transthoracic vagotomy at the conclusion of the abdominal portion of this operation. Another possible alternative is to perform a high (70%) subtotal gastrectomy without a vagotomy. In patients with a history of severe reflux esophagitis, however, there is considerable risk that performing a gastrectomy with Roux-Y gastrojejunostomy but without vagotomy may result in a marginal ulcer because many of these patients tend to have an excessive secretion of gastric acid.

Hemigastrectomy

Follow the procedure described in Chap. 15 for the performance of a Billroth II gastric resection. Close the duodenal stump either by stapling (see Fig. 15–46) or by suturing (see Figs. 15–23 to 15–25).

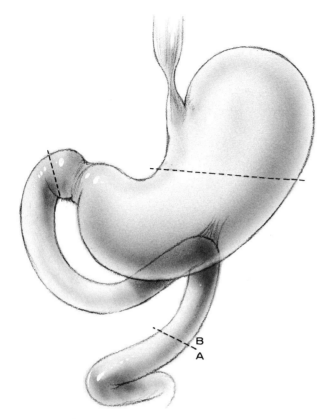

Fig. 71–1

Roux-Y Gastrojejunostomy

Create a Roux-Y limb of jejunum by the technique described in Fig. 19–11. Then perform an end-to-side gastrojejunostomy using either sutures (see Figs. 15–37 to 15–43) or staples (see Figs. 15–45 to 15–50). Position this anastomosis so that it sits about 1 cm proximal to the stapled closed end of the jejunum (see Fig. 15–52). Complete the construction of the Roux-Y segment by anastomosing the proximal cut end of jejunum near the ligament of Treitz to the side of the descending segment of jejunum at a point 60 cm distal to the gastrojejunostomy as shown in Figs. 19–36 to 19–40. Close the defect in the jejunal mesentery by means of interrupted sutures **(Figs. 71–1 and 71–2).**

Closure

Close the abdominal wall without drainage in the usual fashion.

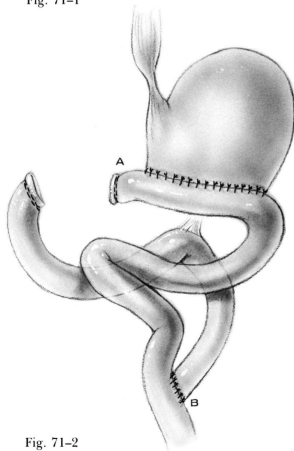

Fig. 71–2

Operative Technique—Bile Diversion Following Esophagogastrectomy

Incision and Exposure

Make a midline incision from the xiphoid to a point somewhat below the umbilicus. Divide the various adhesions subsequent to the previous surgery and expose the pyloroduodenal region. Due to the previous surgery, (esophagogastrectomy, **Fig. 71–3**) this area will now be located 5–8 cm from the diaphragmatic hiatus.

Dividing the Duodenum; Duodenojejunostomy, Roux-Y

Divide the duodenum at a point 2–3 cm beyond the pylorus. Be careful not to injure the right gastric or the right gastroepiploic vessels, as these constitute the entire blood supply of the residual gastric pouch. In order to divide the duodenum, first free the posterior wall of the duodenum from the pancreas for a short distance. If possible, pass one jaw of the TA-55 stapling device behind the duodenum, close the device, and fire the staples. Then divide the duodenum flush with the stapling device. Lightly electrocoagulate the everted mucosa and remove the stapler. This will leave the proximal duodenum open. Leave 1 cm of the posterior wall of the duodenum free (point A, **Fig. 71–4**) in order to construct an anastomosis with the jejunum.

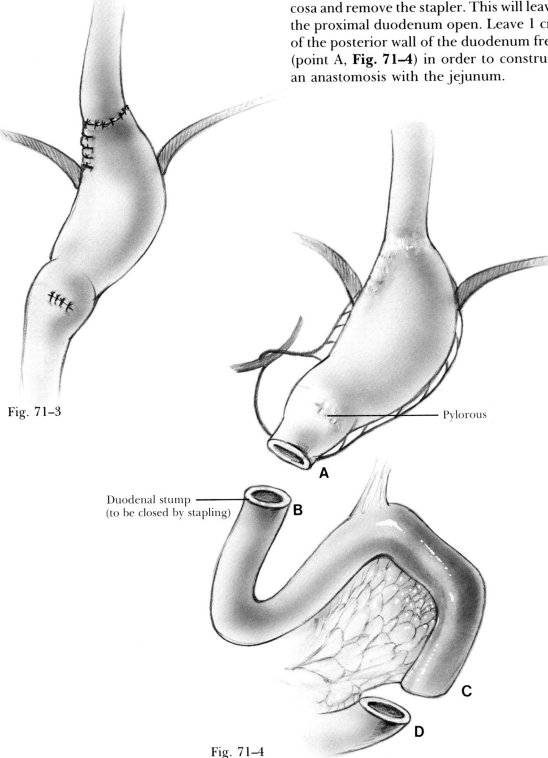

Fig. 71–3

Pylorous

A

Duodenal stump
(to be closed by stapling)

B

C

D

Fig. 71–4

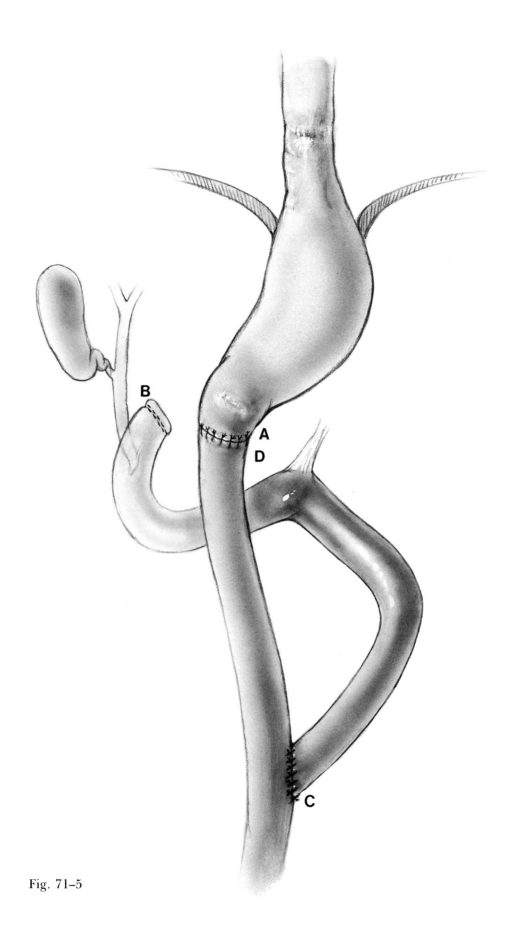

Fig. 71–5

Develop a Roux-Y limb of jejunum by the technique described in Fig. 19–11. Bring the open distal end of the divided jejunum (point D, Fig. 71–2) to the level of the duodenum either in an antecolonic fashion or, in some cases, it may be feasible to bring it through an incision in the mesocolon.

Establish an end-to-end duodenojejunostomy (point A to point D, **Fig. 71–5**) utilizing one layer of interrupted 4–0 cotton for the seromuscular layer and continuous or interrupted sutures of atraumatic 5–0 Vicryl for the mucosal layer (see Figs. 21–2 to 21–10).

Complete the construction of the Roux-Y segment by creating an end-to-side jejunojejunostomy at a point 60 cm distal to the duodenojejunostomy using the technique shown in Figs. 19–36 to 19–40. Close the defect in the jejunal mesentery by means of interrupted sutures.

Closure

Close the abdominal wall without drainage in the usual fashion. Irrigate the operative field intermittently during the procedure with a dilute antibiotic solution.

Postoperative Care

If there is any suspicion that the patient has not had a complete vagotomy, give the patient intravenous cimetidine for the first postoperative week.

Continue nasogastric suction until bowel function resumes.

Postoperative Complications

Marginal ulcer may occur if a complete vagotomy has not been accomplished. Although in some cases a marginal ulcer may respond to conservative management, frequently a transthoracic vagotomy will be necessary for long-term relief. This is true because the secretions in the Roux-Y segment of jejunum lack the buffering capacity of the diverted bile and pancreatic juice.

References

Payne WS (1970) Surgical treatment of reflux esophagitis and stricture associated with permanent incompetence of the cardia. Mayo Clin Proc 45:553

Royston CMS, Dowling BL, Spencer J (1975) Antrectomy with Roux-en-Y anastomosis in the treatment of peptic oesophagitis with stricture. Br J Surg 62:605

Smith J, Payne WS (1975) Surgical technique for management of reflux esophagitis after esophagogastrectomy for malignancy. Further application of Roux-en-Y principle. Mayo Clin Proc 50:588

72 Cricopharyngeal Myotomy and Operation for Pharyngoesophageal (Zenker's) Diverticulum

Concept: When to Perform a Cricopharyngeal Myotomy

Physiology of Swallowing

Normal swallowing begins when the tongue thrusts a bolus of food from the mouth back into the pharynx. When food contacts the pharyngeal mucosa, it initiates afferent impulses to the swallowing center in the medulla. The swallowing center promptly sends an orderly sequence of impulses to the muscles of the pharynx, the esophagus, and the stomach. Forceful contraction of the pharyngeal musculature closes the passageway between the mouth and the nasopharynx to prevent regurgitation into the nose while at the same time the food is propelled forward. At this instant the cricopharyngeal sphincter must relax until the bolus of food has passed into the esophagus where sequential peristaltic contractions carry the food toward the stomach. At the lower end of the esophagus, the lower esophageal sphincter relaxes for a few seconds to permit the food to pass.

In the resting state both the cricopharyngeal and the lower esophageal sphincters are in a state of contraction. In the case of the lower esophageal sphincter, this state of contraction prevents gastroesophageal regurgitation. Since the pressure in the thoracic esophagus during inspiration is lower than it is in the atmosphere, there is a pressure gradient between the mouth and esophagus. In the absence of a closed cricopharyngeal sphincter, air could continuously enter the esophagus. It is notable that the pharyngeal constrictor, the cricopharyngeal, and the cervical esophageal musculature are striated in type. However, these muscles are voluntary only in the sense that a voluntary act of swallowing initiates an ordered series of impulses from the swallowing center to these muscles. It is also notable that the high pressure zone in the area of the cricopharyngeal sphincter measures about 4 cm, a distance which is considerably greater than the anatomical distribution of the cricopharyngeal muscle itself. When the term "cricopharyngeal sphincter" is used physiologically, it must be understood that the functional sphincter includes a few centimeters of the proximal esophagus. Ellis and Crozier prefer to use the term "upper esophageal sphincter" because the physiological sphincter is not in fact confined to the cricopharyngeal muscle.

Operation for Pharyngoesophageal (Zenker's) Diverticulum

For many years it has been theorized by authors like Belsey; Ellis, Schlegel, Lynch, and Payne; and Dohlman and Mattson, that the pharyngoesophageal (or Zenker's) diverticulum bursts through the space between the pharyngeal constrictor muscles and the cricopharyngeus because of "spasm" or achalasia of the cricopharyngeus. However, Ellis and Crozier emphasized that careful manometric studies of the upper esophageal sphincter in patients with pharyngoesophageal diverticula did not demonstrate achalasia (failure of relaxation). Nor did the studies elicit any evidence of spasm or increased pressure in this location. These authors did find, however, that there was an incoordination in the function of the upper esophageal sphincter in that the timing of the relaxation did not coincide with the peak of the pharyngeal contraction. This failure of coordination, they feel, produced repeated stress against the posterior hypopharynx in the weak area where the longitudinal muscles of the pharyngeal constrictors adjoin the transverse fibers of the cricopharyngeus. Repeated stress of this type may result in a pharyngoesophageal diverticulum.

For many years simple diverticulectomy was advocated for patients who had symptomatic pharyngoesophageal diverticula, and generally satisfactory results were reported (Welsh and Payne). However, there are a number of patients, especially those with smaller diverticula, whose dysphagia may persist without much improvement following simple diverticulectomy. While the postoperative X ray may show that the diverticulum was cured by the operation, the patient's symptomatology persists. Persistence or recurrence of symptoms following diverticulectomy has been noted by a number of authors including Siewart and Blum; Worman; and Ellis and Crozier. Belsey emphasized that significant dysphagia often occurs in patients with small diverticula and that these symptoms can be relieved by performing only a myotomy of the upper esophageal sphincter without removing the diverticulum. Worman also noted that the size of the diverticulum is not often related to symptoms and that many patients with small diverticula experience severe dysphagia and aspiration. While primary operations for pharyngoesophageal diverticula are usually safe and straightforward procedures, Huang, Payne, and Cameron reported a 3.2% mortality and a 51.6% morbidity after surgical correction of recurrent diverticula.

In conclusion, it is not wise to perform a diverticulectomy without a concomitant cricopharyngeal and upper esophageal myotomy that is at least 4 cm in length.

Neuromotor Disturbances of the Cricopharyngeal Sphincter

From the above discussion it can be concluded that the pharyngoesophageal diverticulum is simply one manifestation of a functional disorder occurring in the upper esophageal sphincter. A number of observers have reported performing a cricopharyngeal myotomy for patients without any diverticula who suffer from dysphagia secondary to achalasia, delayed relaxation, or persistent elevation in the resting pressure of the cricopharyngeal–upper esophageal sphincter. Palmer and also Ellis and Crozier have published recent reports relevant to this problem. Palmer describes the dysphagia resulting from cricopharyngeal disorders as a sensation that a shelf forms in the throat every time a patient tries to swallow. The patient senses exactly where the dysphagia is located and points just below the larynx. The patient may state that the food catches on a shelf in the throat prior to his developing a choking sensation. Swallowing solid foods may be easier than liquids. The patient may become hoarse and acquire a persistent cough especially at night with some degree of aspiration. The fear of choking may lead to the patient refusing to eat, a fear that is often followed by undernutrition.

Some known causes of this type of dysphagia include extensive resections of oropharyngeal cancers, division of the superior or the recurrent laryngeal nerves, and bulbar palsy (e.g., amyotrophic lateral sclerosis, cerebral vascular accident). Excessively high pressure in the upper esophageal sphincter may be the cause of dysphagia in patients with globus hystericus in some cases. Myotomy of the truly hypertensive upper esophageal sphincter produces excellent results (Ellis and Crozier), when the diagnosis is confirmed by manometry.

The exact role of cricopharyngeal myotomy in the treatment of all of these functional disorders of the upper esophageal sphincter has not yet been delineated. Since the number of these cases is small, few surgeons have acquired any significant experience in managing them. At the present time, patients in this category should be subjected to careful manometric studies in a laboratory experienced in manometry of the cervical esophagus. Only if specific abnormalities, such as persistent elevation of the cricopharyngeal pressure or achalasia, are demonstrated, should a myotomy be performed. Ellis and Crozier found that their patients with bulbar palsy did not respond well to myotomy.

Indications

Pharyngoesophageal diverticulum, symptomatic

Selected cases with functional disorders of the upper esophageal sphincter

Preoperative Care

Patients suffering from pharyngoesophageal diverticula do not require any preoperative diagnostic study other than a barium swallow.

Patients with other functional disorders of the upper esophageal sphincter should have not only X rays but also precise manometric studies of the pharynx and the esophagus.

Pitfalls and Danger Points

Inadequate cricopharyngeal and upper esophageal myotomy

Inadequate closure of cervical esophagus following diverticulectomy with postoperative leak

Damage to recurrent laryngeal nerve

Operative Strategy

Adequate Myotomy

Performing a cricopharyngeal myotomy is not unlike performing a cardiomyotomy. In the first place, it must be recognized that the physiological upper esophageal sphincter is considerably wider than is the anatomical cricopharyngeus muscle. The transverse muscle fibers are only about 2.0–2.5 cm wide while the high pressure zone corresponding to the cricopharyngeus area can measure 4 cm in width. Consequently, a proper cricopharyngeal myotomy should not only transect all of the transverse fibers of the cricopharyngeus muscle but also 1–2 cm of the proximal esophagus so that the myotomy measures 4 cm in length. The incision in the muscle is carried down to the mucosa of the esophagus, which should bulge out through the myotomy after all of the muscle fibers have been divided. Additionally, free the mucosa from the overlying muscle over the posterior half of the esophagus.

Is Diverticulectomy Necessary?

If the pharyngoesophageal diverticulum is a small diffuse bulge measuring no more than 2–3 cm in diameter, we perform only a myotomy and make no attempt to excise any part of the diverticulum because after the myotomy there is only a gentle bulge of mucosa and no true diverticulum. On the other hand, longer, fingerlike projections of mucosa should be amputated because there have been a few case reports of recurrent symptoms due to the persistence of diverticula left behind in patients in whom an otherwise adequate myotomy had been done. Belsey advocated suturing the most dependent point of the diverticulum to the prevertebral fascia in the upper cervical region. This procedure effectively up-ends the diverticulum so that it can drain freely into the esophageal lumen by gravity. He used fine stainless steel wire for the diverticulopexy. We have preferred to amputate diverticula larger than 3 cm rather than to perform a diverticulopexy. With the application of a stapling device, amputation of the diverticulum takes only about 1 minute of additional operating time, and the results have been excellent.

Operative Technique

Incision and Exposure

With the patient's head turned somewhat toward his right, make an incision along the anterior border of the left sternomastoid muscle beginning at a point 2–3 cm above the clavicle **(Fig. 72–1)**. Divide the platysma muscle. Electrocoagulate the bleeding points. Free the anterior border of the sternomastoid muscle and retract it laterally. This will expose the omohyoid muscle crossing the field from medial to lateral. Transect this muscle **(Fig. 72–2)**. The diverticulum will be located deep to the omohyoid muscle. Identify the carotid sheath and the descending hypoglossal nerve. Retract these structures laterally.

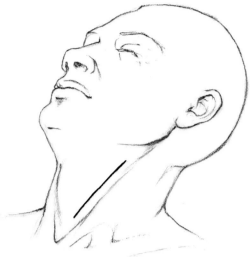

Fig. 72–1

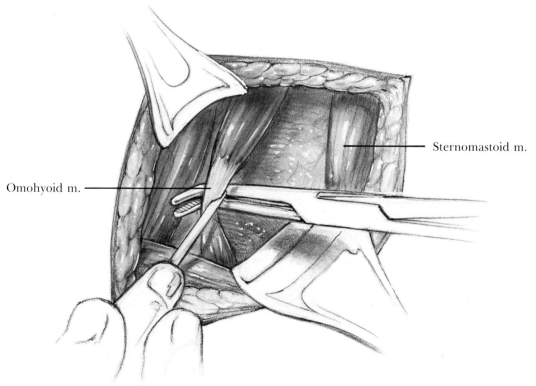

Omohyoid m.

Sternomastoid m.

Fig. 72–2

333

The thyroid gland will be seen in the medial portion of the operative field beneath the strap muscles. Retract the thyroid gland and the larynx in a medial direction. This will reveal, in most cases, a prominent middle thyroid vein **(Fig. 72–3).** Ligate and divide this vein.

Divide the areolar tissue anterior to the carotid artery and identify the inferior thyroid artery and the recurrent laryngeal nerve. In some patients there does not appear to be a true left inferior thyroid artery arising from the thyrocervical trunk. In these patients the lower thyroid is supplied by branches of the superior thyroid artery. In the majority of patients, with the inferior thyroid artery emerging from beneath the carotid artery and crossing the esophagus to supply the lower thyroid (see Fig. 92–8), divide and ligate this vessel after identifying the recurrent laryngeal nerve. After

this step has been completed, retracting the larynx in an anteromedial direction and the carotid artery laterally will expose the lateral and posterior aspects of the cervical esophagus and the pharyngoesophageal junction.

Dissecting the Pharyngoesophageal Diverticulum

The pharyngoesophageal diverticulum emerges posteriorly between the pharyngeal constrictor and the cricopharyngeus muscles. Its neck is at the level of the cricoid cartilage and the dependent portion of the diverticulum descends between the posterior wall of the esophagus and the prevertebral fascia overlying the bodies of the cervical vertebrae. Blunt dissection

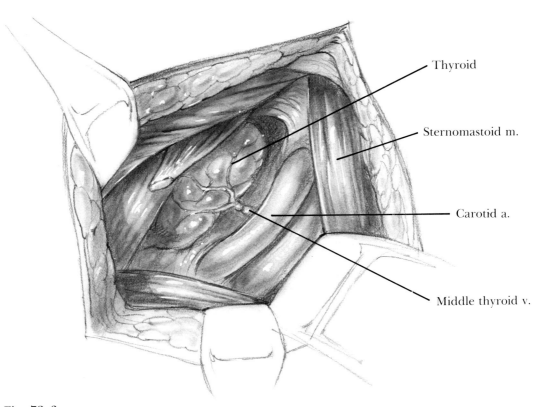

Thyroid

Sternomastoid m.

Carotid a.

Middle thyroid v.

Fig. 72–3

with the index finger or a peanut sponge will generally identify the most dependent portion of the diverticulum. Grasp this with a Babcock clamp and elevate the diverticulum in a cephalad direction. Mobilize the diverticulum by sharp and blunt dissection down to its neck. If there is any confusion about the anatomy, especially in patients who have had previous operations in this area, ask the anesthesiologist to pass a 40F Maloney bougie through the mouth into the cervical esophagus. Guide the tip of the bougie past the neck of the diverticu-

lum so that it enters the esophagus. Now the exact location of the junction between the esophagus and the diverticulum can be identified. There is generally some fibrous tissue overlying the mucosa of the diverticulum. Lightly incise this with a scalpel near the neck of the sac down to the submucosa. At this point the transverse fibers of the cricopharyngeus muscle are easily identified.

Cricopharyngeal and Esophageal Myotomy

Insert a blunt-tipped right-angled hemostat between the mucosa and the tranverse fibers of the cricopharyngeus muscle just distal to the neck of the diverticulum **(Fig. 72–4)**. Elevate the hemostat in the poste-

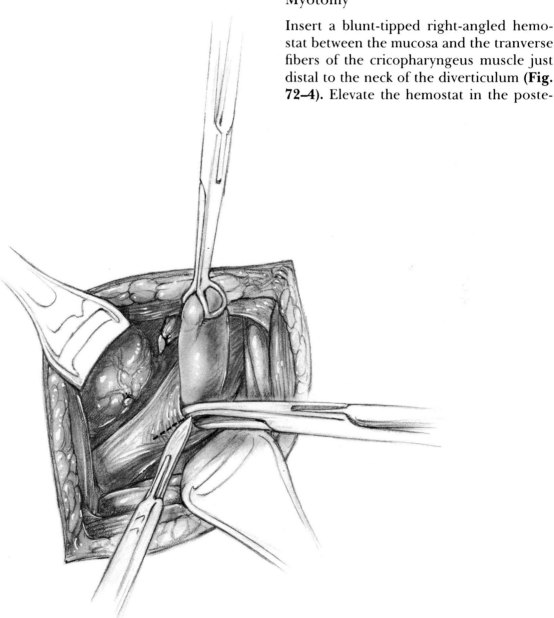

Fig. 72–4

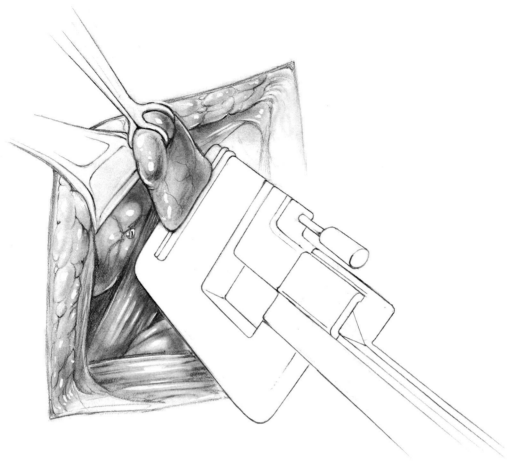

Fig. 72–5

rior midline and incise the fibers of the cricopharyngeus muscle with a scalpel. Continue this dissection down the posterior wall of the esophagus for a total distance of about 4 cm. Now elevate the incised muscles of the cricopharyngeus and the upper esophagus from the underlying mucosal layer over the posterior half of the esophageal circumference by blunt dissection.

After the mucosa has been permitted to bulge out through the myotomy, make a determination as to whether the diverticulum is large enough to warrant resection. If so, apply a TA-30 or a TA-55 stapler with 3.5 mm staples across the neck of the diverticulum. Close the stapler. Fire the staples and amputate the diverticulum flush with the stapling device. Although the stapler is shown applied in a longitudinal

direction in **Fig. 72–5,** Hoehn and Payne prefer to apply staples in a transverse direction. With a 40F Maloney dilator in the lumen of the esophagus, it will not be possible to excise so much mucosa as to cause constriction of the lumen. After removing the stapling device, carefully inspect the staple line and the staples for proper closure. Check for complete hemostasis **(Fig. 72–6).**

An alternative method for performing the myotomy is illustrated in **Fig. 72–7** where the incision is initiated 1 or 1.5 cm cephalad to the cricopharyngeus muscle, in the pharyngeal constrictor muscle. Then it is continued downward for 4–5 cm. The diverticulum is removed in the usual fashion.

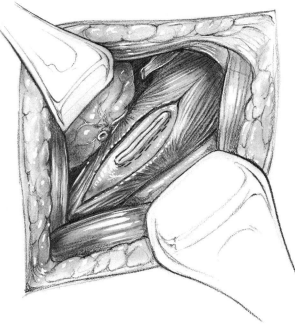

Fig. 72–6

Drainage and Closure

After carefully inspecting the area and assuring complete hemostasis, insert a medium-size latex rubber drain into the prevertebral space just below the area of the diverticulectomy. Bring the drain out through the lower pole of the incision.

Close the incision in layers with interrupted 4–0 PG sutures to the muscle fascia and platysma. Close the skin either by means of a continuous subcuticular suture of 4–0 PG, interrupted nylon sutures, or skin staples.

Postoperative Care

Remove nasogastric suction immediately after operation.

Remove the drain by the 4th postoperative day.

Initiate a liquid diet on the 1st postoperative day and progress to a full diet over the next 2–3 days.

Continue perioperative antibiotics for 24 hours.

Postoperative Complications

Esophageal fistula (When the fistula is small and drains primarily saliva, it will generally close after a week of intravenous feeding if the patient's operative site has been drained as described above.)

Recurrent laryngeal nerve palsy, generally temporary, secondary to excessive traction on the thyroid cartilage or to direct trauma to the nerve

Persistent dysphagia due to inadequate myotomy

References

Belsey R (1966) Functional disease of the esophagus. J Thorac Cardiovasc Surg 52:164

Dohlman G, Mattson O (1960) The endoscopic operation for hypopharyngeal diverticula; a roentgenocinematographic study. Arch Otolaryngol 71:744

Ellis FH Jr, Crozier RE (1981) Cervical esophageal dysphagia; indications for and results of cricopharyngeal myotomy. Ann Surg 194:279

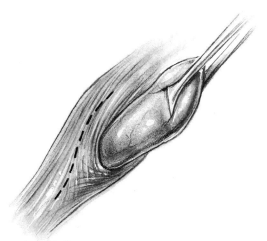

Fig. 72–7

Ellis FH Jr, Schlegel JF, Lynch VP, Payne WS (1969) Cricopharyngeal myotomy for pharyngoesophageal diverticulum. Ann Surg 170:340

Hoehn JG, Payne WS (1969) Resection of pharyngoesophageal diverticulum using stapling device. Mayo Clin Proc 44:738

Huang B, Payne WS, Cameron AJ (1984) Surgical management for recurrent pharyngoesophageal (Zenker's) diverticulum. Ann Thorac Surg 37:189

Palmer ED (1976) Disorders of the cricopharyngeal muscle: a review. Gastroenterol 71:510

Siewart JR, Blum AL (1979) The esophagus. Part I: surgery at the upper esophageal sphincter, tubular esophagus, and lower esophageal sphincter. Clin Gastroenterol 8:271

Welsh GF, Payne WS (1973) The present status of one-stage pharyngoesophageal diverticulectomy. S Clin N Am 53:953

Worman LW (1980) Pharyngoesophageal diverticulum—excision or incision? Surgery 87:236

73 Esophagomyotomy for Esophageal Achalasia and Diffuse Esophageal Spasm

Concept: Which Therapy for Achalasia and Esophageal Spasm

Hydrostatic Dilatation versus Esophagomyotomy

In esophageal achalasia the body of the esophagus is unable to produce organized peristaltic contractions, and the lower esophageal sphincter fails to relax following the act of swallowing. This combination of events results in partial obstruction. The esophagus dilates. The patient suffers from dysphagia, regurgitation, tracheal aspiration, and pneumonitis in advanced cases. Long-term relief from the symptoms of achalasia requires either hydrostatic dilatation of the lower esophagus or an esophagomyotomy. Both procedures result in interrupting the continuity of the circular muscle surrounding the distal esophagus. Sanderson, Ellis, and Olsen report that hydrostatic dilatation has been successful in relieving symptoms in 81% of their cases, of which 3.2% required emergency surgery for esophageal perforation. There were no deaths. On the other hand, Ellis, Kiser, Schlegel, Earlam, and others (1967) feel that surgical esophagomyotomy is the treatment of choice for esophageal achalasia. They experienced one death from malignant hyperthermia in 269 operations. There was only a 3% incidence of symptomatic reflux esophagitis. An additional 3% of cases experienced poor results in the form of either persistent or recurrent symptoms of dysphagia not related to gastroesophageal reflux. A majority of the patients having poor results from esophagomyotomy had previously undergone unsuccessful treatment by hydrostatic dilatation or surgery. Using a similar technique of esophagomyotomy, Okike, Payne, and Newfeld also noted only a 3% incidence of postoperative reflux esophagitis in a study of 200 operations for achalasia done at the Mayo Clinic from 1967 to 1975. These authors report good or excellent results in 90% of their patients.

In the hands of an experienced gastroenterologist, hydrostatic dilatation may achieve satisfactory results. However, we agree with Ellis, that surgical division of the esophageal muscle is a safe and effective procedure for the primary treatment of esophageal achalasia.

Diffuse Esophageal Spasm

Patients with diffuse esophageal spasm suffer from attacks of severe substernal pain, not unlike angina pectoris, as well as from espisodic dysphagia. These symptoms are caused by a severe motor disorder that produces spasm and hypertrophy of the esophageal circular muscle, generally involving the lower two-thirds of the esophagus. The lower esophageal sphincter is usually normal and relaxes well in response to swallowing (Murray). Ellis and associates (Leonardi, Shea, Crozier, and Ellis) recommend a long esophagomyotomy sparing the lower esophageal sphincter if it is normal on manometry. The upper end of the myotomy may have to extend to the level of the aortic arch; the proximal mar-

339

gin of the myotomy is determined by the upper extent of the disordered spastic contractions as shown on preoperative manometric measurements.

If there is achalasia of the lower esophageal sphincter as well as diffuse spasm of the esophagus, then the esophagomyotomy will have to include the lower esophagus. In these cases, Henderson and Ryder perform a very narrow (0.5 cm) Nissen fundoplication to prevent reflux without creating a functional obstruction at the lower end of an esophagus that no longer is capable of any peristalsis.

Indications

Esophageal achalasia as demonstrated by typical symptoms and esophageal X rays

Diffuse esophageal spasm, confirmed by esophageal manometry, if severe and unresponsive to medication

Preoperative Care

Do an esophagoscopy with biopsy of the narrowed portion of distal esophagus in patients diagnosed as suffering from achalasia.

Take esophagram X rays.

In advanced cases, lavage the dilated esophagus with a Levine tube and warm saline for 1–2 days prior to operation to evacuate retained food particles. This should be combined with a liquid diet.

Pass a nasogastric tube into the esophagus the morning of operation.

Administer perioperative antibiotics for 24 hours.

Preoperative esophageal manometry is indicated in patients who have achalasia and experience severe chest pain, since vigorous achalasia may be accompanied by diffuse esophageal spasm. This cannot be diagnosed by

any means other than manometry. Simply dividing the lower esophageal musculature will not be adequate for those patients having diffuse esophageal spasm involving a long segment of the esophagus.

Pitfalls and Danger Points

Extending the myotomy too far on the stomach

Perforating the esophageal mucosa

Performing an inadequate circumferential liberation of the mucosa

Creating a hiatus hernia

Operative Strategy

Length of Myotomy for Achalasia

Ellis, Gibb, and Crozier (1980) attribute their low incidence of postoperative gastroesophageal regurgitation (3%) to the fact that the myotomy terminates only a few millimeters beyond the esophagogastric junction. At the esophagogastric junction, several veins run in a transverse direction just superficial to the esophageal mucosa. One does not encounter any other transverse vein of this size during the myotomy of the more proximal esophagus. Once these veins are encountered, terminate the myotomy. In no case should more than 1 cm of gastric musculature be divided. Continue the myotomy in a cephalad direction for 1–2 cm beyond the point at which the esophagus begins to dilate. In early cases, where no significant esophageal dilatation is evident, the length of the myotomy should be 5–8 cm.

Avoiding the Creation of a Hiatus Hernia

Perform the esophagomyotomy through a thoracotomy incision and do not dissect the esophagus away from the hiatus as this dissection will result in division of the phrenoesophageal ligaments. If the esophagogastric junction is liberated, a potential hiatus hernia will be created. If the esophagomyotomy is performed transabdominally, it is obvious that the phrenoesophageal ligaments will have to be transected to expose enough of the lower esophagus. This approach will increase the likelihood of producing a hiatus hernia. Those patients, in whom a hiatus hernia is already present, should undergo some type of repair of the hiatal defect. Special care must be taken to avoid obstructing the esophagus in patients with achalasia, since these patients do not have normal peristaltic propulsion of food.

Is an Antireflux Procedure Necessary?

While Ellis and associates experienced reflux esophagitis in only 3% of their patients following esophagomyotomy, Skinner advocates adding a modified (loose) Belsey Mark IV type of partial fundoplication. If this procedure is added to the operation for achalasia, the myotomy can be extended onto the stomach further than is shown in Fig. 73–4, a step that, he argues, will eliminate the persistence of achalasia after esophagomyotomy.

On the other hand, Murray, Battaglini, Keagy, Starek et al. advocate adding a fundoplication only in selected cases of achalasia, for example, patients with preexisting reflux esophagitis or hiatus hernia and patients who experienced mucosal perforations during esophagomyotomy. Patients requiring repeat myotomy for recurrent achalasia require extension of the myotomy well onto the gastric wall to provide a patulous opening into the stomach, followed by an antireflux procedure. In general, our views concur with those of Murray and associates.

When a Belsey fundoplication is added to the esophagomyotomy, Skinner emphasizes that it should be looser than usual and that it should encompass only 180° of esophagus.

Mucosal Perforation

In the series reported by Ellis and colleagues (1967), the mucosa was perforated in 10% of the cases during the performance of the esophagomyotomy. In each case, the perforation was closed by interrupted sutures. Empyema developed postoperatively in three patients, in only one of whom was a mucosal perforation recognized at the time of operation. It is advisable for the surgeon to test the integrity of the mucosal layer following myotomy by having the anesthesiologist insert 100–200 ml of a methylene blue solution through the nasogastric tube. When a mucosal perforation is identified during the operation, careful suturing of the mucosa will generally avoid further difficulty. It should be noted that Ellis routinely sutures the incision in the mediastinal pleura following the esophagomyotomy. This will buttress a sutured perforation of the mucosa with a flap of pleura (also see Figs. 74–1 to 74–3).

Operative Technique

Incision and Exposure

Position the patient so that he lies on his right side. Make a skin incision along the course of the 7th intercostal space. Incise the serratus and latissimus muscles with the electrocautery. Then make an incision along the upper border of the 8th rib through the intercostal musculature (see Figs. 69–1 to 69–3). Open the pleura for the length of the 8th rib. Insert a Finochietto retractor and gradually increase the space between the 7th and 8th ribs. Divide the inferior pulmonary ligament and retract the left lung in a cephalad and ante-

Fig. 73–1

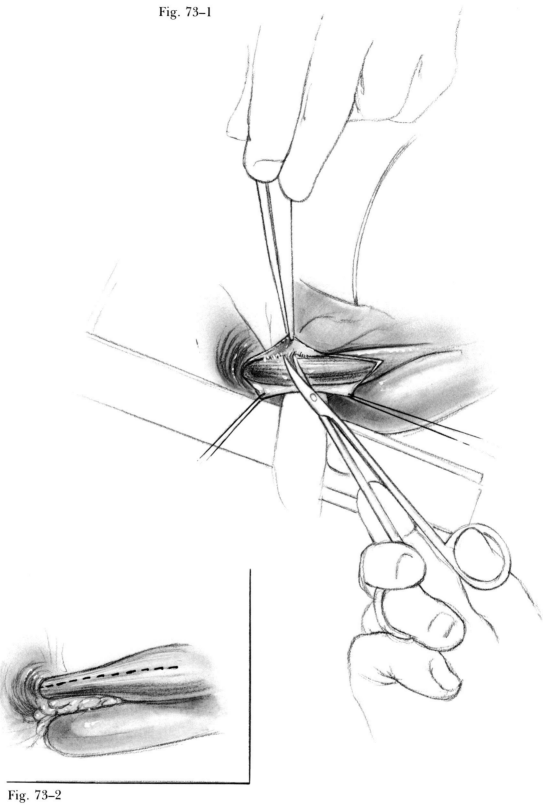

Fig. 73–2

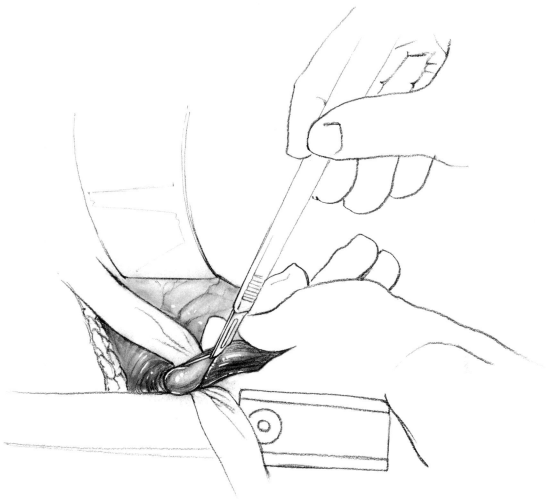

Fig. 73–3

rior direction using large moist gauze pads and Harrington retractors. Make an incision in the mediastinal pleura overlying the distal esophagus **(Fig. 73–1)**. Then gently encircle the esophagus with the index finger. This is facilitated by the indwelling nasogastric tube. Encircle the esophagus with a 2-cm latex drain. Be careful to identify and preserve the vagus nerves. Free the esophagus from surrounding structures down to the level of the diaphragm, but no lower **(Fig. 73–2)**.

Esophagomyotomy for Achalasia

Place the left index finger beneath the distal esophagus. Make a longitudinal incision through both the longitudinal and circular muscle layers of the esophagus until the muscosal surface is exposed **(Fig. 73–3)**. Continue this incision in a cephalad direction for a distance of about 2 cm above the point where the esophagus begins to dilate, or at least 5–7 cm.

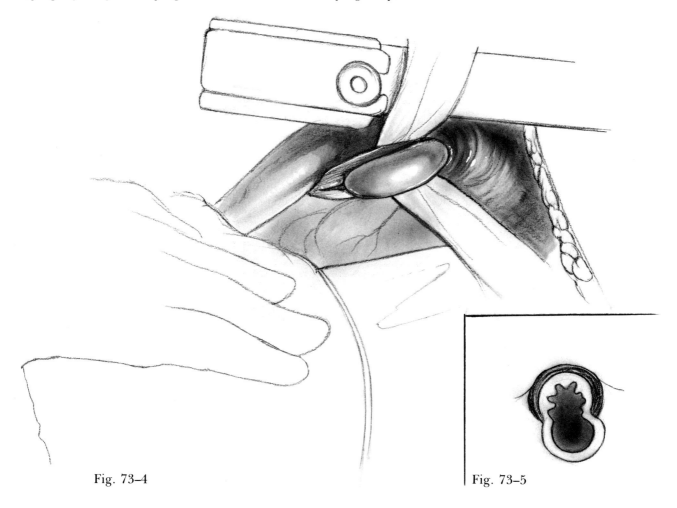

Fig. 73–4

Fig. 73–5

Continue the myotomy in a caudal direction as far as the esophagogastric junction **(Fig. 73–4).** This junction can be identified by noting one or two veins crossing transversely over the mucosa deep to the musculature. Do not continue the incision more than 1 cm into the gastric musculature. Another way of confirming the location of the esophagogastric junction is the fact that the gastric musculature differs from that of the esophagus.

In order to prevent the reuniting of the muscle fibers, it is important to free at least 50% of the circumference of the mucosa from its muscular coat. This may be accomplished by using the Metzenbaum scissors to elevate the circular muscle from the underlying mucosa going both medial and then lateral to the initial longitudinal myotomy until the mucosa bulges out as seen in cross section in **Fig. 73–5.** Achieve complete hemostasis by cautious electrocoagulation and fine suture–ligatures, especially in the incised esophageal muscle.

If the mucosa has been inadvertently incised, carefully repair the laceration with one or more 4–0 nonabsorbable sutures. At this point, ask the anesthesiologist to inject a solution of methylene blue into the esophagus in order to prove that there is no mucosal perforation.

Esophagomyotomy for Diffuse Esophageal Spasm

The technique of performing a myotomy for diffuse spasm does not differ from that described for achalasia except in the length of the myotomy. If the lower esophageal sphincter can relax normally when swallowing occurs, then do not extend the myotomy down to the terminal esophagus. The preoperative manometric assessment of the patient's esophageal contractions will determine how far the esophagomyotomy should be extended.

Closure and Drainage

Bring a 30F plastic catheter out of the chest cavity through a stab wound in the ninth intercostal space in the anterior axillary line. Approximate the ribs with 2 or 3 pericostal sutures of No. 2 PG. Close the remainder of the wound in layers as illustrated in Figs. 8–40 to 8–42.

Postoperative Care

Remove the nasogastric tube the day following surgery.

Initiate oral intake of liquids on the 1st or 2nd postoperative day, if tolerated.

Remove the thoracic drainage tube as soon as the drainage becomes minimal, about the 3rd or 4th postoperative day.

Postoperative Complications

Persistent Dysphagia.   In some cases an inadequate myotomy for achalasia may fail to completely relieve the patient's dysphagia. In these cases, about 2 weeks following operation, the insertion of graduated Maloney dilators through the esophagogastric junction may relieve this complaint.

Recurrent Dysphagia Following Initial Relief of Symptoms.   It is possible that in these cases there has been a reuniting of the muscular tissues. A trial of Maloney bougienage up to size 50F may prove successful. It should be noted, that there appears to be an increased incidence of esophageal carcinoma in patients who have had long-standing esophageal achalasia. Consequently, patients with recurrent dysphagia following a symptom-free interval after esophagomyotomy should have complete study by X ray, esophagoscopy, and biopsy to rule out carcinoma.

Reflux Esophagitis.   Although most patients with symptoms of reflux may be handled conservatively, an antireflux operation will be required in severe cases.

Diaphragmatic Hernia

Empyema

References

Ellis FH Jr, Kiser JC, Schlegel JF, Earlam RJ et al. (1967) Esophagomyotomy for esophageal achalasia: experimental, clinical, and manometric aspects. Ann Surg 166:640

Ellis FH Jr, Gibb SP, Crozier RE (1980) Esophagomyotomy for achalasia of the esophagus. Ann Surg 192:157

Henderson RD, Ryder DE (1982) Reflux control following myotomy in diffuse esophageal spasm. Ann Thorac Surg 34:230

Leonardi HK, Shea JA, Crozier RE, Ellis FH Jr (1977) Diffuse spasm of the esophagus: clinical, manometric, and surgical considerations. J Thorac Cardiovasc Surg 74:736

Murray GF (1980) Operation for motor dysfunction of the esophagus. Ann Thorac Surg 29:184

Murray GF, Battaglini JW, Keagy BA, Starek PJK et al. (1984) Selective application of fundoplication in achalasia. Ann Thorac Surg 37:185

Okike N, Payne WS, Newfeld DM et al. (1979) Esophagomyotomy versus forceful dilatation for achalasia of the esophagus: results in 899 patients. Ann Thorac Surg 28:119

Sanderson DR, Ellis FH Jr, Olsen AL (1970) Achalasia of the esophagus: results of therapy by dilatation 1950–1967. Chest 58:116

Skinner DB (1984) Myotomy and achalasia. Ann Thorac Surg 37:183

74 Operations for Esophageal Perforations and Anastomotic Leaks

Concept: Choice of Therapy

Options in Selecting Therapy

Conservative Management

Although several retrospective studies of esophageal perforations have identified groups of patients who survived with conservative therapy, it must be emphasized that these patients must be carefully selected. When a patient sustains a small perforation of the cervical esophagus following elective esophagoscopy and has minimal symptoms, both local and systemic, nonoperative management by means of antibiotics and intravenous feeding may prove successful. On the other hand, a spontaneous perforation of the thoracic esophagus following a bout of retching in a gourmand with a full stomach should always be treated by prompt operation. Otherwise, a fulminating necrotizing mediastinitis will develop because the chest has been flooded by the powerful digestive ferments of the stomach and duodenum. Nonoperative management is acceptable only in patients who have experienced a contained leak with minimal symptoms and no sign of systemic sepsis. In the thoracic esophagus the presence of fluid or air in the pleural cavity is a contraindication to conservative treatment.

Surgical Drainage

Proper drainage implies a surgical incision followed by the insertion of adequate drains down to the point of perforation, whether in the neck or in the thorax. This is accompanied by proximal decompression with nasogastric suction, antibiotics, and intravenous feeding.

Some surgeons have advocated inserting a large T-tube into the esophageal perforation, bringing the long end of the rubber tube out through the chest (Abbot, Mansour, Logan et al.). At least one instance of erosion of the thoracic aorta has occurred following the use of this method (Goldstein and Thompson).

Local drainage without suturing the opening is generally used in the cervical esophagus where the perforation may sometimes not be identified or may be located in an inaccessible position. Also, in operations performed after a delay of 12–24 hours the quality of the esophageal tissue may be such that suturing is not possible.

Suture Repair and Drainage

Ideally, when a perforation is diagnosed and explored within 12 hours of injury in the absence of a violent inflammatory response, accurate closure of the perforation with two layers of interrupted fine sutures may result in primary healing. In all cases, place a drain down to the vicinity of the repaired perforation. As above, utilize proximal nasogastric suction, antibiotics, and intravenous feeding. Gastrostomy may be performed to accomplish the removal of gastric and duodenal secretions.

Suture Repair with Buttress

Grillo and Wilkins achieved excellent results when they wrapped their sutured thoracic esophageal perforations with a pedicle flap of parietal pleura. Other surgeons have advocated using pedicles of diaphragm or intercostal muscle to buttress the esophageal suture line. When a perforation of the distal esophagus has been repaired, it may be buttressed by performing a Nissen fundoplication or a Thal operation. A pleural or pericardial flap appears to be the most widely applicable buttress because of its flexibility.

Surgical Drainage with Proximal Diversion and Distal Occlusion

For patients with perforations of the thoracic esophagus accompanied by a serious degree of mediastinitis, Urschel advocated performing a cervical esophagostomy to accomplish the proximal diversion of saliva. He performed a thoracotomy both to provide adequate local drainage and to occlude the lower esophagus by means of a strip of Teflon felt. A gastrostomy was also performed. During the early postoperative period, the gastrostomy was used to evacuate digestive secretions. Later on, the same channel was employed for tube feeding.

Although in one retrospective review (Michel, Grillo, and Malt) the diversion-exclusion operation appeared to have a higher mortality rate than conservative management, it is obvious that diversion-exclusion is generally employed in the sickest patients. In many cases the thoracic esophagus will have to be sacrificed and replaced by means of a colon bypass from the neck to the stomach at a later date. Nevertheless, further progress in reducing the mortality from late esophageal perforations and leaks will come when the indications for the pleural wrap and the diversion-exclusion operations have been expanded to include some of the patients who are now failures following more conservative methods of treatment.

The most effective method of assuring proximal diversion is to perform a total thoracic esophagectomy with an end cervical esophagostomy and a closure of the proximal stomach.

Concept: Management of Esophageal Perforations at Various Anatomical Levels

Cervical Esophagus

The cervical esophagus may be perforated during endoscopy, endotracheal intubation, swallowing a foreign body, or by external trauma. Although endoscopic perforations accompanied by minimal symptoms and signs may be treated conservatively, patients who are febrile or have swelling and tenderness in the neck should have prompt exploration and drainage of the retroesophageal space, as well as suture repair of the perforation when possible.

Thoracic Esophagus

Perforation by Endoscopy or Bougienage Esophageal perforation following endoscopy or instrumentation occurred in 0.15% of patients (mortality rate 0.02%) at the Massachusetts General Hospital (Michel et al.) and in 0.2% of 19,600 procedures (0.005%) at the Mayo Clinic (Sarr, Pemberton, and Payne). In an excellent review of 47 endoscopic or instrumental perforations Sarr and colleagues found that the fiberoptic endoscope had been used in 7 patients and the rigid scope in 12; 14 patients sustained perforations when the esophagus was being dilated through a rigid esophagoscope. Twelve patients experienced perforations during instrumental dilatation without endoscopy and one each during endotracheal intubation and instrumental dilatation of achalasia.

Pain was the most frequent complaint (95%) following esophageal perforation; fever and leukocytosis were noted in about two-thirds of the cases. In cervical perforations crepitation was noted in 63% by palpation and 95% on X ray. This finding usually required 4–12 hours to develop. Mediastinal emphysema was present in only 30%–40% of patients with disruptions of the thoracic esophagus, but extravasation of the contrast medium proved to be diagnostic in over 90% of X ray esophagrams.

In selecting the proper treatment for a patient with an iatrogenic perforation of the thoracic esophagus diagnosed within a few hours of the accident, remember that the patient may look quite well during the first few hours and then collapse 24 hours later due to fulminating mediastinitis. We agree with Sarr and associates that when perforation becomes evident early, treatment should include primary surgical drainage with closure of the perforation. We would add a pleural or pericardial flap to buttress the suture line in most cases. Sarr and associates experienced no hospital mortality in 13 cases treated by surgical closure of the perforation with drainage.

When a perforation of the thoracic esophagus is diagnosed later than 24 hours after the event and the patient meets the criteria for conservative management enunciated by Cameron, Keiffer, Hendrix, Mehigan, and others, nonoperative therapy may be acceptable. These authors identified a limited subgroup of patients with the following characteristics: (1) perforation of the thoracic esophagus, (2) late presentation, (3) minimal symptoms, (4) no signs of generalized sepsis, (5) all perforations contained locally within the mediastinum, (6) each perforation able to drain back into the esophagus, and (7) no communication with the pleural space. If the patient has minimal symptoms 24 hours after an intrathoracic perforation and the constrast esophagram demonstrates localization of the leak, the patient has probably passed the danger period during which he is susceptible to fulminating mediastinitis from the reflux of gastric and duodenal juices. In this group, treatment with proximal suction by means of a nasoesophageal tube combined with antibiotics and intravenous feeding was successful in all five patients reported on by Sarr and associates.

Performing a closed thoracostomy to provide drainage of a major thoracic esophageal perforation is an exercise in futility. Michel and associates reported three deaths in patients who were treated by closed thoracostomy after suffering esophageal perforations secondary to bougienage, passage of a Celestin tube, or passage of a Levine tube. They noted only one additional case who survived following this type of therapy, which brings the mortality rate from closed thoracostomy to 75%. The same authors had good results with primary suture repair and drainage of thoracic perforations, but they note that two additional patients, both of whom sustained esophageal perforation by a Sengstaken-Blakemore tube, died following persistent esophageal leakage after suture repair. It is possible that this type of perforation would fare better with a diversion-exclusion operation.

Perforations of the Obstructed Thoracic Esophagus

Perforations produced during endoscopy or dilatation of the obstructed esophagus require simultaneous relief of the obstruction or else a sutured repair is doomed to failure. In the case of an early operation following perforation of an esophagus obstructed by achalasia, it may be possible to combine suture of the perforation with an esophagomyotomy to relieve the obstruction, as advocated by McKinnon and Ochsner and by Skinner, Little, and DeMeester. On the other hand, in the report of Sarr and associates, six patients underwent distal esophagectomy with primary esophagogastric anastomosis for the removal of both the perforated esophagus and the obstructing lesion. Three of these patients died of complications related to anastomotic failure. Two of the three fatal cases came into the hospital with benign strictures and were operated upon more than 8 hours after perforation. Another patient in this series, with perforation of a distal esophageal stricture, underwent a total thoracic esophagectomy, an end cervical esophagostomy, closure of the esophagogastric junction, and a feeding gastrostomy. He was discharged in good health 13 days later. This patient underwent a successful colon interposition operation 2 months later. While it may be necessary to resect a perforated esophagus together with the obstructing lesion in some cases, a primary esophagogastric anastomosis is *contraindicated* in the presence of acute mediastinitis or any significant degree of inflammation of the organs being anastomosed. Closing the upper end of the stomach and bringing normal esophagus out in the neck is a much safer procedure in the presence of inflammation.

Postemetic Perforation (Boerhaave's Syndrome)

In general, postemetic perforations of the thoracic esophagus are dangerous because they often occur in a patient with a full stomach, which floods the mediastinum with food and digestive secretions. Fulminating mediastinitis occurs rapidly. Good results can be expected only if the operation is done within the first 8–24 hours. In the report of Michel and associates eight patients with Boerhaave's syndrome underwent primary sutured repairs with or without a pleural flap. All were successful except for one case. This patient had a primary repair buttressed by a pleural flap but operation was performed more than 24 hours after the perforation and the patient died. When operating upon a patient in whom the diagnosis is made late, and the mediastinal tissues are very inflamed, a diversion-exclusion operation is indicated.

Anastomotic Leaks following Esophagogastrostomy

Patients who develop leaks following an esophagogastric anastomosis *in the neck* respond well to simple drainage, especially if the drain has been placed at the time of surgery. Although a stricture may appear at the site of the anastomosis secondary to the leak, systemic and mediastinal sepsis is unusual and recovery may be anticipated.

Small, contained nonsymptomatic leaks may be identified on the postoperative contrast X ray of the *thoracic* esophagus. These may resemble a perianastomotic diverticulum. Since they drain back into the lumen of the esophagus, the only required treatment is continued nasoesophageal suction and intravenous feeding if the patient has no sign of sepsis. Repeat esophageal X rays will generally show complete healing within a short period of time. We have generally resumed oral feeding if the patient remained nonsymptomatic for a period of 1 week after detecting the contained leak. None of this is meant to imply that a postoperative anastomotic leak is very often a minor complication. Triggiani and Belsey reported a 43% mortality rate from postoperative leaks following esophageal resection with intrathoracic anastomosis. Wilson, Stone, Scully, Ozeran, and others, in a review of leaks following esophagogastrectomy, stated that "anastomotic leaks cause a major portion of the morbidity after esophageal resection, accounting for up to three-fourths of the serious complications. Further, leaks are the most important cause of death: 54 to 100% of patients with anastomotic complications die." These authors reported 19 leaks (11.3%) and 4 deaths (2.4%) after 167 esophagogastrectomies. In their series there were 12 patients with serious anastomotic leaks accompanied by either an intrathoracic fluid collection, an esophagopleurocutaneous fistula, or an anastomotic dehiscence. Most of these patients were treated by continued nasogastric suction, total parenteral nutrition, and "aggressive and accurate replacement of the chest tube" by multiple closed thoracostomies. Chest X rays were obtained daily to be sure that there were no loculations. One patient underwent secondary thoracotomy to accomplish complete drainage of a mediastinal abscess; another patient, who developed anastomotic dehiscence, underwent a diversion-exclusion procedure successfully. Four of these 12 patients died because of uncontrolled sepsis 7–45 days postoperatively. Some of these deaths could probably have been prevented by the more aggressive employment of diversion-exclusion operations or by total thoracic esophagectomy with end cervical esophagostomy and closure of the proximal end of the gastric pouch, accompanied by tube gastrostomy.

Recurrent Sepsis after Operation to Suture and Drain the Perforated Thoracic Esophagus

If a patient has undergone a thoracotomy for the closure of an esophageal perforation combined with drainage of the mediastinum and sepsis has persisted or recurred, this is a definite indication for another thoracotomy to improve the drainage and to accomplish diversion by cervical esophagostomy, with or without a total thoracic esophagectomy, and exclusion by closure of the upper stomach combined with tube gastrostomy.

It should be remembered that any abdominal or thoracoabdominal operation for gastric carcinoma produces some bacterial contamination of the peritoneal as well as the thoracic cavity. A left subphrenic abscess is not a rare complication of esophagogastrectomy for carcinoma. The possibility of a left subphrenic abscess should be kept in mind if sepsis occurs after surgery for gastric cancer.

Abdominal Esophagus

Perforation of the abdominal esophagus may occur following endoscopy or instrumental dilatation in patients with achalasia. Additionally, the esophagus may be perforated during the course of abdominal vagotomy or hiatus hernia repair. It is extremely important to identify this type of perforation during the course of the laparotomy so that prompt repair can be accomplished. An Upper Hand or "chain" retractor to elevate the sternum will provide adequate exposure in most cases. If the exposure is inadequate for a meticulous repair of the esophageal laceration,

do not hesitate to extend the incision into the chest. If there is any question as to the adequacy of the repair, buttress the sutures with the gastric wall by performing a Nissen fundoplication or a Thal operation.

In the series reported by Michel and associates, one patient, who sustained a perforation of the lower esophagus during vagotomy, experienced a 24-hour delay before surgery. This patient died with a persistent esophageal leak, indicating the serious potential of this complication. In patients with advanced sepsis or a failed repair of a perforation of the abdominal esophagus, radical surgery will be necessary to salvage the patient. Divide and close the distal esophagus above the perforation. Close the upper stomach. Perform a Stamm gastrostomy and drain the left subhepatic space with sump and latex drains. Utilize a cervical esophagostomy for proximal diversion.

Any patient suspected of a perforated abdominal esophagus should have a prompt Hypaque contrast esophagram. If there is any leakage into the abdomen, prompt surgery is indicated.

Indications

(See discussion above under "Concept")

Preoperative Care

Confirm perforation with diagnostic studies: chest X ray; in suspected cervical perforations, lateral neck films in hyperextension; contrast esophageal X rays.

Administer nasoesophageal suction proximal to perforation of thoracic esophagus.

Maintain fluid resuscitation.

Administer appropriate systemic antibiotics.

Insert appropriate central venous or pulmonary artery pressure monitors.

351

Pitfalls and Danger Points

Delay in diagnosing the perforation

Inadequate surgery to control continuing contamination

Inadequate drainage

Depending on sutured closure of inflamed esophagus

Suturing a perforated esophagus proximal to an obstruction

Operative Strategy

Be certain to explore an esophageal perforation thoroughly. What appears to be a 1-cm perforation may prove to be three or four times that length after it is mobilized from the mediastinal pleura. Debride necrotic material around the perforation if suturing is anticipated. When the defect appears to be too large or the tissues too inflamed for suturing, it may be possible to apply a roof patch consisting of a flap of pleura or pericardium that is sutured over the perforation. Otherwise, a diversion-exclusion operation or thoracic esophagectomy will be necessary.

Other points of strategy are discussed above under "Concept."

Operative Technique—Pleural Flap Repair of Thoracic Esophageal Perforation

Incision

Make an incision in the left or right thoracic cavity depending on which side the perforation appears to present on the contrast esophageal X ray. Generally, the lower half of the esophagus will be approached through a left 6th or 7th intercostal space thoracotomy. The uncommon perforations of the upper esophagus are better approached through the right chest.

Exposure; Locating the Perforation

Incise the mediastinal pleura above and below the area of suspected perforation. Otherwise, free the mediastinal pleura from the esophagus so that it may be elevated from its bed for thorough exploration. If the perforation is not immediately apparent, ask the anesthesiologist to instill a solution of methylene blue into the naso-esophageal tube. Sometimes the perforation is obscured by a layer of necrotic tissue. The area of perforation will generally be accurately identified by the methylene blue dye.

Repair

When operation is performed soon (8 hours) after perforation, it may be possible to debride the tissues around the esophagus if marked edema and inflammation have not yet occurred. Then close the mucosal layer with interrupted sutures of 5–0 Vicryl. Approximate the muscular layer with interrupted Lembert sutures of 4–0 silk or Prolene. Cover the suture line with a pleural flap. If the perforation is located in the lateral aspect of the esophagus, a simple rectangular flap of pleura is elevated and brought over the suture line. Use many interrupted 4–0 nonabsorbable sutures (Grillo and Wilkins used silk) to fix the pleural flap around the sutured perforation.

When the perforation is not suitable for a sutured closure due to marked edema and inflammation, employ the pleural flap as a roof patch over the open defect in the esophagus. First debride the obvious necrotic tissue around the perforation.

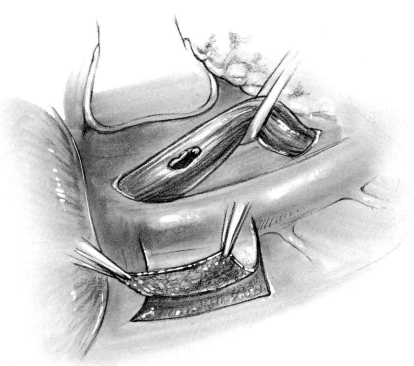

Fig. 74–1

With an extensive defect in the esophagus or one that is located on the posterior surface, outline a large rectangular flap of pleura as illustrated in **Fig. 74–1.** In the presence of mediastinitis, the pleura will be thickened and easy to mobilize from the posterior thoracic wall. Leave the base of the pedicle attached to the adjacent aorta. Slide the pedicle flap beneath the esophagus **(Fig. 74–2)** so as to surround the entire organ. Insert multiple 4–0 interrupted

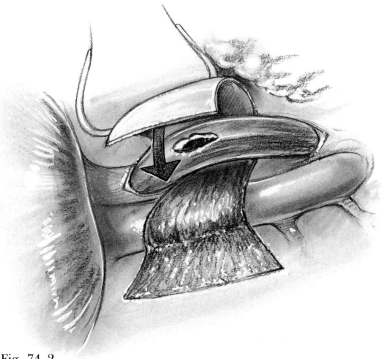

Fig. 74–2

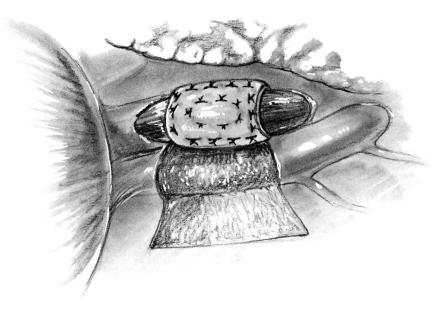

Fig. 74–3

nonabsorbable sutures deep enough to catch the submucosa of the esophagus around the entire circumference of the perforation as well as the entire circumference of the esophagus above and below the perforation as illustrated in **Fig. 74–3.**

Drainage

Place the tip of a 36F multiperforated drainage tube near the site of the esophageal perforation. Suture it to the mediastinal tissues with a catgut stitch. Bring this tube out through a small incision through the 9th or 10th interspace in the anterior axillary line. If desired, place a smaller multiperforated catheter in the posterior portion of the apex of the chest and bring this out through a second stab would. Attach both to some type of underwater drainage device.

Operative Technique— Esophageal Diversion by Cervical Esophagostomy

Incision and Exposure

With the patient's head turned toward the right, make an incision along the anterior border of the sternomastoid muscle beginning 2–3 cm below the level of the mandibular angle and continuing down to the clavicle (see Fig. 7–27). Liberate the anterior border of the sternomastoid muscle. Divide the omohyoid muscle if it crosses the operative field. Retract the sternomastoid muscle and carotid sheath laterally and retract the prethyroid muscles medially, exposing the thyroid gland (see Fig. 7–29). Carefully divide the areolar tissue between the thyroid gland and the carotid sheath to expose the inferior thyroid artery and the recurrent laryngeal nerve. In some cases it may be necessary to divide the inferior thyroid artery. Preserve the recurrent nerve. Identify the tracheoesophageal groove. Then encircle the esophagus with the index finger, but keep the plane of dissection very close to the esophagus. Other-

354

wise, it will be possible to traumatize the *opposite* recurrent laryngeal nerve. After the esophagus has been encircled, pass a latex drain around the esophagus for purposes of traction. Mobilize the esophagus from the level of the hypopharynx down to the upper mediastinum.

Suturing the Esophagostomy

After mobilization is satisfactory, suture the sternomastoid muscle back in place by means of several interrupted 4–0 Vicryl stitches. Close the platysma muscle with interrupted sutures of the same material, leaving sufficient space to suture the esophagostomy to the skin. Then insert interrupted 4–0 PG subcuticular sutures to close the skin leaving a 3–4 cm gap in the closure for the esophagostomy.

Now make a transverse incision across the anterior half of the circumference of the esophagus. Suture the full thickness of the esophagus to the subcuticular layer of skin with interrupted 4–0 Vicryl sutures **(Fig. 74–4)**.

In one case we found that despite thorough mobilization of the esophagus, the incised esophagus could not be sutured to the skin without tension. A subtotal thyroid lobectomy was carried out. Then the incised esophagus was sutured to the platysma muscle with interrupted sutures leaving the skin in this area open. This produced a satisfactory result.

If it has been elected to perform a total thoracic esophagectomy, deliver the specimen into the neck. Transect the esophagus at the level of the sternal notch

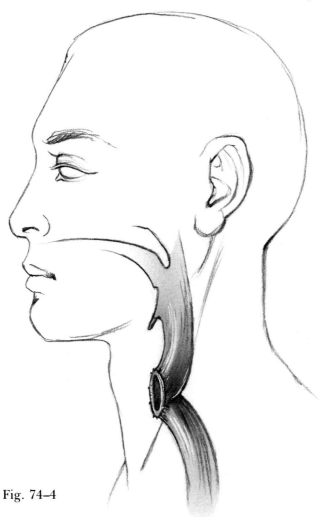

Fig. 74–4

and suture the end of the proximal esophagus to the subcuticular layer of the skin as above.

Operative Technique— Occluding the Lower Esophagus

Perform a thoracotomy as described for the pleural flap operation. Incise the mediastinal pleura and liberate the esophagus from its bed **(Fig. 74–5).** The perforation may be sutured or covered with a pleural flap.

Then free the esophagus around its entire circumference distal to the perforation. Urschel, Razzuk, Wood, Galbraith, and others occluded the esophagus by surrounding it with a strip of Teflon that was sutured to itself to form a circumferential constricting band. Do not make this band so tight that it will strangulate the tissue. An umbilical tape may be passed around the Teflon band and tied to assure the proper degree of constriction. Try to avoid including the vagus nerves in the constricting band.

Alternative methods of occluding the lower esophagus include ligating it with a Silastic tube, such as the Jackson-Pratt catheter **(Figs. 74–6 and 74–7).** This material appears to be less irritating to the tissues than Teflon or umbilical tape.

Another alternative is to use the TA-55 stapling device with 4.8 mm staples to occlude the lower esophagus. When applying the staples, separate the vagus nerves from the esophagus so that they will not be trapped in the staple line. Use staples only if the esophagus is not markedly thickened or inflamed. Otherwise, the thickened tissues may be strangulated by the staples. Then place proper drainage tubes to the area of perforation and close the thoracic incision. At first, all of these patients require a tube gastrostomy, generally of the Stamm type (see Figs. 17–1 to 17–5), to decompress the stomach; after the esophageal perforation has healed, the gastrostomy tube is used for purposes of feeding.

Postoperative Care

Most of these patients will require ventilatory support for several days as well as careful cardiodynamic monitoring.

Insert a small sump-suction drain through the cervical esophagostomy into the proximal esophagus to evacuate saliva. After the esophageal perforation has healed, paste a small drainage bag or ileostomy bag over the esophagostomy to collect the saliva. In patients without an esophagostomy, maintain nasoesophageal suction postoperatively until the leak is controlled as confirmed by a Hypaque swallow esophagram.

Most of these patients will require intensive antibiotic treatment, depending on bacterial cultures of the mediastinum.

Do not remove the thoracotomy drainage tubes until drainage has ceased.

Total parenteral nutrition will be necessary until the gastrostomy tube can be used for feeding.

Perform frequent chest X rays in the search for loculated collections of pus.

Postoperative Complications

Esophagocutaneous fistula
Uncontrolled sepsis including empyema or mediastinal abscess
Subphrenic abscess
Limited expansion of lung, requiring surgical decortication after active infection has subsided.

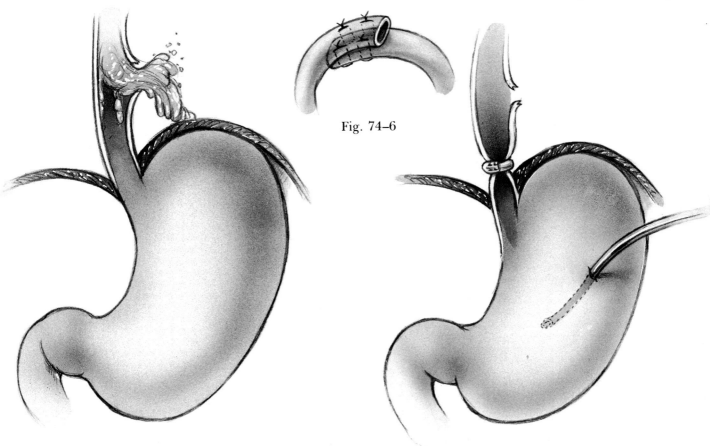

Fig. 74–6

Fig. 74–5

Fig. 74–7

References

Abbott OA, Mansour KA, Logan WD Jr et al. (1970) Atraumatic so-called "spontaneous" rupture of the esophagus: a review of 47 personal cases with comments on a new method of surgical therapy. J Thorac Cardiovasc Surg 59:67

Cameron JL, Keiffer RF, Hendrix TR, Mehigan DG et al. (1979) Selective nonoperative management of contained intrathoracic esophageal disruptions. Ann Thorac Surg 27:404

Goldstein LA, Thompson WR (1982) Esophageal perforations: a 15 year experience. Am J Surg 143:495

Grillo HC, Wilkins EW Jr (1975) Esophageal repair following late diagnosis of intrathoracic perforation. Ann Thorac Surg 20:387

McKinnon WMP, Ochsner JL (1974) Immediate closure and Heller procedure after Mosher bag rupture of the esophagus. Am J Surg 127:115

Michel L, Grillo HC, Malt RA (1981) Operative and nonoperative management of esophageal perforations. Ann Surg 194:57

Sarr MG, Pemberton JH, Payne WS (1982) Management of instrumental perforations of the esophagus. J Thorac Cardiovasc Surg 84:211

Skinner DB, Little AG, DeMeester TR (1980) Management of esophageal perforation. Am J Surg 139:760

Thal AP, Hatafuku T (1964) Improved operation for esophageal rupture. JAMA 188:826

Triggiani E, Belsey R (1977) Oesophageal trauma: incidence, diagnosis, and management. Thorax 32:241

Urschel HC Jr, Razzuk MA, Wood RE, Gailbraith N et al. (1974) Improved management of esophageal perforation: exclusion and diversion in continuity. Ann Surg 179:587

Wilson SE, Stone R, Scully M, Ozeran L et al. (1982) Modern management of anastomotic leak after esophagogastrectomy. Am J Surg 144:94

Abdominal Wall

75 Concept: Which Operation for Inguinal Hernia

Pathogenesis of Inguinal Hernia

Indirect inguinal hernia, even in adult life, is probably caused by the persistence of a patent processus vaginalis and can therefore be classified as a congenital lesion. A patient with this type of hernia is not born with a muscular or aponeurotic weakness; instead, as the neck of the indirect hernia enlarges over a period of years, pressure may produce weakness of the adjacent transversalis fascia. In the geographical area in which we practice, the ready availability of good pediatric care and pediatric surgeons has resulted in the detection and repair of many indirect inguinal hernias during infancy and childhood. Consequently, the majority of our adult hernias are direct in nature, their most probable cause being wear and tear. In the region of Hasselbach's triangle the only structures between the peritoneum and the skin are the transversalis fascia and the external oblique aponeurosis. Once the transversalis fascia becomes attenuated and stretched, a direct hernia will bulge through the external inguinal ring. The attenuated portion of the transversalis fascia is of no use in the repair. Along the superior and medial margins of the weak area, one may use the uninjured portion of the transversalis fascia together with the aponeurosis of the transversus abdominis muscle. On the inferolateral aspect of the weak area, a rim of transversalis fascia, called the iliopubic tract by Nyhus and Condon, is generally intact and useful in the repair. If this is not the case, either the shelving edge of the inguinal ligament or Cooper's ligament is available.

Indirect Hernia

In a child with an indirect inguinal hernia, where the neck of the sac is narrow and the diameter of the internal ring is normal, high ligation of the sac constitutes adequate surgery. Those patients, usually adults, whose internal ring has been forcibly dilated by the indirect hernia, have suffered a defect in the floor of the inguinal canal equivalent to a direct hernia. In this situation, after removing the sac, a procedure should be employed to repair the floor of Hasselbach's triangle. We prefer the Shouldice operation in most cases of this type.

Direct Hernia—Anterior Transversalis Repair (Shouldice)

With respect to the direct hernia, many surgical procedures have been proposed. The Halsted technique is simple, but positioning the new external ring directly over the internal ring results in a high incidence of recurrences at this site. McVay's repair utilizing Cooper's ligament is elegant in concept, but in the hands of many surgeons this repair leaves a weak area in the vicinity of the iliac vein at the medial margin of the new internal inguinal ring because the iliopubic tract or femoral sheath in this area may be attenuated. The preperitoneal repair popularized by Nyhus is valuable when repairing an incarcerated femoral hernia. When used to repair direct hernias, the Nyhus preperitoneal operation has been followed by an excessive recurrence rate (17%–35%, Nyhus and Condon p. 227). The Bassini operation has achieved worldwide popularity owing to its simplicity. The integrity of the Bassini repair depends on attaching the "conjoined tendon" to the shelving edge of the inguinal ligament with one layer of sutures. If any one of these sutures should break or cut through the tissue, recurrence would seem to be inevitable. The defect in the transversalis fascia itself and the internal inguinal ring are not specifically repaired. Followup studies by Berliner, Burson, Katz, and Wise have demonstrated a recurrence rate of 11.5% for this operation.

For the past 10 years at our institution, patients who have had direct or combined indirect-direct inguinal hernia and undergone the Shouldice repair have achieved excellent results, as demonstrated by the thorough studies of our colleagues Berliner and co-workers. The Shouldice technique requires a complete dissection of Hasselbach's triangle with incision of the attenuated transversalis fascia from the internal inguinal ring to the pubic tubercle. All of the preperitoneal structures including the bladder and the deep inferior epigastric artery and vein are dissected away from the transversalis fascia prior to initiating any suturing. Four layers of continuous suture material are utilized so that not only is the defect in the transversalis fascia repaired, but there is also successive attachment of the transversus abdominis arch and the internal oblique muscle to the iliopubic tract, the inguinal ligament, and the undersurface of the external oblique aponeurosis. The attenuated transversalis is *excised* and the healthy tissue is sutured. The effect of the succeeding layers of sutures is to weave into position a "roof patch" of external oblique aponeurosis over Hasselbach's triangle. The continuous nature of the suture permits tension to be equally distributed throughout the area, thus allowing the use of fine suture materials. At the same time

the extensive dissection guarantees that the surgeon will see and evaluate each structure in the inguinal region.

In approximately 1%–2% of our patients with very large direct or sliding hernias we have felt that the area of weakness was so extensive, or in some cases so infiltrated with adipose tissue, as to require a technique other than the Shouldice. In these situations we have inserted polypropylene mesh (Marlex). Although Lichtenstein reported good results with Marlex mesh in the *routine* repair of direct inguinal hernia, we have restricted its use to those cases where the Shouldice operation was not suitable.

Direct Hernia—Cooper's Ligament Repair (McVay)

In McVay's method of repairing the floor of the inguinal canal in a direct (or a large indirect) hernia, all the attenuated transversalis fascia is excised and the aponeurosis of the transversus abdominis muscle (transversus arch) is sutured down to Cooper's ligament and the anterior femoral sheath. This requires careful dissection so that the femoral sheath may be identified. The operation cannot be performed unless a long relaxing incision is made in the posterior leaflet of the anterior rectus sheath. When this operation has been properly executed, excellent results have been reported by Halverson and McVay and by Rutledge. The McVay operation resembles that of Shouldice in that all of the structures deep to the damaged inguinal floor are carefully dissected out and exposed. Both techniques use the transversus arch for the cephalad margin of the repair. Whereas the Shouldice repair uses the iliopubic tract, the femoral sheath, and the inguinal ligament for the lower sutures, McVay employs Cooper's ligament and the femoral sheath. Because we do not have a large experience with the Cooper's ligament repair, the operative technique described below is that of McVay.

362

Inguinal Hernia Repair in Women—Modifications of Technique

In the absence of spermatic vessels and a vas, repairing an inguinal hernia in a woman is much simpler than a man. The round ligament that is found in women in place of the spermatic cord is easily excised together with the sac, if a sac is present. If there is a weak area in the transversalis fascia, perform a standard Shouldice repair. If there is not a significant area of weakness, you can simply close the inguinal floor by inserting interrupted sutures of 2–0 cotton or Tevdek to approximate the "conjoined tendon" to the shelving edge of the inguinal ligament. Then close the incision in the external oblique aponeurosis in the usual fashion. The recurrence rate following the repair in women is generally reported to be lower than in men.

In repairing a femoral hernia, the technique used is identical in both women and men.

Sliding Hernia—Shouldice or McVay Repair

Sliding inguinal hernias generally emerge lateral to the deep inferior epigastric artery and are therefore indirect in nature. Unlike other indirect hernias, the sliding hernia is not the result of a congenital sac. In a sliding hernia the sac is purely coincidental. The pathogenesis here is a large defect in the transversalis fascia that permits colon to slide through the abdominal wall, dragging some peritoneum along with it as an appendage. Consequently, excision of all or part of the sac *is not an essential part of the repair.* The sliding hernia should be treated as a direct hernia after the herniated colon and sac have been reduced. The sac may be opened to confirm the nature of the pathology, but amputation of the sac is not necessary unless the sac is very redundant. One then proceeds with either the typical Shouldice or McVay repair. Ryan reported a recurrence rate of only 1% after repairing 313 sliding hernias by these principles. Our observations confirm his results.

Incarcerated and Strangulated Hernia—Modifications in Anesthesia and Incision

There is no significant variation in technique for these two complications of inguinal hernia, other than the use of general anesthesia in most cases. Do not hesitate to perform an additional midline laparotomy incision if it is necessary to achieve adequate exposure when resecting strangulated bowel.

When repairing a strangulated inguinal hernia contaminated by gangrenous bowel, we use monofilament steel wire to repair the hernia in order to prevent the development of suture granulomata and sinuses postoperatively.

References

Berliner S, Burson L, Katz P, Wise L (1978) An anterior transversalis fascia repair for adult inguinal hernias. Am J Surg 135:633

Halverson K, McVay CB (1970) Inguinal and femoral hernioplasty: a 22-year study of the author's methods. Arch Surg 101:127

Lichtenstein IL (1970) Hernia repair without disability. Mosby, St. Louis

Nyhus LM, Condon RE (eds) (1978) Hernia, 2nd edn. Lippincott, Philadelphia

Rutledge RH (1980) Cooper's ligament repair for adult groin hernias. Surgery 87:601

Ryan EA (1956) An analysis of 313 consecutive cases of indirect sliding hernias. Surg Gynecol Obstet 102:45

76 Anterior Transversalis Repair of Inguinal Hernia (Shouldice)

Indications

All indirect and sliding inguinal hernias should be repaired because of the significant incidence of strangulation.

With the use of local anesthesia, systemic disease is rarely so serious as to constitute a contraindication to operating. Small, nonsymptomatic direct inguinal hernias in elderly, poor-risk patients do not require surgery because they almost never produce strangulation. Direct hernias that produce symptoms, on the other hand, should be repaired.

Preoperative Care

Persuade obese patients to lose weight prior to surgery. Fat interposed between sutured layers of fascia impedes healing.

Pitfalls and Danger Points

Injury to femoral vessels during suturing

Injury to bladder (especially in sliding hernia)

Injury to colon (especially in sliding hernia)

Injury to deep inferior epigastric vessels with postoperative retroperitoneal bleeding

Operative Strategy

Anesthesia

For inguinal hernia repair, local field block anesthesia is preferred. Patients are ambulatory the afternoon of operation and are able to resume a normal diet the same evening. Overdistension of the anesthetized bladder by intravenous fluids often follows the use of general anesthesia. This is a major cause of postoperative urinary retention. Relief of this complication requires bladder catheterization that may, in some cases of borderline prostatism, necessitate a prostatectomy after the hernia repair. Urinary retention is avoided with local anesthesia because it does not obtund the patient's sensation of a full bladder or his ability to urinate.

The addition of small doses of Valium has alleviated the restlessness that some patients experience even in the absence of pain. Local anesthesia does not mean that no attention is paid to the patient by anyone other than the operating team. We require that either an anesthesiologist or a nurse sit at the head of the table to monitor the vital signs.

Although local anesthesia can manage some incarcerated hernias successfully, general anesthesia with endotracheal intubation is indicated whenever strangulation of bowel is suspected.

Avoiding Injury

The iliac or femoral vein may be injured by blindly inserting a suture too deep through the iliopubic tract or the inguinal ligament in the lateral portion of the repair. If this should occur, cut the suture and remove it. Then apply pressure to the vein for 5–10 minutes. This maneuver will often avoid the need to expose the iliac vein and suture the bleeding point.

Occasionally, postoperative preperitoneal hemorrhage of serious nature has been produced by injuring one of the deep inferior epigastric vessels with a deep suture. In the Shouldice technique, this can be prevented by complete dissection of the transversalis fascia away from these structures after dividing the external spermatic vessels.

The bladder may be injured in attempting to amputate a sac in a sliding inguinal hernia. Overenthusiastic dissection on the medial aspect of an indirect sac, in the mistaken notion that the higher the ligation the better, may also traumatize the bladder. If a laceration of the bladder has been identified, close the defect by suturing the full thickness of the bladder wall with a continuous 3–0 PG atraumatic suture. Then invert this layer of stitches with a second continuous or interrupted layer of 3–0 PG Lembert-type sutures. Be sure that the bladder remains decompressed for the next 8–10 days by means of constant drainage with an adequate indwelling Foley catheter.

Colon as well as bladder may be injured if the sliding nature of an inguinal hernia is not diagnosed early in the course of operation. Whenever a bulky inguinal hernia is not accompanied by a thin-walled, transparent sac, the presence of a sliding component should be suspected.

All of these inadvertent injuries can be avoided by taking advantage of the extensive exposure that may be attained by the long incision in the transversalis fascia when using the Shouldice method. The deep inferior epigastric vessels and their branches, the iliac vessels, the peritoneum, and, in case of a sliding hernia, the colon are all easily identified. Visualizing these structures is the best way to prevent damage.

Avoiding Postoperative Wound Infections

Of the patients who suffer a postoperative wound infection, 40%–50% will develop a recurrent hernia. Although the incidence of postoperative infection in all "clean" wounds in our institution has been about 1%, even this figure is excessive. The rate of infection can be minimized in hernia repair if the entire operation is performed with careful, sharp dissection. Also important is meticulous hemostasis, which is sometimes neglected in this area of surgery. Finally, the operative site should be irrigated with aliquots of 0.3% kanamycin solution containing 50,000 units of bacitracin in 300 ml of saline solution. This irrigation appears to have contributed to the complete elimination of postoperative infection in 1,200 consecutive herniorrhapy operations (Berliner).

Operative Technique

Local Anesthesia

Use a mixture of equal parts of 0.5% Marcaine and 2% Nesacaine. Create a field block by injecting into the subcutaneous tissues along the lines shown in **Fig. 76–1.** Inject also along the line of the incision. This will require a total of 40–50 ml of anesthetic solution.

After making the skin incision and exposing the external oblique aponeurosis, inject another 10 ml just beneath this layer. Also inject the abdominal musculature along a line 5 cm cephalad to the inguinal canal. This will improve muscle relaxation for the repair. Later, when the peritoneal sac is exposed, inject 5 ml into the sac. Not only will this technique of local block eliminate pain, but it also produces *surprisingly good muscle relaxation.*

Incision

Start the incision in the skin at a point 2.5 cm medial to the anterior superior spine of the ilium. Continue in an oblique fashion to the point where the external ring adjoins the pubic tubercle.

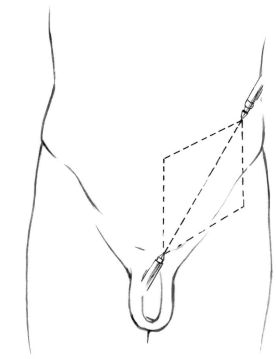

Fig. 76–1

Exposure

By sharp scalpel dissection, clear the external oblique aponeurosis of fat and areolar tissue; continue inferiorly beyond the point where the external oblique aponeurosis becomes the inguinal ligament and curves posteriorly in the upper thigh. Expose the external inguinal ring as well as the spermatic cord emerging from this ring. Ligate the bleeding points with 4–0 PG. Do not depend on electrocoagulation to obtain hemostasis in the fatty subcutaneous layer; doing so will result in more frequent postoperative ecchymoses and hematomas than using ligatures for hemostasis. Reserve electrocoagulation for the bleeding points in the nonfat tissues. Incise the external oblique aponeurosis along the line of its fibers so that the incision will join the external inguinal ring at its *cephalad* margin **(Fig. 76–2)**.

Identify the ilioinguinal nerve and dissect it free. Occasionally, the ilioinguinal nerve runs with the spermatic cord, closely approximated to the cremaster muscle. Retract the lateral leaflet of the external oblique in a caudal direction and expose its junction with the pubic tubercle. It is important now to elevate the medial leaflet of external oblique aponeurosis from the underlying transversus muscle for a distance of at least 3–4 cm. The medial leaflet is then retracted in a cephalad direction by inserting one fork of the self-retaining Farr retractor beneath this leaflet, while the other fork is inserted in the subcutaneous tissue of the lateral skin flap.

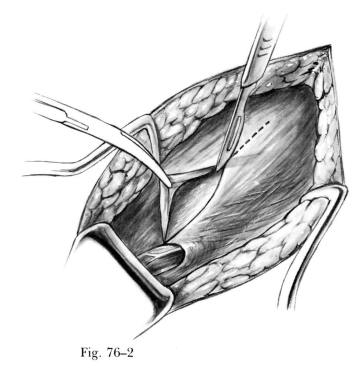

Fig. 76–2

Excising Cremaster Muscle

Free the spermatic cord from surrounding attachments at a point medial to the pubic tubercle. An attempt to underrun the cord lateral to this point may result in traumatizing the structures enclosed in a direct hernia. In the medial location there is much less difficulty freeing the cord from surrounding structures. Remember that in patients with a direct hernia, the hernia sac remains behind when the spermatic cord is encircled. Use a latex tape for purposes of traction.

Transect attachments between the spermatic cord and the underlying tissues. This can be accomplished with the electrocautery. Resect lipomas and adipose tissue. In order to reduce the diameter of the cord, excise the *entire cremaster muscle* from that portion of the spermatic cord which will remain in the inguinal canal. This will permit the surgeon to minimize the diameter of the internal inguinal ring when it is reconstructed. Be sure to remove all of the cremaster muscle fibers from their attachments to the iliopubic tract, the femoral sheath, and the transversalis fascia **(Figs. 76–3 and 76–4).** Only after accomplishing the removal of all these fibers will the visualization of these important structures be clear. Positive identification must be made of both the vas deferens and the internal spermatic vessels prior to resecting the cremaster.

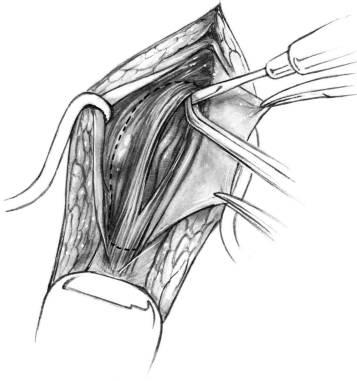

Fig. 76–3

Excising Indirect Sac

At this point, place the left index finger behind the cord near the internal ring and dissect out the cord structures in order positively to rule out the presence in the cord of an indirect sac. If an indirect sac is identified and the patient has a combined indirect and direct hernia, do not employ Hoguet's maneuver of attempting to convert the direct hernia into an indirect type as it is useless. Simply free the indirect sac

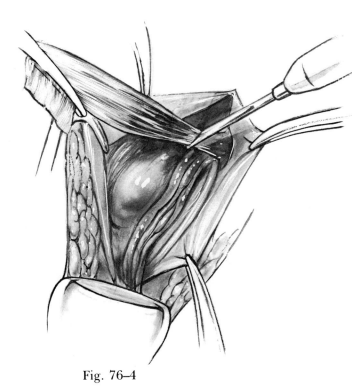

Fig. 76–4

to its neck; explore the sac **(Fig. 76–5)**; transfix it with a single suture-ligature **(Fig. 76–6a)**; and amputate the redundant portion **(Fig. 76–6b).** It is important to free the neck of the sac from surrounding structures so that the stump of ligated sac may retract into the abdomen. The hemostat retracting the lateral leaflet of the external oblique aponeurosis is now removed. This removal permits the cord to be placed lateral to this leaflet together with the ilioinguinal nerve, after which the hemostat is replaced as in **Fig. 76–7.**

Transversalis Dissection

Attention is directed to the bulge in Hasselbach's triangle, which constitutes the direct "sac." Identify the *external* spermatic vessels, which branch off the deep inferior epigastric artery and vein and lie superficial

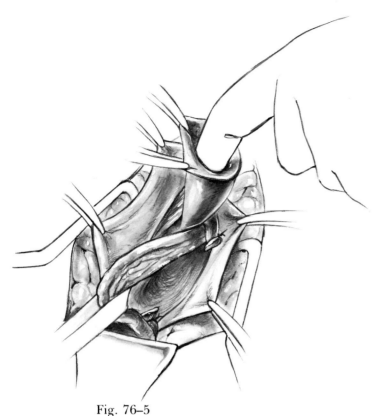

Fig. 76–5

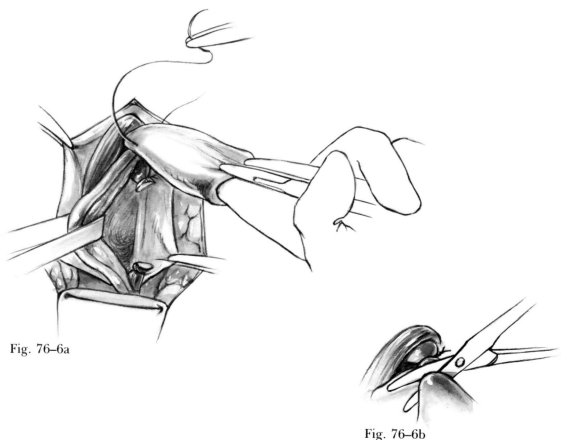

Fig. 76–6a

Fig. 76–6b

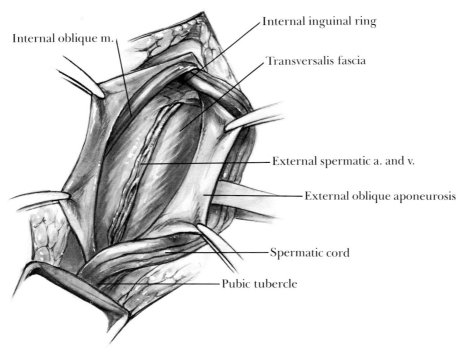

Internal oblique m.

Internal inguinal ring

Transversalis fascia

External spermatic a. and v.

External oblique aponeurosis

Spermatic cord

Pubic tubercle

Fig. 76–7

to the transversalis fascia (Fig. 76–7). Resect the external spermatic vessels between two ligatures of 2–0 PG, one at their junction with the deep inferior epigastric vessels and the other at the pubic tubercle **(Fig. 76–8).** Occasionally a small branch of the genitofemoral nerve runs along the floor of the inguinal canal together with the external spermatic vessels. Excise this nerve together with the vessels. These steps will clear the entire floor of Hasselbach's triangle. Make a scalpel incision through the bulging attenuated transversalis fascia from the pubic tubercle to a point just medial to the deep inferior epi-

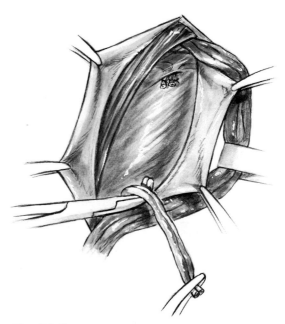

Fig. 76–8

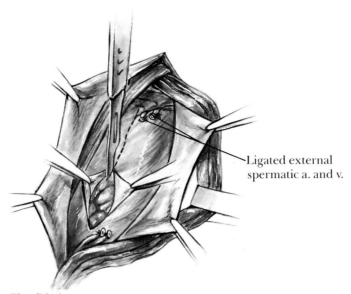

Ligated external
spermatic a. and v.

Fig. 76–9

gastric vessels **(Fig. 76–9).** When lobules of preperitoneal fat bulge through the scalpel incision, the remainder of the incision may be accomplished with a Metzenbaum scissors if preferred. If one is in the proper plane of dissection, the deep inferior epigastric vessels will have been entirely cleared of areolar tissue; Cooper's liga-

ment will be clearly visible laterally, and the preperitoneal fat will be easily separated from the deep surface of the transversalis fascia in a cephalad direction **(Fig. 76–10).** If any branches of the deep inferior epigastric vessels join the deep surface of the transversalis fascia, carefully divide and ligate them so that the epigastric vessels can be pushed down away from the repair. Otherwise, retroperitoneal bleeding may be caused by inadvertently piercing these

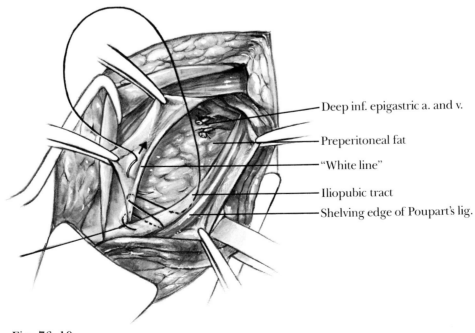

Deep inf. epigastric a. and v.

Preperitoneal fat

"White line"

Iliopubic tract

Shelving edge of Poupart's lig.

Fig. 76–10

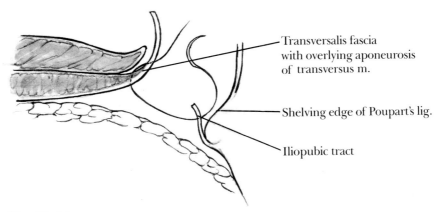

Transversalis fascia
with overlying aponeurosis
of transversus m.

Shelving edge of Poupart's lig.

Iliopubic tract

Fig. 76–11

vessels with a needle while suturing the transversalis layer. Excise the attenuated portions of transversalis fascia and apply straight hemostats to the free cut edge of the medial leaflet of the transversalis fascia for purposes of traction. Apply a moist gauze sponge in a sponge-holder to the preperitoneal fat and bladder in order to push these structures posteriorly.

Shouldice Repair: Layer #1

Anchor the initial stitch (3–0 Tevdek on a C-5 atraumatic needle) by catching lacunar ligament and pubic periosteum in one bite and the undersurface of the medial flap of transversalis with overlying rectus fascia in the other. Tie this stitch. Apply upward traction on the straight clamps holding the medial leaflet of transversalis fascia; this will reveal a "white line" of fibrous tissue on the undersurface of the transversalis fascia. The "white line" represents the aponeurosis of the transversus muscle as seen through the transversalis fascia. This aponeurosis of the transversus abdominis muscle is thought by McVay and Halverson and by Nyhus and Condon to be the most important tissue involved in inguinal hernia repair. This arch of aponeurotic tissue becomes muscular as it approaches the internal inguinal ring. In-

clude the "white line" in the continuous stitch that attaches the cut lateral edge of the transversalis fascia to the undersurface of the medial leaf of the transversalis (Fig. 76–10). Insert the needle into the lateral leaflet of transversalis fascia near the point where this layer appears to attach to the inguinal ligament **(Fig. 76–11).** This condensation of the caudal margin of the transversalis fascia is identical to what Nyhus and Condon call the iliopubic tract. Be sure to remove all the cremaster muscle fibers that cover the iliopubic tract and femoral sheath. Otherwise it is not possible to identify these structures accurately for proper suturing.

Each stitch should contain 4–6 mm of tissue. Continue the suture in a lateral direction until the newly constructed internal ring has been closed snugly around the spermatic cord so that only the tip of a Kelly hemostat will fit loosely between the cord and the internal ring.

Shouldice Repair: Layer #2

Excise the attenuated portion of the transversalis fascia. Then, use the same continuous strand of suture material as in Layer #1 and sew the free cut edge of the medial leaflet of transversalis fascia with adjacent internal oblique muscle to the anterior aspect of the iliopubic tract. One can include 2–3 mm of the shelving edge of the inguinal ligament in the continuous suture

371

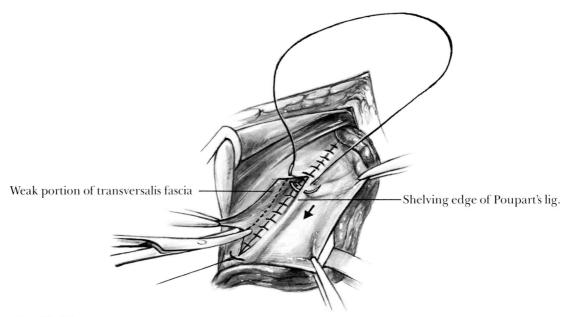

Fig. 76–12

going medially **(Figs. 76–12 and 76–13).** Continue this suture to the pubic tubercle. Devote special attention to insert the last stitch into the pubic periosteum. At this point, terminate the suture by knotting it to its tail. Excise fatty tissue if present in the internal oblique muscle layer prior to suturing. A worthwhile modification of the Shouldice technique is to excise the lower 2 cm of the internal oblique muscle to expose the underlying aponeurosis of the transversus muscle. This step is, in fact, an integral part of McVay's method of hernia repair as shown in Fig. 77–1. After accomplishing this step, one can insert the sutures for Shouldice's layer #3 into the

transversus aponeurosis instead of into the fleshy, internal oblique muscle.

Shouldice Repair: Layer #3

Use a new strand of 3–0 Tevdek to begin this layer. Take a bite of internal oblique muscle or "conjoined tendon" and another of the shelving edge of the inguinal ligament and tie the suture, beginning this time at the medial margin of the newly constructed internal ring. If the internal oblique muscle is flimsy, resect the muscle and sew to the underlying aponeurosis of the transversus muscle. Insert this suture continuously in a medial direction **(Figs. 76–14 and 76–15)** as far as the pubic tubercle. Do not leave any gap in the suture line near the pubic tubercle as this oversight is a common cause of recurrent hernia adjacent to the pubis.

Shouldice Repair: Layer #4

Use the same continuous suture to create a fourth layer by taking first a bite of internal oblique muscle just cephalad to the previous layer and then a 4-mm bite of the undersurface of external oblique apo-

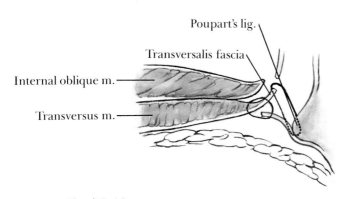

Fig. 76–13

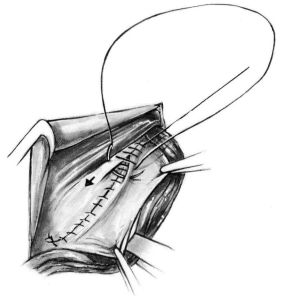

Fig. 76–14

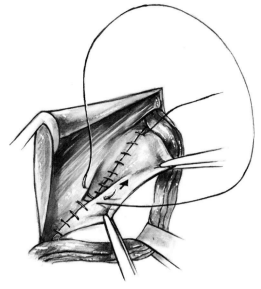

Fig. 76–16

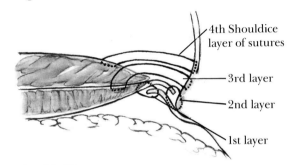

Fig. 76–17

neurosis just anterior to the previously inserted layer (**Figs. 76–16 and 76–17**). Continue this suture until it approaches its point of origin at the internal ring, where the suture is terminated by being tied to its tail.

Shouldice Repair: Layer #5

Carry out a meticulous inspection of the cord and obtain complete hemostasis by a combination of fine ligatures and electrocoagulation. Replace the cord in the canal, which is now displaced somewhat in a cephalad direction. Elevate the medial portion of the external oblique aponeurosis to provide adequate space for the spermatic cord. Suture together the two leaflets of external oblique aponeurosis by utilizing a continuous atraumatic 2–0 PG suture (**Fig. 76–18**). At the new external inguinal

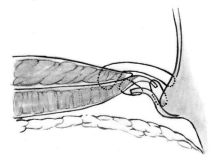

Fig. 76–15

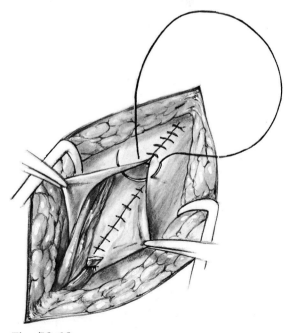

Fig. 76–18

373

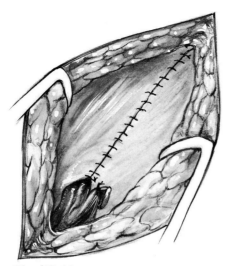

Fig. 76–19

ring include in the last bite of this suture the proximal cut edge of cremaster muscle **(Fig. 76–19)**. This will prevent the testis from descending to an abnormally low point in the scrotum as a consequence of resecting the cremaster muscle. There is no virtue in creating a tight external ring. Rather, allow a 2-cm opening for the spermatic cord.

At intervals during the operation, irrigate the field with a dilute antibotic solution of kanamycin and bacitracin, see p. 365.

Approximate Scarpa's fascia with several 3–0 PG sutures. Accomplish the skin closure by interrupted fine nylon sutures or, as preferred by the author, a continuous subcuticular suture of 4–0 PG, supplemented by strips of sterile adhesive to the skin (Steri-strip).

Postoperative Care

Begin active ambulation the afternoon of the operation. Analgesia will require aspirin or Tylenol and codeine for the next 3 days. Terminate the intravenous infusion in patients who have undergone local anesthesia when they leave the recovery room. This generally takes place from 1–3 hours following completion of surgery.

Laxatives should be given on the night of the first postoperative day in order to avoid patient discomfort at defecation.

Discharge the patient on the 3rd postoperative day, although young patients may leave the hospital on the day of surgery.

Postoperative Complications

Systemic complications of a pulmonary, cardiac, or urological nature are extremely rare.

Wound infections should be rare. Treat them promptly by opening the skin and subcutaneous tissues for adequate drainage and by ordering appropriate antibiotics.

Hematomas may occur in the wound and are generally treated expectantly. Some degree of superficial ecchymosis may be secondary to the injection of the agents for local anesthesia.

Testicular swelling is generally due to vascular obstruction. Although this may sometimes be due to excessive constriction of the newly reconstructed internal ring, it is more often the result of trauma, or hematoma, or inadvertent ligature of the internal spermatic vessels in the inguinal canal. Although this complication may lead to testicular atrophy or necrosis, in most cases satisfactory results may be anticipated from expectant therapy.

For a discussion of the incidence, the causes, and the treatments of recurrent inguinal hernia, see Chap. 78.

References

Berliner S (1984) Personal communication

McVay CB, Halverson K (1980) Inguinal and femoral hernias. In: Beahrs RW, Beart RW (eds) General Surgery. Houghton Mifflin, Boston

Nyhus LM, Condon RE (eds) (1978) Hernia, 2nd ed. Lippincott, Philadelphia

77 Cooper's Ligament Herniorrhapy (McVay)

Operative Technique for Direct or Large Indirect Inguinal Hernia

Incision and Exposure

Make a skin incision over the region of the external inguinal ring and continue laterally to a point about 2 cm medial to the anterior superior iliac spine. Open the external oblique aponeurosis with an incision along the line of its fibers from the external inguinal ring laterally for a distance of about 5–7 (see Fig. 76–2). Mobilize the spermatic cord. Excise the *entire* cremaster muscle from the area of the inguinal canal (see Fig. 76–3). Also remove any lipomas of the cord. Explore the cord carefully for the presence of the indirect sac. If a sac is present, dissect it from the cord. Open the sac, explore it, close the sac at its neck with a suture-ligature, amputate the sac, and permit the stump to retract into the abdominal cavity. Identify the *external* spermatic vessels at the point where they emerge from the transversalis fascia (see Fig. 76–7). Divide and ligate them at this point and remove about 4–5 cm of the vessels and ligate them again at the pubic tubercle (see Fig. 76–8).

In patients with an indirect inguinal hernia, identify the margins of the transversalis fascia around the internal inguinal ring. If the internal inguinal ring is only slightly enlarged, close the ring by means of several sutures between the healthy transversalis fascia along its cephalad margin and the anterior femoral sheath at its caudal margin. If the hernia has eroded more than 2 cm of posterior inguinal wall, a complete reconstruction will be necessary. In this case, incise the transversalis fascia with a scalpel beginning at a point just medial to the pubic tubercle (see Fig. 76–9). Carry the incision laterally with a scalpel or Metzenbaum scissors, taking care not to injure the underlying deep inferior epigastric vessels. The incision must be continued until the transversalis fascia has been incised all the way to the internal inguinal ring. Sweep the preperitoneal fat away from the under surface of the transversalis fascia. Free the deep inferior epigastric vessels so that they may be retracted posteriorly together with the preperitoneal fat. A few small branches may have to be divided and ligated.

If you follow McVay's procedure, excise the iliopubic tract adjacent to Cooper's ligament. Then apply two identifying hemostats to the cephalad cut edge of the transversalis fascia and elevate. This will expose the aponeurosis of the transversus muscle. Excise the fleshy portion of the internal oblique muscle overlying the fi-

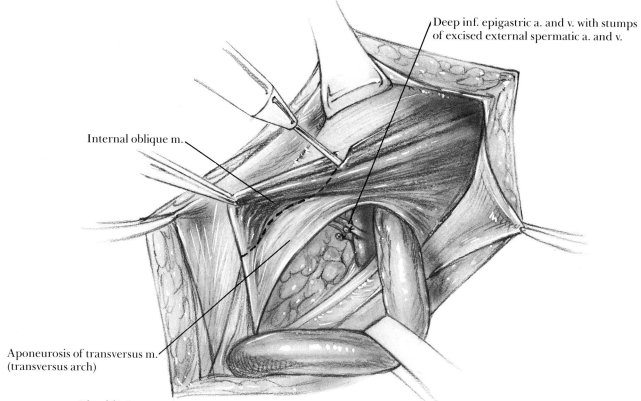

Deep inf. epigastric a. and v. with stumps
of excised external spermatic a. and v.

Internal oblique m.

Aponeurosis of transversus m.
(transversus arch)

Fig. 77–1

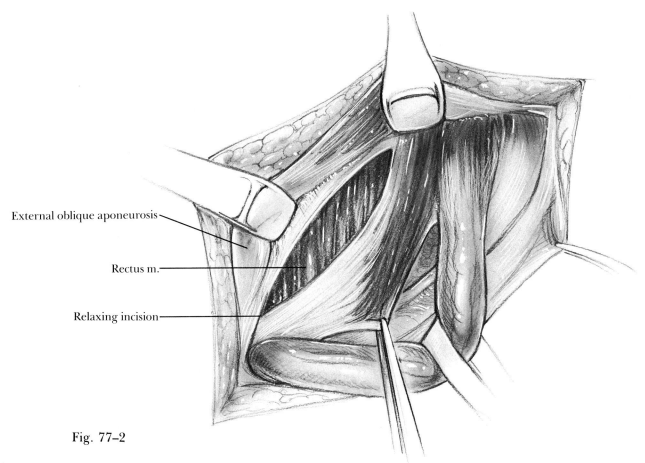

External oblique aponeurosis

Rectus m.

Relaxing incision

Fig. 77–2

brous transversus arch to improve the exposure **(Fig. 77–1)**.

Identify the anterior femoral sheath by gently inserting the back of a scalpel handle between the shelving edge of Poupart's ligament and the femoral sheath overlying the external iliac artery and vein. Then identify the anterior surface of the external iliac vein and artery and retract them gently in a posterior direction with a peanut sponge dissector. This will separate these vessels from the femoral sheath. In order to see the femoral sheath clearly, be certain to excise 100% of the overlying cremaster muscle fibers.

Making the Relaxing Incision

A relaxing incision is essential to prevent tension on the suture line. Elevate the medial portion of the external oblique aponeurosis and dissect it bluntly away from the internal oblique muscle and from the anterior rectus sheath. Make a 7–8 cm incision beginning about 1.5 cm above the pubic tubercle and continue this incision in a cephalad fashion just lateral to the point where the external oblique aponeurosis fuses with the anterior rectus sheath. This will constitute a vertical line that curves laterally as it continues in a superior direction. The anterior belly of the rectus muscle will be exposed as downward traction is applied to the transversus arch **(Fig. 77–2)**.

Inserting the Cooper's Ligament Sutures

Suture the transversus arch to Cooper's ligament using atraumatic 2–0 silk or other nonabsorbable suture material **(Fig. 77–3)**.

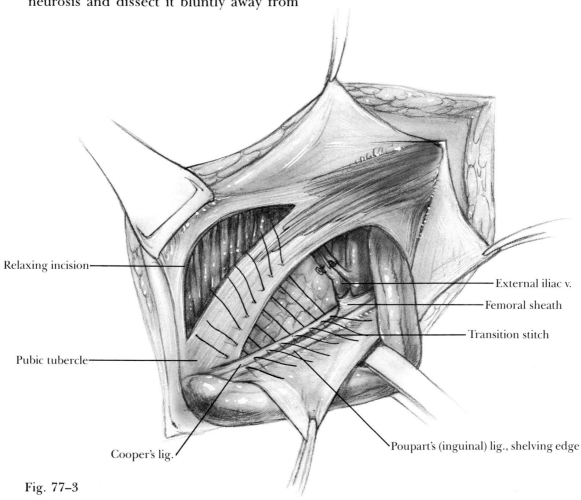

Relaxing incision

Pubic tubercle

Cooper's lig.

External iliac v.

Femoral sheath

Transition stitch

Poupart's (inguinal) lig., shelving edge

Fig. 77–3

377

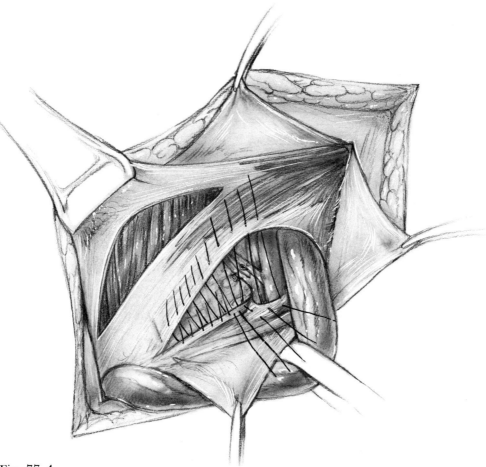

Fig. 77–4

Take substantial bites of both the transversus arch and Cooper's ligament and place the sutures no more than 5 mm apart. Do not tie the sutures until all of them are in place. As the suture line progresses laterally, the external iliac vein will be approached. At this point insert a "transition suture" that penetrates the transversus arch, Cooper's ligament, and then the anterior femoral sheath. Lateral to this suture, sew the transversus arch to the femoral sheath **(Fig. 77–4)**. In his description of Cooper's ligament repair, Rutledge advocates including a bite of the shelving edge of the inguinal ligament together with the anterior femoral sheath. Continue to insert sutures until the internal ring is sufficiently narrowed to admit only a Kelly hemostat alongside the spermatic cord **(Fig. 77–5)**. In effect, the spermatic cord has been transplanted in a lateral direction. Do not insert any sutures lateral to the cord. After all the sutures have been inserted, tie each suture going from medial to lateral **(Fig. 77–6)**.

Suture the incised anterior rectus sheath down to underlying muscle along the lateral aspect of the relaxing incision with a few 3–0 interrupted silk sutures.

Closing the External Oblique Aponeurosis

Replace the cord in the inguinal canal. Check to assure complete hemostasis. Close the external oblique aponeurosis superficial to the cord by inserting interrupted 3–0 silk sutures. Leave a 4–5 mm opening adjacent to the cord in reconstructing the external inguinal ring.

378

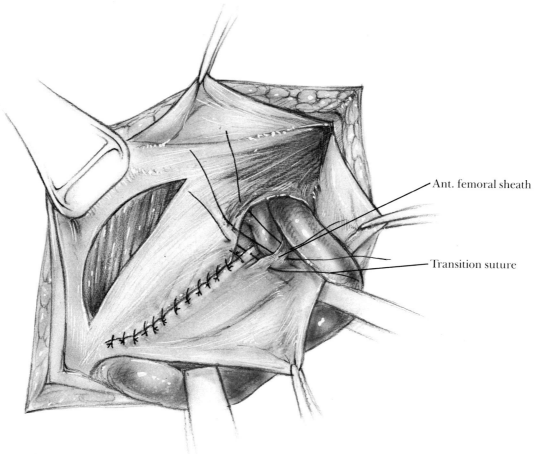

Ant. femoral sheath

Transition suture

Fig. 77–5

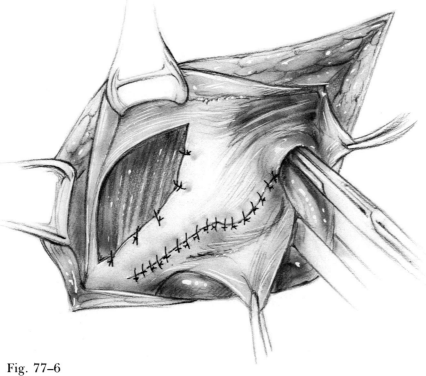

Fig. 77–6

Close Scarpa's fascia with fine interrupted sutures and approximate the skin with interrupted fine nylon or a continuous 4–0 PG subcuticular suture.

Intermittently during the operation, irrigate the operative field with a dilute antibiotic solution of kanamycin and bacitracin.

Postoperative Care
(See Chap. 76.)

Postoperative Complications
(See Chap. 76.)

References

McVay CB, Halverson K (1980) Inguinal and femoral hernias. In: Beahrs OH, Beart RW (eds) General Surgery. Houghton Mifflin, Boston

Rutledge RH (1980) Cooper's ligament repair for adult groin hernias. Surgery 87:601

78 Operations for Recurrent Inguinal Hernia

Concept: Pathogenesis and Prevention of Recurrent Hernia

Scope of Problem

A number of experts with particular interest in the surgical technique of repairing an inguinal hernia have reported a very low postoperative recurrence rate. This is true of Glasgow with respect to the Shouldice technique, Halverson and McVay and Rutledge for the Cooper's ligament technique, and Nyhus for the preperitoneal approach. Depending on the thoroughness and duration of the followup study, the above authors have reported recurrence rates between 0.25% and 3% for the repair of the direct inguinal hernia.

Unfortunately, as Berliner, Burson, Katz, and Wise state, a great proportion of the patients who are lost to a followup study are in fact suffering from a recurrent hernia. As time passes, more and more patients are lost to followup study. For instance, Halverson and McVay's study was able to follow only 76% of patients during the course of the 1–22 year followup. A study of long duration is necessary because only 57% of recurrent direct hernias are detected in the first 5 years, 78% after 10 years, and the remaining 22% between the 10th and 40th year in Postlethwait's report.

Berliner and associates noted an 11.5% failure rate in patients followed for 4–9 years after a Bassini or a Cooper's ligament repair. After devoting special study to the technique of hernia surgery, these authors adopted the Shouldice technique. During a 2–5 year study following 504 primary repairs by this technique, the recur-

rence rate was 1.8%. Following 1,084 cases Berliner noted a personal recurrence rate of 1.1%. Thieme and Quillinan reported recurrence rates of 9% and 10%, respectively, following the repair of groin hernias. With respect to the preperitoneal approach, it appears to be a good method for the repair of a femoral hernia. However, following the use of this approach for the repair of a direct hernia, Dyson and Pierce experienced a 35% recurrence rate, Gaspar and Casberg, 21%, and Ljungdahl, 17%.

On the other hand, repair of a simple indirect hernia with *no direct component* is followed by a low recurrence rate if the sac is completely excised. If there is no transversalis weakness, a complicated repair is not necessary to prevent a recurrence. This is especially true of hernias in children.

Pathogenesis of the Recurrent Groin Hernia

Internal Ring Left Too Large
If the internal ring is not reconstructed so that it admits the spermatic cord plus only 2–3 mm and no more, the risk of recurrence is increased. If the cremaster muscle and lipomata are not removed from the spermatic cord as it passes through the internal ring, then proper narrowing of this ring by suturing transversalis fascia and the transversus arch cannot be accomplished.

Inadequate closure of the internal ring often follows the repair of a large indirect hernia in the adult. Simply removing the sac and then performing a Bassini type of repair by suturing internal oblique muscle to the inguinal ligament are procedures that often fail to accomplish an adequate closure of the internal ring.

Defect at Pubic Tubercle

The second most common location of the hernial defect in a recurrent inguinal hernia is the most medial portion of Hasselbach's triangle adjacent to the pubic tubercle. This is often a localized defect measuring no more than 1–2 cm in diameter. The exact cause of this defect is not clear. It may result if the surgeon does not continue the suture line up to and including the pubic periosteum. Also, tying sutures with excessive tension may play a part in the etiology of this type of defect.

Failure to Suture Transversalis Fascia or Transversus Arch

Perhaps the most commonly utilized technique for repairing an inguinal hernia is some version of the Bassini repair. In the hands of many surgeons this consists of suturing the internal oblique muscle to the shelving edge of the inguinal ligament. Often these sutures fail to catch transversalis fascia or the aponeurosis of the transversus muscle (transversus arch), which are the structures that have the most strength in the region of inguinal hernial defects. In the traditional techniques of hernia repair, no attempt was made clearly to identify these structures prior to inserting sutures.

Failure to Excise Sac

Failure to remove the entire indirect sac has been reported to constitute an important cause of recurrent hernia. Obviously if the surgeon fails to remove the sac, recurrence of the hernia is probable. However, in recent years we have found that the presence of an indirect sac was rather uncommon in the recurrent hernias that we have encountered. Presumably a higher quality of surgery is being practiced, and the average surgeon is sophisticated enough to identify and remove the sac when one is present.

Use of Absorbable Sutures

It has long ago been demonstrated that the use of catgut in repairing an inguinal hernia is followed by an excessive rate of recurrence. Nevertheless, a few surgeons persist in using this suture material, which loses most of its tensile strength within a week or two, a period of time inadequate for the solid healing of an inguinal hernia repair.

Subcutaneous Transplantation of Cord

A significant number of patients present themselves with recurrent inguinal hernias following a Halsted repair in which the spermatic cord is transplanted into the subcutaneous plane by fashioning a new external ring directly superficial to the internal ring. The superimposition, one ring over the other, results in a repair that is weaker than those that preserve the obliquity of the inguinal canal. Following the Halsted repair, a recurrent hernia presents at the point where the spermatic cord exits from the internal-external ring. Generally the two rings appear to have fused together, and the hernia protrudes from this common orifice alongside the cord. Although we are not aware of any statistical studies, it is our impression that the recurrence rate following the Halsted repair is more common than after the Bassini, the Shouldice, or the McVay repairs.

Femoral Recurrence Following Inguinal Hernia Repair

Several authors (McVay and Halverson; Glassow) have emphasized that following the repair of an inguinal hernia, 1%–3% of patients will later develop a femoral hernia on the same side. When operating to repair an inguinal hernia, the surgeon should inspect and palpate the cephalad opening of the femoral canal in search for a small femoral hernia. The normal femoral canal will not admit the surgeon's fingertip. The only circumstances in which this step might be omitted is in the case of a young patient who presents a simple indirect hernia and no weakness of the floor of the inguinal canal.

If a femoral hernia is detected, it should be repaired simultaneously with the inguinal hernia repair. McVay's technique using Cooper's ligament automatically repairs any femoral defect by suturing the transversus arch to Cooper's ligament and the femoral sheath. Glassow recommends exposing the inferior opening of the femoral canal in the groin and repairing it with a few sutures from the lower approach. He then completes the inguinal repair by the Shouldice technique. A "plug" of Marlex mesh may be inserted into the femoral hernial ring from above to repair the femoral hernia.

Infection

Although this has not been discussed in a number of studies of recurrent hernia, our colleague, Dr. Stanley Berliner, noted 10 wound infections in 643 operations for inguinal hernia. Four of these 10 infected patients developed a recurrent hernia. After adopting the practice of irrigating the hernia incisions at intervals during the operation with a solution of kanamycin and bacitracin, he observed no wound infection in over 1,200 cases. Although a 1%–2% incidence of wound infection seems to be an insignificant number, the situation assumes more importance if 40% of the infected patients will develop recurrent hernias. We have been pleased with the results of antibiotic wound irrigation during hernia repairs over the past 8 years.

Prevention of Recurrence

Indirect Inguinal Hernia

In every repair of an indirect hernia free the sac above the internal ring after excising the entire cremaster muscle. Next remove it and carefully identify the margins of the internal ring. In order to do this,

it will be necessary to delineate the transversalis fascia, which forms the medial margin of the internal ring. It is also important to differentiate weak from strong transversalis fascia. By identifying the lateral edge of the transversalis fascia as it joins the internal ring, one can then insert the index finger behind the transversalis layer and evaluate the strength of the inguinal canal's floor.

Although in infants and young children it is rarely necessary to reconstruct the internal ring following removal of the sac, in the adult the indirect hernia has often reached sufficient width to erode the adjacent transversalis fascia and to leave an internal ring with diameter of 2–4 cm. When this has occurred, we prefer to perform a Shouldice repair, similar to that which is done for the direct inguinal hernia.

In both indirect and direct hernia repairs for the adult patient, remove all of the cremaster muscle and adipose tissue surrounding the spermatic cord. If the diameter of the spermatic cord is narrowed, the aperture of the internal inguinal ring can also be made narrow. This will leave an insignificant defect in the floor of the inguinal canal for the potential recurrent hernia.

Direct Inguinal Hernia

A successful repair of a direct hernia requires meticulous dissection and exposure of the transversalis fascia, the aponeurosis of the transversus muscle, and the lateral condensation of the transversalis fascia near the inguinal ligament (iliopubic tract and femoral sheath) prior to suturing the transversus arch–transversalis fascia to the iliopubic tract and the inguinal ligament. Excellent results have been reported following both the Shouldice and the McVay types of repair (Glassow 1978; Berliner et al.; Halverson and McVay; Rutledge). In both operations, each of the above mentioned anatomical structures must be carefully dissected. Each must be evaluated for attenuated portions that are not useful for the repair. The weakened areas must be excised and only strong tissues employed for suturing.

Indications

Strangulation

Incarceration or recent history of incarceration

Symptomatic hernia in good-risk patients

Preoperative Care

If the patient suffers from chronic pulmonary disease, make every effort to achieve optimal improvement. All patients should be encouraged to stop smoking for at least a week before the operation.

Encourage the obese patient to lose weight.

Evaluate elderly male patients for potential prostatic obstruction.

Administer perioperative antibiotics if the use of mesh is anticipated.

Pitfalls and Danger Points

Injuring internal spermatic artery and vein

Injuring vas deferens

Injuring colon (rare)

Injuring bladder (rare)

Using weak tissues for repair

Operative Strategy

Anesthesia

Many operations for a recurrent inguinal hernia can be performed under local anesthesia without undue difficulty. Those patients who have had previous operations for recurrent hernia and have accumulated a great deal of scar tissue are preferably done with general anesthesia. Also, when the preperitoneal approach is used for hernia repair, general anesthesia is necessary.

Selecting the Optimal Technique

Thieme followed 2,163 patients who underwent a primary inguinal hernia repair. He observed a recurrence rate of 8.8%. Of 166 patients operated on for recurrent inguinal hernia and subsequently followed for an average of 9 years, 33.1% of them experienced a second postoperative recurrence! Clear reported that 39% of 53 operations for recurrent hernia, followed for 10 years, had a second recurrence. On the other hand, Halverson and McVay as well as Glassow have reported recurrence rates of 3% or less following operations for recurrent inguinal hernia. These statistics indicate that the traditional approach of exposing the hernial defect and then simply suturing the defect closed is followed by a high incidence of failure.

In an elderly patient who has a recurrent hernia following a primary Halsted repair, it may be permissible to excise the sac and to narrow the fused internal-external ring aperture by means of two or three heavy nonabsorbable sutures, providing all of the surrounding tissues are strong and that there is not excessive tension on the sutures. Also, after opening the external oblique aponeurosis and exposing the floor of the inguinal canal, one may encounter a small (1–2 cm) defect restricted to the medial portion of the floor. *Rarely,* a small defect of this type may be closed by a means of a few interrupted sutures.

Often, this maneuver will require excessive tension. One alternative recommended by Lichtenstein is to insert a small Marlex plug into the defect and to fix it in place with one or two polypropylene sutures. In most other cases the defect in the floor of Hasselbach's triangle will require that the entire transversalis fascia between the internal and external rings be incised and the repair be accomplished by the method of Shouldice or McVay. In many cases of recurrent hernia the primary operation did not include a dissection deep to the transversalis fascia. In these cases, once the transversalis layer is identified and incised, virgin tissues are encountered and a standard repair, similar to that for a direct hernia, may be accomplished.

However, in *many* cases it will not be possible to approximate strong transversalis fascia or transversus arch to the iliopubic tract or Cooper's ligament without excessive tension because too large a portion of these tissues has been destroyed by the previous operation and by the pressure of the enlarging hernia. In these cases there must be no hesitation to substitute, for the absent transversalis layer, one or two layers of prosthetic mesh. We agree with McVay and Halverson that inserting a small segment of mesh and suturing it to the outer margin of the hernial defect is not an adequate operation. These authors have stated, "a small patch of mesh cut to fit the defect and sutured circumferentially in place is an unsatisfactory solution to the problem. We have operated on patients in whom mesh has previously been used in this way and either we could not find the previously inserted mesh or it was rolled up in one portion of the wound." We prefer to use a piece of mesh that is 1.5–2.0 cm larger than the hernial defect along its entire perimeter. Also, we prefer to place the mesh between the peritoneum and the transversalis layer of the abdominal wall rather than to place it superficial to the abdominal musculature. This technique is illustrated below. When this technique is used, we generally make no attempt to suture the two edges of the hernial defect together. In other words, the mesh replaces the defect in the abdominal wall. A small opening is left for the spermatic cord. If possible, the cord is covered by the resutured external oblique aponeurosis. This leaves only the prosthetic mesh and the spermatic cord between the peritoneal and external oblique layers. Only in this fashion can tension be completely eliminated.

An alternative method of inserting the mesh is to use the preperitoneal approach of Nyhus and then to suture the mesh into place behind the abdominal wall. This technique is especially suitable in patients who have had two or more previous operations for recurring hernia. In these cases an anterior approach through the dense scar tissue carries with it a considerable risk of producing postoperative testicular atrophy by traumatizing the spermatic artery and veins. The preperitoneal approach markedly reduces the incidence of postoperative testicular complications. We do not believe that the preperitoneal approach is indicated for patients with primary direct inguinal hernias or for recurrent inguinal hernia unless prosthetic mesh is used to replace the defective transversalis layer of the floor of the inguinal canal.

Technique of Dissection

When the anterior inguinal approach has been selected, remember that the patient may have undergone his previous repair by the Halsted technique. This means that the surgeon should anticipate the possibility of encountering the spermatic cord in the subcutaneous layer of the dissection. Therefore, soon after the skin incision is made, elevate the cephalad skin flap and direct the dissection so that the anterior surface of the external oblique aponeurosis will be exposed at a point 3–5 cm above the inguinal canal. This will be virgin territory that has not been involved in previous surgery. Then carefully direct the dissection in a manner that will not expose the external oblique aponeurosis inferiorly until either subcutaneous spermatic cord or the reconstructed external ring has been exposed. In the absence of a previous Halsted repair, continue the dissection beyond the previous suture line of the external oblique aponeurosis until the junction of the inguinal ligament with the upper thigh has been exposed. If one does encounter the spermatic cord in a subcutaneous location, meticulous dissection is necessary to preserve the fragile spermatic veins.

In the absence of a previous Halsted repair, incise the aponeurosis of the external oblique with caution to avoid traumatizing the cord.

Avoiding Testicular Complications

In the elderly patient with a large recurrent hernia, the repair will be simplified if the patient is willing preoperatively to accept a simultaneous orchiectomy. In most series of recurrent hernia repairs, 10%–15% of cases undergo simultaneous orchiectomy. In younger patients and in those in whom the surgeon wishes to minimize the risk of having a testicular complication, the preperitoneal approach offers a sound alternative to dissecting in a previous operative field. Otherwise, take the time to perform a meticulous dissection of the spermatic vessels and vas. Sometimes the spermatic veins have been spread apart by a large hernia, increasing their vulnerability to operative trauma.

Some surgeons have advocated that the spermatic cord be deliberately divided at some point between the internal and external rings. They claim that if the testis has not been mobilized from its normal location in the scrotum, there will be sufficient collateral circulation for most testes to survive following division of the cord. Heifetz reported that 35% of 112 patients developed definite atrophy of the testis following division of the spermatic cord. Other patients experienced fever, testicular pain, and swelling secondary to interruption of the cord. The high complication

rate following division of the cord without orchiectomy makes this an unacceptable procedure.

When the anterior inguinal approach through the previous incision has been elected for the repair of a recurrent hernia in a young male, it may occasionally appear that preserving the spermatic cord seems to be impossible. In this situation, it is advisable to abandon the anterior approach. In this case, extend the skin incision so that the medial skin flap can be elevated for a distance of 3–5 cm. Then continue the operation by an incision through the abdominal wall using the preperitoneal approach of Nyhus. After dissecting the peritoneum and the sac away from the posterior abdominal wall in the inguinal region, insert a prosthetic mesh. This approach will help avoid testicular complications.

Operative Technique— Inguinal Approach

Incision and Exposure

Enter the operative site by applying the scalpel along the previous operative scar. Alternatively, excise the previous scar. Then dissect the skin flap in a cephalad direction. Be aware of the possibility that at the previous operation the surgeon may have transplanted the spermatic cord into the subcutaneous location. Be careful not to injure the cord during this dissection. After the skin flap has been dissected for a distance of about 2–3 cm, carry the dissection down to the aponeurosis of the external oblique muscle. Accomplish this in an area that is superior to the region of the previous surgery.

Now dissect all of the subcutaneous fat off the anterior surface of the aponeurosis, proceeding in an inferior and lateral direction until the inguinal ligament and the subcutaneous inguinal ring have been cleared.

Repairing Recurrent Hernia Following Previous Halsted Operation without Opening the Inguinal Canal

When a patient has had his spermatic cord transplanted into the subcutaneous plane at the previous operation, the subcutaneous and the deep inguinal rings will be superimposed, one directly upon the other. In this case, the inguinal region is generally quite strong except for a single defect that represents an enlarged common external-internal ring, through which the spermatic cord will pass together with the hernial sac. In these patients it is often extremely difficult to separate the external oblique aponeurosis from the deeper structures, a step that is necessary before accomplishing either a Shouldice or McVay repair. Instead of incising the external oblique aponeurosis in the region between the hernial defect and the pubic tubercle in these patients, it may be more prudent to remove the hernial sac and then to narrow the enlarged common ring with several heavy sutures.

In order to accomplish this, carefully identify and dissect the spermatic cord free from surrounding structures. Isolate the hernial sac. Then, open it and insert the index finger to verify that the floor of the inguinal canal is indeed strong. Dissect the sac away from any attachments at its neck. Close the sac with a single suture ligature of 2–0 PG or nonabsorbable material. Alternatively, a purse-string stitch may be used. Amputate the sac and permit the stump to retract into the abdominal cavity. Dissect areolar tissue, fat, and cremaster from the margins of the hernial defect. Close the defect medial to the point of exit of the spermatic cord, using 2–0 (or heavier) Tevdek or Prolene on an atraumatic needle. In effect, the needle will penetrate, at the medial margin of the ring, 5–6 mm of the external oblique aponeurosis, underlying internal oblique, and transversalis fascia. At the lateral margin of the repair the needle will pierce the external oblique aponeurosis and the shelving edge of the inguinal ligament. Narrow the ring to the extent that a Kelly hemostat can be passed into the revised inguinal ring alongside the spermatic cord. Making the ring smaller than this will increase the risk of testicular complications.

If the hernial defect is large (over 2–3 cm in diameter) and closing it with sutures requires a significant degree of tension, then apply a patch consisting of a double layer of Marlex or Prolene mesh to cover the defect. Suture the mesh to the edge of the hernial defect by using large bites of interrupted or continuous 2–0 atraumatic Prolene. Leave an opening for the exit of the spermatic cord along the lateral margin of the repair.

Dissecting the Inguinal Canal

Most patients presenting with a recurrent inguinal hernia will have had their previous repair performed by some variety of the Bassini technique with the spermatic cord remaining in its normal location deep to the external oblique aponeurosis. In these cases, make an incision in the external oblique aponeurosis along the lines of its fibers, aimed at the cephalad margin of the external inguinal ring, as described above. Perform a patient, meticulous dissection of the spermatic cord in order to avoid traumatizing the delicate spermatic veins. After mobilizing the spermatic cord, identify the hernial sac. In our experience the most common location of a recurrence is in the floor of Hasselbach's triangle medial to the deep inferior epigastric vessels. The previous surgeon will probably not have identified the transversalis fascia and the aponeurosis of the transversus muscle. If this area is virgin territory, repair the recurrent hernia by the classical Shouldice technique described in Chap. 76. This re-

387

pair is also suitable in patients who have a recurrence of an indirect nature since these patients will almost always also have considerable weakness of the inguinal canal. Of course, the indirect sac must be excised.

Repairing a Localized Defect in the Inguinal Floor

A number of patients with recurrent hernia suffer from a relatively small (1.5 cm or less) defect in the inguinal canal floor just medial to the pubic tubercle. Simple suturing of this defect may produce excessive tension. The standard repair calls for an incision through the floor of the inguinal canal followed by a definitive Shouldice or McVay reconstruction. In order to avoid this extensive dissection, Lichtenstein has recommended that this defect be repaired by inserting a plug of rolled-up Marlex mesh and suturing it in place with one or two stitches of 2–0 Prolene as described in the repair of a femoral hernia (see Fig. 79–7).

Prosthetic Mesh Repair

In many cases of recurrent hernia, following the dissection of the inguinal canal, it will be found that the remaining tissues are simply not strong enough to assure a successful result in suturing the hernial defect. By far the most common error made by surgeons repairing a recurrent hernia is to misjudge the strength of the tissues being sutured. Attenuated scar tissue sutured under tension will not produce a successful long-term repair. Do not hesitate to excise these weakened tissues. Then, if the defect cannot be repaired by suturing, even with a relaxing incision, make no attempt to close the defect by sutures. Rather, insert prosthetic mesh. This can be inserted to replace the defect without any tension at all.

Complete the dissection of the inguinal canal through the layer of the transversalis fascia (see Figs. 76–2 to 76–10) so that the peritoneum, Cooper's ligament, and the aponeurosis of the transversus muscle have all been exposed. Separate the peritoneum from the transversalis fascia for a distance of at least 2 cm around the perimeter of the inguinal defect. Trim away attenuated tissues. Now take a double layer of Marlex or Prolene mesh and cut a patch in the shape of an ellipse that is 2 cm–4 cm larger in diameter than is the defect. Place the double thickness of mesh behind the abdominal wall between the peritoneum and the transversalis fascia. Suture the mesh in place by means of 2–0 atraumatic Prolene stitches through the entire abdominal wall in a mattress fashion as seen in **Fig. 78–1a.** Continue to insert these interrupted mattress sutures around the perimeter of the defect and to penetrate external oblique, internal oblique, transversus muscles, and transversalis fascia. Along the medial aspects of the hernial defect, the sutures penetrate the anterior rectus sheath, the rectus muscle, and the transversalis fascia. Along the lateral margin of the defect, suture the mesh to Cooper's ligament with interrupted 2–0 Prolene stitches going from the pubic tubercle laterally to the region of the femoral canal. Lateral to this point, suture the mesh to the femoral sheath and the shelving edge of Poupart's ligament. Cut a small section out of the lateral portion of the mesh so as to avoid constricting the spermatic cord **(Fig. 78–1b).** In most cases, it has not been possible to suture the layers of the abdominal wall together over the mesh without creating excessive tension. After irrigating the operative area thoroughly with a dilute antibiotic solution, close Scarpa's fascia with 3–0 PG and close skin with a continuous 4–0 PG subcuticular suture.

A closed suction drain, such as the flat Jackson-Pratt, may be brought out from the area of the mesh through a puncture wound of the skin. Suction is maintained until drainage volume becomes insignifi-

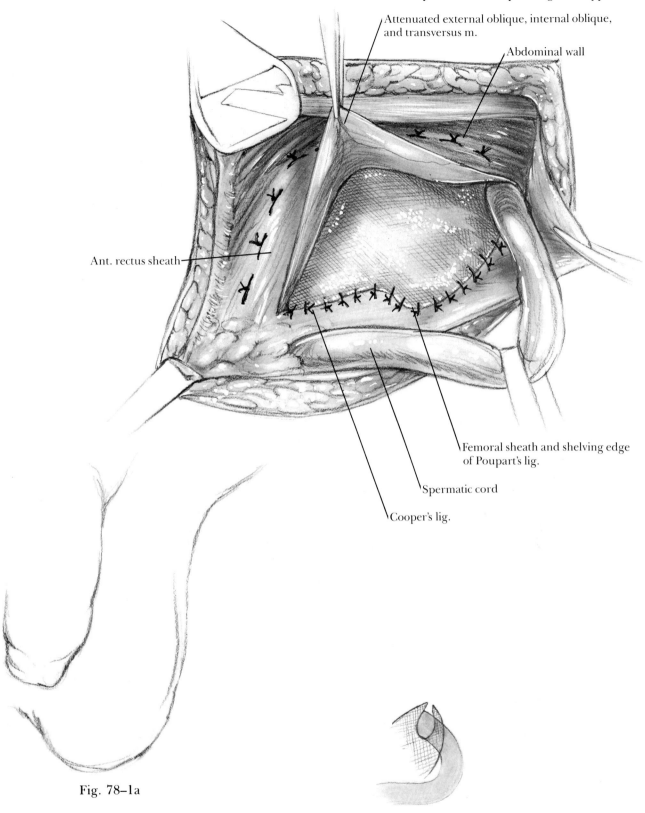

Attenuated external oblique, internal oblique, and transversus m.

Abdominal wall

Ant. rectus sheath

Femoral sheath and shelving edge of Poupart's lig.

Spermatic cord

Cooper's lig.

Fig. 78–1a

Fig. 78–1b

cant in a few days. If the mesh can be covered by external oblique aponeurosis, the drain may be omitted.

Abandoning the Anterior Approach

In rare cases of recurrent inguinal hernia it may be apparent during the dissection of the spermatic cord, that there is such dense fibrosis as to endanger preservation of the cord. When these conditions are encountered, especially in young patients, simply abandon the anterior approach. Elevate the cephalad skin flap and make an incision through the abdominal wall down to the peritoneum, as described below for the preperitoneal approach to the repair of a recurrent hernia. Dissecting peritoneum away from the posterior wall of the inguinal canal via the preperitoneal approach does not endanger the spermatic cord because this dissection is carried out in territory free of scar tissue.

Operative Technique— Preperitoneal Approach Using Mesh Prosthesis

The technique described below is derived in many aspects from the contributions of Notaras, Calne, McVay and Halverson, and Ponka. It is indicated for a large right recurrent inguinal hernia.

Incision and Exposure

Enter the abdominal cavity by making a transverse incision in the right lower quadrant, at a level that will be at least 3 cm above the upper margin of the hernial defect. Start the skin incision near the abdominal midline approximately two fingerbreadths above the pubic symphysis and proceed laterally for a distance of about 10 cm, aiming at a point just above the anterior superior spine of the ilium. Expose the external oblique aponeurosis and the anterior rectus sheath. Identify the ex-

ternal inguinal ring. Incise the anterior rectus sheath about 2–3 cm cephalad to the ring. Expose the rectus muscle. Continue the incision laterally along the line of the fibers of the external oblique aponeurosis, again ascertaining that the incision will be about 3 cm cephalad to the upper margin of the hernial defect (see Fig. 79–9). Incise the fibers of the internal oblique and transversus abdominis muscles and expose the underlying transversalis fascia. Carefully incise the transversalis fascia and identify the preperitoneal fat. The presence of this fat as well as the deep inferior epigastric vessels confirms the fact that the proper plane has been entered. Do not open the peritoneal layer. If this has been done inadvertently, suture the peritoneal laceration.

Apply a small Richardson retractor to the lower margin of the incision and sweep the peritoneum away from the lower abdominal wall using a moist gauze sponge in a sponge-holder.

Dissecting the Hernial Sac

In the process of sweeping the peritoneum away from the pelvic floor, the location of the sac will become apparent (see Fig. 79–10). If there is fibrosis in the region of the hernia due to multiple previous repairs, identify the deep inferior epigastric artery as it enters the posterior rectus sheath. Divide and ligate the epigastric vessels at this point. Grasp the distal cut edge of the epigastric vessels and trace the course of these vessels down to their point of origin from the external iliac artery and vein. The recurrent inguinal hernia will invariably be just medial to this junction point. If the hernial sac comes away from the cord without difficulty, then sweep it in a cephalad fashion together with the peritoneal envelope. If the sac remains adherent to the cord, make no attempt to dissect it free. Rather, identify the neck of the sac and incise the peritoneum at this point. Free the peritoneum from the circumference of the sac and then close the defect in the pelvic peritoneum with a continuous atraumatic 3–0 PG suture. Avoid damaging the

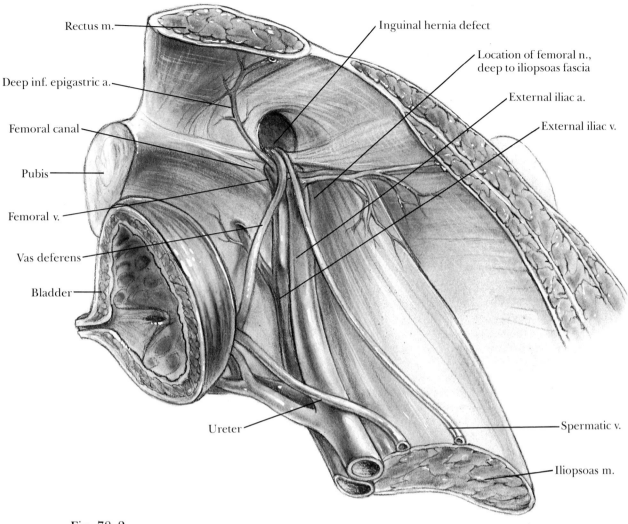

Rectus m.

Deep inf. epigastric a.

Femoral canal

Pubis

Femoral v.

Vas deferens

Bladder

Ureter

Inguinal hernia defect

Location of femoral n.,
deep to iliopsoas fascia

External iliac a.

External iliac v.

Spermatic v.

Iliopsoas m.

Fig. 78–2

bladder, which may be adherent to the medial margin of the hernial sac.

At the conclusion of this dissection, the entire posterior wall of the pelvis should be visible including the external iliac vessels, the spermatic cord, the superior pubic ramus (Cooper's ligament), the vas deferens, the iliopsoas fascia along the iliopectineal line lateral to the iliac vessels, and the femoral nerve just lateral and deep to the external iliac artery. **Fig. 78–2** illustrates the anatomy of structures encountered in this preperitoneal dissection on the *right* side of the patient.

Suturing the Mesh

Cut two squares of Marlex or Prolene mesh sufficiently large to provide a double layer of prosthesis that will reach from the abdominal incision (cephalad) to Cooper's ligament and to the iliopsoas fascia (caudad), and from the midrectus region medially to the anterior superior iliac spine laterally.

In cases of recurrent hernia repaired by this approach, do not attempt to close the hernial defect by suturing it because the tension will be excessive and the tissues are generally not strong enough to hold sutures. Use 2–0 atraumatic Prolene

391

swaged on a stout needle and take substantial bites of strong tissue to assure that the mesh will remain permanently in place. Do not expect that the ingrowth of fibrous tissue into the mesh will assure fixation since the polypropylene is relatively inert and substantial fibrous ingrowth does not always take place. Place the first suture in the ligamentous tissue adjacent to the pubic symphysis. We use a double layer of mesh. Continue the suture line laterally, passing interrupted 2–0 atraumatic Prolene sutures through the double layer of mesh deep into Cooper's ligament along the pubic ramus. At the femoral ring, suture the mesh to the femoral sheath and the shelving edge of the inguinal ligament. When the internal inguinal ring is reached, leave a space for the spermatic cord to exit from the abdominal cavity in the male patient. Lateral to the external iliac artery carry the suture line in a posterior direction and attach the mesh to the iliopsoas fascia going laterally. Take deep bites into this fascia after identifying and protecting the femoral nerve, which runs just below the fascia. Continue the suture line in the iliopsoas fascia laterally towards the anterior superior iliac spine until the lateral margin of the abdominal incision is reached. In the female patient, suturing the mesh to the femoral sheath and the iliopsoas fascia will completely obliterate the internal inguinal ring, although this operation, using mesh to repair a large recurrent inguinal hernia, will rarely be necessary in a woman.

Attach the medial margin of the double layer of mesh to the medial portion of the rectus muscle. Accomplish this by dissecting the subcutaneous fat off the anterior rectus sheath down to the pubis. Then insert the 2–0 Prolene sutures by taking the bite, first through the anterior rectus sheath, next through the body of the rectus muscle, and then through the two layers of mesh in the abdomen. Return the

same suture as a mattress by taking a bite through the mesh, through the body of the rectus muscle, and finally through the anterior rectus sheath. After tying the stitch, the knot will be on the anterior rectus sheath. Continue this suture line up to the level of the transverse abdominal incision. **Fig. 78–3** depicts the appearance of the mesh, sutured in place.

Intermittently during the operation, irrigate the operative site with a dilute antibiotic solution. By this point in the operation, the mesh has been sutured into place medially, caudally, and laterally; only the cephalad margin is left unattached. Trim the mesh so that this cephalad margin terminates evenly with the inferior margin of the transverse abdominal incision. Because of the irregular nature of the surface that has been covered by the flat patch of mesh, there will be a surplus of mesh in the lateral portion of the incision. Correct this by making a vertical fold in the mesh, as necessary, to include the mesh in the closure of the abdominal incision.

Prior to inserting many of the sutures, it will be necessary either to ligate and divide or to coagulate a number of blood vessels in the region of Cooper's ligament and the femoral sheath so that inserting the sutures will not produce bleeding.

Closing the Abdominal Incision

Insert a flat Jackson-Pratt closed-suction drain through a puncture wound above the lateral margin of the incision. Place the tip of the drain along the medial portion of the pelvis behind the patch of mesh.

Close the anterior rectus sheath with interrupted nonabsorbable sutures. Lateral to the rectus muscle, close the abdominal incision by using the Smead-Jones technique of 0 or 2–0 interrupted Prolene sutures that grasp a width of at least 1.5 cm of the abdominal wall, including the external oblique aponeurosis, the internal oblique and transversus muscles, the transversalis fascia *and the proximal edge of the mesh* in the caudal margin of the incision, and the same layers on the cephalad margin

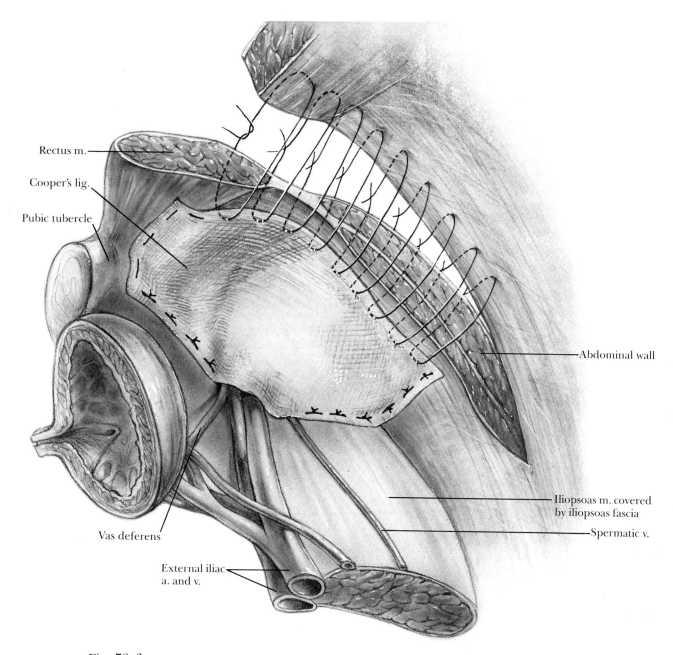

Rectus m.

Cooper's lig.

Pubic tubercle

Abdominal wall

Iliopsoas m. covered
by iliopsoas fascia

Spermatic v.

Vas deferens

External iliac
a. and v.

Fig. 78–3

except for the mesh. Close the skin with
a continuous 4–0 PG subcuticular stitch.
Fig. 78–3 illustrates the completed incision
suture line.

Postoperative Care

Ambulate the patient the day of the
operation or on the following day.

Continue perioperative antibiotics effective against staphylococci by the
parenteral route for 24 hours in patients who have had a mesh prosthesis
inserted.

Postoperative Complications

Testicular swelling and/or atrophy

Urinary retention in males

Wound hematoma

Wound sepsis

(When infection develops in patients who have had the insertion of a mesh prosthesis, it is not always necessary to remove this foreign body in order to remedy the infection as the mesh is made up of monofilament fibers. In most patients, wide drainage of the skin incision accompanied by parenteral antibiotics with, perhaps, local antibiotic irrigation may prove effective. We have had no experience in managing a pelvic infection after the insertion of a mesh prosthesis in the pelvis by the preperitoneal route. We would subject a patient of this type to a trial of conservative therapy after opening the incision to explore the pelvis and to insert indwelling irrigating catheters and sump-suction drains.)

Recurrence of hernia

References

Berliner S (1984) Personal communication

Berliner S, Burson L, Katz P, Wise L (1978) An anterior transversalis fascia repair for adult inguinal hernias. Am J Surg 135:633

Calne RY (1974) Repair of bilateral hernia with Mersilene mesh behind rectus abdominis. Arch Surg 109:532

Clear J (1951) Ten-year statistical study of inguinal hernias. Arch Surg 62:70

Dyson WL, Pierce WS (1965) Changing concept of inguinal herniorrphaphy; experience with preperitoneal approach. Arch Surg 91:971

Gaspar MR, Casberg MA (1971) An appraisal of preperitoneal repair of inguinal hernia. Surg Gynecol Obstet 132:207

Glassow F (1970) Femoral hernia following inguinal herniorrhaphy. Can J Surg 13:27

Glassow F (1978) The Shouldice repair for inguinal hernia, In: Nyhus LM, Condon RE (eds) Hernia (see below)

Halverson K, McVay CB (1970) Inguinal and femoral herniorrhaphy: a 22-year study of the author's methods. Arch Surg 87:601

Heifetz CJ (1971) Resection of the spermatic cord in selected inguinal hernias. Arch Surg 102:36

Lichtenstein IL (1982) A two-stitch repair of femoral and recurrent inguinal hernias by a "plug" technique. Contemp Surg 20:35

Ljungdahl I (1978) [comment] In: Nyhus LM, Condon RE (eds) Hernia (see below) p. 239

McVay CB, Halverson K (1980) Inguinal and femoral hernias, In: Beahrs OH, Beart RW (eds) General surgery, Houghton Mifflin, Boston

Notaras ML (1974) Experience with Mersilene mesh in abdominal wall repair. Proc R Soc Med 67:1187

Nyhus LM, Condon RE (eds) (1978) Hernia, 2nd ed. Lippincott, Philadelphia

Ponka JL (1980) Hernias of abdominal wall, Saunders, Philadelphia

Postlethwait RW (1971) Causes of recurrence after inguinal herniorrhaphy. Surgery 69:772

Quillinan RH (1969) Repair of recurrent inguinal hernia. Am J Surg 118:593

Rutledge RH (1980) Cooper's ligament repair for adult groin hernias. Surgery 87:601

Thieme ET (1971) Recurrent inguinal hernia. Arch Surg 103:238

79 Femoral Hernia Repair

Concept: Choice among Low Groin, Preperitoneal, or Inguinal Approaches

In most cases of femoral hernia the diameter of the femoral canal, through which the femoral hernia protrudes, is quite narrow, often measuring less than 1.5 cm. By approaching the hernia from below, it is simple to free the sac, open it, reduce the hernia, and amputate the sac. Following this step, the ring is obliterated by means of 2–4 sutures attaching the inguinal ligament to Cooper's ligament and the pectineus fascia. An even simpler method has been suggested by Lichtenstein and Shore. They roll up a length of Marlex mesh into the form of a cigarette whose diameter is equal to the diameter of the femoral ring. After inserting this Marlex "cigarette" into the femoral ring, they fix it in place with 1–2 sutures through the inguinal ligament, the Marlex, and the ligament of Cooper. In the low approach, local anesthesia works well and the entire procedure takes only 20–30 minutes. Reducing the stress of the operation and the anesthesia is desirable because most of these operations are performed in elderly patients under emergency conditions.

Good results following the low groin approach have been reported by Glassow, by Ponka, by Tanner, and by Monro.

When strangulated bowel is encountered in a low groin incision, do not attempt a resection and anastomosis by this approach. A secondary laparotomy incision should be made in the middle of the lower abdomen. When this is done, general anesthesia will be required. In those patients in whom strangulation of bowel is suspected prior to initiating the operation, the preperitoneal approach of Henry or Nyhus has several advantages. Through the low abdominal incision of this method, the peritoneum is swept away from the cephalad surface of the femoral canal to expose the hernial sac from above as it enters the femoral ring. The ring may be opened under direct vision and the bowel reduced into the abdominal cavity where resection and anastomosis are easily performed. The hernia is repaired by suturing the inguinal ligament to Cooper's ligament medial to the iliac vein, which is easily seen from above. The disadvantages in using the preperitoneal approach routinely are that general anesthesia is required and that the operation is more complex than the low groin procedures.

We prefer to use the inferior approach in most cases of femoral herniorrhaphy, reserving the preperitoneal exposure for the younger patient and for the patient suspected of suffering bowel strangulation. When the low groin approach has been erroneously selected for patients who suffer strangulation of intestine, make a midline abdominal incision for reduction of the strangulated bowel and subsequent resection. Using these criteria, over 85% of patients can be done by the low groin approach.

Some surgeons use an inguinal incision followed by incision of the external oblique aponeurosis and the transversalis fascia in order to expose the cephalad entrance to the femoral canal. After removing the sac, the hernia is corrected by suturing transversalis fascia and conjoined tendon down to Cooper's ligament and the femoral sheath. Although surgeons like McVay have mastered this operation and achieved excellent results, others who do not regularly use the Cooper's ligament operation will find that the McVay operation is more difficult to perform than is the low groin repair.

Indications

As strangulation is common in patients with femoral hernia, it is advisable to operate on all patients who suffer from this condition unless their medical status is so precarious that it contraindicates even an operation under local anesthesia.

Preoperative Care

If there are signs of intestinal obstruction, initiate nasogastric suction.

When a patient has symptoms suggestive of a femoral hernia but lacks definitive physical findings, request a sonogram of the groin. This study may reveal a small incarcerated femoral hernia. Sonography is also helpful in diagnosing symptomatic Spigelian and other interstitial hernias of the abdominal wall.

Pitfalls and Danger Points

Injuring or constricting femoral vein

Transecting aberrant obturator artery

Operative Strategy

Low Groin Approach

After the sac has been opened and its contents reduced, the sac is amputated. It is not necessary to close the neck of the sac with sutures (Ferguson). It is important, however, to clear the femoral canal of any fat or areolar tissue so that the sutures can bring the inguinal ligament in direct contact with Cooper's ligament and the pectineus fascia. This will obliterate the femoral canal but will leave an opening of 6–8 mm adjacent to the femoral vein. Equally good results can be obtained if the femoral canal is obliterated by inserting a plug of Marlex mesh.

To reduce an incarcerated femoral hernia, an incision may be made to divide the constricting neck of the hernial sac. This should be done on the medial aspect of the hernial ring. Although we have never observed the phenomenon, a number of texts warn that an anomalous obturator artery may follow a course that brings it into contiguity with the neck of the hernial sac and thus makes it vulnerable to injury when the constricted neck is incised. This accident will *rarely* occur if the neck of the sac is incised on its medial aspect. If hemorrhage is indeed encountered during this maneuver and the artery cannot be ligated from below, then control the bleeding by finger pressure and rapidly expose the inner aspect of the pelvis by the Henry approach, which involves a midline incision from the umbilicus to the pubis, after which the peritoneum is swept in a cephalad direction to expose the femoral canal from above. With this exposure a bleeding obturator artery can be easily ligated. It should be emphasized that this complication is so rare that it does not constitute a significant disadvantage of the low approach to femoral herniorrhaphy.

If the sutures drawing the inguinal ligament down to Cooper's ligament have to be tied under excessive tension, abandon this technique and insert a plug of Marlex mesh to obliterate the femoral canal, as described below.

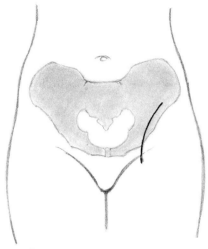

Fig. 79–1

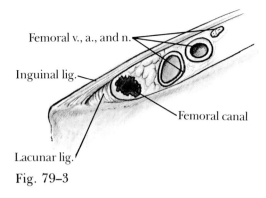

Femoral v., a., and n.

Inguinal lig.

Femoral canal

Lacunar lig.

Fig. 79–3

Operative Technique

Low Groin Approach for Left Femoral Hernia

Make an oblique incision about 6 cm in length along the groin skin crease curving down over the femoral hernia **(Fig. 79–1)**. Carry the incision down to the external oblique aponeurosis and the inferior aspect of the inguinal ligament. Identify the hernial sac as it emerges deep to the ingui-

nal ligament in the space between the lacunar ligament and the common femoral vein **(Fig. 79–2)**. Dissect the sac down to its neck using Metzenbaum scissors.

Grasp the sac with two hemostats and incise with a scapel. Often the peritoneum is covered by two or more layers of tissue, each of which may resemble a sac. These consist of preperitoneal tissues and fat. This is especially true when intestine is incarcerated in the sac.

When the bowel or the omentum remains incarcerated after opening the sac, incise the hernial ring on its medial aspect by inserting a scapel between the sac and the lacunar ligament **(Figs. 79–3 and 79–**

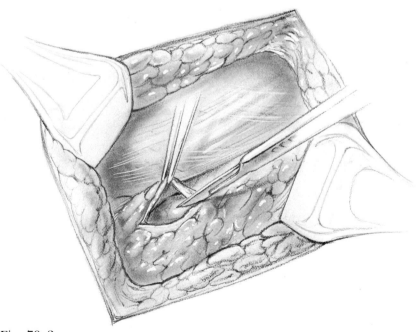

Fig. 79–2

397

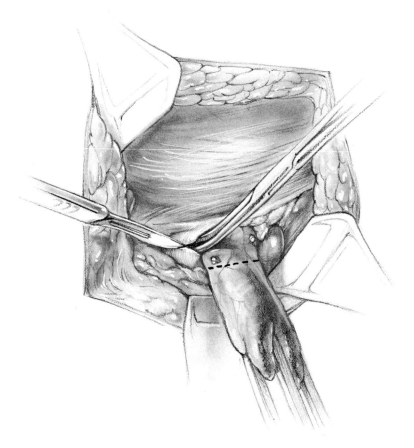

Fig. 79–4

4). After returning the bowel and the omentum to the abdominal cavity, amputate the sac at its neck. It is not necessary to ligate or suture the neck of the sac, but this step may be accomplished if desired **(Fig. 79–5).** Using a peanut sponge, push any remaining preperitoneal fat into the abdominal cavity, thus clearing the femoral canal of all extraneous tissues.

Repair the hernial defect by suturing the inguinal ligament down to Cooper's ligament using interrupted 2–0 sutures of Prolene on a heavy Mayo needle. Often this can be accomplished if the inguinal ligament is pressed down and cephalad towards Cooper's ligament with the index finger. Then the needle is passed through the inguinal ligament and through Cooper's ligament in one simultaneous motion. Cooper's ligament is indistinguishable from the periosteum overlying the cephalad aspect of the pubic ramus. An alternative method involves placing the stitch first through the inguinal ligament, then placing a narrow retractor in the femoral canal in order to take a bite of Cooper's ligament and pectineus fascia. No more than 2–4 sutures are generally necessary. Identify the common femoral vein where it emerges from beneath the inguinal ligament. Leave a gap of 4–6 mm between the femoral vein and the lateralmost suture of hernia repair **(Fig. 79–6).**

Close the skin of the groin incision with either a continuous 4–0 PG subcuticular suture or interrupted 4–0 nylon sutures.

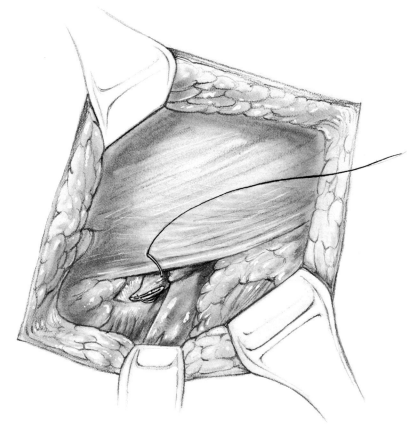

Fig. 79–5

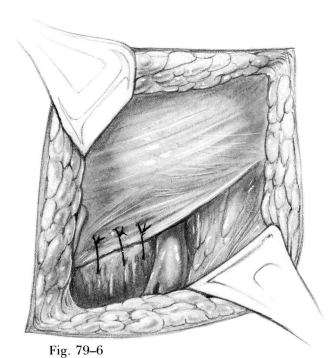

Fig. 79–6

If strangulated bowel requiring resection is encountered after opening the hernial sac, make a second incision in the midline between the umbilicus and the pubis. Separate the two rectus muscles and identify the peritoneum. Do not incise the peritoneum. By blunt dissection elevate the peritoneum from the pelvis until the iliac vessels and the femoral hernial sac are identified. At this point, open the peritoneum just above the sac. Incise the constricting neck of the femoral canal on its medial aspect and reduce the strangulated bowel. After resecting the bowel, irrigate the femoral region with a dilute antibiotic solution and repair the femoral ring from below as already described, but use 2–0 stainless steel wire sutures instead of Prolene to avoid a postoperative suture sinus in a contaminated wound. Irrigate the abdomen and close the abdominal incision in routine fashion.

399

Low Groin Approach Using Prosthetic Mesh "Plug"

If approximating the inguinal to the Cooper's ligament by sutures requires excessive tension, then modify the technique. Monro, who strongly favored the low groin approach, emphasized that the sutures should be tied loosely so that they form a lattice of monofilament nylon. This technique serves to occlude the defect without producing any tension. The same end can be accomplished even more simply by inserting a rolled up plug of Marlex mesh as advocated by Lichtenstein and Shore.

Cut a strip of Marlex mesh about 2 cm by 8 cm. Roll the Marlex strip in the shape of a cigarette, 2 cm in length. After the hernial sac has been eliminated and all the fat has been cleared out of the femoral canal, insert this Marlex plug into the femoral canal. The diameter of the plug may be adjusted by using a greater or lesser length of Marlex, as required. When the properly sized plug is snug in the femoral canal with about 0.5 cm of the plug protruding into the groin, fix the Marlex in place by inserting 1 or 2 sutures of 2–0 atraumatic Prolene **(Fig. 79–7).** Insert the needle first through the inguinal ligament, then through the Marlex plug, and finally into the pectineus fascia or Cooper's ligament. After the two sutures have been tied, the plug should fit securely in the canal. After irrigating the wound with a dilute antibiotic solution, check for complete hemostasis and then close the skin incision without drainage. If the patient accumulates serum in the incision postoperatively, aspirate the fluid occasionally with a needle.

Preperitoneal Approach for Right Femoral Hernia (Nyhus)

Anesthesia
Almost all practitioners of the preperitoneal approach believe that general anesthesia with good relaxation is a prerequisite for this type of hernia repair.

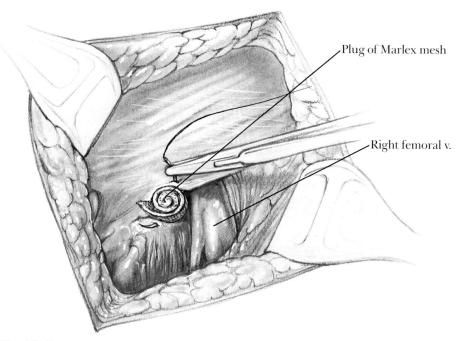

Plug of Marlex mesh

Right femoral v.

Fig. 79–7

the anterior rectus sheath and the external oblique aponeurosis. Elevate the caudal skin flap sufficiently to expose the external inguinal ring.

Make a transverse incision in the anterior rectus sheath at a level about 1.5 cm cephalad to the upper margin of the external inguinal ring for a distance of about 5 cm in a direction parallel to the inguinal canal **(Fig. 79–9).** Retract the rectus muscle medially and deepen the incision through the full thickness of the internal oblique and transversus abdominis muscles. This will expose the transversalis fascia. Carefully make a transverse incision in this layer, but do not incise the peritoneum.

Apply a Richardson retractor against the lateral margin of the incised abdominal wall. Use blunt dissection to elevate the peritoneum out of the pelvis.

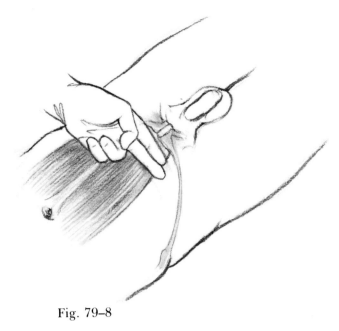

Fig. 79–8

Incision

Start the skin incision at a point 2 fingerbreadths above the symphysis pubis **(Fig. 79–8)** and about 1.5 cm lateral to the abdominal midline. Carry the incision laterally for a distance of 8–10 cm and expose

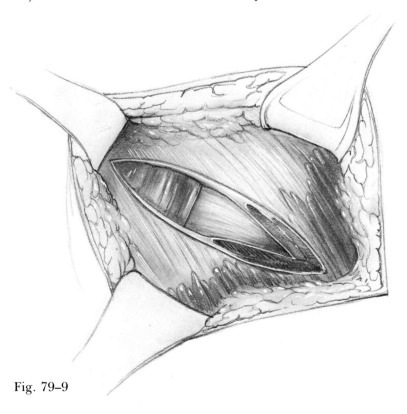

Fig. 79–9

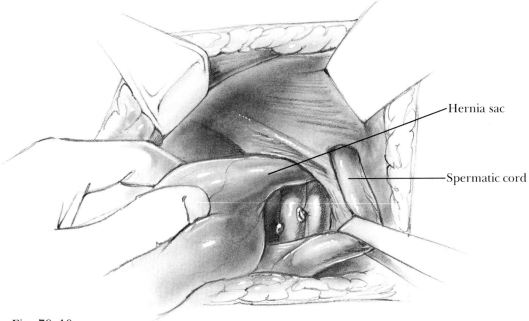

Fig. 79–10

Mobilizing the Hernial Sac
If the femoral hernia is incarcerated, it will be possible to mobilize the entire pelvic peritoneum except for that portion which is incarcerated in the femoral canal (**Fig. 79–10**). If the hernia cannot be extracted by gentle blunt dissection around the femoral ring, then incise the medial margin of the femoral ring and extract the hernial sac by combining traction plus external pressure against the sac in the groin.

Although the presence of an aberrant obturator artery along the medial margin of the femoral ring is a rarity, there may be one or two small venous branches that will require suture-ligation prior to incising the medial margin of the ring.

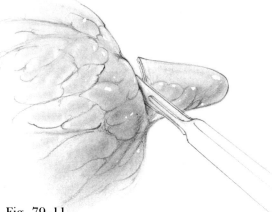

Fig. 79–11

Open the sac (**Fig. 79–11**). Evaluate the condition of the bowel. If strangulation mandates bowel resection, enlarge the incision enough so that adequate exposure for a careful intestinal anastomosis may be guaranteed. If bowel has been resected, change gloves and instruments before initiating the repair. Also irrigate the incision with a dilute antibiotic solution. Avoid using any nonabsorbable suture material for the closure of the ring and of the abdominal incision, other than monofilament stainless steel wire. Excise the peritoneal sac and close the defect with continuous 3–0 PG.

Suturing the Hernial Ring
The superficial margin of the femoral ring consists of the iliopubic tract and the femoral sheath. These structures are just deep to the inguinal ligament. The deep margin of the femoral ring is Cooper's ligament, which represents the reinforced periosteum of the superior ramus of the pubis. In repairing the hernial defect, suture the strong tissue situated in the superficial margin of the femoral ring to Cooper's ligament with several interrupted sutures of 2–0 Tevdek or Prolene (**Figs. 79–12 and 79–13**). Whether the suture catching the

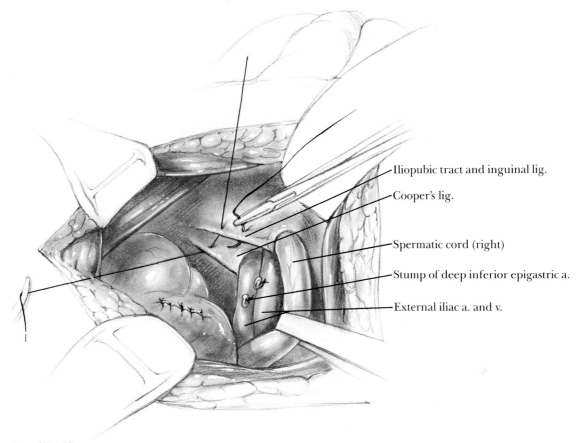

Iliopubic tract and inguinal lig.

Cooper's lig.

Spermatic cord (right)

Stump of deep inferior epigastric a.

External iliac a. and v.

Fig. 79–12

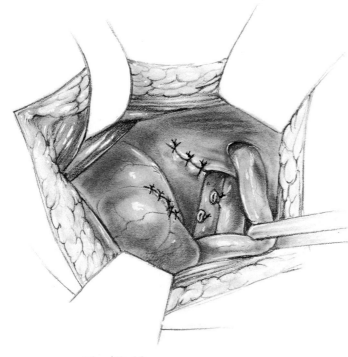

Fig. 79–13

superficial margin of the femoral ring contains only iliopubic tract or whether it also catches a bite of inguinal ligament is immaterial so long as there is not excessive tension when the knot is tied. If closing the ring by approximating strong tissues will result in excessive tension, then it is preferable, in these rare cases, to insert a small "cigarette" of Marlex by the technique of Lichtenstein and Shore as described above with the inferior approach.

In any case, do not permit the closure of the femoral ring to impinge upon the iliac vein because obstructing the venous flow may result in thrombosis and pulmonary embolism.

Closure of Abdominal Wall
Check the pelvis for the presence of a direct inguinal hernia. If present, this may be repaired by suturing the superior edge of the hernial defect (transversus abdominis aponeurosis) to the iliopubic tract be-

403

low. Ascertain complete hemostasis. Irrigate the cavity with a solution of 1,000 ml of saline containing 1 gram of kannamycin and 50,000 units of bacitracin.

Close the anterior rectus sheath with interrupted 3–0 Tevdek. Close the remaining layers of the abdominal wall with interrupted nonabsorbable sutures in layers. Alternatively, we have closed this portion of the abdominal wall using modified Smead-Jones stitches of interrupted 1 PDS. Close the skin with a few 4–0 PG sutures to the subcutaneous fascia and a continuous subcuticular suture of 4–0 PG. No drain is necessary.

Postoperative Care

Early ambulation and discharge from the hospital by the 3rd postoperative day is our usual practice in routine cases.

Perioperative antibiotics are employed in patients with intestinal obstruction or those who have had bowel resection for strangulation. Use nasogastric suction in patients with intestinal obstruction or bowel resection.

Postoperative Complications

Deep vein thrombosis has been reported secondary to constriction of the femoral vein by suturing.

Wound infections (rare)

Ventral hernia following preperitoneal approach to femoral hernia repair

Recurrent hernia appears to be in the 1% range in the hands of Nyhus for the preperitoneal operation. Using the low groin approach, Ponka reported a 3% recurrence rate and Glassow, 2%. We are not aware of any followup studies of Lichtenstein's repair, but our experience with it has been very favorable.

References

Ferguson DJ (1978) In: Nyhus, LM, Condon, RE (eds) Hernia, 2nd ed. Lippincott, Philadelphia

Glassow F (1966) Femoral hernias: review of 1143 consecutive repairs. Ann Surg 163:227

Lichtenstein IL, Shore JM (1974) Simplified repair of femoral and recurrent inguinal hernia by a "plug" technique. Am J Surg 128:439

Monro A (1964) In: Nyhus LM, Harkins HN (eds) Hernia, 1st ed. Lippincott, Philadelphia

Ponka JL (1980) Hernias of the abdominal wall, Saunders, Philadelphia

Tanner NC (1978) In: Nyhus LM, Condon RE (eds) Hernia, 2nd ed. Lippincott, Philadelphia

80 Operations for Large Ventral Hernia

Concept: Pathogenesis of Incisional Hernia

Sepsis

Infection of the postoperative abdominal wound not uncommonly leads to an incisional hernia at a later date, especially if the infection was not detected and drained widely early in the course of its development. Blomstedt and Welin-Berger studied 279 patients for 8–24 months after cholecystomy. In the absence of a wound infection, 6% developed an incisional hernia. Of the patients suffering postoperative wound infections, 31% had incisional hernias.

A postoperative wound infection may be nosocomial in origin or it may be the result of endogenous contamination during the course of the abdominal operation. The prevention of infection following the contamination of an abdominal wound is discussed in Vol. I, Chap. 2.

Occult Wound Dehiscence

When a large ventral hernia appears within the first few months following an abdominal operation, a likely cause of the hernia is the dehiscence of the fascial and muscular layers of the abdominal wall during the early postoperative course in a patient whose skin incision has remained intact. For this reason, the wound dehiscence may be undetected by the surgeon until he notes a large hernia in the scar when the patient returns for a followup visit a month or two later. The prevention of postoperative wound dehiscence is discussed in Vol. I, Chap. 5.

Making Too Large a Drain Wound

When the stab wound for a latex drain is made too large, a postoperative hernia is likely to occur. Generally, if the stab wound admits only one finger, a postoperative hernia is unlikely. When drainage is designed to facilitate the escape of necrotic tissue (e.g., necrotizing acute pancreatitis), large drainage wounds are required despite the risk of developing a hernia.

Transverse versus Vertical Incision

As discussed in Vol. I, Chap. 5, we have not detected an increased incidence of incisional hernia or wound dehiscence when comparing the midline vertical incision with transverse or oblique subcostal incisions, provided that the midline incision has been closed with sutures that encompass large bites of abdominal wall, such as the Smead-Jones stitch.

405

Technique of Suturing

Type of Suture Material

Goligher, Irvin, Johnston, deDombal, and associates demonstrated that closing an abdominal incision with catgut resulted in a larger number of wound dehiscences and incisional hernias than was experienced with nonabsorbable sutures, unless the catgut closure was supplemented by multiple large retention sutures. Also in the repair of inguinal and ventral hernias, suturing with catgut is followed by a larger number of recurrences than is the case with nonabsorbable suture material.

Whether the new and more slowly absorbable suture materials (e.g., Vicryl, Dexon, and PDS) retain their strength long enough to equal the performance of nonabsorbable sutures is a question that has not yet been settled. We have performed over 400 consecutive closures of midline abdominal incisions with interrupted #1 PG or PDS Smead-Jones sutures without experiencing a single wound dehiscence. We are aware of one fairly large and three quite small incisional hernias, but a complete followup study of these patients has not been performed. While we have confidence in these suture materials for the closure of a primary abdominal incision, we do not believe that their use has yet been validated in hernia repair.

Size of Tissue Bites

We agree with the findings of Jenkins that the width of tissue included in each suture is an important determinant of the incidence of wound dehiscence or incisional hernia, regardless whether a continuous or interrupted technique is used. Sutures, that contain small bites of tissue, tend to cut through in response to muscle tension. We believe that *at least* 2 cm of musculofascial tissue on each side of the incision should be included in the stitch.

Tension with Which Suture Should Be Tied

When a stitch in an abdominal incision is tied with strangulating force, no matter how large a bite of tissue the stitch contains, strangulation will cause the stitch to cut through the abdominal wall. This error will manifest itself by the appearance of a small hernia, 1–2 cm lateral to the scar several months following operation. The hernial ring will often be no more than 1.0–1.5 cm in diameter when first detected. This phenomenon is somewhat more likely to occur when using monofilament stainless steel wire than Prolene. The diameter of a 2–0 wire suture is considerably less than that of 1 PDS or 0 Prolene. For this reason it has a greater tendency to cut the tissue and must be tied without tension. In using Prolene for closing the abdominal wall, it is easy to tie the knot with excessive tension because the suture material is slippery. Consequently, as the surgeon applies an additional throw to the knot, the entire knot slips and tightens the suture. In any case, it is not necessary to tie the knot in an abdominal closure with any greater tension than one would apply to a suture in a bowel anastomosis. Insisting that the anesthesiologist provide adequate relaxation of the abdominal wall will facilitate the surgeon's effort to apply the proper tension to each suture.

Intercurrent Disease

Cirrhosis and ascites

Long-term high-dose steriod treatment

Marked obesity

Severe malnutrition

Abdominal wall defects secondary to tumor resection

(Defects in the abdominal wall, secondary to resection for tumor, may be managed by insertion of a prosthetic mesh as described below for ventral hernia repair, provided that adequate coverage of the mesh with viable skin and subcutaneous fat is possible. Otherwise, a full thickness pedicle skin flap will have to be designed to cover the mesh.)

Indications

Good-risk patients should have an elective repair of a ventral hernia that has a defect of more than 1–2 cm. Early repair of the small hernia is a simple procedure. Nonoperative therapy is almost always followed by gradual enlargement of the hernial ring over a period of time. Not only does this make the repair more difficult, but there is a significant incidence of intestinal obstruction due to the incarceration of intestines in the hernia.

Preoperative Care

Nasogastric tube prior to operation for large hernias

Perioperative antibiotics for 12–24 hours in patients with hernias large enough to require prosthetic mesh

Pitfalls and Danger Points

Sewing tissues that are too weak to hold sutures

Excessive tension on the suture line

Postoperative sepsis

Failure to achieve complete hemostasis

Operative Strategy

Identifying Strong Tissues

Every ventral hernia is characterized by a defect, small or large, in the tissue of the abdominal wall. In the hope of facilitating the approximation of the edges of the defect, the surgeon is often tempted to preserve and to insert sutures into weak scar tissue instead of carrying the dissection be-

yond the edge of the hernial ring to expose the normal musculoaponeurotic tissue of the abdominal wall. Depending on scar tissue to hold sutures for the repair of a hernia leads to a high recurrence rate. Carry the dissection for a width of 2–3 cm beyond the perimeter of the hernial ring on all sides and clearly expose the anterior surface of the muscle fascia. *Often an incisional hernia is accompanied by additional smaller hernias 3–5 cm away from the major defect.* These secondary hernias occur because more than one suture, inserted at the previous repair, has cut through the tissue leaving additional small defects. If the additional defects are close to the large hernial ring, incise the tissue bridges and convert the several defects into one large hernial ring.

Some surgeons advocate separating the abdominal wall into its component layers, namely peritoneum, muscle, and fascia. Then they suture each layer separately. We believe that in most cases it is preferable to insert the suture by taking a large bite of the entire abdominal wall in each stitch, following the principle of the Smead-Jones technique, rather than splitting the abdominal wall and closing each layer separately. By the same token, we have not used relaxing incisions through the aponeurosis of the external oblique layer to expedite hernial closure because we have observed subsequent herniation through the area of the relaxing incision. Other surgeons have advocated making a flap out of the anterior rectus sheath on each side and then bridging the hernial defect by suturing one fascial flap to the other. Our experience suggests that this technique will not be successful in repairing an incisional hernia larger than a few centimeters in diameter.

Avoiding Tension in the Repair

By far the most dangerous threat to long-term success in hernial repair is excessive *tension on the suture line.* While all surgeons

407

agree with this principle, there is a wide variation in each surgeon's perception of what comprises "excessive" tension. We believe that *any* degree of tension is "excessive" because this judgment is always made with the patient under anesthesia. Even local anesthesia produces muscle relaxation in the area of anesthesia, so that any degree of tension will be magnified when the effects of anesthesia have disappeared.

Although it is sometimes possible under anesthesia to approximate abdominal wall defects 6–8 cm in width without appearing to have produced excessive tension, *many* of these patients will return with recurrent hernias if they are followed for 4–5 years or more. Unfortunately, to our knowledge there are no long-term followup studies of a large number of patients who have undergone incisional hernia repair. Berliner also has noted in his experience that ventral hernias of substantial size repaired by traditional techniques are followed by a very high rate of recurrence if the patient is observed for more than a few years subsequent to the operation. Ponka reported a 9% recurrence rate after 794 incisional herniorrhaphies, only 53% of which could be followed for up to 5 years.

In the case of smaller ventral hernias, 3–4 cm in diameter, success may be anticipated if the weakened tissues are excised and the remaining defect in the abdominal wall is simply approximated by the use of the Smead-Jones technique, just as one would close a primary abdominal incision (see Vol. I, Chap. 5). While it is important to excise all of the attenuated tissues, it is not necessary to remove the condensation of fibrous tissue that often forms a firm ring and separates the hernial defect from the normal tissues of the abdominal wall. Using the Smead-Jones stitch, simply insert the sutures 2–3 cm beyond the hernial ring through all the layers of the abdominal wall including peritoneum. If a

circular defect can be closed in a transverse direction, this may be preferable to a vertical closure, but the main consideration is to select the direction that produces least tension.

Role of Prosthetic Mesh

If there is tension on the proposed suture line, do not close the defect at all. Rather, bridge the defect with one or two layers of a prosthetic mesh. With this technique no attempt is made to close the defect. The defect is *replaced* by the mesh, which is sutured in place by means of 2–0 or 0 Prolene mattress sutures that penetrate the full thickness of the abdominal wall. Although there are certain disadvantages to the use of a permanent prosthesis in the abdominal wall, the monofilament polypropylene (Prolene or Marlex) mesh has proved to be safe in our hands, although we have not accumulated a very large series of patients at this time. Unfortunately, this technique, first described by Usher, has not yet been validated by published long-term followup studies.

Cerise, Busuttil, Craighead, and Ogden have demonstrated a statistically significant increase in the bursting pressure of abdominal incisions in rats when a sheet of polyester mesh is sutured as an onlay patch over the abdominal closure prior to suturing the skin. Nevertheless, it is not at all clear that closing a ventral hernia with sutures under significant tension and then placing an onlay patch of mesh will result in long-term success. It would seem that tension would still cause the primary abdominal sutures to cut through the tissues over a period of time, leaving the mesh as the only barrier to a recurrent hernia. It is possible that merely the presence of the mesh patch will stimulate fibrosis and prevent this type of recurrence, but this fact *has not yet been established* in humans. For this reason, when there is a defect in the abdominal wall that would require sutures to be tied with any significant degree of tension, we have preferred to leave the defect open and to use the mesh as a replacement for this portion of the abdominal wall. Whether this judgment is the correct one will require a complex randomized study to determine.

Since the mesh is composed of monofilament fibers, the patient will often tolerate a wound infection without the necessity of removing the mesh. Opening the skin widely for drainage will generally prove sufficient and, in most cases, avoid the need to remove the mesh.

The most serious complication following the use of prosthetic mesh arises when dense adhesions sometimes form between the small intestine and the fabric of the mesh. If intestinal obstruction in this situation requires a subsequent laparotomy, it may prove impossible to separate the mesh from the bowel without extensive intestinal damage. Prolene mesh seems less prone to this complication than Marlex (Stone, Fabian, Turkleson, and Jurkiewicz). Although this complication is uncommon and we have not personally encountered it, it is important to take the precaution of interposing omentum between the mesh and the intestines whenever possible. In cases where omentum is not available for this purpose, one may preserve the hernial sac and interpose this tissue between the intestines and the mesh, which is then sutured as an onlay patch over the defect. Although using an onlay patch mechanically does not result in so strong a repair as inserting stitches through the entire abdominal wall to fasten the mesh, it may be preferable to taking the risk of producing excessive intestinal adhesions.

Marlex versus Prolene Mesh

Although the Marlex (Davol) and the Prolene (Ethicon) meshes are both composed of the identical chemical, namely polypropylene monofilament fibers that are knitted into a mesh, Prolene appears to be somewhat more pliable than Marlex. As mentioned above, Stone and associates found that when they used Prolene mesh in complicated cases of abdominal wall defects subsequent to trauma and sepsis, there were fewer long-term complications than when they used Marlex mesh in similar circumstances. We are not aware of any other reports at this time that contradict their published followup experience with these two products.

Use of Pneumoperitoneum prior to Repair of Large Ventral Hernia

Another method of avoiding tension in the repair of large ventral hernias is to induce pneumoperitoneum, as suggested by Moreno in 1947. This is especially recommended for use in patients having a hernia so large that it has lost its right of domicile in the abdominal cavity. Although Connolly and Perri could find published reports of only 22 cases of adult hernia patients prepared for surgery by pneumoperitoneum in the American literature prior to 1969, Moreno reported that he personally performed 500 operations using this modality with excellent results and only 3 fatalities. Moreno described the following contraindications to the use of pneumoperitoneum: (1) advanced age combined with poor general condition; (2) cardiac decompensation; (3) hernias in which there is a danger of gangrene. In the latter case, emergency surgery would be indicated; this would not allow time for preoperative pneumoperitoneum. To this list of contraindications we would add the condition of acute intestinal obstruction. We have seen one case of a huge incarcerted inguinal hernia where the induction of pneumoperitoneum resulted in transection of the ileum requiring emergency surgery to salvage the patient. Incarceration of bowel in a huge hernia is not itself a contradiction. Most of the giant hernias for which Moreno recommended pneumoperitoneum were not reducible. In the absence of intestinal obstruction, the gradual induction of pneumoperitoneum not only enlarged the abdominal girth by stretching the abdominal muscles in a manner similar to that which takes place during pregnancy, but air also entered the hernial sac and stretched whatever adhesions existed between the intestines and the sac. This made subsequent dissection technically easy. Patients, who have hernias with small rings, should receive pneumoperitoneum cautiously. Moreno recommended starting with perhaps four daily "test doses" of 500 ml of air prior to instituting the routine pneumoperitoneum in patients who had small rings and a previous history of intermittent intestinal obstruction, as well as those whose general condition was borderline. If the test doses cannot be tolerated, pneumoperitoneum is contraindicated.

The technique of instituting pneumoperitoneum, as described by Moreno, was based on inserting a spinal needle into the abdomen at the midpoint of a line running from the anterior superior iliac spine to the umbilicus after an intradermal injection of a local anesthetic agent. Obviously, avoid inserting the needle in the vicinity of a previous abdominal scar. Steichen modified this technique by using an Intracath intravenous catheter and inserting it into the abdominal cavity. The advantage of the catheter is that it can remain in place for the entire duration of the pneumoperi-

toneum (7–21 days). Forrest used an indwelling peritoneal dialysis catheter inserted into the abdomen under local anesthesia and left in place until the course of intra-abdominal air injections had been completed. We have used a #20 gauge Angiocath, which consists of a plastic catheter fitted around a metal needle. When the Angiocath is in its proper location, remove the needle and leave the plastic catheter in place. Then suture the plastic catheter to the skin and attach a bacterial air filter to the catheter. Attach a 3-way stopcock to the air filter.

While Moreno injected 1,000–2,000 ml of air into the abdominal cavity every 2–3 days, we and others (Forrest) have injected 500–2,000 ml daily. In administering the pneumoperitoneum each day, we use a disposable sterile 50 ml syringe. With the aid of the 3-way stopcock, inject increments of air until the patient experiences significant abdominal discomfort or dyspnea, at which time the injection of air is discontinued for the day. Moreno measured the pressure of air in the abdominal cavity at the conclusion of each day's dose. He found that a pressure of 30–40 cm of water was generally as much as the average patient could tolerate. Moreno also measured the patient's vital capacity every 2–3 days. Remarkably enough, he noted that despite the cumulative injection of 20–30 liters of air, the patient's vital capacity at the end of the course of treatment was consistently greater than it was before pneumoperitoneum was instituted. He felt that this increase in vital capacity was one indication that the patient was ready for surgery. The usual patient with a giant ventral or scrotal hernia requires 10–21 days of preparation with the cumulative injection of 12–20 liters of air prior to operation.

Surprisingly, there have been no reported instances of air embolism following the use of pneumoperitoneum. The actual repair of the giant hernia has generally been relatively simple because of the extreme degree of stretching that the abdominal musculature has undergone. The postoperative course in these patients has been remarkably smooth because the abdominal cavity has been stretched sufficiently to receive the contents of the large hernia, yet allowing for abdominal closure with no tension.

Our experience with pneumoperitoneum in giant hernias has been limited to a small number of cases, but these results have confirmed the favorable reports by Moreno and others. What is not clear from the published literature and our own observations is the question whether the stretched abdominal wall will soon contract to its previous state of tension, and whether this tension will result in recurrence of the hernia in an unacceptable number of patients. None of the published reports includes a proper followup study to determine the exact rate of recurrence.

At this time, pneumoperitoneum would appear to be the best method of approaching a patient with a giant ventral or giant scrotal hernia, where the hernial contents appear to have forfeited their right of domicile in the abdominal cavity. In these cases, there is often no other satisfactory method of approaching the patient.

In past years, excision of a large segment of the small intestine and the omentum was performed to reduce the bulk of the abdominal contents. Closure of the hernia was then often followed by extreme respiratory distress owing to the excessive pressure in the abdominal cavity.

In other cases of large abdominal hernias, it is not clear whether the use of pneumoperitoneum combined with primary suture of the defect under mild tension will prove superior to the use of prosthetic mesh without tension, when the patients are followed up for 5–10 years subsequently.

Myocutaneous Flap

The recent increased interest in the myocutaneous flap has resulted in the development of techniques that facilitate the rotation of large flaps of muscle covered by skin and subcutaneous fat into defects of the abdominal wall with retention of excellent blood supply to the flap. The tensor fascia lata muscle is one example of such a myocutaneous flap that can be used to bridge defects in the abdomen. A number of such flaps has been described by Mathes and Nahai. The exact role of this modality as compared to prosthetic mesh in replacing abdominal defects is still under study. It should be emphasized, however, that a split-thickness skin graft cannot consistently be expected to survive if it is placed over a layer of mesh, even if the mesh has been covered by healthy looking granulation tissue. In many cases, the mesh must be covered either by a pedicle flap of skin and subcutaneous tissue or the mesh must be replaced by means of a myocutaneous flap.

Summary

While many papers have been written describing the virtues of various techniques of repairing a ventral hernia, we are not aware of any definitive publication that describes a careful 5-year followup study of patients subjected to various types of ventral hernia repair. Consequently, our operative strategy is based on our clinical experience and not on statistically validated data. After proper dissection to identify normal tissues around the ring, we would close a small hernia with large bites of Smead-Jones stitches, using heavy Prolene suture material, provided that the tissues could be approximated *without tension*.

In patients with larger hernias or multiple defects, suturing under tension has in our experience resulted in frequent recurrences. It is quite possible that one reason for the failure of the *initial* abdominal closure was some deficiency in the quality of the patient's collagen deposition. In these cases excellent results can be achieved by the proper use of polypropylene mesh to *replace* the defective section of abdominal wall and thereby to avoid tension.

Operative Technique—Elective Ventral Hernia Repair

Dissecting the Hernial Sac

Make an elliptical incision in the skin along the axis of the hernial ring and carry the incision down to the sac **(Figs. 80–1 and 80–2).** Dissect the skin away from the sac on each side until the area of the hernial ring itself has been exposed in its entire circumference **(Fig. 80–3).** Now retract the skin flap away from the sac and make a scalpel incision down to the anterior muscle fascia. Continue to dissect the normal muscle fascia, using either scalpel or Metzenbaum scissors, until at least a 2-cm width of fascia has been exposed around the entire circumference of the hernial defect. This dissection will generally leave some residual subcutaneous fat attached to the area where the sac meets the hernial ring. Using a scissors, remove this collar of fat from the base of the hernia.

Resecting the Hernial Sac

Now make an incision along the apex of the hernial sac and divide all of the adhesions between intestine and sac **(Figs. 80–**

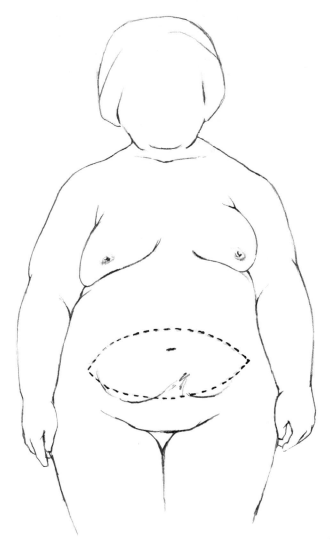

Fig. 80–1

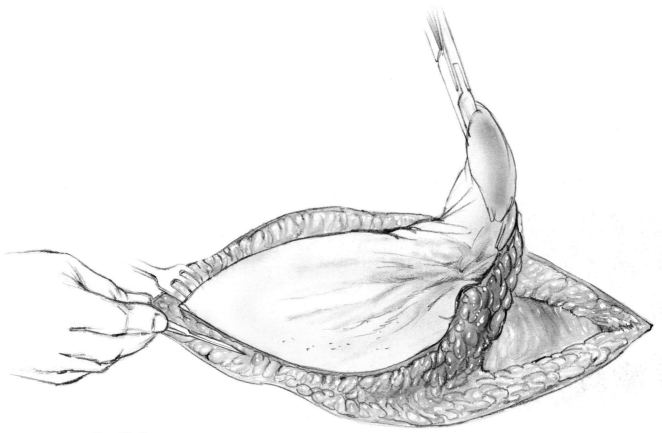

Fig. 80–2

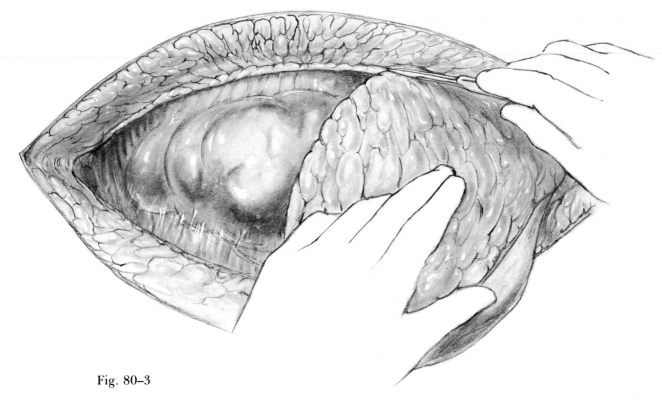

Fig. 80–3

4 and 80–5), reducing the intestines into the abdominal cavity **(Fig. 80–6).** Expose the circumference of the hernial defect so that the neck of the sac and a width of peritoneum of 2–3 cm are freed of all adhesions around the entire circumference of the hernia. Irrigate the wound with a

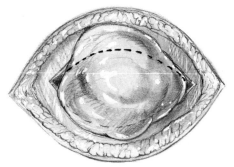

Fig. 80–4

dilute antibiotic solution intermittently **(Fig. 80–7).**

With the bowel reduced into the abdominal cavity and kept in position by means of moist gauze pads, evaluate the size of the defect. Apply Allis clamps to the edge of the defect and attempt to approximate the two edges of the hernia tentatively, in both vertical and in horizontal positions.

If the diameter of the defect is no more than 3–4 cm, and the edges can be approximated without tension, then a primary closure may be attempted. After this decision is made, excise the hernial sac down to its neck.

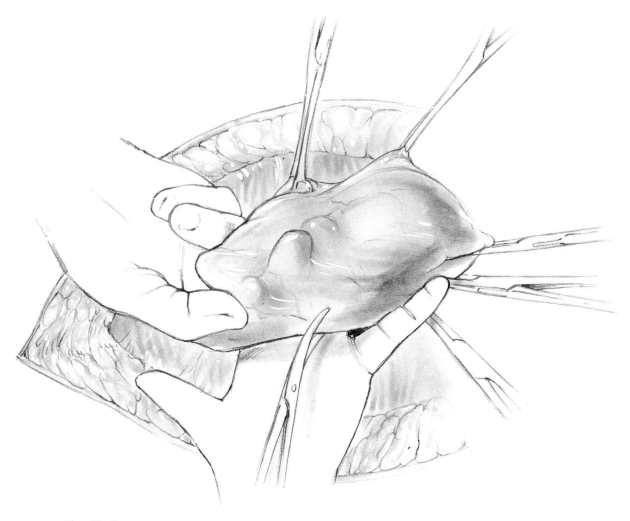

Fig. 80–5

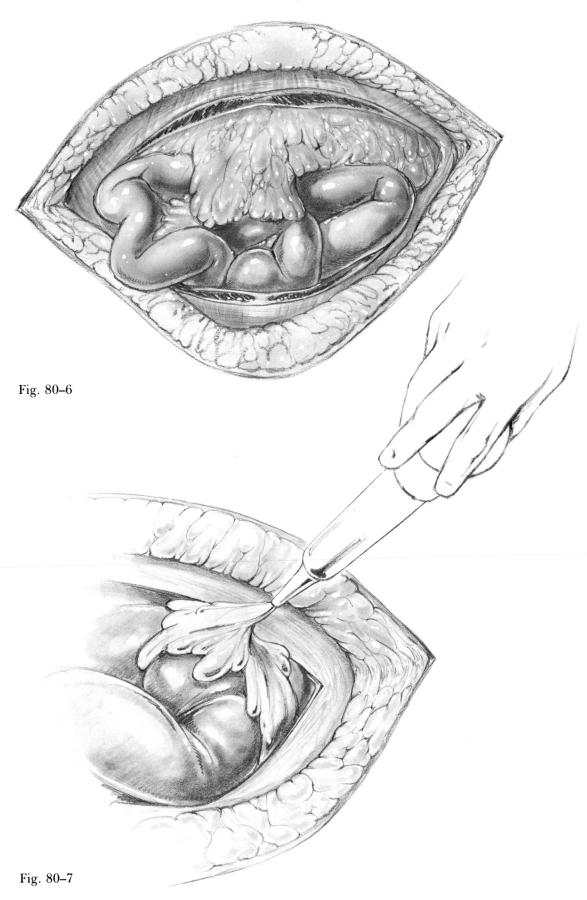

Fig. 80-6

Fig. 80-7

Smead-Jones Repair of Ventral Hernia

In the absence of tension, close the defect by the same technique that one would use for the primary closure of the abdominal incision. Use interrupted sutures of 2–0 monofilament stainless steel wire or 0 sutures of one of the nonabsorbable synthetic materials, such as Tevdek or Prolene, as described in Vol. I, Chap. 5. We have not used heavy PG or PDS suture material for the repair of ventral hernias because there are no data to indicate that these absorbable sutures retain their tensile strength for a sufficient period of time to permit firm healing in these hernia cases.

Achieve *complete* hemostasis by means of both electrocoagulation and fine PG ligatures since a postoperative hematoma will increase the incidence of postoperative infection, and infection will increase the incidence of postoperative wound failure.

Trim away any excess skin and close the skin incision without drainage, in routine fashion.

Mesh Repair of Ventral Hernia

Sandwich Repair

The "sandwich repair" was first described by Usher. Two identical sheets of polypropylene mesh are cut from a large sheet. Each piece of mesh should be 2 cm larger than the hernial defect. One sheet is placed inside the abdominal cavity and the other makes contact with the fascia around the hernial ring. The two sheets are held by sutures that go through the top sheet, then through the full thickness of the abdominal wall, and then through the deep sheet of mesh. The stitch then returns as a mattress stitch penetrating the deep sheet of mesh, the full thickness of abdominal wall, and, finally, the superficial sheet of mesh before being tied with a knot located in the subcutaneous layer **(Fig. 80–8)**. In the ideal situation, the deep layer of mesh should be separated from the bowel by the omentum. In the absence of a satisfactory layer of

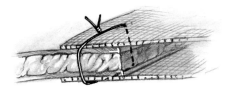

Fig. 80–8

omentum, it may be preferable to omit the intraperitoneal layer of mesh and to preserve enough hernial sac so that the sac, after being trimmed and sutured closed, can be retained as a protective layer to separate the intestines from the mesh, which is now used as an onlay patch, as described in the next section (p. 419).

Application of the sandwich technique to a large recurrent ventral hernia in an obese patient is illustrated beginning with **Fig. 80–9**. After the skin flaps have been elevated, exposing healthy fascia around the entire circumference of the hernial defect, make certain that there are no additional hernial defects above or below the major hernia. If there are additional hernias, combine them into one large defect by incising the bridge of tissue between them. Excise the sac down to its point of attachment to the hernial ring and excise subcutaneous fat around the hernial ring. Then insert one sheet of mesh inside the abdominal cavity and the other over the rectus fascia. Place the mattress sutures through the mesh at a point about 2 cm away from the hernial ring to be certain the sutures engage normal abdominal muscle and aponeurosis. A horizontal mattress suture penetrates first the superficial layer of mesh, next the entire abdominal wall, and then the deep layer of mesh. In returning the suture, the width of the bite of mesh must be less than the width of the bite in

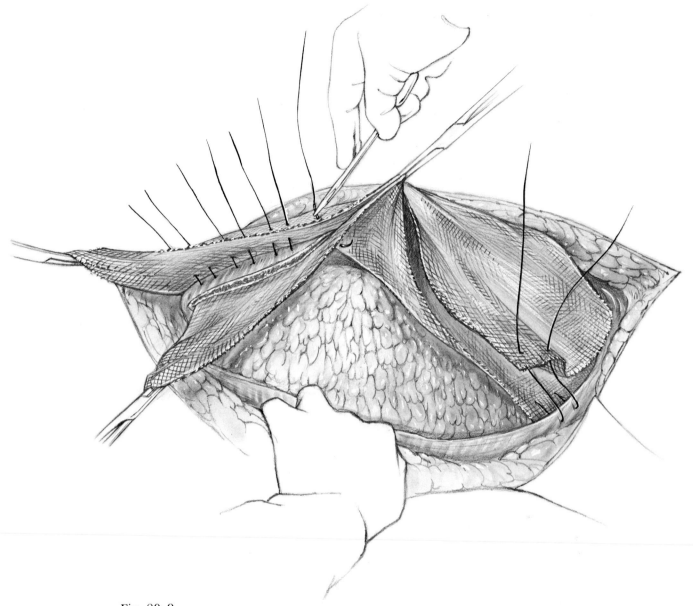

Fig. 80–9

the abdominal wall. Otherwise, the mesh will tend to bunch together when the stitch is tied rather than lying flat. Therefore, when returning the stitch through the deep layer of mesh, select a spot that will encompass only 7 mm of mesh while including a 1-cm width of abdominal wall. After penetrating the anterior rectus fascia, pass the needle through the anterior layer of mesh again at a point 7 mm away from the tail of the stitch. Tie the suture. We use the 3-1-2 knot (see Vol. I, Fig. B–28), supple-

mented by a few additional throws. The suture material used is 2–0 Prolene on an atraumatic needle. Insert additional mattress sutures of the same material at intervals of about 1.0–1.5 cm until half of the sutures have been inserted and tied. Then insert the remaining sutures, but do not tie any of them until all have been properly inserted. After tying all of the sutures,

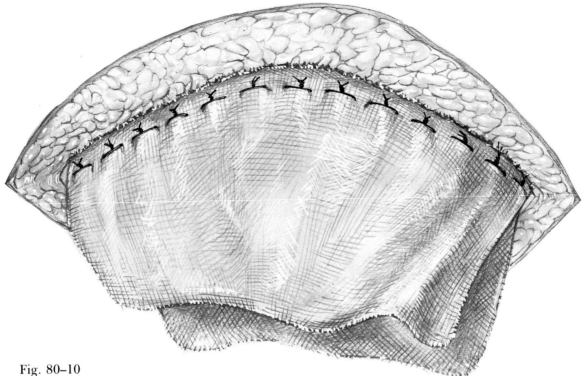

Fig. 80–10

check for any possible defects in the repair **(Figs. 80–10 and 80–11).**

When a hernial defect borders on the pubis, include the periosteum of the pubis in the sutures attaching the mesh to the margins of the defect.

Be certain to achieve complete hemostasis with electrocoagulation and fine PG ligatures. Insert two multiperforated closed-suction catheters through small puncture wounds in the skin. Lead the

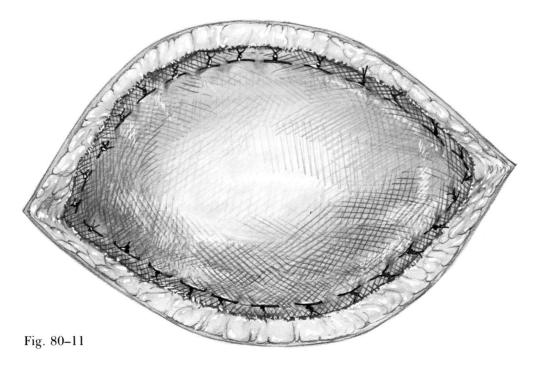

Fig. 80–11

catheters across the superficial layer of the mesh. Attach the catheters to a Hemovac-type closed-suction device. Approximate the skin with fine interrupted nylon sutures. Apply a sterile pressure dressing.

Onlay Patch Mesh Repair

As mentioned above, this repair is suitable when there is no layer of omentum available to be interposed between the intestines and the mesh. Here the hernial sac is preserved. Trim away the excess sac leaving enough tissue so that it may be closed without tension by means of a continuous 2–0 atraumatic PG suture **(Fig. 80–12)**. This will serve as a viable layer that hopefully will avoid the development of adhesions between the bowel and the mesh. The drawback to this technique is that its sutures, compared with those of the sandwich technique, are weaker because the bites of tissue are not equivalent to those of large mattress sutures that penetrate the entire abdominal wall. With this method only the peritoneum of the hernial sac is sutured to cover the defect. Then a piece of Prolene mesh is cut, 2–3 cm larger on all sides than the diameter of the hernial defect. If the patient is young and vigorous and has a large defect, we will use a double thickness of mesh. The first stitch of 0 Prolene starts at the caudal margin of the defect and catches the fascia overlying the hernial ring. Tie the stitch and then proceed with a continuous stitch fixing the mesh to the dense fibrous tissue at the margin of the hernial defect. When the cephalad edge of the hernial defect is reached, insert a second stitch and tie it. Anchor the first stitch by tying it to the tail of the second one. The second stitch runs in a continuous fashion along the opposite margin of the hernia and is terminated at the caudal edge of the hernial defect.

Using a similar technique, stitch the *edge* of the mesh to the anterior layer of

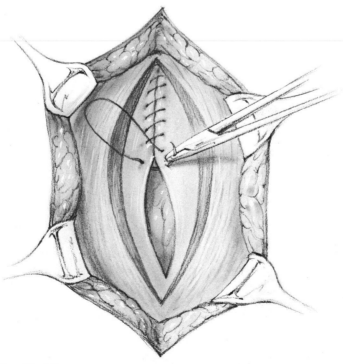

Fig. 80–12

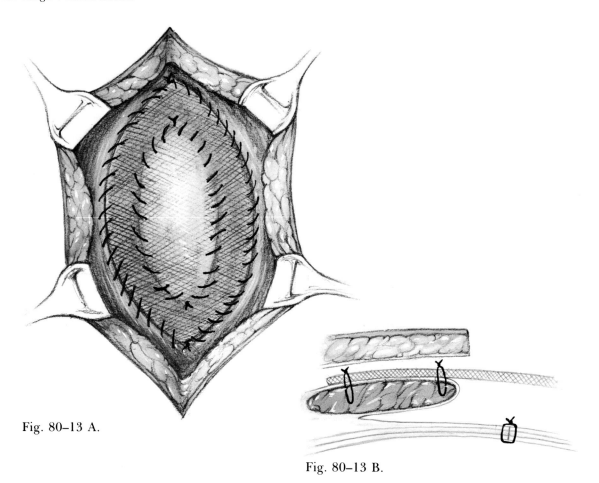

Fig. 80–13 A.

Fig. 80–13 B.

muscle fascia in a continuous fashion, using atraumatic 2–0 Prolene in **Figs. 80–13a and 80–13b.**

Insert 1 or 2 closed-suction catheters through puncture wounds and close the skin in routine fashion.

Postoperative Care

Remove the suction drains 5–7 days following operation.

Continue perioperative antibiotics for 12–24 hours for the ventral hernias repaired with mesh.

Institute early ambulation promptly on recovery from anesthesia.

Postoperative Complications

Wound Infection

With proper precautions wound infection should be rare following the elective repair of a ventral hernia. If an infection of the subcutaneous wound does occur, it is not generally necessary to remove the mesh. Because of its monofilament nature, polypropylene mesh with monofilament Prolene sutures will resist infection if the skin incision is promptly opened widely for drainage. Change the moist gauze packing daily until clean granulations have formed over the mesh. Then permit the skin to heal by secondary intention.

Hematoma

Most hematomas, unless large, can be treated expectantly.

References

Berliner S (1984) Personal communication

Blomstedt B, Welin-Berger T (1972) Incisional hernias. Acta Chir Scand 138:275

Cerise EJ, Busuttil RW, Craighead CC, Ogden WW II (1975) The use of Mersilene mesh in repair of abdominal wall hernias: a clinical and experimental study. Ann Surg 181:728

Connolly DP, Perri FR (1969) Giant hernias managed by pneumoperitoneum. JAMA 209:71

Forrest J (1979) Repair of massive inguinal hernia with pneumoperitoneum and without using prosthetic mesh. Arch Surg 114:1087

Goligher JC, Irvin TT, Johnston D, deDombal FT et al. (1975) A controlled clinical trial of three methods of closure of laparotomy wounds. Br J Surg 62:823

Jenkins TPN (1976) The burst abdominal wound—a mechanical approach. Br J Surg 63:873

Mathes SJ, Nahai F (1979) Clinical atlas of muscle and musculocutaneous flaps. Mosby, St. Louis

Moreno IG (1947) Chronic eventrations and large hernias: preoperative treatment by progressive pneumoperitoneum. Surgery 22:945

Ponka JL (1980) Hernias of the abdominal wall. Saunders, Philadelphia, p. 393

Steichen FM (1965) A simple method for establishing, maintaining, and regulating surgically induced pneumoperitoneum in preparation for large hernia repairs. Surgery 58:1031

Stone HH, Fabian TC, Turkleson ML, Jurkiewicz MJ (1981) Management of acute full-thickness losses of the abdominal wall. Ann Surg 193:612

Usher FC (1970) The surgeon at work: the repair of incisional and inguinal hernias. Surg Gynecol Obstet 131:525

81 Operations for Necrotizing Fasciitis of Abdominal Wall and Infected Abdominal Wound Dehiscence

Concept: Diagnosis and Management of Necrotizing Fasciitis

Necrotizing fasciitis that involves the *superficial fascia* of the abdominal wall produces necrosis primarily of the subcutaneous fat. The appearance of the overlying skin may be deceptively normal. A small area of apparent skin necrosis may be accompanied by an extensive (5–10 cm) area of necrotic subcutaneous fat. The underlying musculoaponeurotic layer often remains intact. The bacterial organisms are generally beta-hemolytic streptococci, staphylococci, or Gram-negative rods combined with anaerobes. Therapy requires the prompt excision of all of the subcutaneous fat and overlying skin until the surgeon encounters subcutaneous fat and skin that bleeds upon being incised. Take multiple samples of tissue and/or pus for culture and immediate Gram's stain studies. Aitken, Mackett, and Smith advise serial studies of muscle compartment pressures (wick catheter, Sorensen Research Co., Sandy, Ohio) in patients with necrotizing diseases of the extremities. Elevated compartmental pressure recordings constitute an indication for fasciotomy, biopsy, and debridement.

A far more dangerous problem is the necrotizing fasciitis that attacks the fascia or the aponeurosis overlying the abdominal muscles (Dellinger). The infection in these cases may result in necrosis of the full thickness of the abdominal wall. While this type of necrotizing fasciitis may occur after some type of trauma, it is more often seen in the patient who has had several laparotomies for peritonitis or abdominal abscesses. Often the patient has a deficient immune mechanism or is diabetic. The first manifestations of necrotizing fasciitis in these patients may be moderate edema of the previous laparotomy wound and (perhaps) a small area of skin necrosis. This is followed by liquefaction of the fascia and muscle layers of the abdominal wall and dehiscence of the abdominal incision.

If detected in its early stages, the infection may be aborted prior to dehiscence of the abdominal incision by removing all of the skin sutures, opening the skin widely, debriding all of the necrotic tissues, and administering appropriate systemic antibiotics. If the patient's previous incision was closed with through-and-through retention sutures, which included the skin within the confines of the stitches, then these retention sutures must be removed without hesitation in the treatment of necrotizing fasciitis, despite the likelihood of causing a wound dehiscence.

Preoperative Care

Administer therapeutic doses of systemic intravenous antibiotics that are effective against Gram-negative rods, enterococci, and anaerobes, including the clostridia, until definitive bacterial cultures and sensitivity studies are available. This will require an aminoglycoside, ampicillin or penicillin, and

422

clindamycin (or metronidazole or chloramphenicol). Third- and fourth-generation cephalosporins may also prove effective in these cases.

Since intra-abdominal sepsis is a frequent companion, if not the cause, of the necrotizing infection, many of these patients will require total parenteral nutrition.

Nasogastric suction

In the elderly and the critically ill patient, monitor the fluid requirements and cardiorespiratory function by means of pulmonary artery pressures, cardiac output determinations, and frequent blood gas determinations.

Pitfalls and Danger Points

Inadequate debridement of devitalized tissue

Failure to identify and drain intra-abdominal abscesses

Operative Strategy

Wide Debridement

Unhesitatingly cut away all devitalized tissue and continue the scalpel dissection until bleeding is encountered from the cut edge of the tissue. If even a small remnant of devitalized fat or other tissue is left, there will be a haven for the bacteria to proliferate and to destroy more of the abdominal wall.

Managing the Abdominal Wall Defect

If there is a small defect, less than 4–6 cm in diameter, simply place a layer of Adaptic gauze over the defect and cover it with moist gauze packing. Change the moist gauze twice a day until granulation tissue has covered the exposed abdominal viscera. Then the granulation tissue can be covered with a split-thickness skin graft. The resulting incisional hernia can be re-paired at a time of election after the patient has made a complete recovery.

Do not, under any condition, try to achieve closure of the defect by suturing the edges together after debriding an area of necrotizing fasciitis. If you do, infection and liquefaction of the abdominal wall is very likely to recur. Stone, Fabian, Turkelson, and Jurkiewicz found that out of 13 patients managed by debridement and primary closure *under tension*, dehiscence of the abdominal wound occurred in each case. The mortality rate in this group was 85%.

After debriding an infected abdominal wound that leaves a defect of more than 4–6 cm in diameter, replace the defect with a sheet of Prolene mesh. Do not use the same technique that has been described in Chap. 80 for the elective repair of large ventral hernias since this method consumes more operating time. Use one of the simpler techniques described below to suture a single layer of Prolene mesh to the edges of the wound by means of an interrupted or continuous suture of 2–0 Prolene. Apply daily dressings of moist saline gauze over the mesh until clean granulation tissue has formed. You may then elect to apply a split-thickness graft to the granulating surface. Voyles, Richardson, Bland, Tobin, and others found that in nine cases where split-thickness grafts were applied over Marlex mesh, in each case the mesh eventually extruded. Prolene mesh appears to be preferable in this respect (Stone et al.).

Alternatively, after the wound is clean and granulation tissue has formed, one may remove the Prolene mesh. Then apply a split-thickness graft directly to the granulation tissue overlying the intestinal viscera. This will provide a temporary cover until an elective repair of the massive abdominal defect can be performed after the patient has completely recovered and after any intestinal stomas have been closed.

423

This may require a waiting period of 4–6 months. The eventual definitive repair may consist of a myocutaneous graft, such as the tensor fascia lata flap. Alternatively, after excising the split-thickness graft, the large abdominal hernia may be repaired with a Prolene mesh sandwich. The mesh should then be covered by skin and subcutaneous fat. If an adequate layer of skin cannot be dissected from the area adjacent to the hernial defect, a large pedicle skin flap of some type should be rotated to provide a permanent cover for the mesh. Owing to the paucity of followup reports, it is not clear how often long-term success can be achieved by applying a simple split-thickness graft to a layer of Prolene mesh that has been covered with granulation tissue.

Repeat Laparotomy for Recurrence of Abdominal Sepsis

After successfully debriding an infected abdominal incision and repairing the defect with Prolene mesh, subsequent clinical observation may disclose the necessity to reexplore the abdomen for recurrent sepsis between the loops of small bowel, the pelvis, the subhepatic or subphrenic spaces or elsewhere. If necessary, it is generally simple to make an incision through the Prolene mesh, perform the abdominal exploration, and then repair the mesh with a continuous 2–0 Prolene suture. Stone and associates noted that adhesions between bowel and Prolene mesh were much less marked then when Marlex mesh was used. In some cases, where Marlex has been used and a layer of omentum has not been interposed between the mesh and the intestines, dense adhesions have formed between the small bowel and the Marlex mesh. When a patient, who suffers from this condition, requires laparotomy, entering the abdomen in the vicinity of the Marlex mesh may prove to be impossible without extensive damage to the bowel.

In some cases, placing the patient in a position facedown will encourage drainage of abdominal infections through the pores of the mesh.

Management of Intestinal Stomas and Fistulas

When a patient who is taken to the operating room for debridement of an infected abdominal incision also requires the exteriorization of an intestinal fistula or requires a colostomy, do not perform a loop colostomy or a loop enterostomy. Ostomies of the loop type are difficult to control. Consequently, secretions from these stomas will tend to contaminate continuously the layer of mesh and the open abdominal wound. Preferably, create matured end stomas of the small bowel or colon and bring them out at sites well away from the open abdominal wound if at all possible.

Operative Technique

In surgery for large abdominal defects, that remain after wide debridement of infected abdominal incisions, we do not recommend the technique described in Chap. 80. In order to expedite the operation in these acutely ill patients, we prefer to use a single layer of Prolene mesh. Cut the mesh so that it is only 1 cm larger than the size of the abdominal defect. Be certain that all intra-abdominal abscesses have been evacuated. Make an attempt to place a layer of omentum between the mesh and the underlying bowel. In no case should a bowel *anastomosis* ever be left in contact with synthetic mesh. Then use atraumatic sutures of 2–0 Prolene to attach the cut end of the mesh to the undersurface of the abdominal wall. In most cases these sutures will be of the interrupted type, but in the extremely ill patient, continuous sutures may be employed. The technique described either by Markgraf (**Fig. 81–1**) or that of Boyd (**Fig. 81–2**) may be employed. In both cases, take a larger bite of abdomi-

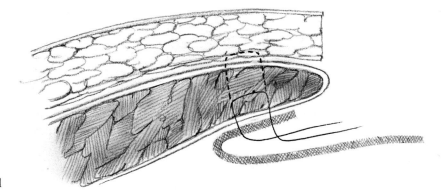

Fig. 81–1

nal wall than of the mesh. Otherwise the mesh will wrinkle. Apply slight tension to the mesh in inserting these sutures so that it will lie as flat as possible. Markgraf made the recommendation that when inserting sutures into the abdominal wall below the semicircular line, it is helpful to insert the suture through the entire thickness of the rectus muscle including the *anterior* rectus fascia. Otherwise the muscle and peritoneum may have inadequate holding power.

After the mesh has been sutured in place, apply gauze packing moistened with isotonic saline. In some cases, it may be appropriate to moisten the gauze with an antibiotic solution for the first 24 hours after debriding the wound.

Postoperative Care

Continue therapeutic dosages of appropriate antibiotics.

Change the gauze packing over the mesh every 8–12 hours until it is ascertained that there has been no extension of the necrotizing fasciitis.

Thereafter, inspect the wound and change the dressing daily.

Observe the patient carefully for recurrent abdominal sepsis and take appropriate diagnostic, therapeutic, and surgical measures to correct this sepsis.

After the wound is clean and granulation has formed, it is possible, if the defect is small, that epithelization may proceed spontaneously. In most cases, as abdominal distension disappears, wrinkling of the mesh will preclude spontaneous healing. In these cases, remove the mesh when the wound is clean and the patient's condition has stabilized, preferably around the 20th postoperative day. Then apply a split-thickness graft over the granulations covering the intestinal viscera. Delay definitive repair of a large abdominal hernia until a later date. (See the discussion above under Operative Strategy.)

Fig. 81–2

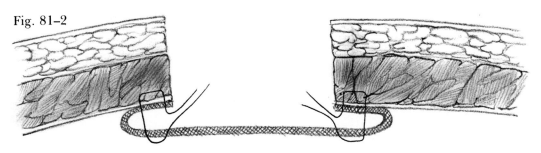

References

Aitken DR, Mackett MCT, Smith LL (1982) The changing pattern of hemolytic streptococcal gangrene. Arch Surg 117:561

Boyd WC (1977) Use of Marlex mesh in acute loss of the abdominal wall due to infection. Surg Gynecol Obstet 144:251

Dellinger EP (1981) Severe necrotizing soft-tissue infections: multiple disease entities requiring a common approach. JAMA 246:1717

Markgraf WH (1972) Abdominal wound dehiscence: a technique for repair with Marlex mesh. Arch Surg 105:728

Stone HH, Fabian TC, Turkelson ML, Jurkiewicz MJ (1981) Management of acute full-thickness losses of the abdominal wall. Ann Surg 193:612

Voyles CR, Richardson JD, Bland KI, Tobin GR et al. (1981) Emergency abdominal wall reconstruction with polypropylene mesh: short-term benefits versus long-term complications. Ann Surg 194:219

Anus and Rectum

82 Rubber Band Ligation of Internal Hemorrhoids

Concept: When to Band a Hemorrhoid

Hemorrhoids, although extremely common, require treatment only when they are symptomatic. Symptoms consist of bleeding, discomfort due to protrusion, and pain generally due to thrombosis. Although painful thrombosis most often occurs in external hemorrhoids, the source of symptoms in most patients is the internal hemorrhoid. Surgical treatment for most cases of symptomatic internal hemorrhoids can be carried out in the office without anesthesia by utilizing rubber band ligation, by injecting sclerosing solution, or by applying cryosurgery. This last method, however, produces an excessive amount of drainage during the postoperative period, and because it has no compensating advantages, it is uncommonly used at the present time. If the proper guidelines are followed in the technique of rubber band ligation, this technique achieves satisfactory results over the long term in more cases than does the injection of sclerosing solution. The modern method of rubber band ligation was introduced by Barron. It involves the application of a strangulating rubber band ligature to an internal hemorrhoid, with the rubber band being placed above the mucocutaneous junction to avoid grasping sensory nerve endings. Nivatvongs and Goldberg point out that a hemorrhoid is caused by downward displacement of the anal cushion. Therefore, they advocate applying the rubber band to the redundant rectal mucosa above the hemorrhoid rather than to the hemorrhoid itself. When the banded segment of mucosa shrivels up into fibrous tissue, the hemorrhoid is eliminated. This method has the advantage of avoiding the sensitive tissues at the dentate line and thus minimizing pain. Alexander-Williams and Crapp experienced excellent results with this technique. This method is suitable for most patients with second-degree, and for many with third-degree, hemorrhoids.

When a patient's complaints are due to the prolapse of large hemorrhoidal masses of the combined external-internal type or when the neck of an internal hemorrhoid proves to be painful if pinched by a forceps, rubber band ligation is contraindicated. For large third-degree hemorrhoids, surgical excision may be necessary. For the smaller bleeding internal hemorrhoid that seems to be supplied with nerve endings or for the patient who is extremely apprehensive, then either injection with a sclerosing solution or surgery is the preferred procedure.

Rudd encountered only two patients in 1,000 who could not be treated by rubber band ligation. These two had extremely large external hemorrhoids. Rudd claims that his patients experienced recurrence of hemorrhoids in less than 4% of cases after banding.

Indication

Symptomatic (often bleeding) internal hemorrhoids situated above the area in the anal canal that is innervated by sensory nerves

Pitfall and Danger Point

Applying a rubber band in an area supplied by sensory nerves

Operative Strategy

In order to avoid postoperative pain, apply the rubber band to a point at least 5–6 mm above the dentate line. In some patients a margin of 5–6 mm is not sufficient to avoid pain. These patients can be identified by pinching the mucosa at the site of the proposed application of the band by using the curved Allis tissue forceps supplied with the McGivney rubber band applicator. If the patient has pain when the mucosa is pinched, apply the band at a higher level where the mucosa is not sensitive, or else abandon the rubber-banding procedure.

If the patient has severe pain after the rubber band has been applied, it is possible to remove the rubber band by using a fine-tipped forceps and a sharp pointed scissors. If the removal of the rubber band is attempted some hours after the application, the surrounding edema will often make this procedure difficult if not impossible without anesthesia and without causing bleeding.

Operative Technique

Perform sigmoidoscopy to rule out other possible sources of rectal bleeding.

With the patient in the knee-chest position, insert a fenestrated anoscope (e.g., Hinkel-James type) that permits the internal hemorrhoid to protrude into the lumen of the anoscope. Inspect the circumference of the anal canal. Try to identify the hemorrhoid that caused the bleeding. If this is not possible, identify the largest internal hemorrhoid. Insert the curved Allis tissue forceps into the anoscope and pinch the mucosa around the base of the hemorrhoid

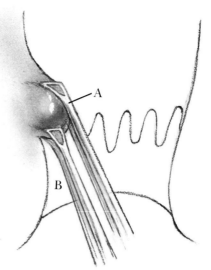

Fig. 82–1

in order to identify an insensitive area. Ask the assistant to hold the anoscope in a steady position. Now inspect the McGivney rubber band applicator. Be sure that two rubber bands have been inserted into their proper position on the drum of the applicator. Ask the patient to strain. With the left hand pass the drum up to the *proximal* portion of the hemorrhoid. Insert the angled tissue forceps through the drum.

In grasping the rectal mucosa, be sure to grasp it along the cephalad surface of the hemorrhoid at point A, not point B, in **Fig. 82–1.** If this is done, then the rubber band will not encroach upon the sensitive tissue at the dentate line. Draw the mucosa into the drum, which is simultaneously pressed against the wall of the rectum (**Fig. 82–2).** When the McGivney applicator is in the proper position, compress the handle of the applicator. Remove the tissue forceps and the McGivney applicator from the anoscope. The result should be a round purple mass of hemorrhoid, about the size of a cherry, strangulated by the two rubber bands at its base.

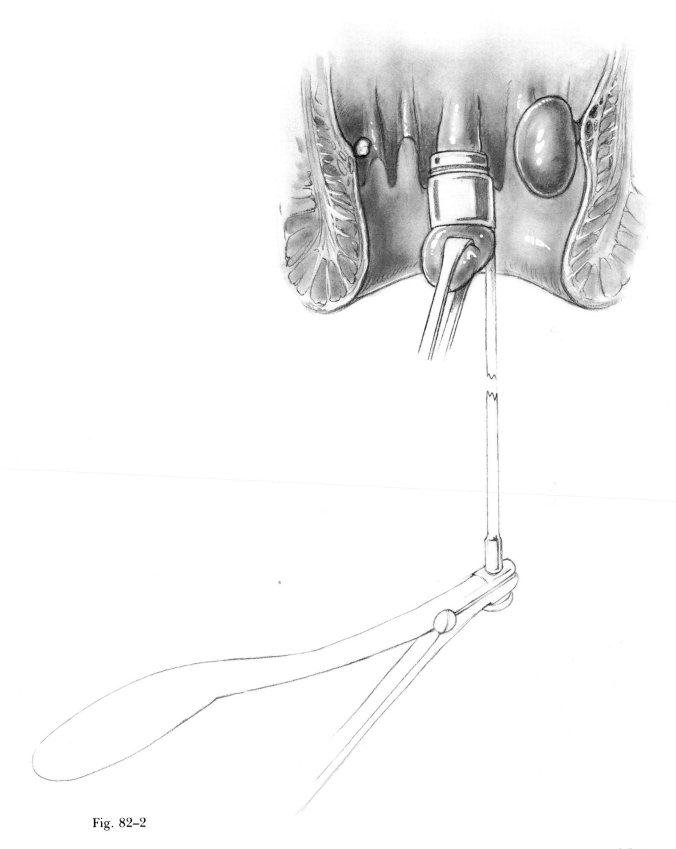

Fig. 82-2

Tchirkow, Haas, and Fox have recommended injecting 1–2 ml of a local anesthetic (we use 0.25% bupivacaine or lidocaine with epinephrine 1:200,000), using a 25-gauge needle, into the banded hemorrhoid. This appears to lessen some of the postoperative discomfort and may accelerate sloughing of the strangulated mass.

When employing the method advocated by Nivatvongs and Goldberg, insert the slotted anoscope and ask the patient to strain. The redundant rectal mucosa just proximal to the hemorrhoid will bulge into the slot of the anoscope. Grasp this mucosa with the tissue forceps. Draw the tissue into the McGivney ligator and release the rubber bands.

In general, treat only one hemorrhoid at each office visit. Have the patient return in about 3 weeks for the second application. Rarely are more than 3 applications necessary. Applying 2 or 3 bands at one sitting will often cause significant discomfort.

Postoperative Care

Inform the patient that postoperatively he or she may feel a vague discomfort in the area of the rectum accompanied by mild tenesmus, especially for 1–2 days after the procedure. Mild analgesic medication should be prescribed. Apprehensive patients do well if this medication is supplemented by a tranquilizer like diazepam.

Also warn the patient prior to the procedure that on rare occasions sometime between the 7th and 10th postoperative day, when the slough separates, there may be active bleeding into the rectum. A serious degree of bleeding requiring hospitalization occurs in no more than 1%–2% of cases.

Prescribe a stool softener like Colace. For constipated patients, Senokot-S, 2 tablets nightly, constitutes a medication that helps to keep the stool soft and also stimulates colonic peristalsis.

Patients may return to their regular occupation if they so desire.

Postoperative Complications

Pain. If *severe* pain occurs upon application of the band, remove the band promptly before the patient leaves the office. A *mild* degree of vague discomfort is treated with medication.

Bleeding. If the patient sustains a mild degree of blood spotting in the stool when the slough separates a week or 10 days after the banding, this may be treated expectantly. In case of a major bleed, proctoscope the patient. Suction out all the clots. Identify the bleeding point. If there is a significant amount of blood in the rectum or the patient has lost more than a few hundred milliliters, admit the patient to the hospital. In some cases, the bleeding point may be grasped with the Allis tissue forceps and a rubber band again applied to this area. Alternatively, under general or local anesthesia, either use the electro-coagulator or a suture to control the bleeding.

References

Alexander-Williams J, Crapp AR (1975) Conservative management of hemorrhoids. I. injection, freezing and ligation. Clin Gastroenterol 4:595

Barron J (1963) Office ligation treatment of hemorrhoids. Dis Colon Rectum 6:109

Rudd WWH (1973) Ligation of hemorrhoids as an office procedure. Can Med Assoc J 108:56

Tchirkow G, Haas PA, Fox TA Jr (1982) Injection of a local anesthetic solution into hemorrhoidal bundle following rubber band ligation. Dis Colon Rectum 25:62

Nivatvongs S, Goldberg SM (1982) An improved technique of rubber band ligation of hemorrhoids. Am J Surg 144:379

83 Hemorrhoidectomy

Concept: Selecting the Appropriate Treatment for Symptomatic Hemorrhoids

Hemorrhoids are known to have afflicted mankind for centuries, yet their pathogenesis remains obscure. Histologically, hemorrhoids do not differ significantly from normal anorectal submucosa; they resemble cushions of thickened submucosa. These cushions contains a vascular complex that includes arteriovenous communications. The submucosal cushions are normally located, even in children, in the left midlateral, the right anterolateral, and the right posterolateral positions in the anal canal. Thomson postulated that hemorrhoids represent normal anal submucosal cushions that, for some reason, have been displaced in a downward direction. The cause of this displacement may be constipation combined with chronic straining during defecation, although proof for this hypothesis is lacking.

The mere presence of nonsymptomatic hemorrhoids, internal or external, on routine physical examination cannot be considered a pathological finding. Treatment for nonsymptomatic hemorrhoids is not indicated. Hemorrhoids are best identified on physical examination by using an anoscope that has an opening on one side. This opening will permit a hemorrhoidal mass to protrude into the opening as the anoscope is rotated.

Bleeding, discomfort, and protrusion are the symptoms caused by hemorrhoids.

Severe pain is not a symptom caused by hemorrhoids unless there has been an acute thrombosis. More commonly, painful defecation is due to an anal fissure. Persistent protrusion of a hemorrhoid accompanied by continuous discharge of mucous may cause excoriation of the perianal skin, resulting in chronic discomfort. Medical management of these symptoms should aim to correct chronic constipation and strain on defecation by adding unprocessed bran to the patient's diet to increase the bulk of the stool while simultaneously softening it. Hydrophilic laxatives like psyllium seed (Metamucil) is also helpful in this regard. When this type of management fails, some manipulative therapy is indicated. For the bleeding internal hemorrhoid, that is situated above the dentate line and is not supplied with sensory nerves that carry pain impulses, the rubber band technique is an excellent choice (Chap. 82). It can be carried out as an office procedure without anesthesia. If the neck of the hemorrhoid is innervated by pain fibers, and the hemorrhoid can be classified as first or second degree in severity, it may be treated by the submucosal injection of 2–3 ml of a sclerosing solution like 5% phenol in oil. This is injected just proximal to each of the three usual locations of the internal hemorrhoidal masses near the anorectal ring (the proximal margin of the anal canal where the puborectalis muscle is situated). Injecting the sclerosing solution at these three sites presumably thromboses the hemorrhoidal veins and produces submucosal fibrosis that fixes the mucosa to the underlying internal sphincter muscle. Bleeding from small, nonpro-

433

truding hemorrhoids is almost always controlled by this technique, one which is very popular in Great Britain. Be sure to inject into the submucosal plane as an injection into the mucosa will produce necrosis. For the vast majority of internal hemorrhoids, however, we prefer the rubber band ligation technique.

External hemorrhoids do not cause symptoms except in the case of acute thrombosis. In this situation, if the patient presents within 24–48 hours of the onset of symptoms, excision of the thrombosed hemorrhoid under local infiltration anesthesia may result in prompt relief of symptoms. In general, if the patient reports to the physician later in the course of this disease, local surgery is not effective in relieving pain. In these cases, conservative management with analgesic medication and the local application of moist heat appears to give results equally satisfactory as excisional therapy.

When a symptomatic hemorrhoid appears to be innervated by sensory nerves, the patient generally has combined internal and external hemorrhoids. Often this is a large second- or third-degree hemorrhoidal mass. If symptoms persist, a formal hemorrhoidectomy may be required for relief. When a large protruding hemorrhoidal mass develops acute thrombosis, spasm of the internal sphincter muscle often results, which produces strangulation necrosis of the hemorrhoidal mass. In previous years, it was feared that excisional surgery for strangulated hemorrhoids might introduce sepsis into the portal venous system and that, consequently, emergency hemorrhoidectomy was contraindicated for strangulated hemorrhoids. It has since been shown that prompt hemorrhoidectomy for strangulated hemorrhoids produces rapid relief of symptoms and is followed by a smooth postoperative course.

A widely adopted technique of hemorrhoidectomy was introduced at St. Mark's Hospital, London, by Miles and modified by Milligan and Morgan in 1934 (see Goligher). This method involves the dissection of each of the three major hemorrhoidal masses off the internal sphincter muscle, followed by transfixion of the hemorrhoidal "pedicle" with a suture-ligature. The hemorrhoid is excised distal to the ligature. The defect in the anoderm and rectal mucosa is not reapproximated by suturing. Various modifications of this technique are in widespread use. Properly performed, open hemorrhoidectomy gives highly satisfactory results although several weeks are necessary before the wound is completely healed. It is *essential* that a bridge of undisturbed anoderm be left intact between each of the three hemorrhoid excisions. Otherwise, anal stenosis is likely to occur.

In a "closed" hemorrhoidectomy, the defect in the mucosa and anoderm is closed with sutures in a technique first popularized by Ferguson and Heaton and more recently by Goldberg, Gordon, and Nivatvongs. In this technique, only narrow widths of anoderm and mucosa are excised, and the hemorrhoidal tissue is dissected from underneath the adjacent mucosa whenever necessary. In this fashion, sufficient tissue has been retained to permit primary suturing of the hemorrhoidectomy incisions without narrowing the anus or rectum. Advocates of this technique claim that the patients have less postoperative pain, more rapid healing, and a smoother postoperative course. In fact, many of these hemorrhoidectomy suture lines separate during the postoperative period and heal by secondary intention. Nevertheless, it appears that following closed hemorrhoidectomy, total time elapsed between the operation and complete healing is generally less than following open hemorrhoidectomy. Properly performed, either the open or the closed method gives satisfactory results (Goligher).

It must be emphasized that the vast majority of patients with symptomatic hemorrhoids can be managed by an office procedure (see Chap. 82) without anesthesia or surgery. The few patients who require surgery have large, prolapsing hemorrhoids with a large component of external hemorrhoids. This advanced stage of disease is often accompanied by what appears to be a circumferential prolapse of anoderm and rectal mucosa together with the hemorrhoids. The usual methods of hemorrhoidectomy do not efficiently correct the pathology in those patients who have a circumferential mucosal prolapse. For this group of patients we have employed the modified open method of hemorrhoidectomy described below.

In Great Britain, surgeons perform hemorrhoidectomy under general anesthesia in the lithotomy position, often supplementing the general anesthesia with a local block to achieve better relaxation of the sphincter muscles. In the United States, the prone position with the hips elevated on a rolled-up sheet or sandbag, has achieved well-deserved popularity. Hemostasis is easier to achieve because the blood flows away from the field by gravity. Also, the surgeon and his first assistant can assume positions that allow for much greater operative efficiency than can be achieved when the patient is placed in the lithotomy position. With the patient lying prone, general anesthesia requires endotracheal intubation. Using exclusively local anesthesia for hemorrhoidectomy has the disadvantage that the initial injection of the anesthetizing agent is followed by considerable pain. Consequently, general anesthesia with endotracheal intubation, followed by local perianal anesthesia, has been recommended by Goldberg and associates for hemorrhoidectomy and similar anal canal operations.

Nivatvongs has recently described a technique for local anesthesia that he claims will avoid the pain of the initial injection and therefore preclude the necessity for general anesthesia. We have found this method to be simple and effective.

Indications and Contraindications

Persistent bleeding, protrusion, or discomfort

Symptomatic second- and third-degree (combined internal-external) hemorrhoids

Symptomatic hemorrhoids combined with mucosal prolapse

Strangulation of internal hemorrhoids

Early stage of acute thrombosis of external hemorrhoid

Preoperative Care

A sodium phosphate packaged enema (Fleet) is adequate cleansing for most patients.

Sigmoidoscopy and/or colonoscopy as indicated by the patient's symptoms

Routine preoperative blood coagulation profile (partial thromboplastin time, prothrombin time, and platelet count)

Preoperative shaving of the perianal area is preferred by some surgeons, but is not necessary.

Pitfalls and Danger Points

Narrowing the lumen of the anus and thus inducing anal stenosis

Trauma to sphincter

Failing to identify associated pathology (e.g., inflammatory bowel disease, leukemia, portal hypertension, coagulopathy, or squamous carcinoma of anus)

Operative Strategy

Avoiding Anal Stenosis

The most serious error in performing hemorrhoidectomy is the failure to leave adequate bridges of mucosa and anoderm between each site of hemorrhoid excision. If a minimum of 1.0–1.5 cm of viable anoderm is left intact between each site of hemorrhoid resection, there need be no fear of the patient developing postoperative anal stenosis. Preserving viable anoderm is much more important than is the removal of all external hemorrhoids and redundant skin.

Achieving Hemostasis

Traditionally, surgeons have depended on mass ligature of the hemorrhoid "pedicle" for achieving hemostasis. This policy ignores the fact that small arteries penetrate the internal sphincter and enter the operative field. Also numerous vessels are divided when incising the mucosa to dissect the pedicle. In fact, the concept of a "pedicle" as being the source of a hemorrhoidal mass is largely erroneous. A hemorrhoidal mass is not a varicose vein situated at the termination of the portal venous system. It is, indeed, a vascular complex with multiple channels that is not fed predominantly by a large single vessel in the pedicle. Therefore it is important to control bleeding from each of the many vessels that are transected during the operation. A convenient method of accomplishing this is with careful and accurate application of the coagulating electrocautery. As pointed out by Goldberg and associates, most of the vessels come from the incised mucosa. Before suturing the defect following hemorrhoid excision, perfect hemostasis should be achieved.

Associated Pathology

Even though hemorrhoidectomy is a minor operation, a complete history and physical examination are necessary to rule out important systemic diseases like leukemia. Leukemic infiltrates in the rectum can cause severe pain and can mimic hemorrhoids and anal ulcers. Operating erroneously on an undiagnosed acute leukemia patient is fraught with the dangers of bleeding, failure of healing, and sepsis. Crohn's disease must also be ruled out by careful local examination and sigmoidoscopy, as well as biopsy in doubtful situations.

Another extremely important condition, that is sometimes overlooked during the course of hemorrhoidectomy, is squamous cell carcinoma of the anus. This may resemble nothing more than a small ulceration on what appears to be a hemorrhoid. Any suspected hemorrhoid that demonstrates a break in the continuity of the overlying mucosa should be suspected of being a carcinoma, as should any ulcer of the anoderm, except for the classical anal fissure located in the posterior commissure. Prior to scheduling a hemorrhoidectomy, biopsy all ulcerations and atypical lesions of the anal canal.

Operative Technique—Closed Hemorrhoidectomy

Local Anesthesia

Choosing an Anesthetic Agent
A solution of 0.5% lidocaine (maximum dosage 80 ml) or 0.25% bupivacaine (maximum dosage 80 ml), combined with epinephrine 1:200,000 and 150–300 units of hyaluronidase, is an anesthetic agent that is effective and has an extremely low incidence of toxicity.

Since the perianal injection of these agents is painful, the patient is generally premedicated with an intramuscular injection 1 hour before the operation of some combination of a narcotic and a sedative (e.g., Demerol and a barbiturate, or Innovar, 1–2 ml). Alternatively, diazepam in a dose of 5–10 mg, may be given intravenously just before the perianal injection.

Techniques of Local Anesthesia

In the technique originally introduced by Kratzer, the anesthetic agent is placed in a syringe with a 25-gauge needle. The needle should be at least 5 cm in length. Initiate the injection at a point 2–3 cm lateral to the middle of the anus. Inject 10–15 ml of the solution in the *subcutaneous* tissues surrounding the right half of the anal canal including the area of the anoderm at the anal verge. Warn the patient that this injection may be quite painful. Repeat this maneuver through a needle puncture site to the left of the anal canal. After placing a slotted anoscope in the anal canal, insert the needle into the tissues just beneath the anoderm and into the plane between the submucosa and the internal sphincter 3–4 cm deep into the anal canal **(Fig. 83–1)**. If the injection creates a wheal in the mucosa similar to that seen in the skin after an intradermal injection, then the needle is in too shallow a position. An injection into the proper submucosal plane will produce no visible change in the overlying mucosa. Inject 3–4 ml of anesthetic solution in the course of withdrawing the needle. Make similar injections in each of the four quadrants until the subdermal and submucosal tissues of the anal canal have been surrounded with anesthetic agent. This should require a total of no more than 30–40 ml of anesthetic solution. Satisfactory relaxation of the sphincters will be achieved without the necessity of directly injecting solution into the muscles or of attempting to block the inferior hemorrhoidal nerve in the ischiorectal space. Wait 5–10 minutes for complete relaxation and anesthesia.

Nivatvongs, in a recent publication, described a technique that he claims avoids pain. Insert a small anoscope into the anal canal. Make the first injection into the *submucosal* plane 2 mm *above* the dentate line. Since the mucosa above the dentate line lacks sensory innervation, this step is free of pain, unlike the initial injection of the Kratzer technique of inducing local anesthesia. Inject 2–3 ml of anesthetic solution. Inject an equal amount of solution in each of the remaining three quadrants of the anus. Then remove the anoscope and insert a well-lubricated index finger into the anal canal. Use the tip of the index finger to massage the anesthetic agent from the submucosal area down into the

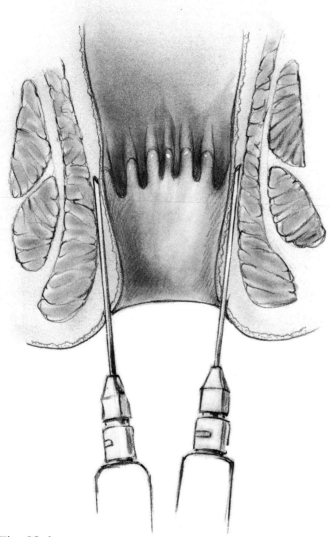

Fig. 83–1

tissues beneath the anoderm. Repeat this maneuver with respect to each of the four injection sites. By spreading the anesthetic agent distally, this maneuver will serve to anesthetize the very sensitive tissues of the anoderm just distal to the dentate line. When this has been accomplished, make another series of injections 2 mm *distal* to the dentate line. Inject 2–3 ml of solution beneath the anoderm and the subcutaneous tissues in the perianal region through four sites, one in each quadrant of the anus. Then use the index finger again to massage the tissues of the anal canal in order to spread the anesthetic solution circumferentially around the anal and perianal area. In some cases additional anesthetic agent may be necessary for complete circumferential anesthesia. An average of 20–25 ml of solution is required. Nivatvongs states that this technique will provide excellent relaxation of the sphincters and permit operations like hemorrhoidectomy to be accomplished without general anesthesia. For a lateral internal sphincterotomy, it is not necessary to anesthetize the entire circumference of the anal canal when using this technique. Inject only the area of the sphincterotomy.

Intravenous Fluids

Since local anesthesia has a minimum of systemic effects, it is not necessary to administer a large volume of intravenous fluid during the operation. In fact, if large volumes of fluid are administered during a hemorrhoidectomy or even during an inguinal hernia repair, the bladder becomes rapidly distended. In the presence of general anesthesia or even heavy sedation during local anesthesia, the patient is not sufficiently alert to have the desire to void. By the time the patient is alert, the bladder muscle has been stretched and may be too weak to empty the bladder, especially if the patient also has some degree of prostatic hypertrophy. This can be the cause of postoperative urinary retention, requir-

ing catheterization. All of this can be prevented by avoiding general anesthesia and heavy premedication and, in addition, by limiting the dosage of intravenous fluids to 100–200 ml during and after hemorrhoidectomy.

Positioning the Patient

We prefer to place the patient in the semiprone jacknife position with either a sandbag or rolled-up sheet under the hips and a small pillow to support the feet. It is not necessary to shave the perianal area; if the buttocks are hirsute, shave this area. Then apply tincture of benzoin. When this solution has dried, apply wide adhesive tape to the buttock and attach the other end of the adhesive strap to the operating table. In this fashion lateral traction is applied to each buttock, affording excellent exposure of the anus.

Incision and Dissection

Gently dilate the anal canal so that it admits two fingers. Insert a bivalve speculum like the Parks retractor or a medium size Hill-Ferguson retractor. One advantage of using the medium Hill-Ferguson retractor is that it approximates the diameter of the normal anal canal. If the defects remaining in the mucosa and anoderm can be sutured closed with the retractor in place following hemorrhoid excision, then no narrowing of the anal canal will occur. By rotating the retractor and applying countertraction to the skin of the opposite wall of the anal canal, each of the hemorrhoidal masses can be identified. Generally three hemorrhoidal complexes will be excised, one in the left midlateral position, another in the right anterolateral, and the third in the right posterolateral location. Avoid placing incisions in the anterior or posterior commissures. Grasp the most dependent portion of the largest hemorrhoidal mass in a Babcock clamp. Then make an incision in the anoderm outlining the distal extremity of the hemorrhoid (**Fig. 83–2**) using a No. 15 (Bard-Parker) scalpel. If the hemor-

438

rhoidal mass is unusually broad (more than 1.5 cm), do not excise all of the anoderm and mucosa overlying a hemorrhoid of this type. If each of the hemorrhoidal masses is equally broad, excising all of the anoderm and mucosa overlying each of the hemorrhoids will result in inadequate tissue bridges between the sites of hemorrhoid excision. In such a case, incise the mucosa and anoderm in an elliptical fashion overlying the hemorrhoid. Then initiate a submucosal dissection using small, pointed scissors to elevate the mucosa and anoderm from that portion of the hemorrhoid that still remains in a submucosal location. Carry the dissection of the hemorrhoidal mass down to the internal sphincter muscle **(Fig. 83–3).** After incising the mucosa and anoderm, draw the hemorrhoid away from the sphincter, using blunt dissection as necessary, to demonstrate the lower border of the internal sphincter. This muscle has whitish muscle fibers that run in a transverse direction. A thin bridge of fibrous tissue will often be seen connect-

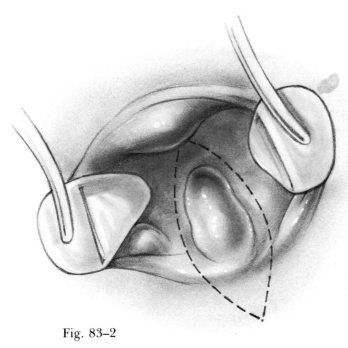

Fig. 83–2

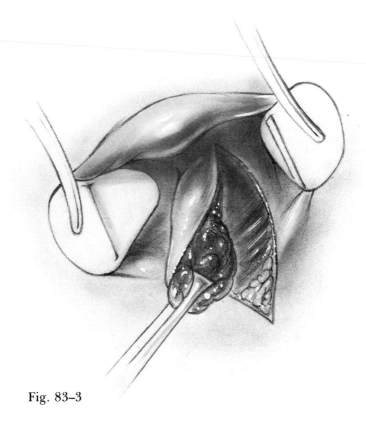

Fig. 83–3

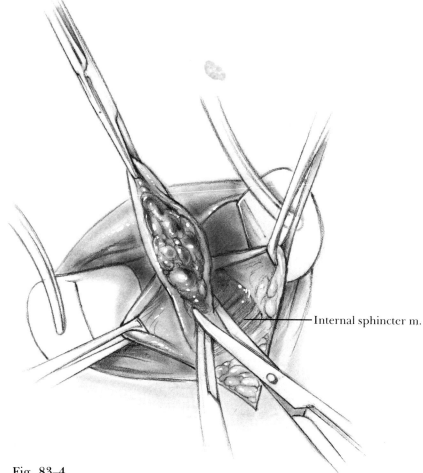

Internal sphincter m.

Fig. 83–4

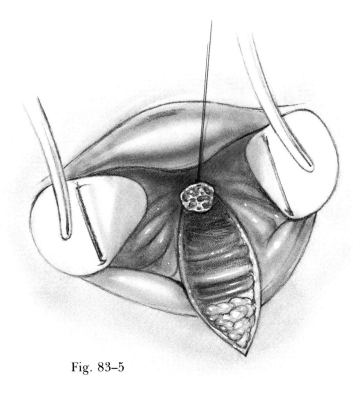

Fig. 83–5

ing the substance of the hemorrhoid to the internal sphincter. Divide these fibers with a scissors **(Fig. 83–4)**. Dissect the hemorrhoidal mass for a distance of about 1–2 cm above the dentate line where it may be divided with the electrocoagulator. Remove any residual internal hemorrhoids from beneath the adjacent mucosa. Achieve complete hemostasis, primarily with careful electrocoagulation. It is not necessary to clamp and suture the hemorrhoidal "pedicle," but many surgeons prefer to do so **(Fig. 83–5)**. Although it is helpful to remove all the internal hemorrhoids, we do not attempt to extract fragments of external hemorrhoids from beneath the anoderm as this step does not appear to be necessary. Most of these small

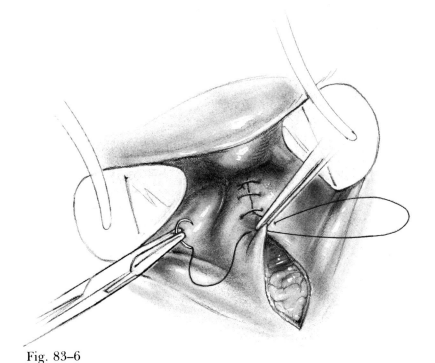

Fig. 83–6

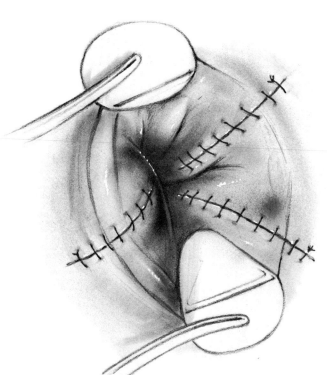

Fig. 83–7

external hemorrhoids will disappear spontaneously following internal hemorrhoidectomy.

After complete hemostasis has been achieved, insert an atraumatic 5–0 Vicryl suture into the apex of the hemorrhoidal defect. Tie the suture and then close the defect with a continuous suture taking 2–3 mm bites of mucosa on each side (**Fig. 83–6**). Also include a small bit of the underlying internal sphincter muscle with each pass of the needle. This will serve to force the mucosa to adhere to the underlying muscle layer and thereby help prevent mucosal prolapse and recurrent hemorrhoids. Continue the suture line until the entire defect has been closed.

Now repeat the same dissection for each of the other two hemorrhoidal masses. Close each of the mucosal defects by the same technique (**Fig. 83–7**). Be certain not to constrict the lumen of the anal canal. To avoid this complication, remem-

441

ber that the ellipse of mucosa–anoderm, which is excised with each hemorrhoidal mass, must be relatively narrow. Also, remember that if the tissues are sutured under tension, the suture line will undoubtedly break down.

A few patients prior to surgery will suffer some degree of anal stenosis together with their hemorrhoids. Under these conditions, rather than forcibly dilating the anal canal at the onset of the operation, perform a lateral internal sphincterotomy to provide adequate exposure for the operation. This is also true for patients who have a concomitant chronic anal fissure.

For those surgeons, who prefer to keep the skin unsutured for drainage, it is possible to modify the above operative procedure by discontinuing the mucosal suture line at the dentate line, thereby leaving the defect in the anoderm unsutured. It is also permissible not to suture the mucosal defects at all after hemorrhoidectomy (see above).

Operative Technique—Radical Open Hemorrhoidectomy

Incision

This operation is restricted to patients who no longer have three discreet hemorrhoidal masses, but in whom all of the hemorrhoids and prolapsing rectal mucosa seem to have coalesced into an almost circumferential mucosal prolapse. For these patients the operation will excise the hemorrhoids, both internal and external, the redundant anoderm, and prolapsed mucosa from both the left and right lateral portions of the anus, leaving 1.5 cm bridges of intact mucosa and anoderm at the anterior and posterior commissures. With the patient in the prone position, as described above for the closed hemorrhoidectomy, outline the incision on the left side of the anus as shown in **Fig. 83–8.**

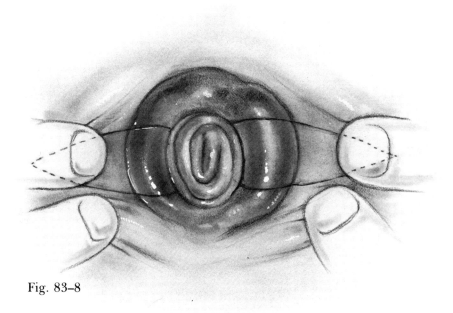

Fig. 83–8

Excising the Hemorrhoidal Masses

Elevate the skin flap together with the underlying hemorrhoids by sharp and blunt dissection until the lower border of the internal sphincter muscle has been unroofed **(Fig. 83–9)**. This muscle can be identified by the transverse whitish fibers. Now elevate the anoderm above and below the incision in order to enucleate adjacent hemorrhoids that have not been included in the initial dissection **(Fig. 83–10)**. This will permit the removal of almost all the hemorrhoids and still permit an adequate bridge of anoderm in the anterior and posterior commissures.

After the mass of hemorrhoidal tissue with overlying mucosa has been mobilized to the level of the normal location of the dentate line, amputate the mucosa and hemorrhoids with the electrocoagulator at the level of the dentate line. This will leave a free edge of rectal mucosa. Suture this mucosa to the underlying internal sphincter muscle with a continuous 5–0 atrau-

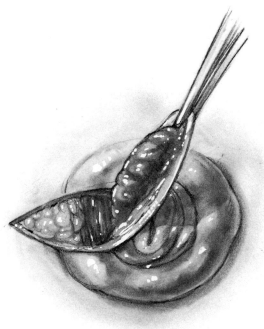

Fig. 83–9

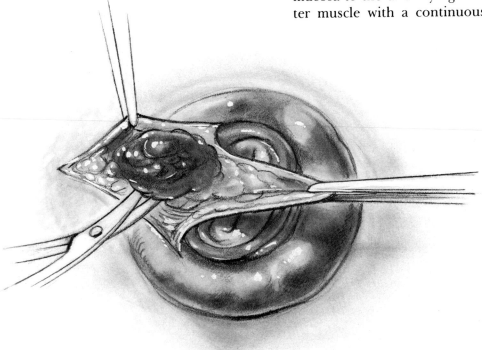

Fig. 83–10

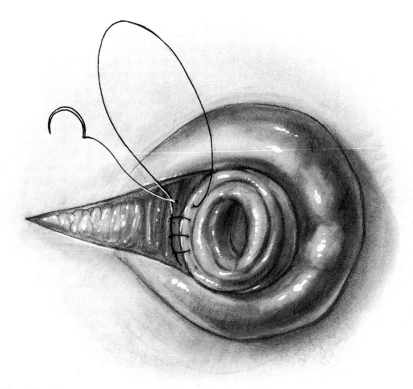

Fig. 83–11

matic Vicryl suture as illustrated in **Fig. 83–11.** This will recreate the dentate line at its normal location. Do not bring the rectal mucosa down to the area that is normally covered by anoderm or skin, because this will cause continuous secretion of mucous that will irritate the perianal skin.

Execute the same dissection to remove all of the hemorrhoidal tissue between one and 5 o'clock on the right side and reattach the free cut edge of rectal mucosa to the underlying internal sphincter muscle as depicted in **Fig. 83–12.** There may be some redundant anoderm together with some external hemorrhoids at the anterior or the posterior commissure of the anus. Do not attempt to remove every last bit of external hemorrhoid because this will jeopardize the viability of the anoderm in the commissures. Unless viable bridges, about 1.5 cm each in width, are preserved in the anterior and posterior commissures,

the danger of a postoperative anal stenosis far outweighs the ill effect of leaving behind a skin tag or an occasional external hemorrhoid.

Be certain that hemostasis is complete, using the electrocoagulator and occasional suture-ligatures of fine PG or chromic catgut. Then insert into the anus a small piece of rolled up Gelfoam. This roll should not be more than 1 cm in thickness. It will serve to apply gentle pressure and will encourage coagulation of minor bleeding points that may have been overlooked. The Gelfoam need not be removed since it will dissolve when the patient starts having his sitz baths postoperatively. Apply a sterile dressing to the perianal area.

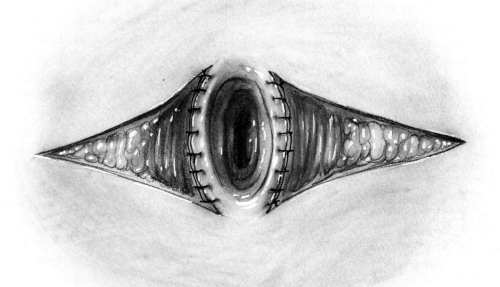

Fig. 83–12

Postoperative Care

Encourage ambulation the evening of operation.

Prescribe analgesic medication.

Prescribe Senokot-S, Metamucil, or mineral oil, while the patient is in the hospital. After discharge, limit the use of cathartics because the passage of a well-formed stool is the best guarantee that the anus will not become stenotic. In patients with severe chronic constipation, some type of laxative or stool softener will be necessary following discharge from the hospital.

Order warm sitz baths several times a day, especially following each bowel movement.

Discontinue intravenous fluids as soon as the patient returns to his room and initiate a regular diet and oral fluids as desired.

Discharge the patient on the 3rd or 4th postoperative day if he has had the first bowel movement without undue difficulty. Young, good-risk patients will tolerate hemorrhoidectomy as ambulatory outpatients.

Postoperative Complications

Bleeding during the period of hospitalization is rare if complete hemostasis has been achieved in the operating room. However, when it does occur, the patient should probably be returned to the operating room in order to have the bleeding point suture-ligated, as the majority of patients who experience major bleeding after discharge from the hospital had experienced a minor degree of bleeding before discharge (Buls and Goldberg). About 1% of patients will present with hemorrhage severe enough to require reoperation for hemostasis, generally 8–14 days following operation.

If, for some reason, the patient is not returned to the operating room for the control of bleeding, it is possible to achieve at least temporary control by inserting a 30 ml Foley catheter into the rectum. Then blow up the Foley balloon and apply downward traction to the catheter. Reexploration of the anus for surgical control of bleeding is far preferable.

Infection is rare.

Skin tags follow hemorrhoidectomy in 6–10% of cases. Although no treatment is required, for cosmetic purposes a skin tag may be excised under local anesthesia as an office procedure when the operative site has healed completely.

References

Buls JG, Goldberg SM (1978) Modern management of hemorrhoids. S Clin N Amer 58:469

Ferguson JA, Heaton JR (1959) Closed hemorrhoidectomy. Dis Colon Rectum 2:176

Goldberg SM, Gordon PH, Nivatvongs S (1980) Essentials of anorectal surgery. Lippincott, Philadelphia

Goligher JC (1980) Surgery of the anus, rectum and colon, 4th ed. Balliere Tindall, London

Kratzer GL, (1974) Improved local anesthesia in anorectal surgery. Am Surg 40:609

Nivatvongs S (1982) An improved technique of local anesthesia for anorectal surgery. Dis Colon Rectum 25:259

Thomson WHF (1975) The nature of hemorrhoids. Br J Surg 62:542

84 Anorectal Fistula and Pelvirectal Abscess

Concept: Pathogenesis and Treatment of Anorectal Fistulas

Anorectal Anatomy

The muscles of the pelvic floor assume the anatomical configuration of two cylinders, one within the other. The inner cylinder consists of the lower rectum and anal canal, which contains mucosa and submucosa as well as the circular and the longitudinal muscle layers. In the anal canal the circular muscle layer is very well developed and constitutes the internal sphincter muscle, an involuntary sphincter made up of smooth muscle. The outer cylinder consists of the external sphincter and the puborectalis muscles. At its proximal extremity the outer cylinder fans out in the shape of a funnel since it is continuous with the levator ani muscles that form the pelvic diaphragm. The inner visceral muscle cylinder and the outer somatic cylinder are separated by the intersphincteric space **(Fig. 84–1).** It is striking that in the course

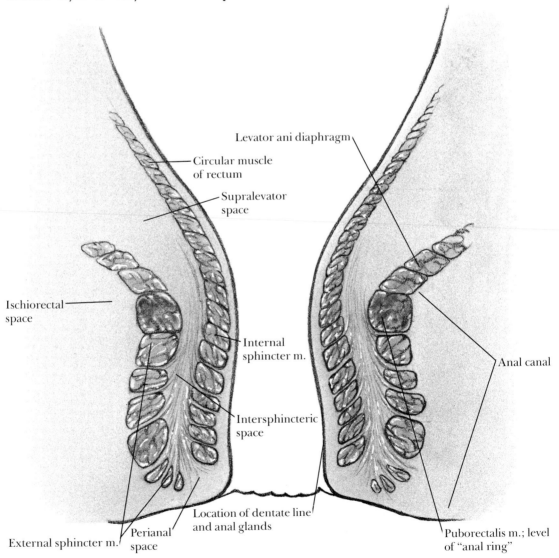

Levator ani diaphragm

Circular muscle of rectum

Supralevator space

Ischiorectal space

Internal sphincter m.

Anal canal

Intersphincteric space

External sphincter m.

Perianal space

Location of dentate line and anal glands

Puborectalis m.; level of "anal ring"

Fig. 84–1. Anatomy of Anorectal Region

of a low anterior resection, if the surgeon dissects the rectum down to the puborectalis level, it is possible to insert a finger or an instrument along the outer wall of the rectum all the way down to the perianal skin without dividing any structure. This passage takes place in the intersphincteric space external to the internal sphincter muscle and internal to the external sphincter. This fact is important in understanding the spread of infection and the formation of anal fistulas.

Above the levator ani muscle diaphragm is the pararectal or pelvirectal space that is the site of the supralevator abscess. Distal to the levator diaphragm is the ischiorectal space, the location of the common perirectal abscess (see Fig. 84–1).

Normal fecal continence requires, among other elements, the presence of a functional anorectal ring. The anorectal ring consists of the voluntary muscles at the proximal margin of the anal canal, primarily the puborectalis. When an index finger is inserted into the posterior segment of the anal canal, it is easy to identify the anorectal ring because this is the proximal margin of the external sphincter musculature, a point about 4.0–4.5 cm above the anal verge. What the finger is palpating is the proximal margin of the powerful puborectalis sling. If the finger is directed anteriorly, the proximal margin of the anal canal (the anorectal ring) will be more difficult to identify because the puborectalis sling does not encircle the anterior wall of the rectum. Before dividing any portion of the external sphincter muscle during the course of an anal fistulotomy, be certain to leave the proximal portion of this sphincter (anorectal ring) intact. This can be accomplished by inserting a probe into the fistula while the patient is awake with the index finger in the canal. If the internal opening of the fistula is at the midpoint of the anal canal, well below the anorectal ring, complete division of the portion of the internal and external sphincters distal to the midpoint will not be followed by fecal incontinence in most patients. In certain aged individuals, with marked weakness of the sphincter muscles, division of even half the internal and external sphincters will interfere with normal fecal continence.

Pathogenesis of Anorectal Abscesses and Fistulas

The following discussion of pathogenesis, classification, and treatment of anorectal abscesses and fistulas is based primarily on two excellent reports by Parks, Hardcastle, and Gordon and by Parks and Stitz, as well as the earlier work of Eisenhammer. Anorectal sepsis is believed to arise in the small anal glands situated in the intersphincteric space. These glands have ducts that discharge into the anus at a point close to the mucocutaneous junction or dentate line. After one of these glands has become infected, a small abscess forms in the intersphincteric space at the midpoint of the anal canal. Pus from a chronic intersphincteric abscess may then track in multiple directions to form various types of anal fistulas. A Type 1 fistula develops when the track extends from the intersphincteric abscess down the intersphincteric space to the perianal skin (see Fig. 84–3). In the Type 2 fistula the intersphincteric abscess erodes directly through the external sphincter muscle and the track then continues to the skin of the buttock (see Fig. 84–8). A Type 3 fistula (extremely rare) travels in a proximal direction in the intersphincteric plane, enters the supralevator space, erodes through the levator ani muscle, and continues in a distal direction to the skin of the buttock. Since this fistula encircles the entire external sphincter muscle, Parks calls it a suprasphincteric fistula (see Fig. 84–10).

The type 4 extrasphincteric fistula (extremely rare) does not arise from an intersphincteric abscess. This type of fistula reaches from the orifice in the skin of the buttock up through the ischiorectal space, through the levator ani muscle, through the supralevator space, and through the wall of the rectum above the levator diaphragm (see Fig. 84–11). Many extrasphincteric fistulas are secondary to trauma, Crohn's proctocolitis, or diverticulitis with perforation and abscess formation.

Parks, Hardcastle, and Gordon summarize the pathogenesis of anal fistula in this fashion.

> The present concept of pathogenesis strongly suggests that both abscess and fistula are one and the same disease: abscess is the acute phase, fistula the chronic . . . the epithelial channel between the anal crypt and intersphincteric gland may become blocked. In this case a fistula in the true sense of the word no longer exists; a sinus is present down to an infected primary (intersphincteric) abscess.

Treatment of Fistulas

Although Eisenhammer proposed that successful treatment of a chronic anal fistula could comprise an incision of the internal sphincter muscle in the region of the intersphincteric abscess, thus presumably eliminating the cause of the fistula, most authorities advocate identifying the site from which the fistula arose and then performing either an excision of the fistulous tract or a fistulotomy. Actually, there is no evidence that it is necessary to excise the infected anal gland that presumably gave rise to the fistula. Simple fistulotomy appears to be curative. Also, there is no data to demonstrate that excising a fistulous tract is more beneficial than simply incising it and laying it open. On the other hand, some patients present with anal pain owing to an *intersphincteric abscess* that has not yet developed into a fistula. After identifying the point of maximal tenderness in these patients, perform an internal sphincterotomy over this point (or the point of fluctuation, if present) to drain the abscess and relieve the patient's symptoms.

When a fistula appears to be suprasphincteric (Type 3) in nature, under no conditions should the surgeon divide the entire external sphincter during the fistulotomy. Since this type of fistula is extremely rare, patients suffering from this condition should be referred to a specialist. One method of management is to lay the fistula open and divide only the distal half of the sphincter mechanism. Then insert a seton of heavy silk into the portion of the tract that goes above the puborectalis muscle. Parks and Stitz left the seton in place an average of 5.4 months in these cases in order to stimulate fibrosis and permit adequate drainage of the supralevator infection. At the end of this period of time, in some cases the seton could be removed and satisfactory healing followed, but in most cases the muscles enclosed in the seton were divided to complete the operation. Most patients maintained good fecal continence after this sequence of procedures.

Parks and associates emphasized that the 400 cases included in their study were not typical of the unselected patients who would appear in the practice of a general surgeon, since many of these patients were specifically referred to the authors because of their acknowledged expertise in this area. They estimated that in an unselected series the following distribution would be more likely: intersphincteric fistulas 70%, transsphincteric 23%, suprasphincteric 5%, and extrasphincteric 2%.

Indications

> When the diagnosis of an anorectal abscess is made, operation is indicated. There is no role for conservative management because severe sepsis can develop and spread before fluctuation and typical physical findings appear. This is especially true in diabetic patients.
>
> When patients have recurrent or persistent drainage from a perianal fistula, operation is indicated.

449

Having weak anal sphincter muscles constitutes a relative contraindication to fistulotomy, especially in the unusual cases in which the fistulotomy must be performed through the anterior aspect of the anal canal. In the anterior area of the canal the absence of the puborectalis muscle explains why the sphincter mechanism is already weaker in this location.

Preoperative Care

Cathartic the night before operation and saline enema on the morning of operation

Preoperative anoscopy and sigmoidoscopy

Barium colon enema, small bowel X-ray series, or both when Crohn's enteritis or colitis is suspected

Pitfalls and Danger Points

Failing to diagnose anorectal sepsis and to perform early incision and drainage

Failing to diagnose or to control Crohn's disease

Failing to rule out anorectal tuberculosis or acute leukemia

Inducing fecal incontinence by excessive or incorrect division of the anal sphincter muscles

Operative Strategy

Localizing Fistulous Tracts

Goodsall's Rule

When a fistulous orifice is identified in the perianal skin posterior to a line drawn between 3 o'clock and 9 o'clock, the internal opening of the fistula will almost always be found in the posterior commissure in a crypt approximately at the dentate line. Goodsall's rule also states that if a fistulous tract is identified anterior to the 3 o'clock—9 o'clock line, its internal orifice is likely to be located along the course of a line connecting the orifice of the fistula to an imaginary point exactly in the middle of the anal canal. In other words, a fistula that is draining in the perianal area at 4 o'clock, in a patient lying prone, is likely to have its internal opening situated at the dentate line at 4 o'clock. There are exceptions to this rule. For instance, a horseshoe fistula may drain anterior to the anus but continue in a posterior direction and terminate in the posterior commissure.

Physical Examination

First, attempt to palpate the course of the fistula in the perianal area. Frequently the fibrosis along the tract can be identified in this fashion. Second, insert a bivalve speculum into the anus and try to identify the internal opening by gentle probing at the point indicated by Goodsall's rule. If the internal opening is not readily apparent, do not make any false passages. The most accurate method of identifying the direction of the tract is to gently insert a silver probe into the fistula with the index finger in the rectum. In this fashion it may be possible to identify the internal orifice by palpating the probe with the index finger in the anal canal.

Injection of Dye or Radiopaque Material

On rare occasions the injection of a blue dye may help identify the internal orifice of a complicated fistula. Some surgeons have advocated the use of milk instead of a blue dye. The injection of a radiopaque liquid followed by X-ray studies can be valuable for the extrasphincteric fistulas leading high up into the rectum, but it does not appear to be helpful for the usual type of fistula.

Preserving Fecal Continence

As mentioned in the discussion above, the puborectalis muscle (anorectal ring) must be functioning normally in order to preserve fecal continence following fistulotomy. It is important to identify this muscle accurately before dividing the anal sphincter muscles during the course of a fistulotomy. Use light general anesthesia without muscle relaxants whenever possible for the operation of fistulotomy. If the fistulous tract can be identified with a probe *preoperatively*, the surgeon's index finger in the anal canal can identify the anorectal ring without difficulty, especially if the patient is asked to tighten the voluntary sphincter muscles.

If there is any doubt about the identification of the anorectal ring (the proximal portion of the anal canal), then do not complete the fistulotomy but rather insert a heavy silk or braided polyester ligature through the remaining portion of the tract. Tie the ligature loosely with 5–6 knots without completing the fistulotomy. When the patient is examined in the awake state, it will be simple to determine whether the upper border of the seton has encircled the anorectal ring or whether there is sufficient puborectalis muscle (1.5 cm or more) above the seton to complete the fistulotomy by dividing the muscles enclosed in the seton, at a later stage. If no more than half of the external sphincter muscles in the anal canal have been divided, fecal continence will be preserved except in those patients who had a weak sphincter muscle prior to operation.

Fistulotomy versus Fistulectomy

In performing surgery for the cure of an anal fistula, most authorities are satisfied that incising the fistula along its entire length constitutes adequate therapy. Others have advocated the actual excision of the fibrous cylinder that constitutes the fistula, leaving only surrounding fat and mus-cle tissue behind. The latter technique leaves a larger open wound, which takes much longer to heal. Much more bleeding is encountered during a fistulectomy than a fistulotomy. There is no evidence to indicate that excising the wall of the fistula has any advantages.

Combining Fistulotomy with Drainage of Anorectal Abscess

Some surgeons have advocated, in patients with an acute ischiorectal abscess, that the surgical procedure include a fistulotomy simultaneous with drainage of the abscess. After the pus has been evacuated, a search is first made for the internal opening of the fistulous tract; then the tract is opened. This combination of operations is contraindicated for two reasons. First, 40%–50% of our patients who undergo simple drainage of an abscess never develop a fistula. It is likely that the internal orifice of the anal duct has become occluded before the abscess is treated. These patients do not require a fistulotomy. Second, acute inflammation and edema surrounding the abscess make accurate detection and evaluation of the fistulous tract extremely difficult. There is great likelihood that the surgeon will create false passages that may prove so disabling to the patient that any time saved by combining the drainage operation with a fistulotomy is insignificant.

Operative Technique—Anorectal and Pelvirectal Abscess

Perianal Abscess

In draining an anorectal abscess, it is important to excise a patch of overlying skin so that the pus will drain freely. Do not depend on packing or indwelling drains, since it is difficult to keep these drains in place unless the patient is at complete rest. The typical perianal abscess is located fairly close to the anus. Treatment consists of excising, often under local anesthesia, an ellipse of overlying skin combined with evacuation of the pus. Generally no indwelling pack is necessary if the bleeding points have been controlled by ligature or electrocoagulation.

Ischiorectal Abscess

The ischiorectal abscess is generally larger than the perianal, develops at a greater distance from the anus, and may be deep seated. Fluctuation on physical examination may be a late sign. Early drainage is indicated. Under general anesthesia, make a cruciate incision over the apex of the inflamed area. Excise enough of the overhanging skin to permit free drainage and evacuate the pus. Explore the abscess for loculations.

Intersphincteric Abscess

Many physicians fail to diagnose an intersphincteric abscess until the abscess ruptures into the ischiorectal space and forms an ischiorectal abscess. A patient who complains of persistent anal pain should be suspected of harboring an intersphincteric abscess. This is especially true if, on inspecting the anus with the buttocks spread apart, the physician can rule out the presence of an anal fissure. In order to confirm the diagnosis of an intersphincteric abscess, examination under anesthesia may be necessary, although digital examination in the unanesthetized patient may indicate at which point in the anal canal the abscess is located. Parks and Thomson found that 61% of the intersphincteric abscesses occurred in the posterior quadrant of the anal canal. In half their patients a small mass could be palpated in the anal canal with the index finger inside the canal and the thumb just outside. Occasionally an internal opening that is draining a few drops of pus can be identified near the dentate line. Rarely, a patient may have both an anal fissure as well as an intersphincteric abscess.

Under a local or general anesthesia, carefully palpate the anal canal. Then insert a bivalve speculum and inspect the circumference of the anus to identify a possible fissure or an internal opening of the intersphincteric abscess. After identifying the point on the circumference of the anal canal that is the site of the abscess, perform an internal sphincterotomy by the same technique as described in Chap. 85 for an anal fissure. Place the internal sphincterotomy directly over the site of the intersphincteric abscess. Explore the cavity, which is generally small, with the index finger. If the abscess has been properly unroofed, simply reexamine the area daily with an index finger for the first week or so postoperatively. Uneventful healing can be anticipated unless the abscess has already penetrated the external sphincter muscle and created an undetected extension in the ischiorectal space.

Pelvirectal Supralevator Abscess

An abscess above the levator diaphragm is manifested by pain (gluteal and perineal), fever, and leukocytosis; it often occurs in patients with diabetes or other illnesses. Pus can appear in the supralevator space by extension upward from an intersphincteric fistula, by penetration through the levator diaphragm of a transsphincteric fistula, or by direct extension from an abscess in the rectosigmoid area. When there is obvious infection in the ischiorectal fossa, secondary to a *transsphincteric* fistula, as manifested by local induration and tenderness, make an incision at the dependent point of the ischiorectal infection **(Fig. 84-2)**. Make the incision large enough to explore the area with the index finger. It may be necessary to incise the levator diaphragm from below and to enlarge this opening with a long Kelly hemostat in order to provide adequate drainage of the supralevator abscess. After thoroughly irrigating the area, insert gauze packing.

In those pelvirectal abscesses arising from an *intersphincteric* fistula, one will often be able to palpate the fluctuant abscess by

452

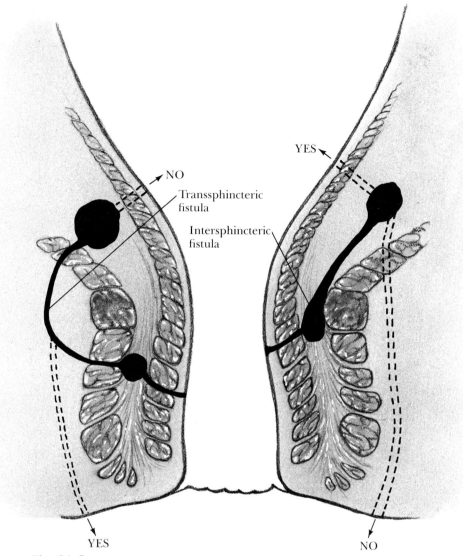

NO

Transsphincteric
fistula

Intersphincteric
fistula

YES

YES

NO

Fig. 84–2

inserting the index finger high up in the rectum. Under general anesthesia, aspirate the region of fluctuation. If pus is obtained, make an incision in the rectum with the electrocautery and drain the abscess through the rectum (Goldberg, Gordon, and Nivatvongs) (see Fig. 84–2).

Under no condition should one drain a supralevator abscess through the rectum if the abscess has its origin in an *ischiorectal* space infection (see Fig. 84–9). This error may result in a high extrasphincteric fistula. Similarly, if the supralevator sepsis has arisen from an intersphincteric ab-

scess, draining the supralevator infection through the ischiorectal fossa also leads to a high extrasphincteric fistula, and this error should also be avoided (see Fig. 84–6).

Operative Technique— Anorectal Fistula

Intersphincteric Fistula

Simple Low Fistula
When dealing with an unselected patient population, simple low fistula occurs in perhaps half of all patients presenting with

453

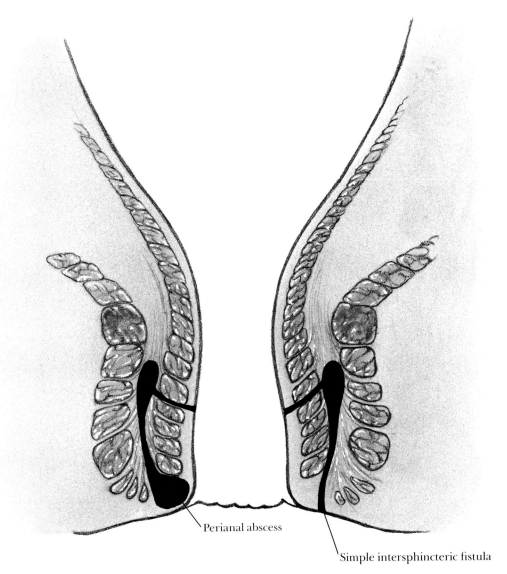

Perianal abscess

Simple intersphincteric fistula

Fig. 84–3

anorectal fistulas. Here the infected anal gland burrows distally in the intersphincteric space to form either a perianal abscess or a perianal fistula as illustrated in **Fig. 84–3.** Performing a fistulotomy in this type of case requires only the division of the internal sphincter and overlying anoderm up to the internal orifice of the fistula approximately at the dentate line. This will divide the distal half of the internal sphincter, rarely producing any permanent disturbance of function.

High Blind Track (Rare)
In this type of fistula the midanal infection burrows in a cephalad direction between the circular internal sphincter and the longitudinal muscle fibers of the upper canal and lower rectal wall to form a small *intramural* abscess above the levator diaphragm **(Fig. 84–4).** This abscess can be palpated by digital examination. The infection will probably heal if the primary focus

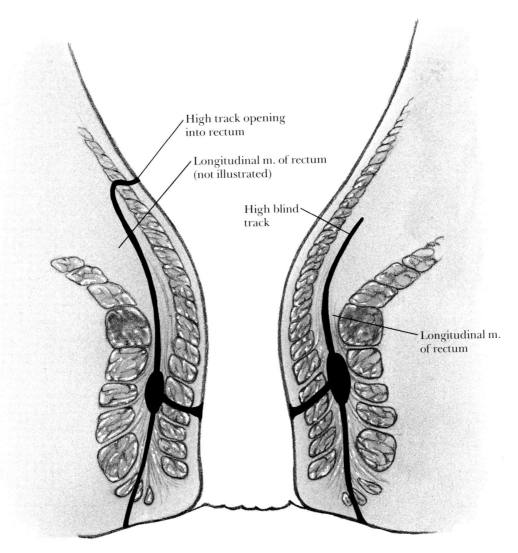

High track opening into rectum

Longitudinal m. of rectum (not illustrated)

High blind track

Longitudinal m. of rectum

Fig. 84–4. High Intersphincteric Fistulas

is drained by excising a 1 cm × 1 cm square of internal sphincter at the site of the internal orifice of this "fistula." Parks, Hardcastle, and Gordon state that even if the entire internal sphincter is divided in laying open this high blind track by opening the internal sphincter from the internal orifice of the track to the upper extension of the track, little disturbance of continence will develop because the edges of the sphincter are held together by the fibrosis produced as the track develops.

High Track Opening into Rectum (Rare)
In this type of fistula, a probe inserted into the internal orifice will continue upward between the internal sphincter and the longitudinal muscle of the rectum. The

probe will open into the rectum at the upper end of the fistula (see Fig. 84–4). If the surgeon recognizes, by palpating the probe, that this fistula is quite superficial and is located deep only to the circular muscle layer, the tissue overlying the probe can be laid open without risk. On the other hand, if the probe does in fact go deep to the *external* sphincter muscle prior to reentering the rectum (see Fig. 84–11) this constitutes a type of extrasphincteric fistula, one which is extremely difficult to manage (see below). If the surgeon has any doubt about the true nature of this type of fistula, the patient should be referred to a specialist who can employ an electromyographic needle, inserted into the tissue just deep to the track. This device can distinguish between the longitudinal muscle of the rectal wall and the voluntary external sphincter muscle.

High Track with No Perineal Opening (Rare)

In this unusual intersphincteric fistula the infection begins in the midanal intersphincteric space and burrows upward in

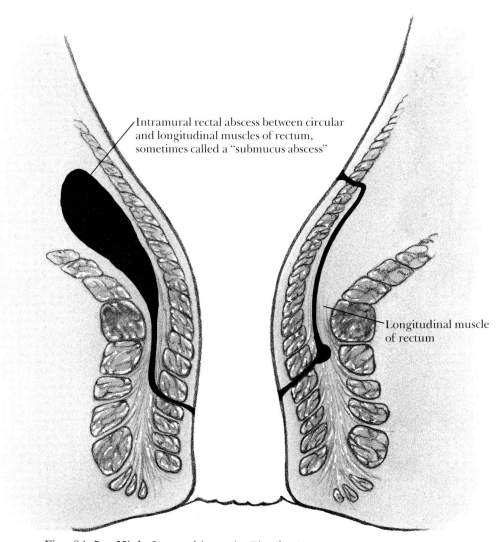

Intramural rectal abscess between circular and longitudinal muscles of rectum, sometimes called a "submucus abscess"

Longitudinal muscle of rectum

Fig. 84–5. High Intersphincteric Fistula (or abscess) with no perineal openings

456

the rectal wall, reentering the lower rectum through a secondary opening above the anorectal ring **(Fig. 84–5)**. There is no downward spread of the infection and no fistula in the perianal skin. To treat this fistula it is necessary to lay the track open from its internal opening in the midanal canal up into the lower rectum. Parks and associates emphasize that the lowermost part of the track in the midanal canal must be excised because this contains the infected anal gland that is the primary source of the infection. Leaving it behind may result in a recurrence. If a fistula of this type presents in the acute phase, it resembles a "submucus abscess," but this is an erroneous term because the infection is indeed deep not only to the mucosa but also deep to the circular muscle layer (see Fig. 84–5). This type of abscess is drained by incising the overlying mucosa and circular muscle of the rectum.

High Track with Pelvic Extension (Rare)
In this case the infection spreads upward in the intersphincteric space, breaks through the longitudinal muscle, and enters the pelvis (supralevator) **(Fig. 84–6)**.

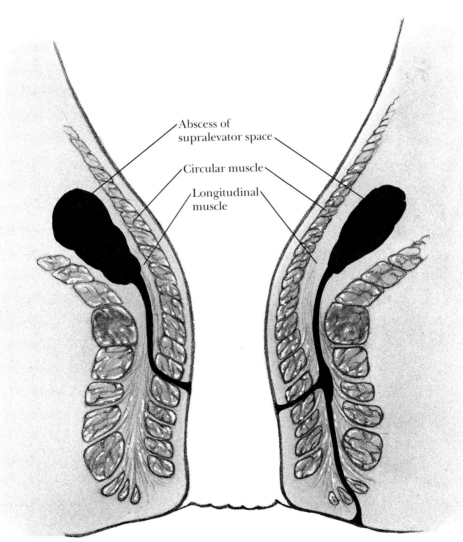

Fig. 84–6.   High Intersphincteric Tracks (with supralevator abscesses)

457

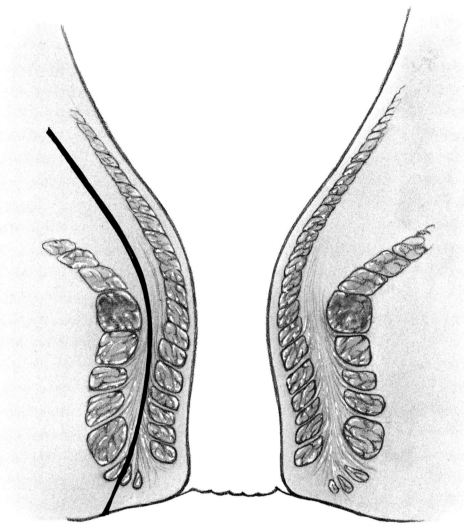

Fig. 84–7. High Intersphincteric Track (*secondary* to pelvic sepsis)

Proper treatment requires that the fistulous track be laid open by incising the internal sphincter together with the overlying mucosa or anoderm, up into the rectum for 1–3 cm, and draining the pelvic collection through this incision, the drain exiting into the rectum.

High Track Secondary to Pelvic Disease (Rare)

As mentioned above, the intersphincteric plane "is a natural pathway for infection from the pelvis to follow should it track downwards" (Parks, Hardcastle, and Gordon). This type of fistula **(Fig. 84–7)** does not arise from anal disease and does not require perianal surgery. Treatment consists of removing the pelvic infection by abdominal surgery.

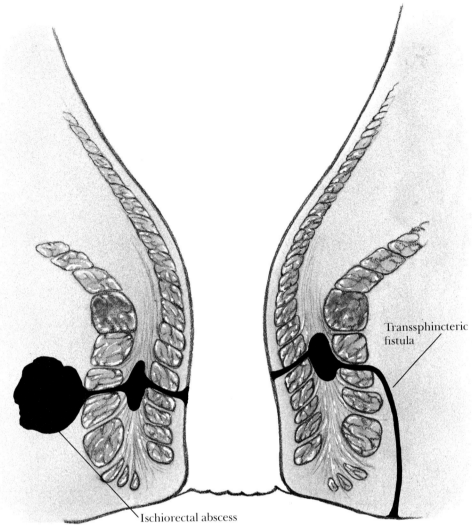

Fig. 84–8. Transphincteric Fistula and Ischio-rectal Abscess

Transsphincteric Fistula

Uncomplicated

As illustrated in **Fig. 84–8,** the fairly common uncomplicated transsphincteric fistula arises in the intersphincteric space of the midanal canal, and then the infection burrows laterally directly through the external sphincter muscle. There it may form either an abscess or a fistulous track down through the skin overlying the ischiorectal space. If a probe is passed through the fistulous opening in the skin and along the track until it enters the rectum at the internal opening of the fistula, all of the overlying tissue may be divided without serious functional disturbance because only the distal half of the internal sphincter and the distal half of the external sphincter will have been transected. Occasionally one of these fistulas crosses the external sphincter closer to the puborectalis muscle than is illustrated. In this case, if there is doubt that the entire puborectalis can be left intact, the external sphincter may be divided in two stages. Divide the distal half in the first stage. Insert a seton through the remaining fistula, around the remaining muscle bundle, and leave it intact for 2 or 3 months before dividing the remainder of the sphincter.

459

High Blind Track

In this group of patients, the fistula burrows through the external sphincter, generally at the level of the midanal canal. Then the fistula not only burrows downward to the skin but also in a caphalad direction to the apex of the ischiorectal fossa **(Fig. 84–9).** Occasionally the fistula burrows through the levator ani muscles into the pelvis. Parks, Hardcastle, and Gordon point out that when a probe is passed into the external opening, it will generally go directly to the upper end of the blind track and that the internal opening in the midanal canal may be difficult to delineate by this type of probing. Occasionally there is localized induration in the midanal canal to indicate the site of the infected anal gland that initiated the pathological process. Probing of this area should indicate the internal opening. By inserting the index finger into the anal canal, one can often feel, above the anorectal ring, the indu-

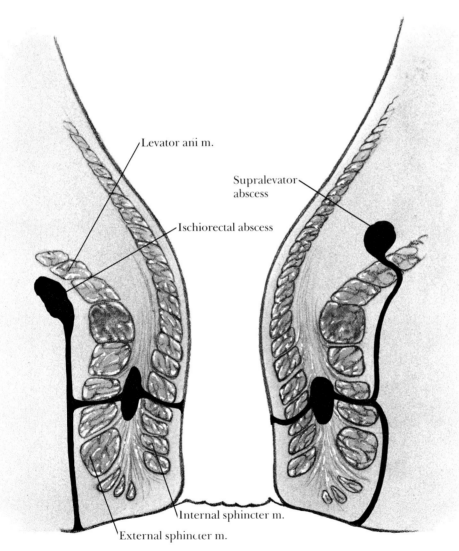

Levator ani m.

Supralevator abscess

Ischiorectal abscess

Internal sphincter m.

External sphincter m.

Fig. 84–9. Transsphincteric Fistulas (with high blind tracks)

ration that is caused by the supralevator extension of the infection. With the index finger the surgeon can often feel the probe in the fistula. The probe may feel close to the rectal wall. Parks emphasizes that it is dangerous to penetrate the wall of the rectum with this probe or to try to drain this infection through the upper rectum. If this should be done, an extrasphincteric fistula would be created with grave implications for the patient. The proper treatment for this type of fistula, even with a supralevator extension, is to transect the mucosa, the internal sphincter, the external sphincter, and the perianal skin from the midanal canal down to the orifice of the track in the skin of the buttock. The upper extension will heal with this type of drainage.

Suprasphincteric Fistula (Extremely Rare)

This type of fistula originates, as usual, in the midanal canal in the intersphincteric space where its internal opening can generally be found. The fistula extends upward in the intersphincteric plane above the puborectalis muscle into the supralevator space, where it often causes a supralevator abscess. Then the fistula penetrates the levator diaphragm and continues downward in the ischiorectal space to its external orifice in the perineal skin (**Fig. 84–10**). This type of supralevator infection must not be

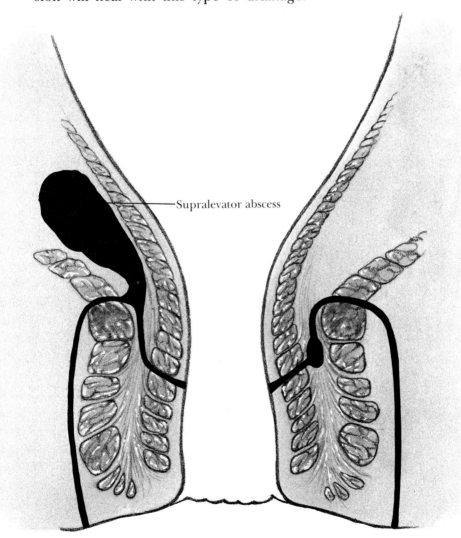

—Supralevator abscess

Fig. 84–10.   Suprasphincteric Fistulas

drained through an incision in the rectum. Parks and Stitz recommend an internal sphincterotomy from the internal opening of the fistula distally and an excision of the abscess in the intersphincteric space, if present. They then divide the lower 30%–50% of the external sphincter muscle. Continue this incision laterally until the lower portion of the fistulous track has been opened down to its external opening in the skin. This will leave the upper half of the external and internal sphincter muscles intact, as well as the puborectalis muscle. Insert a seton of heavy braided nylon through the fistula as it surrounds the muscles. Tie the seton with 5–6 knots, but keep the loop in the seton loose enough so it does not constrict the remaining muscles at this time. Insert a drain into the supralevator abscess, preferably in the intersphincteric space between the seton and the remaining internal sphincter muscle. Once adequate drainage has been established, remove this drain as the heavy seton will prevent the lower portion of the wound from closing prematurely. Parks does not remove these setons for at least 3 months. It is often necessary to return the patient to the operating room 10–14 days following the initial operation to examine the situation carefully and to ascertain that no residual pocket of infection has remained undrained. Examination under anesthesia may be necessary on several occasions before complete healing has been achieved. In the majority of cases, after 3 or more months have passed, the supralevator infection will have healed completely, and it will not be necessary to divide the muscles enclosed in the seton. In these cases, simply remove the seton and permit the wound to heal spontaneously. If after 3–4 months there is lingering infection in the upper reaches of the wound, it will be possible to divide the muscles contained in the seton because the long-standing fibrosis will not permit these muscles to retract significantly and they will generally heal with restoration of fecal continence.

Extrasphincteric Fistula (Extremely Rare)

Secondary to Transsphincteric Fistula

In this unusual situation a transsphincteric fistula after entering the ischiorectal fossa travels not only downward to the skin of the buttocks but also in a cephalad direction penetrating the levator diaphragm into the pelvis and then through the entire wall and mucosa of the rectum (**Fig. 84-11**). If this fistula were to be completely laid open surgically, the entire internal and entire external sphincter together with part of the levator diaphragm would have to be divided. The result would be total fecal incontinence. The proper treatment here consists of a temporary diverting colostomy combined with a simple laying open of the portion of the fistula that extends from the midanal canal to the skin. After the defect in the rectum heals, the colostomy can be closed.

Secondary to Trauma

A traumatic fistula may be caused by a foreign body penetrating the perineum, the levator ani muscle, and then the rectum. Also, a swallowed foreign body, such as a fish bone, may perforate the rectum above the anorectal ring and be forced through the levator diaphragm into the ischiorectal fossa. An infection in this space may then drain out through the skin of the perineum to form a complete extrasphincteric fistula. In either case, treatment consists of removing any foreign body, establishing adequate drainage, and performing a temporary colostomy. It is not necessary to divide any sphincter muscle because the anal canal is not the cause of the patient's pathology.

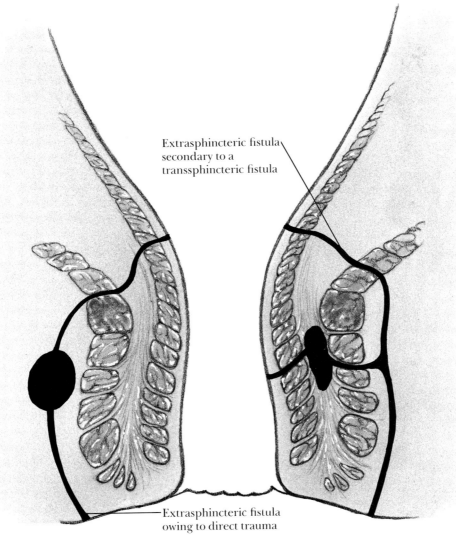

Extrasphincteric fistula
secondary to a
transsphincteric fistula

Extrasphincteric fistula
owing to direct trauma

Fig. 84–11. Extrasphincteric Fistulas

Secondary to Specific Anorectal Disease
Conditions such as ulcerative colitis, Crohn's disease, and carcinoma may produce unusual and bizarre fistulas in the anorectal area. These are not usually amenable to local surgery. The primary disease must be remedied, often requiring total proctectomy.

Secondary to Pelvic Inflammation
A diverticular abscess of the sigmoid colon or Crohn's disease of the terminal ileum or a perforated pelvic appendicitis may result in perforation of the levator diaphragm with the infection tracking downwards to the perineal skin. In making the proper diagnosis, performing an X-ray sinogram by injecting an aqueous iodinated contrast medium into the fistula may demonstrate its supralevator entrance into the rectum. Therapy in this type of fistula consists of eliminating the pelvic sepsis by abdominal surgery. There is no need to cut any of the anorectal sphincter musculature.

463

Technical Hints in Performing Fistulotomy

Position

We prefer the prone position with the patient's hips elevated on a small pillow, with the patient under light general anesthesia.

Exploration

In accordance with Goodsall's rule, search the suspected area of the anal canal after inserting a Parks bivalve retractor. The internal opening should be located in a crypt near the dentate line, most often in the posterior commissure. If an internal opening has been identified, insert a probe to confirm this fact. Then, insert a probe into the external orifice of the fistula. In a simple fistula, in which the probe goes directly into the internal orifice, simply make a scalpel incision dividing all of the tissues superficial to the probe. In this maneuver, a grooved directional probe is helpful.

In complex fistulas the probe may not pass through the entire length of the track. In some cases gentle maneuvering with various sizes of lacrimal probes may be helpful. If these maneuvers are not successful, Goldberg and associates suggest the injection of a dilute (1:10) solution of methylene blue dye into the external orifice of the fistula. Then incise the tissues over a grooved director along that portion of the track that the probe enters easily. At this point it is generally easy to identify the probable location of the fistula's internal opening. For those fistulas in the posterior half of the anal canal, this opening will be located in the posterior commissure at the dentate line. If a patient has multiple fistulas, including a horseshoe fistula, the multiple tracks generally enter into a single posterior track that leads to an internal opening at the usual location in the posterior commissure of the anal canal. In patients with multiple complicated fistulas, Goldberg and associates recommend a preoperative fistulagram X ray to help delineate the pathology.

Marsupialization

In order to accelerate healing in cases where fistulotomy results in a large gaping wound, Goldberg and associates suggested that the wound be marsupialized by suturing the outer walls of the laid-open fistula to the skin by means of a continuous absorbable suture.

In any case, curet all of the granulation tissue away from the wall of the fistula that has been laid open.

Postoperative Care

Administer a bulk laxative, such as Metamucil daily. For the first bowel movement, an additional stimulant, such as Senokot-S, 2 tablets, may be necessary.

See that the patient begins a regular diet.

For patients who have had operations for fairly simple fistulas, warm sitz baths, 2–3 times daily, may be initiated beginning on the first postoperative day, after which no gauze packing may be necessary.

For patients who have complex fistulas, a light general anesthesia may be required for the removal of the first gauze packing on the 2nd or 3rd postoperative day.

In the early postoperative period, check the wound every day or two to be sure that healing takes place in the depth of the wound before any of the more superficial tissues heal together. Later on, check the patient once or twice weekly.

When a significant portion of the external sphincter has been divided, warn the patient that for the first week or so there will be some degree of fecal incontinence.

In the case of the rare types of fistula with high extension and a deep wound, Parks and Stitz recommend that the patient be taken to the operating room at intervals for careful examination under anesthesia.

Perform a weekly anal digital examination and dilatation, when necessary, in order to avoid an anal stenosis secondary to the fibrosis that takes place during the healing of a fistula.

Postoperative Complications

Urinary retention

Postoperative hemorrhage

Fecal incontinence

Sepsis including cellulitis and recurrent abscess

Recurrent fistula

Thrombosis of external hemorrhoids

Anal stenosis

References

Eisenhammer S (1958) A new approach to the anorectal fistulous abscess based on the high intermuscular lesion. Dis Colon Rectum 106:595

Goldberg SM, Gordon PH, Nivatvongs S (1980) Essentials of anorectal surgery. Lippincott, Philadelphia

Parks AG, Hardcastle JD, Gordon PH (1976) A classification of fistula-in-ano. Br J Surg 63:1

Parks AG, Stitz RW (1976) The treatment of high fistula-in-ano. Dis Colon Rectum 19:487

Parks AG, Thomson JPS (1973) Intersphincteric abscess. Br Med J 2:537

85 Lateral Internal Sphincterotomy for Chronic Anal Fissure

Concept: Pathogenesis and Treatment of Anal Fissure

A typical anal fissure presents in its acute stage as a linear superficial tear, always distal to the dentate line and in 90% of cases in the posterior commissure of the anus. It is believed to result from the trauma of passing an inspissated stool. In the acute stage, conservative management aimed at softening the stool, combined with the local application of an anesthetic ointment may reverse the pathology in less than a week's time. When the narrow linear fissure becomes chronic, it resembles an ulcer with slightly thickened sides, measuring perhaps 1–2 mm in thickness, and the fissure widens for a distance of 3–6 mm. Characteristically, the base of a chronic anal fissure demonstrates transverse muscle fibers of the circular muscle that constitutes the internal sphincter. Further along in the development of a chronic anal fissure, a sentinel pile develops. This is an inflammatory thickening of the skin situated at the distal margin of the fissure. Once the anal fissure has reached a chronic stage, it is theorized that spasm of the internal sphincter prevents healing, while at the same time the spasm produces the intense pain on defecation that constitutes the patient's chief complaint.

In past years the surgical treatment for a chronic anal fissure consisted of excising the chronic ulcer together with a few millimeters of surrounding normal tissue, combined with the division of some part of the internal sphincter in the posterior commissure. Ferguson divided only the superficial fibers of the distal margin of the internal sphincter and achieved excellent results with the excision technique. Other authors found that, perhaps because a deeper incision was made in the internal sphincter, a keyhole deformity occurred in the posterior commissure, causing annoying seepage of stool at the point of this deformity. Eisenhammer in 1959 suggested that this problem could be averted by placing the internal sphincterotomy in the lateral aspect of the anal canal. Comparative study by a number of authorities (Goligher; Abcarian) confirmed that the results of a lateral internal sphincterotomy are superior to the older techniques. Notaras developed the method of performing the lateral internal myotomy with a sharp cataract knife through a tiny incision in the perianal skin.

When planning surgery for chronic anal fissure, be certain to rule out the possibility that this "fissure" may represent Crohn's disease, ulcerative colitis, or even a syphilitic chancre. Occasionally multiple fissures of the anus are caused by the trauma of per anal sexual intercourse. None of these conditions requires a sphincterotomy.

Indication

Chronic anal fissure

Preoperative Care

Many patients with anal fissure will not tolerate a preoperative enema due to excessive pain. Consequently, a mild cathartic the night before operation constitutes the only preoperative care necessary.

Pitfalls and Danger Points

Injury to external sphincter
Inducing fecal incontinence by overly extensive sphincterotomy
Bleeding, hematoma

Operative Strategy

Accurate identification of the lower border of the internal sphincter is essential to the successful completion of an internal sphincterotomy. Placing a bivalved speculum (like a Parks retractor) into the anal canal and opening the speculum for a distance of about two fingerbreadths will place the internal sphincter on stretch. At this time palpation will disclose a distinct groove between the subcutaneous external sphincter and the lower border of the tense internal sphincter. Palpating this groove serves to identify accurately the lower bor-

der of the internal sphincter. Optionally, the surgeon may make a radial incision through the mucosa directly over this area to identify visually the lower border of the internal sphincter, but we have not found this step to be necessary.

Operative Technique

Anesthesia

A light general or a local anesthesia are both satisfactory for this procedure.

Closed Sphincterotomy

Place the patient in the lithotomy position. (If local anesthesia is used, the prone position is also satisfactory.) Insert a Parks retractor with one blade placed in the anterior and the other in the posterior aspect of the anal canal. Open the retractor about two fingerbreadths. Now, at the right or left lateral margin of the anal canal, palpate the groove between the internal and external sphincter. Once this has been clearly identified, insert a cataract knife into this groove **(Fig. 85–1).** During this insertion keep the flat portion of the blade parallel

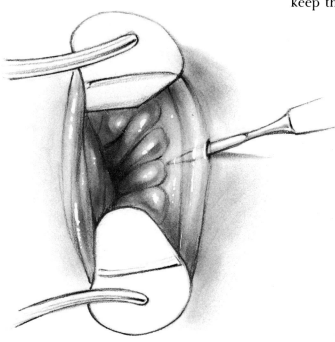

Fig. 85–1

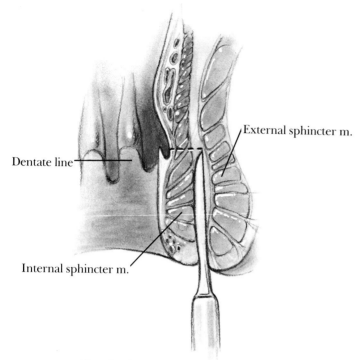

Fig. 85–2

to the internal sphincter. When the blade has reached the level of the dentate line (about 1.5 cm), rotate the blade 90° so that its sharp edge rests against the internal sphincter muscle **(Fig. 85–2).** Insert the left index finger into the anal canal opposite the scalpel blade. Then, with a gentle sawing motion transect the lower portion of the internal sphincter muscle. There is a gritty sensation while the internal sphincter is being transected, followed by a sudden "give" when the blade has reached the mucosa adjacent to the surgeon's left index finger. Remove the cataract knife and palpate the area of the sphincterotomy with the left index finger. Any remaining muscle fibers will be ruptured by lateral pressure exerted by this finger. In the presence of bleeding, apply pressure to this area for at least 5 minutes. It rarely will be necessary to make an incision in the mucosa for the identification and coagulation of a bleeding point.

An alternative method of performing the subcutaneous sphincterotomy is to insert the cataract knife between the mucosa and the internal sphincter. Then turn the cutting edge of the blade so that it faces laterally and cut the sphincter in this fashion. This approach has the disadvantage of possibly lacerating the external sphincter if excessive pressure is applied to the blade. Do not suture the tiny incision in the anoderm.

Open Sphincterotomy

In this variation, a radial incision is made in the anoderm just distal to the dentate line and carried across the lower border of the internal sphincter in the midlateral portion of the anus. Then the lower border of the internal sphincter is identified as is the intersphincteric groove. The fibers of the internal sphincter have a whitish hue. Divide the lower portion of the internal sphincter up to a point level with the dentate line. Achieve hemostasis with the electrocautery, if necessary. The skin wound may be left open and a dressing applied.

Removal of the Sentinel Pile

If the patient has a sentinel pile more than a few millimeters in size, simply excise it with a scissors. Leave the skin defect unsutured. Nothing more elaborate need be done for this condition.

If, in addition to the chronic anal fissure, the patient has symptomatic internal hemorrhoids that require surgery, hemorrhoidectomy may be performed simultaneously with the lateral internal sphincterotomy. If the patient has large internal hemorrhoids, and hemorrhoidectomy is not performed simultaneously, then it is possible that a lateral internal sphincterotomy operation may induce prolapse of these hemorrhoids.

Postoperative Care

Apply a simple gauze dressing to the anus. Remove this the following morning.

Discharge patients either the same day or the day following operation. Generally, there is dramatic relief of the patient's pain promptly after sphincterotomy.

Administer a mild cathartic (e.g., Senokot-S, 2 tablets) the night of the operation and repeat nightly until normal soft stools can be achieved without medication.

Prescribe a mild analgesic in case the patient has some discomfort in the operative site.

Postoperative Complications

Hematoma or bleeding (rare)

Perianal abscess (rare)

Flatus and fecal soiling. (Some patients complain that they have less control over the passage of flatus following sphincterotomy than they had before operation, or they may have some fecal soiling of their underwear, but generally both these complaints are temporary and rarely last more than a few weeks.)

References

Abcarian H (1980) Surgical correction of chronic anal fissure: results of lateral internal sphincterotomy vs fissurectomy—midline sphincterotomy. Dis Colon Rectum 23:31

Eisenhammer S (1959) The evaluation of the internal anal sphincterotomy operation with special reference to anal fissure. Surg Gynecol Obstet 109:583

Ferguson JA, MacKeigan JM (1978) Hemorrhoids, fistulae and fissures: office and hospital management—a critical review. In: Rob C (ed) Advances in surgery, Vol 12, Yearbook Medical Publishers, Chicago

Goligher JC (1980) Surgery of the anus, rectum and colon, 4th edn. Balliere Tindall, London

Notaras MJ (1971) The treatment of anal fissure by lateral subcutaneous internal sphincterotomy—a technique and results. Br J Surg 58:96

86 Anoplasty for Anal Stenosis

Concept: Operations for Anal Stenosis

Although most cases of anal stenosis appear to follow a previous hemorrhoidectomy, we have encountered a number of elderly patients, especially women, who developed this condition without having had any prior surgery. The etiology in these cases is not clear. However, in most cases of anal stenosis the stricture appears to be limited to the superficial layer of the anal canal without much involvement of the sphincter musculature. Because of this fact, it is not difficult to dissect the anoderm and rectal mucosa away from the muscle, making enlargement of the anal orifice possible by the simple application of the Heineke-Mikulicz principle. We have been pleased with this technique except for severe cases. When marked fibrosis occurs, construct a sliding skin flap to fill in the defect.

Indication

Symptomatic fibrotic constriction of the anal canal not responsive to simple dilatation

Preoperative Care

Preoperative saline enema

Pitfalls and Danger Points

Fecal incontinence
Slough of flap
Inappropriate selection of patients

Operative Strategy

Some patients have a tubular stricture where the fibrosis involves not only the anoderm but also the mucosa and the anal sphincters. This type of condition, frequently following inflammatory bowel disease, is not susceptible to local surgery. In other cases of anal stenosis, elevating the anoderm and mucosa in the proper plane will succeed in freeing these tissues from the underlying muscle and permitting the formation of sliding pedicle flaps to resurface the denuded anal canal subsequent to dilating the stenosis.

Fecal incontinence is avoided by performing only a gradual dilatation of the anal canal to 2–3 fingerbreadths and performing, when necessary, a lateral internal sphincterotomy.

Patients with milder forms of anal stenosis may respond to a simple internal sphincterotomy.

Operative Technique—Sliding Mucosal Flap

Incision

With the patient in the prone position and the buttocks retracted laterally by means of adhesive tape, make an incision at 12

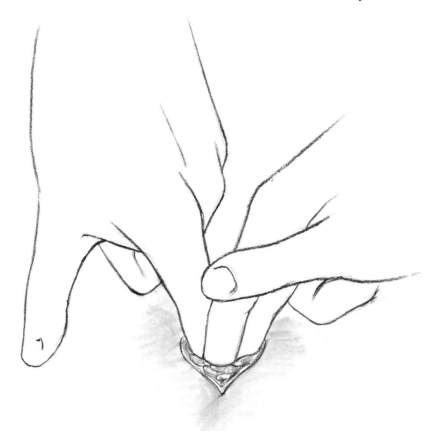

Fig. 86–1

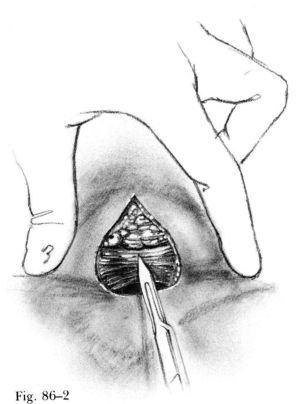

Fig. 86–2

o'clock. This incision should extend from the dentate line outward into the anoderm for about 1.5 cm, as well as internally into the rectal mucosa for about 1.5 cm. This will result in a linear incision about 3 cm in length. Elevate the skin and mucosal flaps for about 1 to 1.5 cm to the right and to the left of the primary incision. Gently dilate the anus **(Fig. 86–1)**.

Internal Sphincterotomy

Insert the bivalved Parks or a Hill-Ferguson retractor into the anal canal after gently dilating the anus. Identify the groove between the external and internal sphincter muscles. If necessary, incise the distal portion of the internal sphincter muscle, no higher than the dentate line **(Fig. 86–2)**. This should permit dilatation of the anus to a width of 2–3 fingers.

471

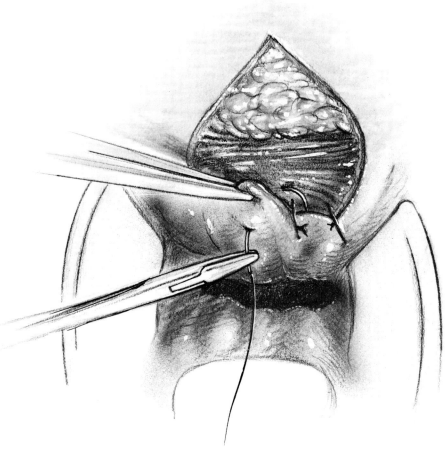

Fig. 86–3

Advancing the Mucosa

Complete the elevation of the flap of rectal mucosa. Then advance the mucosa so that it can be sutured circumferentially to the sphincter muscle **(Fig. 86–3)**. This suture line should fix the rectal mucosa near the normal location of the dentate line. Advancing the mucosa too far will result in an ectropion with annoying chronic mucus secretion in the perianal region. Use fine chromic catgut or PG for the suture material. It is not necessary to insert any sutures into the perianal skin. In a few cases of severe stenosis it may be necessary to repeat this process and create a mucosal flap at 6 o'clock **(Figs. 86–4** and **86–5).**

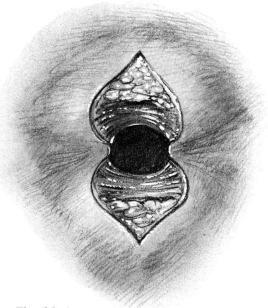

Fig. 86–4

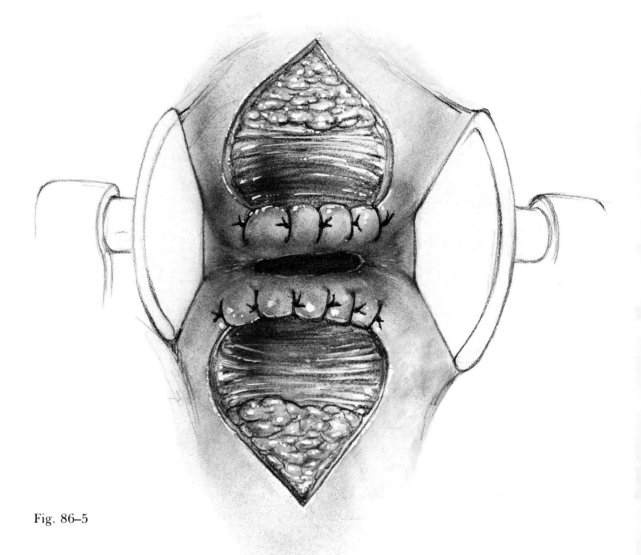

Fig. 86–5

Hemostasis should be complete following the use of accurate electrocoagulation and fine ligatures. Insert a small Gelfoam pack into the anal canal.

Operative Technique—Sliding Anoderm Flap

Incision

After gently dilating the anus so that a small Hill-Ferguson speculum may be inserted into the anal canal, make a vertical incision at the posterior commissure, beginning at the dentate line and extending upward in the rectal mucosa for a distance of about 1.5 cm. Then make a "Y" extension of this incision on to the anoderm as

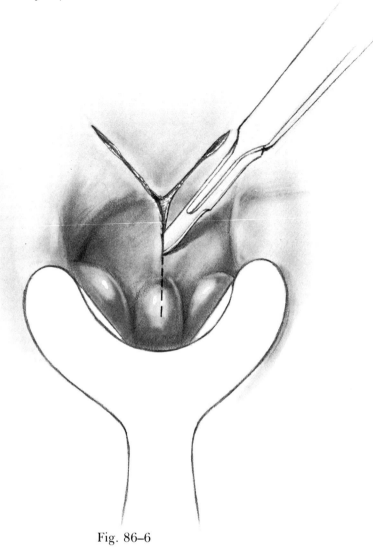

Fig. 86–6

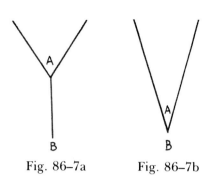

Fig. 86–7a   Fig. 86–7b

in **Fig. 86–6.** Be certain that the two limbs
of the incision in the anoderm are separated by an angle of at least 90° (angle A
in **Fig. 86–7a).** Now by sharp dissection,
gently elevate the skin and mucosal flaps
for a distance of about 1–2 cm. Take special
care not to injure the delicate anoderm
during the dissection. When the dissection
has been completed, it will be possible to
advance point A on the anoderm to point
B on the mucosa **(Fig. 86–7b)** without tension.

Internal Sphincterotomy

In most cases enlarging the anal canal will
require division of the distal portion of the
internal sphincter muscle. This may be performed through the same incision at the
posterior commissure. Insert a sharp scalpel blade in the groove between the internal and external sphincter muscles. Divide
the distal 1.0–1.5 cm of the internal sphincter. Then dilate the anal canal to a width
of 2–3 fingers.

Advancing the Anoderm

Using continuous sutures of 5–0 atraumatic Vicryl, advance the flap of anoderm
so that point A meets point B (Fig. 86–
7b and **Fig. 86–8)** and suture the anoderm
to the mucosa with a continuous suture
that catches a bit of the underlying sphincter muscle. When the suture line has been
completed, the original "Y" incision in the
posterior commissure will resemble the
"V" as illustrated in Fig. 86–7b and **Fig.
86–9.** Insert a small Gelfoam pack into the
anal canal.

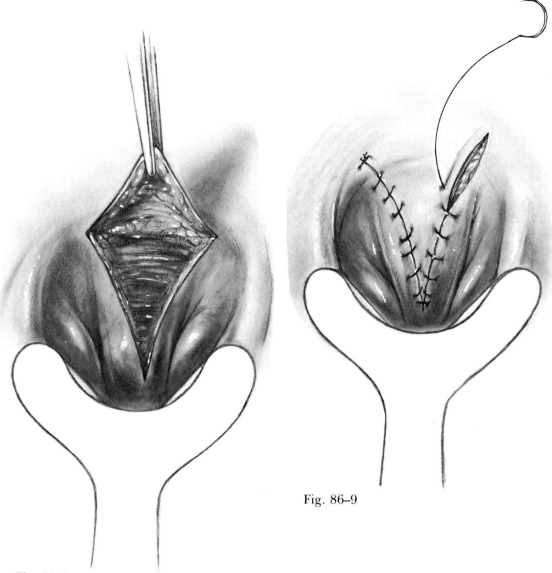

Fig. 86–9

Fig. 86–8

Postoperative Care

Remove the gauze dressings from the anal wound. It is not necessary to mobilize the Gelfoam because it will tend to dissolve in the sitz baths that the patient should initiate 2 or 3 times daily on the day following the operation.

Regular Diet
Mineral oil (45 ml) nightly for the first 2 or 3 days. Thereafter a bulk laxative, such as Metamucil, is prescribed for the remainder of the postoperative period.

Discontinue all intravenous fluids in the recovery room if there has been no untoward postanesthesia complication. This will reduce the incidence of postoperative urinary retention.

Postoperative Complications

Urinary Retention

Hematoma

Anal ulcer and wound infection (quite rare)

87 Operation for Rectal Prolapse (Thiersch)

Concept: When to Perform a Thiersch Operation

Prolapse of the rectum is, in fact, a form of intussusception with the proximal rectum and the sigmoid colon sliding through the anal canal to the outside. The concept behind the Thiersch operation is to prevent this intussusception by narrowing the diameter of the anal canal. This may be accomplished by encircling the anal sphincters with a heavy No. 20 SWG silver wire. By tying the encircling ligature with sufficient tension, intussusception and prolapse is prevented. Unfortunately, in patients who have large prolapses the wire either breaks, producing a recurrence of the prolapse, or the wire cuts through the tissues, causing an infection (Goligher). In the latter case the wire must be removed. It is uncommon for the wire repairs to last more than 1–2 years subsequent to operation.

In an attempt to prolong the successful result of the Thiersch operation, surgeons have used materials other than silver wire for the encircling ligature, such as heavy nylon, stainless steel wire, or strips of synthetic fabric, such as Prolene mesh. Lomas and Cooperman have used a four-ply strip of Marlex mesh 1.5 cm wide to encircle the anal canal in 50 patients with excellent results in 47. This modification of the Thiersch operation appears to us to be the method of choice. The great advantage of the Thiersch operation is its basic simplicity. It can be performed rapidly with minimal risk even in patients who suffer from serious concurrent disease. For good-risk patients, the Ripstein operation, described in Chap. 42, has a superior record of successful long-term followup.

Indications

The Thiersch operation is indicated in poor-risk patients who have prolapse of the full thickness of rectum. (See Vol. I Chap. 42.)

Preoperative Care

Since many patients with rectal prolapse suffer from severe constipation, cleanse the colon over a period of a few days with cathartics and enemas. Initiate an antibiotic bowel preparation 18 hours prior to scheduled operation, as for colon resection. (See Vol. I, Chap. 25.)

Pitfalls and Danger Points

Tying the encircling ligature too tight so that it cuts through the tissues

Wound infection

Injury to vagina or rectum

Operative Strategy

Selecting Proper Suture or Banding Material

We have preferred the technique of Lomas and Cooperman who recommend that the anal canal be encircled by a 4-ply layer of polypropylene mesh. Since the band is 1.5 cm in width, the likelihood that it will cut through the tissues is minimized.

Achieving Proper Tension of the Encircling Band

Although some surgeons advocate that the encircling band be adjusted to fit snugly around a Hegar dilator, we have not found this technique to be satisfactory. If the surgeon will insert an index finger into the anal canal and have his assistant adjust the tension of the encircling band so that it fits snugly around the index finger, proper tension can be achieved. If the band is too loose, prolapse will not be prevented.

Placing the Encircling Band

In order to avoid erosion of the synthetic mesh through the skin, it is important that the encircling band be placed around the anal canal approximately at its midpoint.

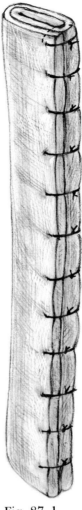

Fig. 87–1

Operative Technique—Thiersch Procedure Using Polypropylene Mesh

Fabricating the Encircling Band of Mesh

Although Lomas and Cooperman prefer Marlex mesh, we believe that Prolene mesh is preferable because of the reasons discussed in Chap. 81. Cut a rectangle of Pro-lene mesh 6 × 20 cm. Then fold the mesh over and over until one has achieved a 4-ply strip measuring 1.5 × 20 cm. Apply straight hemostats to each end of the strip in order to maintain the position. Then insert interrupted sutures at 1-cm intervals along the open end of the mesh band using 2–0 or 3–0 Prolene sutures, as illustrated in **Fig. 87–1.** Remove the two hemostats.

Incision and Position

This operation may be done either in the prone jackknife or lithotomy position, under general or regional anesthesia. We prefer the prone position. Make a 2-cm ra-

477

dial incision at 10 o'clock starting at the lateral border of the anal sphincter muscle and continue laterally. Make a similar incision at 4 o'clock. Make each incision about 2.5 cm deep.

Inserting the Mesh Band

Insert a large curved Kelly hemostat or a large right-angled clamp into the incision at 4 o'clock and gently pass the instrument around the external sphincter muscles so that it emerges from the incision at 10 o'clock. Insert one end of the prepared Prolene mesh strip into the jaws of the hemostat and draw the mesh through the upper incision and extract it from the incision at 4 o'clock. Then pass the hemostat through the 10 o'clock incision around the other half of the circumference of the anal canal until it emerges from the 4 o'clock incision. Insert the end of the mesh into the jaws of the hemostat and draw the hemostat back along this path **(Fig. 87–2)** so that it delivers the end of the mesh band into the posterior incision. At this time the entire anal canal has been encircled by the band of mesh and both ends protrude through the posterior incision. In this ma-

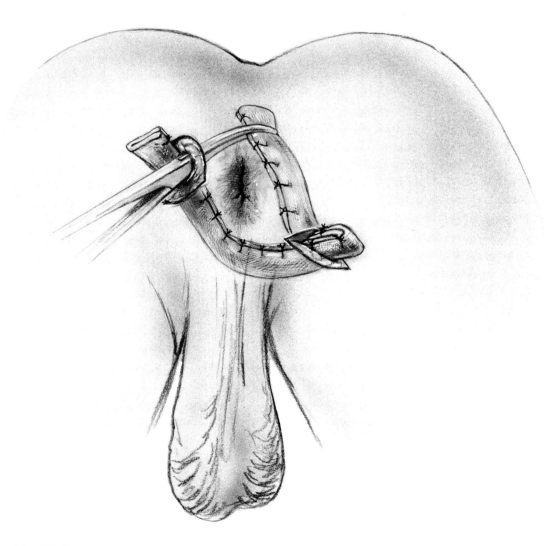

Fig. 87–2

478

nipulation be careful not to penetrate the vagina or the anterior rectal wall. Also, do not permit the mesh to become twisted during its passage around the anal canal. Keep the band flat.

Adjusting Tension

Apply a second sterile glove on top of the previous glove on the left hand. Insert the left index finger into the anal canal. Apply a hemostat to each end of the encircling band. Ask the assistant to gradually increase the tension by overlapping the two ends of mesh. When the band feels snug around the index finger, ask the assistant to insert a 2–0 Prolene suture to maintain this tension. After the suture has been inserted, recheck the tension of the band. Then remove the index finger and remove the contaminated glove. Insert 3–4 additional 2–0 Prolene interrupted sutures to approximate the two ends of the mesh and amputate the excess length of the mesh band. The patient should now have a 1.5 cm wide band of mesh encircling the external sphincter muscles at the midpoint of the anal canal with sufficient tension to be snug around an index finger in the rectum (**Fig. 87–3**).

Closure

Irrigate both incisions thoroughly with a dilute antibiotic solution. Close the deep perirectal fat with interrupted 4–0 PG interrupted sutures in both incisions. Close the skin with interrupted or continuous subcuticular sutures of the same material. Apply collodion over each incision.

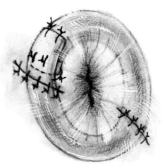

Fig. 87–3

Postoperative Care

Continue perioperative antibiotics for 3 doses.

Prescribe a bulk-forming laxative like Metamucil, plus any additional cathartic that may be necessary to prevent fecal impaction.

Initiate sitz baths after each bowel movement and two additional times daily for the first 10 days.

Postoperative Complications

If the patient develops a wound infection, it may not be necessary to remove the band. First, open the incision to obtain adequate drainage and treat the patient with antibiotics. If the infection heals, it will not be necessary to remove the foreign body.

References

Goligher JC (1980) Surgery of the anus, rectum and colon, 4th ed. Balliere Tindall, London

Lomas ML, Cooperman H (1972) Correction of rectal procidentia by use of polypropylene mesh (Marlex). Dis Colon Rectum 15:416

88 Operations for Pilonidal Disease

Concept: Pathogenesis and Selection of Optimal Operation

In past decades it was thought that a pilonidal sinus was the result of a congenital remnant of epithelium or an invagination of skin. The presence of hair in the pilonidal cyst was explained by the persistence of hair follicles in the invaginated epithelium. If this hypothesis were true, corrective surgery would require a complete excision of the congenital lesion. Consequently, wide excision of a large elliptical segment of skin down to the sacral fascia was advocated. This often left a large skin defect which could not generally be closed per primam. Consequently, complicated operations, such as sliding flaps of gluteal muscle or broad-based sliding skin flaps, were devised to close the defect. Despite the extensive surgery, primary healing was not uniformly achieved, and recurrences were not uncommon. If the wound was left open after a radical excision, healing by granulation tissue and contraction often required 6–12 months.

Evidence against the congenital theory is the fact that in 90% or more of cases, a pilonidal cyst or sinus is lined by dense fibrous tissue, and no epithelium or hair follicles can be identified (Patey and Scarff). Rather than resulting from a congenital remnant, it appears much more likely that the pilonidal sinus is an acquired disease. One mechanism, especially in the hirsute male, is the penetration of the skin by hairs in the midgluteal cleft. This apparently can take place when twisted hair is stimulated by the rolling action of the but-

tocks during the process of walking, resulting in a drilling action that permits the hair to penetrate the skin. When the hair accumulates in the subcutaneous fat, it acts as a foreign body. When the area has been contaminated by bacteria, chronic recurrent infection, abscess formation, and persistent drainage is perpetuated by the presence of the foreign body (hair). This theory of pathogenesis easily explains the presence of pilonidal sinuses in the interdigital clefts of barbers.

Whether or not the hypothesis that the entry of hair beneath the skin explains the origin of pilonidal disease, it is certainly true that the entry of hair into the healing wound following excision of a pilonidal cyst is a common cause of a recurrence.

After a histological study of excised pilonidal specimens, Bascom came to the conclusion that almost all pilonidal disease begins with an infected hair follicle in the midgluteal cleft. The infection follows the occlusion of the follicle's orifice with keratin. Then the infection ruptures through the deep side of the follicle into the subcutaneous fat, creating a pilonidal abscess. If this is a virulent infection, an acute abscess becomes the presenting complaint of the patient. In other cases a chronic pilonidal abscess with intermittent purulent drainage may occur. Eventually the abscess burrows laterally, forming additional sinuses. Based on this hypothesis of pilonidal pathogenesis, Bascom has designed a therapy based on local excision of each of

480

the dilated hair follicles (sinus pits) located in the midgluteal cleft. These are left unsutured. Drainage of the pilonidal cyst or sinus is then accomplished by a lateral incision. Granulation tissue and hair is carefully evacuated through this lateral incision. Bascom performs this surgery under local anesthesia on an ambulatory outpatient basis. He never performs definitive surgery in the presence of an acute abscess. Rather, the acute abscess is drained through a lateral incision and the definitive operation performed 5–7 days later. Bascom treated 50 consecutive cases by these principles. The mean disability was no more than 1 day. Average time for complete healing of the wounds was 3 weeks. After 24 months' followup, recurrence was noted in 8%. Each recurrence was healed within 3 weeks after similar outpatient surgery. There were no second recurrences. Although we do not have sufficient personal experience with this technique to confirm Bascom's excellent results, his basic principles appear to be sound and the results excellent. The principle of avoiding a midline incision, one that is notoriously slow to heal, may prove to be an important contribution to conservative surgery for pilonidal disease.

When a patient has a midline chronic sinus following the rupture of an infected follicle into the deep fat, hair is sucked into the depth of the sinus. The presence of loose hair in the midgluteal cleft is due to inadequate hygiene. When the patient is in a sitting position the pilonidal cyst is collapsed, but when the patient assumes the erect position, air and loose hair are sucked into the sinus as the cavity reforms when the overlying skin is no longer pressed against the sacrum.

Although none of these theories completely explains all of the manifestations of pilonidal disease, the evidence against the congenital nature of this condition encourages the trend towards conservatism in therapy. It is not necessary to perform radical excision to cure a pilonidal sinus.

In the presence of chronic infection, conservative excision of a narrow strip of skin will unroof the pilonidal cyst, will also eliminate the pits, and will permit the surgeon to remove all of the hair and chronic granulation tissue. This leaves behind the fibrous base of the pilonidal cyst. Healing of the defect can be accelerated if the opening is marsupialized by suturing the skin to the cut edge of the cyst. As the fibrous tissue contracts, the skin edges will be brought into approximation, generally within a period of 3–6 weeks. During this time, careful cleansing of the area and weekly shaving of the skin around the cyst will prevent the ingress of hair into the healing wound. Abramson has reported excellent results with this method.

Excision of pilonidal disease with primary suture of the skin is an operation that can be successfully accomplished only in carefully selected patients. Operation must be done at a time when infection is quiescent. The ideal patient for this operation will not have more than one lateral sinus tract. Preferably, the entire diseased area can be encompassed by excising a width of no more than 1.0–1.5 cm of skin and underlying fat. Plan the operation so that the dissection encompasses the pilonidal sinus tract without entering into the diseased area. If this can be accomplished by a conservative excision, then the resulting defect can be reconstructed by suturing the fat in one layer and the skin in a second layer *without excessive tension*. Simply suturing the skin together and leaving a large subcutaneous empty space will often result in postoperative infection. Similarly, closures that require large retention sutures to be tied under tension will also lead to an unacceptable number of wound failures. When a primarily sutured pilonidal wound develops a secondary wound infection that requires open drainage, the time required for eventual healing will be much longer than if a simple marsupialization operation

481

were performed in the first instance. Consequently, good judgment will restrict primary suture to those patients in whom primary healing can be assured. Holm and Hulten noted primary healing in 94% of 48 operations by this method.

Indication

Recurrent symptoms of pain, swelling, and purulent drainage

Pitfalls and Danger Points

Unnecessarily radical excision

Operative Strategy

Acute Pilonidal Abscess

If an adequate incision can be made, and all of the granulation tissue and hair removed from the cavity, a cure may be accomplished in a number of patients with acute abscesses.

Marsupialization

In this procedure a narrow elliptical incision is made unroofing the length of the pilonidal cavity. Do not excise any significant width of the overlying skin but only enough to remove the sinus pits. If this is accomplished, one can approximate the lateral margin of the pilonidal cyst wall to the subcuticular layer of the skin with interrupted sutures. At the conclusion of this procedure, there should be no subcutaneous fat visible in the wound. Healing of exposed subcutaneous fat tends to be very slow. On the other hand, the fibrous tissue lining the pilonidal cyst tends to contract fairly rapidly. This produces approximation of the marsupialized edges of skin during a period of only several weeks. There is no necessity to excise a width of skin more than 0.8–1.0 cm. Conservative skin excision is followed by more rapid healing.

Of course, all granulation tissue and hair must be curetted away from the fibrous lining of the pilonidal cyst.

Excision with Primary Suture

Successful accomplishment of primary healing requires that the pilonidal disease be encompassed by the excision of a narrow strip of skin including the sinus pits and a patch of subcutaneous fat not much more than 1 cm in width. If this can be achieved without entering the diseased area, closing the relatively shallow and narrow wound will not be difficult. Perform the dissection with the electrocautery because hemostasis must be perfect if the surgeon is to be certain that he has not transected some part of the pilonidal sinus resulting in an incomplete excision and possible contamination of the wound. If this technique has been successfully accomplished, the postoperative convalescence is quite short.

It is not necessary to carry the dissection down to the sacrococcygeal ligaments in order to assure the successful elimination of the pilonidal sinus. In essence, the surgeon is simply excising a chronic granuloma surrounded by a fibrous capsule and covered by a strip of skin containing the pits that constituted the original portal of entry of infection and hair into the abscess. For primary excision, the operation should be timed some months after an episode of acute infection so that the bacterial content of the pilonidal complex is minimal. Primary healing following this excision will require that the surgeon achieve the principles of good wound architecture. If a large segment of subcutaneous fat is excised, simply approximating the skin over a large dead space may result in temporary healing in the absence of bacteria, but eventually the wound is likely to separate. Unless the surgeon is willing to construct extensive sliding skin flaps or a Z-plasty, the operation of excision with primary closure should be restricted to those cases in whom wide excision is not necessary.

Operative Technique

Acute Pilonidal Abscess

Although it is sometimes possible under local anesthesia to excise the midline sinus pits, and to evacuate the pus and hair through this incision, in most cases the abscess points in an area away from the gluteal cleft and complete extraction of the hair will prove to be too painful to the patient. Consequently, in most cases, evacuate the pus during the initial drainage procedure and postpone a definitive operation until the infection has subsided.

Infiltrate the skin overlying the abscess with 1% lidocaine containing 1:200,-000 epinephrine. Make a scalpel incision of sufficient size to evacuate the pus and necrotic material. Whenever possible,

avoid making the incision in the midline. If it is possible to extract the loose hair in the abscess, do so. Otherwise, simply insert loose gauze packing.

Marsupialization Operation

This operation, first described by Buie in 1944, begins with the insertion of a probe or grooved director into the sinus. Then incise the skin overlying the probe with a scalpel. Do not carry the incision beyond the confines of the pilonidal cyst. If the patient has a tract leading in a lateral direction, insert the probe into the lateral sinus and incise the skin over it. Now excise no more than 3–5 mm of the skin edges on each side to include the epithelium of all of the sinus pits along the edge of the skin wound **(Fig. 88–1)**. This will expose a narrow band of subcutaneous fat between the

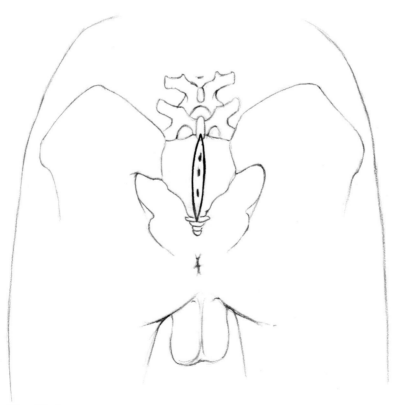

Fig. 88–1

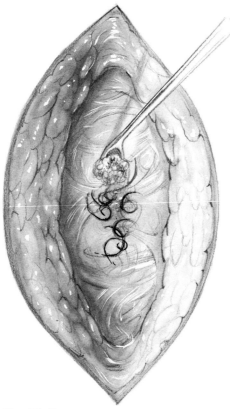

Fig. 88–2

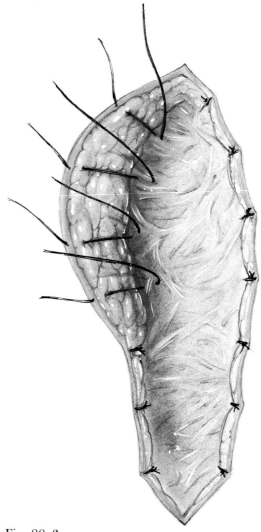

Fig. 88–3

lateral margins of the pilonidal cyst and the epithelium of the skin. Achieve complete hemostasis by carefully electrocoagulating each bleeding point.

Upon unroofing the pilonidal cyst, remove all granulation tissue and hair, if present, by using dry gauze, the back of a scalpel handle, or a large curet to wipe clean the posterior wall of the cyst **(Fig. 88–2).**

Then approximate the subcuticular level of the skin to the lateral margin of the pilonidal cyst with interrupted sutures of 3–0 or 4–0 PG **(Fig. 88–3).** Ideally, at the conclusion of this procedure there will be a fairly flat wound consisting of skin attached to the fibrous posterior wall of the pilonidal cyst, with no subcutaneous fat being anywhere visible. In the quite rare situation where the pilonidal cyst wall is covered by squamous epithelium, the marsupialization operation will be just as effective as in the great majority of cases where the wall consists only of fibrous tissue.

Although we usually perform this operation with the patient in the prone position with the buttocks retracted laterally by adhesive straps under general anesthesia, Abramson advocates local field block anesthesia for his modification of the marsupialization operation.

Pilonidal Excision with Primary Suture

Use either caudal, general, or local field block anesthesia. Place the patient in the prone position with a pillow under the hips and the legs slightly flexed. Apply adhesive strapping to each buttock and retract each

each side of the pilonidal sinus **(Fig. 88–4)**. Use the electrocoagulator for the dissection to achieve complete hemostasis. Otherwise, the presence of blood will prevent the accurate visualization that is necessary to avoid entering one of the potentially infected pilonidal tracts. Dissect the specimen away from the underlying fat without exposing the sacrococcygeal periosteum or ligaments. Remove the specimen and check for complete hemostasis. The specimen should not measure more than 5 x 1.5 x 1.5 cm in size. This makes it possible to approximate the subcutaneous fat with interrupted 3–0 or 4–0 PG sutures without tension **(Fig. 88–5)**. Insert

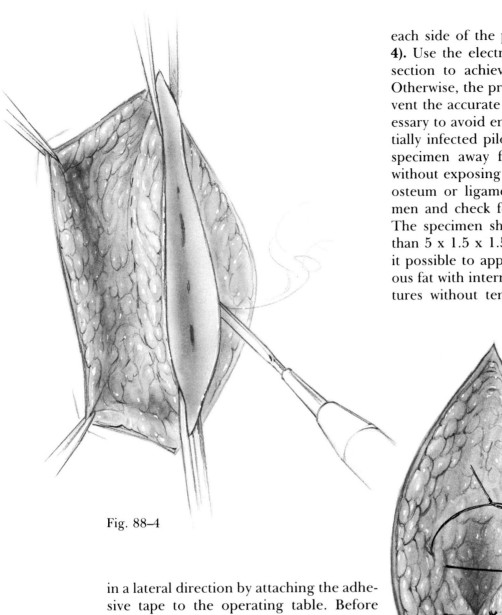

Fig. 88–4

Fig. 88–5

in a lateral direction by attaching the adhesive tape to the operating table. Before scrubbing, in preparation for the surgery, insert a sterile probe into the pilonidal sinus and gently explore the dimensions of the underlying cavity in order to confirm the fact that it is not too large for excision and primary suture.

After shaving, cleansing, and preparing the area with an iodophor solution, make an elliptical incision only of sufficient length and width to encompass the underlying pilonidal sinus and the sinus pits in the gluteal cleft (see Fig. 88–1). In properly selected patients, this will require the excision of a strip of skin no more than 1.0–1.5 cm in width. Deepen the incision on

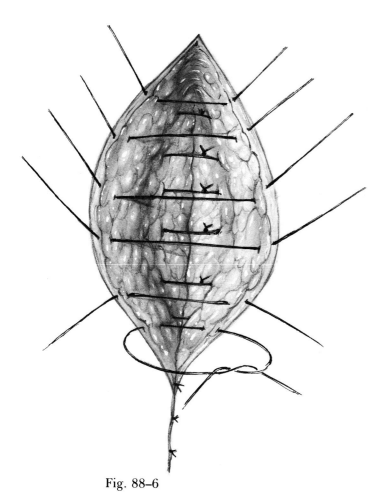

Fig. 88–6

interrupted subcuticular sutures of 4–0 PG **(Fig. 88–6)** or close the skin with interrupted nylon vertical mattress sutures. Avoid leaving any dead space in the incision. If at some point in the operation the pilonidal cyst has been inadvertently opened, irrigate the wound with a dilute antibiotic solution and complete the operation as planned unless frank pus has filled the wound. In the latter case, simply leave the wound open and insert gauze packing without any sutures.

Excision of Sinus Pits with Lateral Drainage

In Bascom's modification of Lord and Millar's operation, only the sinus pits **(Fig. 88–7)** are excised in the midgluteal cleft. This may be accomplished with a pointed #11 scalpel blade **(Fig. 88–8a),** or with the dermatologist's round skin biopsy punches. These are available in diameters as large as 5 mm. They simply represent cork borers whose ends have been sharpened to a cutting edge. Most of the pits are simply

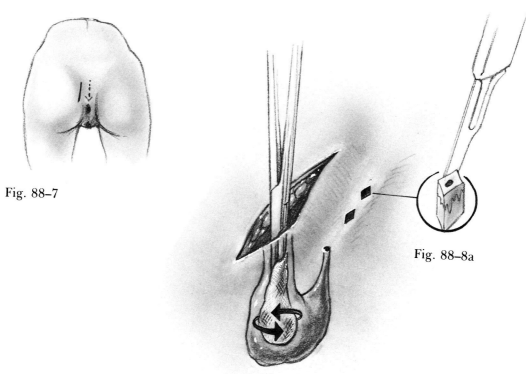

Fig. 88–7

Fig. 88–8a

Fig. 88–8b

epithelial tubes going down toward the pilonidal cyst for a distance of a few millimeters. Leave unsutured the resulting wounds from the pit excisions.

Insert a probe into the underlying pilonidal cavity to determine its dimensions. Then make a vertical incision parallel to the long axis of the pilonidal cavity. Make this incision about 1.5 cm lateral to the midgluteal cleft **(Fig. 88–8b).** Open the pilonidal cyst through this incision. Curet out all of the granulation tissue and hair. Achieve complete hemostasis with the electrocoagulator. A peanut gauze dissector is also useful in this step. Bascom does not insert any drains or packing. Occasionally three or more enlarged follicles (pits) are so close together in the midgluteal cleft that individual excision of each follicle is impossible. In this case Bascom simply excises a narrow strip of skin encompassing all of the pits. If the skin defect in the cleft exceeds 7 mm, he sutures it closed. The lateral incision is always left open. In patients who have lateral extensions of their pilonidal disease, each lateral sinus pit is excised.

Bascom found that occasionally there was an ingrowth of dermal epithelium into the subcutaneous fat forming an epithelial tube resembling a thyroglossal duct remnant. These resemble pieces of macaroni, and Bascom advises excising these epithelial tubes through the lateral incision.

Postoperative Care

Following the drainage of an *acute pilonidal abscess,* remove the gauze packing in 2 days and have the patient shower daily in order to keep the gluteal cleft clean and free of any loose hair.

Shave the skin for a distance of about 5 cm around the midgluteal cleft weekly. In some cases it is possible to use a depilatory cream to achieve the same result. Otherwise, hair will find its way into the pilonidal cavity and act as a foreign body, initiating a recurrence of infection.

Following *excision and primary suture,* remove the gauze dressing on the 2nd day and leave the wound exposed. Initiate daily showering especially after each bowel movement. Discharge the patient from the hospital, generally by the 4th postoperative day. Observe the patient closely 2 or 3 times a week in the office. If evidence of a localized wound infection appears, open this area of the wound and administer appropriate antibiotics, treating the condition in the same way as you would treat an infection in an abdominal incision. If the infection is extensive, it is necessary to lay open the entire incision. With good wound architecture, infection will be uncommon. Also, shave or apply a depilatory cream to the area of the midgluteal cleft for the first two or three postoperative weeks or until the wound is completely healed.

If the patient has undergone *pit excision and lateral drainage,* postoperative care is limited to daily showers and weekly observation by the surgeon to remove any hairs that may have invaded the wound. Bascom applies Monsel's solution to granulation tissue. All of his patients have been operated upon as ambulatory outpatients.

No matter what the operative procedure, patients with pilonidal disease require instruction to always avoid the accumulation of loose hair in the midgluteal cleft. Daily showering with special attention to cleaning this area should prevent recurrence.

Postoperative Complications

Infection may follow the primary suture operation.

Hemorrhage has been reported in the series described by Lamke, Larsson, and Nylen. Of the patients treated by wide excision and packing, 10% experienced postoperative hemorrhage requiring blood transfusion and reoperation. This complication is easily preventable by meticulous electrocoagulation of each bleeding point in the operating room. It is rare following primary suture or marsupialization operations.

In patients followed for a number of years, recurrence of pilonidal disease seems to take place in 15% of cases whether treated by primary suture, excision and packing, or marsupialization. Goligher noted that even the radical excision operation did not seem to prevent recurrence. Consequently, it appears that in most cases recurrence is caused by poor hygiene permitting hair to drill its way into the skin of the midgluteal cleft, rather than inadequate surgery.

There may be a failure to heal. Some patients, especially those who have had a radical excision of pilonidal disease which leaves a large midline defect bounded by sacrococcygeal periosteum in its depths and subcutaneous fat around its perimeter, may sometimes endure failure of healing for a period as long as 2 years (Bascom). In some cases this is due to inadequate postoperative care in which the bridging of unhealed cavities has taken place, or in which loose hair has found its way into the cavity and produced reinfection. Occasionally, even when postoperative care is conscientious in these patients, there appears to be a cessation of the continuing fibrous contracture that brings the lips of the wound together over a period of time. Bascom states that the preferred treatment is to unroof the wound widely followed by packing it with cotton saturated with Monsel's solution once or twice weekly. The patient is permitted to bathe with the packing in place. Because these midline wounds may occasionally take one or more years to heal, Bascom strongly recommends lateral incisions for pilonidal operations and claims never to have had the problem of delayed healing in his experience with the lateral incision.

References

Abramson DJ (1960) A simple marsupialization technique for treatment of pilonidal sinus; long-term follow-up. Ann Surg 151:261

Bascom J (1980) Pilonidal disease: origin from follicles of hairs and results of follicle removal as treatment. Surgery 87:567

Buie LA (1944) Jeep disease (pilonidal disease of mechanized warfare). South Med J 37:103

Goligher JC (1980) Surgery of the anus, rectum and colon, 4th ed. Balliere Tindall, London

Holm J, Hulten L (1970) Simple primary closure for pilonidal disease. Acta Chir Scand 136:537

Lamke LO, Larsson J, Nylen B (1974) Results of different types of operation for pilonidal sinus. Acta Chir Scand 140:321

Lord PH, Millar DM (1965) Pilonidal sinus: a simple treatment. Br J Surg 52:298

Patey DH, Scarff RW (1946) Pathology of postanal pilonidal sinus: its bearing on treatment. Lancet 2:484

Lymph Nodes: Axillary, Inguinal, Pelvic

89 Axillary Lymphadenectomy

Concept: When to Perform Lymphadenectomy for Melanoma

Radical axillary lymphadenectomy requires the removal of all the axillary lymph nodes. In this respect it is identical with the lymphadenectomy of a radical mastectomy. The medial boundary of the dissection is the point at which the axillary vein meets the clavicle and the lateral boundary is the anterior border of the latissimus dorsi muscle.

Lymph flows to the axilla from the skin overlying the shoulders, the upper extremity, the anterior portion of the trunk from the clavicle to the umbilicus anteriorly, and the posterior trunk down to the level of approximately L2–3. Lesions within the 2–3 cm of the midline, anteriorly or posteriorly, may drain into the opposite axilla. Although some squamous cell carcinomas of the skin metastasize to the regional lymph nodes, most regional node dissections are performed for metastases from malignant melanoma of the skin. In patients who do not have distant metastases a regional node dissection is clearly indicated in the therapy of malignant melanoma when clinical examination of the axilla discloses a metastatic node. If the melanoma is in an area contiguous to the axilla, a wide and deep resection of the primary lesion is performed in continuity with the regional node dissection. If the primary lesion is some distance from the axilla, excise the lesion, close the defect by suturing or with a skin graft, and perform the axillary dissection through a separate incision.

Although there is general agreement that a therapeutic regional node dissection is indicated when the diagnosis of a lymph node metastasis is made in the patient with melanoma, considerable controversy still surrounds the concept of a prophylactic node dissection when there is no clinical suspicion of a lymph node metastasis. Balch, Murad, Soong, Ingalls, and others have demonstrated that the thickness of the melanoma, as measured by Breslow's technique, is a direct indication of the incidence of regional lymph nodes metastasis in malignant melanoma patients. In patients whose tumor was less than 0.76 mm in thickness, no lymph node metastases occurred during a 3-year period of observation. For tumors 0.76 to 1.50 mm in thickness, 25% developed metastases; for 1.50 to 3.99 mm lesions, the corresponding figure was 51%; and for lesions greater than 4.0 mm in thickness, 62%. Roses, Harris, Hidalgo, Valensi, and others did not encounter any lymph node metastases in patients with a melanoma less than 1 mm thick. One randomized prospective study by Veronesi, Adamus, Bandiera, Brennhord, and others did not find any significant increase in survival when they compared immediate with delayed node dissection in patients suffering from melanoma of the extremities who had clinically negative regional nodes. On the other hand, Balch and associates, in a retrospective study, noted that the actuarial 5-year survival rate increased from 37% following wide local excision alone to 83% when wide excision was combined with a prophylactic regional node dissection in patients who suffered from melanomas that

491

were 1.50 to 3.99 mm in thickness. A number of other retrospective studies have also concluded that elective regional node dissections were indicated in the higher risk melanoma patient (Breslow; Cohen, Ketcham, Felix, Li et al.; Das Gupta; Holmes, Moseley, Morton, Clark et al.; and Wanebo, Fortner, Woodruff, MacLean et al.). Although increasing thickness of the primary lesion and the number of metastases to the regional nodes are the two most significant factors in worsening the prognosis of a malignant melanoma, other factors contribute to an adverse prognosis: the presence of ulceration in the melanoma, the location of the primary lesion on the trunk as opposed to the extremities; its location in the lower extremity as opposed to the upper; and the sex of the patient (male rather than female).

Some patients present to the physician with a metastatic lymph node when no primary lesion can be detected. It is believed that in these cases the primary melanoma has undergone complete regression. Therapy in such cases consists of performing a regional node dissection, and the prognosis is not worse than the more common situation following wide excision of the primary lesion together with the therapeutic node dissection.

Indications

Palpable lymph node metastases from primary malignancies involving the skin of the upper extremity and shoulder, the skin of the breast and upper trunk

Malignant melanoma involving the skin in the regions listed above, if the depth of invasion is 1.5 mm or more, when lymph nodes are clinically negative

If tylectomy for breast cancer is performed, axillary lymphadenectomy is indicated for purposes both of therapy and staging.

Preoperative Care

Undertake survey to rule out distant metastasis.

Pitfalls and Danger Points

Nerve injury (lateral pectoral nerve, brachial plexus)

Injury to axillary vein

Operative Strategy

Fundamentally, this operation employs the same strategy as that used for the modified radical mastectomy. Adipose and lymphatic tissues anterior and inferior to the axillary vein are excised en bloc from the clavicle to the anterior border of the latissimus muscle. Adequate exposure requires that the arm be flexed on the trunk to relax the major pectoral muscle during the medial part of the dissection; and the minor pectoral muscle must be divided. We generally excise most of the minor pectoral muscle to be certain that all of Rotter's lymph nodes are removed. The long thoracic and thoracodorsal nerves may be preserved if they are not involved with tumor.

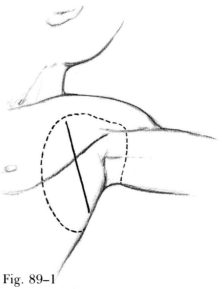

Fig. 89–1

Operative Technique (Also see Chap. 45)

Incision

The skin incision, in a general way, follows the course of the axillary vein. Start the incision over the pectoralis major and continue laterally across the axilla to the level of the latissimus muscle. The area of skin to be dissected is outlined by the dotted line in **Fig. 89–1.** Elevate both the superior and inferior skin flaps leaving no more than 7–8 mm of fat on the skin. The superior dissection will expose the anterior surface of the major pectoral muscle in its medial aspect, the fat overlying the axillary vein and brachial plexus in the middle, and the coracobrachialis and latissimus muscles laterally **(Fig. 89–2).** Dissect the lower flap for a distance of 8–10 cm.

Exposing the Axillary Contents

Incise the fascia overlying the lateral border of the major pectoral muscle. Dissect this fascia away from the undersurface of the muscle. Insert a Richardson retractor beneath the pectoral muscle and expose the coracobrachial muscle. Dissect fat and fascia off the inferior surface of the coracobrachial muscle and continue this dissection toward the coracoid process where the coracobrachial meets the minor pectoral muscle. Encircle the minor pectoral muscle with the index finger and divide it near

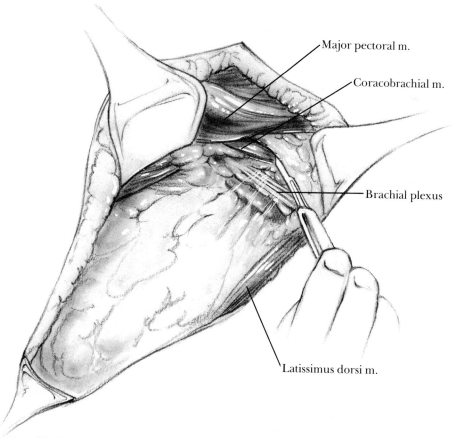

Major pectoral m.

Coracobrachial m.

Brachial plexus

Latissimus dorsi m.

Fig. 89–2

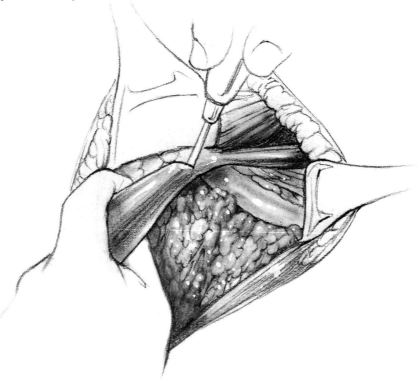

Fig. 89–3

its insertion using the electrocoagulator **(Fig. 89–3)**. Branches of the medial pectoral nerve will be seen entering the minor pectoral muscle near its *lateral* border. Divide these nerves, but take care to *protect the pectoral nerve that emerges along the medial margin of the minor pectoral muscle* because this nerve will largely constitute the innervation of the major pectoral muscle. Freeing the upper half of the pectoralis minor from the chest wall will improve exposure for the axillary dissection.

Incise the fat along the anterior border of the latissimus muscle to identify the lateral boundary of the lymphadenectomy.

Incise the thin layer of costocoracoid ligament at a level calculated to be just cephalad to the course of the axillary vein. Do not skeletonize the nerves of the brachial plexus as this may produce a permanent painful neuritis. After dividing this ligament, sweeping the loose fat in a caudal direction will generally expose the axillary vein.

Clearing the Axillary Vein

Identify the axillary vein in the lateral portion of the axilla. Elevate its adventitia with a Brown-Adson or DeBakey forceps and incise it with a Metzenbaum scissors. Continue this division of the adventitia in a medial direction until the clavicle is reached. Several branches of the lateral anterior thoracic and thoracoacromial nerves and blood vessels will be encountered crossing over the axillary vein. Divide each of these between small Hemoclips.

Dissect the adventitia in a caudal direction exposing the various branches of the axillary vein coming from below. Divide and ligate or clip each of the branches that enters the axillary vein on its inferior surface **(Fig. 89–4)**. Preserve the subscapular vein, which enters the posterior wall of the axillary vein.

Dissecting the Chest Wall

Incise the clavipectoral fascia on a line parallel to and just caudal to the axillary vein beginning at the level of the clavicle and

494

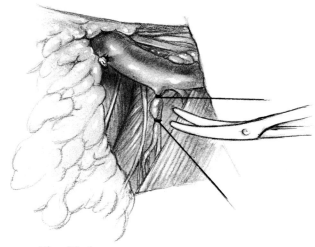

Fig. 89–4

continuing to the subscapular space. Suture a label to the lymph nodes at the apex of the dissection (near the clavicle). Make a vertical incision in the fascia from the apex of the dissection downward for 4–6 cm parallel to the sternum. Now sweep the

lymphatic and adipose tissue in a lateral direction exposing the ribs and intercostal musculature. Bleeding points may be controlled with electrocoagulation. Use the cautery also to excise part of the minor pectoral muscle leaving its proximal half attached to the thorax. Divide the intercostobrachial nerve that emerges from the second intercostal space and enters the specimen.

At this point in the dissection, the anterior and inferior portion of the axillary vein will have been cleared, as well as the upper 6–10 cm of the anterior chest wall.

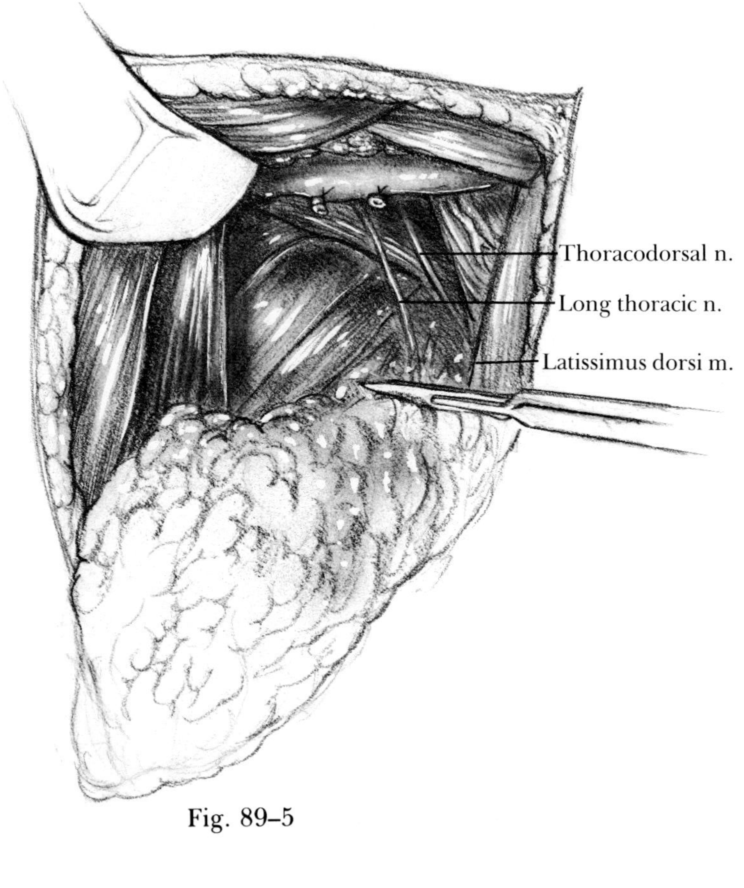

Subscapular Space

In the subscapular space, use a gauze pad to bluntly dissect the loose fat and areolar tissue from above downward to clear the space between the scapula and the lateral chest wall. This will expose the long thoracic nerve which tends to hug the thoracic cage. Identify the thoracodorsal nerve, which crosses the subscapular vein and moves laterally together with the vessels supplying the latissimus muscle (**Fig. 89–5**).

If the anterior border of latissimus muscle was not dissected free during the first step in this operation, liberate this muscle at this time, preserving the thoracodorsal nerve. Now dissect the specimen free of the chest wall after dissecting out and preserving the long thoracic nerve.

Label the lateral margin of the lymph node dissection to orient the pathologist.

Drainage and Closure

Make a puncture wound in the anterior axillary line about 10 cm below the armpit and pass a plastic multiperforated catheter through the puncture wound into the apex of the axillary dissection near the point where the axillary vein goes under the clavicle. It may be necessary to suture the catheter in place with fine catgut.

Thoracodorsal n.

Long thoracic n.

Latissimus dorsi m.

Fig. 89–5

495

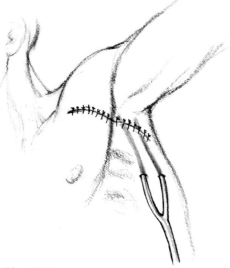

Fig. 89-6

Close the skin incision with interrupted 4–0 nylon sutures or skin staples. Attach the catheter to a closed-suction drainage device **(Fig. 89–6)**.

Postoperative Care

Maintain suction on the catheter till the drainage is less than 30 ml per day. Then remove the catheter.

Limit abduction of the arm during the first postoperative week. Thereafter encourage the patient to exercise the shoulder joint through its entire range of motion.

Encourage the patient to achieve full ambulation on the day following operation.

Later in the postoperative course, a seroma may develop under the skin flap. Aspirate the fluid once or twice weekly as necessary.

Postoperative Complications

Hematoma or seroma
Wound infection

References

Balch C, Murad T, Soong SJ, Ingalls A et al. (1979) Tumor thickness as a guide to surgical management of clinical Stage I melanoma patients. Cancer 43:883

Breslow A (1975) Tumor thickness, level of invasion and node dissection in Stage I cutaneous melanoma. Ann Surg 182:72

Cohen MH, Ketcham AS, Felix EL, Li S-H, et al. (1977) Prognostic factors in patients undergoing lymphadenectomy for malignant melanoma. Ann Surg 186:635

Das Gupta TK (1977) Results of treatment of 169 patients with primary cutaneous melanoma: a five-year prospective study. Ann Surg 186:201

Holmes EC, Moseley S, Morton D, Clark W et al. (1977) A rational approach to the surgical management of melanoma. Ann Surg 186:481

Reintgen DS, McCarty KS, Woodard B, Cox E et al. (1983) Metastatic malignant melanoma with an unknown primary. Surg Gynecol Obstet 156:335

Roses D, Harris M, Hidalgo D, Valensi Q et al. (1982) Primary melanoma thickness correlated with regional lymph node metastases. Arch Surg 117:921

Veronesi V, Adamus J, Bandiera CC, Brennhord ID et al. (1977) Inefficacy of immediate node dissection in Stage I melanoma of the limbs. N Engl J Med 297:627

Wanebo HJ, Fortner JG, Woodruff J, MacLean B et al. (1975) Selection of the optimum surgical treatment of Stage I melanoma by depth of microstage technique (Clark-Breslow). Ann Surg 182:302

90 Inguinal and Pelvic Lymphadenectomy

Concept: When to Perform Inguinal and Pelvic Lymphadenectomy
(See also Chap. 89.)

Groin lymphadenectomy is comprised of two separate lymph node groups: inguinal and pelvic. The inguinal nodes are located in the femoral triangle, based on the inguinal ligament with its apex formed by the crossing of the adductor longus and the sartorius muscles. The pelvic component of the dissection includes the lymph nodes in a triangular area whose apex is formed by the bifurcation of the common iliac artery and whose base is essentially the fascia over the obturator foramen. If the *inguinal* lymphadenectomy specimen is negative for metastases from the primary malignant melanoma or epidermoid carcinoma of the skin of the extremities or lower trunk, performing the *pelvic* dissection is probably unnecessary because the incidence of positive nodes will then be less than 5% (Holmes et al.)

For primary carcinoma of the external genitalia, the vulva, or the vagina, often a combined excision of the primary lesion together with bilateral inguinal lymphadenectomy is carried out. When a patient has a primary epidermoid carcinoma of the anus that is accompanied by metastatic lymph nodes in the groin, radical lymphadenectomy does not appear to influence prognosis and is therefore not indicated. Patients who have epidermoid carcinoma of the skin, in general, are not subjected to prophylactic groin lymphadenectomy, but rather the node dissection is postponed until a suspicious node is palpated. As discussed in Chap. 89, for patients with malignant melanomas 1.5 mm or more in thickness, prophylactic lymphadenectomy is warranted. If a patient has a melanoma of the trunk in the midline or within 2 cm of the midline, tumor emboli may metastasize either to the ipsilateral or the contralateral groin or axilla.

Indications

Metastatic involvement of inguinal lymph nodes secondary to malignant melanoma or epidermoid carcinoma of the skin of the lower extremity, the lower trunk, or the external genitalia.

Preoperative Care

Administer perioperative systemic antibiotics.

Prior to hospitalization, have the patient's lower extremity measured for a fitted elastic stocking to cover the area from the toes to the upper thigh (e.g., Jobst).

Check for distant metastases by performing chest X ray and liver scan.

Pitfalls and Danger Points

Impairing the viability of the skin flaps

Injuring iliofemoral artery or vein, or femoral nerve and its branches

497

Operative Strategy

Preserving Skin Viability

Traditionally, surgeons have used a vertical elliptical incision centered on the femoral vessels and have emphasized a wide dissection of thin skin flaps. This often led to areas of necrosis in the dissected skin. Delayed healing by secondary intention will then cause some degree of subacute cellulitus and occlusion of collateral lymphatic pathways, thus increasing the incidence or severity of postoperative lymphedema of the extremity. It is not necessary to dissect the skin flaps beyond the confines of the femoral triangle. The less the dissection, the less the impairment of blood supply to the skin flaps. Also, we agree with Holmes and associates that a primarily oblique skin incision along the inguinal crease is less prone to loss of viability than is the vertical type of incision.

Exposing the Iliac Region

In exposing the region of the iliac vessels for a pelvic lymphadenectomy, two approaches have commonly been employed. One involves vertical division of the inguinal ligament along the line of the iliofemoral vein with later resuturing of this ligament and the floor of the inguinal canal. In some patients the suture line is insecure and this results in a hernia. Also, patients in whom this approach is employed appear to have an increased number of skin complications. An alternative approach to the pelvis for iliac lymphadenectomy is to perform a second incision in the lower abdomen parallel to and about 3–4 cm cephalad to the inguinal ligament. After this incision has been carried through the transversalis fascia, the peritoneal sac is retracted upward to expose the iliac vessels and their adjacent fat and lymph nodes. Exposure by this approach is adequate and closing the incision is simple.

Operative Technique

Incision and Exposure

Position the lower extremity so that the thigh is mildly abducted and flexed as well as being externally rotated. Support the leg in this position by a firm pillow or sand bag.

Start the incision 2–3 cm cephalad and medial to the anterior superior spine of the ilium. Continue caudally to a point 1–2 cm below the inguinal crease. Continue along the inguinal crease in a medial direction until the femoral vein has been reached. At this point curve the incision gently in a caudal direction for about 5 cm as noted in **Fig. 90–1**. Elevate the cephalad skin flap with rake retractors. Use either the electrocautery with a low cutting current or a scalpel to dissect the skin flap in a superior direction in a plane that leaves 4–5 mm of subcutaneous fat on the skin. In obese patients, we make the plane of dissection somewhat deeper than 4–5 mm; in thin patients, we make the skin flap

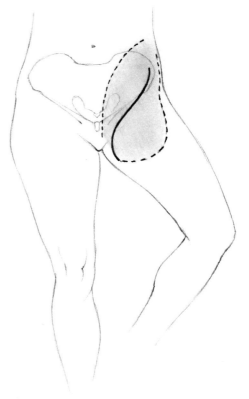

Fig. 90–1

somewhat thinner. As a skin flap is dissected toward the outer margin of the operative field, increase the thickness of the flap in a tapered fashion so that the base of the flap is thicker than its apex. The cephalad margin of the dissection should be 5–6 cm above the inguinal ligament.

Now dissect the inferior skin flap in a similar fashion. Remember that it is not necessary to elevate this skin flap beyond the lower boundaries of the femoral triangle. The lateral boundary consists of the medial border of the sartorius muscle. The lateral aspect of the adductor longus muscle is the medial boundary. The apex of the femoral triangle constitutes the point where the sartorius muscle meets the adductor longus. Dissecting the skin beyond

the femoral triangle has no therapeutic value and may impair the blood supply to the skin.

Exposing the Femoral Triangle

Initiate the dissection along a line parallel and 5–6 cm cephalad to the inguinal ligament. Incise the fat down to the aponeurosis of the external oblique muscle. Then, using a scalpel, dissect the abdominal fat off this aponeurosis down to and beyond the inguinal ligament. In men, identify and preserve the spermatic cord as it emerges from the external inguinal ring **(Fig. 90–2).**

Use a scalpel or Metzenbaum scissors to incise the fat overlying the adductor longus muscle just below the inguinal ligament about 2 cm medial to the pubic tubercle. Expose the muscle fibers of the

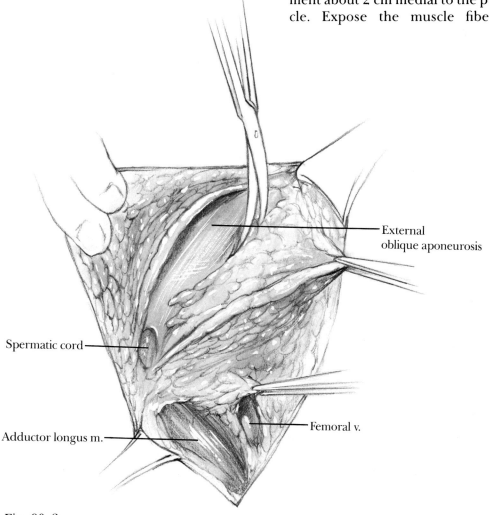

External
oblique aponeurosis

Spermatic cord

Femoral v.

Adductor longus m.

Fig. 90–2

adductor muscle and use a scalpel to dissect the fat and fascia down along the lateral border of this muscle. Continue the dissection along this muscle in a caudal direction to a point where the sartorius muscle crosses the lateral margin of the adductor longus muscle. Sweep the muscle fascia, fat, and lymph nodes in a medial direction **(Fig. 90–3).** At the apex of the femoral triangle, identify, ligate, and divide the internal saphenous vein. Then incise the fascia overlying the sartorius muscle beginning at the apex of the femoral triangle and continuing in a cephalad direction up to the origin of the sartorius muscle at the iliac bone. Sweep the fat, lymphatic tissue, and fascia overlying the sartorius muscle by dissecting in a medial direction.

Dissecting Femoral Artery, Vein, and Nerve

Identify the femoral artery and vein near the apex of the femoral triangle. Using Metzenbaum scissors dissection, elevate the areolar tissue and fat from the anterior surfaces of the femoral vessels proceeding in a cephalad direction (Fig. 90–3). Dissect the specimen from the medial border of the femoral triangle in a lateral direction to expose the medial aspect of the femoral vein. There are no branches on this side of the vein. Identify the entrance of the internal saphenous vein into the anterior surface of the femoral vein. Ligate and divide the saphenous vein. This dissection

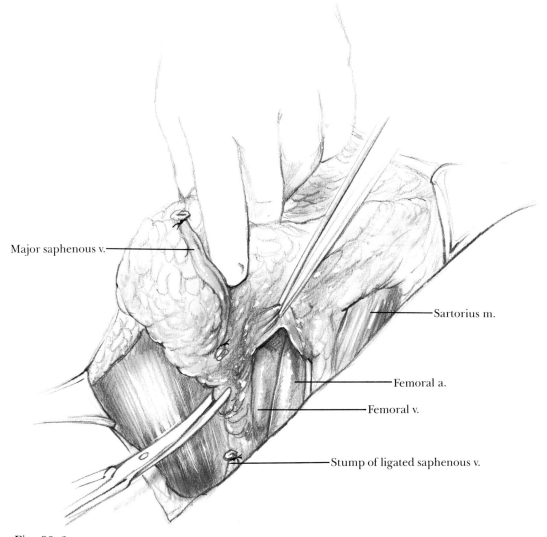

Major saphenous v.

Sartorius m.

Femoral a.

Femoral v.

Stump of ligated saphenous v.

Fig. 90–3

will have exposed the pectineus muscle deep to the femoral vein and medial to the adductor longus muscle. The femoral canal is located deep to the inguinal ligament just medial to the femoral vein. Remove and identify the cephalad lymph node situated in this triangle. Label it for the pathologist. Continue to dissect the specimen laterally exposing the length of the femoral artery. Several small arterial branches going to the specimen have to be divided and ligated before the specimen can be separated from this vessel.

Take note of the fact that the femoral nerve, situated just lateral to the femoral artery, is covered by a thin fibrous layer of the femoral sheath. Carefully incise this layer at a point below the inguinal ligament and lateral to the femoral artery. Identify and preserve the branches of the femoral nerve as it passes deep to the sartorius muscle. After this step, detach the specimen and submit it for frozen section pathological examination to determine the presence of metastatic disease in the lymph nodes.

Irrigate the operative field with a dilute antibiotic solution and achieve complete hemostasis by means of PG ligatures and electrocoagulation. If the inguinal specimen does not contain any metastatic lymph nodes, terminate the operation and omit the pelvic lymphadenectomy. If metastatic lymph nodes are found, proceed to a pelvic lymphadenectomy.

The appearance of the operative field at the conclusion of the inguinal lymphadenectomy is illustrated in **Fig. 90–4.**

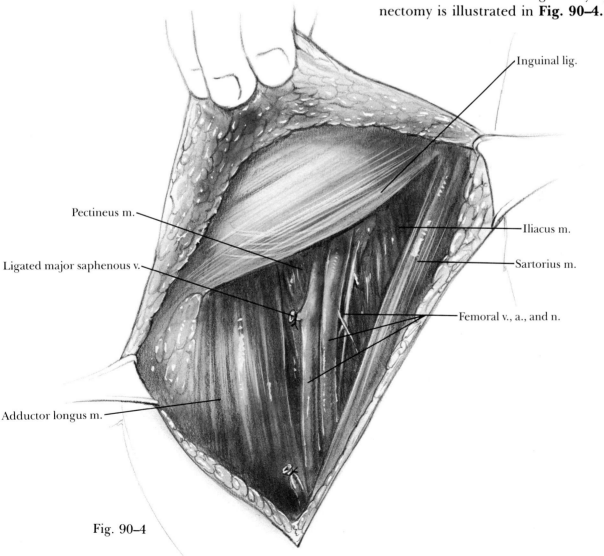

Inguinal lig.

Pectineus m.

Iliacus m.

Ligated major saphenous v.

Sartorius m.

Femoral v., a., and n.

Adductor longus m.

Fig. 90–4

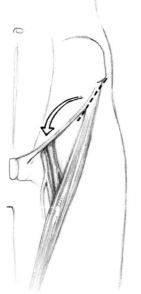

Fig. 90-5

Transposing Sartorius Muscle

In some patients necrosis of the skin overlying the femoral vessels may occur and thus endanger the viability of these structures. In order to protect the femoral artery and vein from the consequences of a possible slough, transpose the sartorius muscle in a medial direction so that it lies over the femoral vessels **(Fig. 90–5).** Transect the sartorius muscle at its insertion by using the electrocoagulating device **(Fig. 90–6).** Free the proximal 6–7 cm of this muscle from underlying attachments and transpose it in a medial direction so that it is now situated in a vertical line overlying the femoral vessels. Suture the cut end of the sartorius muscle to the inguinal ligament using interrupted 3–0 Tevdek sutures **(Fig. 90–7),** prior to closing the skin.

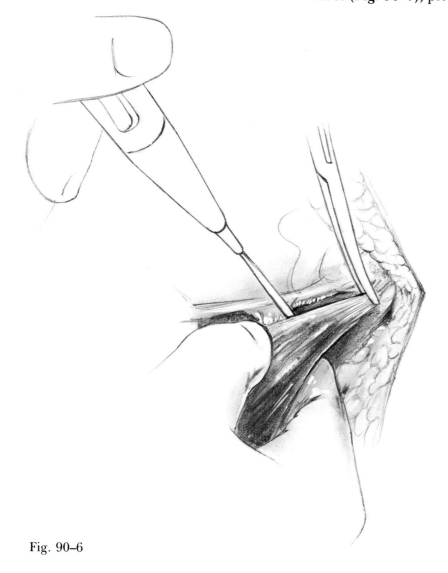

Fig. 90–6

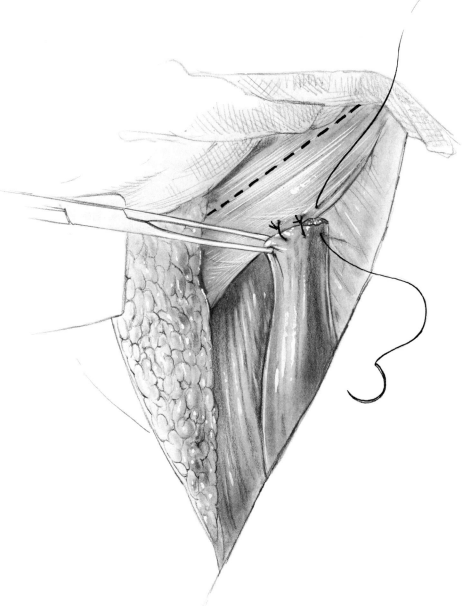

Fig. 90–7

Pelvic Lymphadenectomy

Make an incision with the scalpel in the direction of the fibers of the external oblique aponeurosis at a level about 3–4 cm above the inguinal ligament from the region above the external inguinal ring to the anterior superior spine (Fig. 90–7). Next, divide the underlying internal oblique muscle with the electrocoagulator. Carry the incision through the transversus muscle together with the underlying transversalis fascia but not through the perito-neum. This procedure is similar to that used in Chap. 77 for the exposure required in a Cooper's ligament repair of an inguinal or femoral hernia. Identify the deep inferior epigastric artery and vein arising just above the inguinal ligament from the external iliac artery and vein. Ligate and divide the deep inferior epigastric vessels. Now use gauze dissection to sweep the

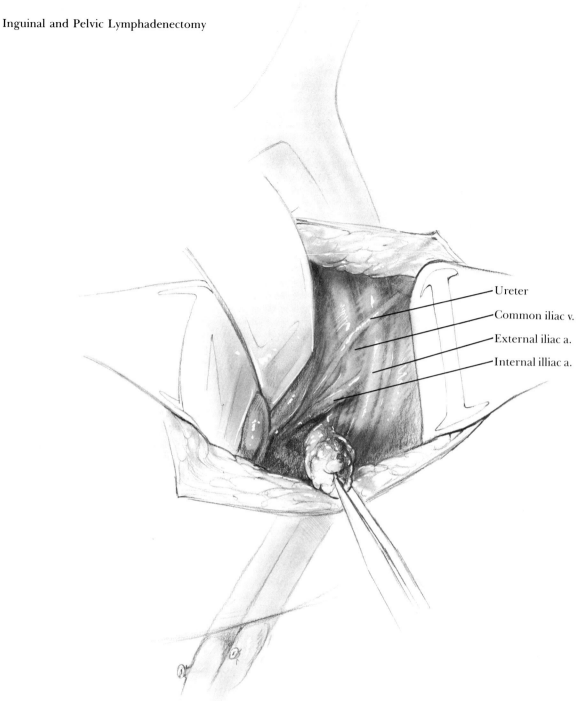

Fig. 90–8

peritoneum together with the abdominal contents in a cephalad direction. Insert a moist gauze pad and a wide deep retractor to elevate these structures out of the pelvic cavity. *Identify and preserve* the ureter. Generally it will remain adherent to the peritoneal layer and will have been elevated out of the pelvis together with the abdominal structures behind the retractor.

The area to be dissected is that contained between the external iliac and the internal iliac vessels down to the obturator membrane overlying the obturator foramen **(Fig. 90–8).**

Initiate the mobilization by dissecting the lymph nodes and fat overlying the external iliac artery and vein beginning at the inguinal ligament and proceeding in a cephalad direction to the junction with the internal iliac vessels. Be careful in clearing fat and lymphatic tissue from the iliac vein since this structure is quite fragile. Lacerations of the vein produce considerable hemorrhage and are difficult to control. After sweeping the fat and lymphatic tissues from the apex of the dissection in a downward direction, identify and preserve the obturator artery and vein. Terminate the dissection at this point and remove the specimen. Hemostasis is achieved in this dissection primarily by careful application of Hemoclips and ligatures. After hemostasis is assured, irrigate the pelvis with a dilute antibiotic solution.

Now close the incision of the lower abdomen in layers by inserting interrupted 2–0 cotton sutures into the transversalis fascia and the overlying aponeurosis of the transversus muscle; then into the internal oblique muscle; and finally into the external oblique aponeurosis. Close the defect in the femoral canal by suturing the inguinal ligament down to either Cooper's ligament or the pectineus fascia from below. No drains are placed in the pelvis.

Skin Closure and Drainage

Drain the area of the femoral triangle by passing two perforated plastic catheters, 3.0 mm in internal diameter, through puncture wounds in the area of the inguinal lymphadenectomy. Attach the catheters to a closed-suction drainage device. Irrigate the operative field again with a dilute antibiotic solution. Trim away any portion of the skin that seems devitalized. Close the skin with interrupted sutures of 4–0 nylon.

Postoperative Care

Continue perioperative antibiotics.

Continue closed-suction drainage until the volume is less than 40 ml per day.

In the operating room, apply the elastic stocking that was manufactured preoperatively to fit this patient's lower extremity.

Keep the patient at bed rest with the extremity elevated for no more than 2 or 3 days. Thereafter, although the patient is permitted to walk, he should not spend much time in a chair. Rather, much of the day should be spent in bed with the leg elevated. After discharge from the hospital, the patient should continue to wear a snug elastic stocking up to the upper thigh for at least 6 months. For the first 6–8 weeks he should lie down with the leg elevated for 1 hour 3 times daily. Otherwise permanent lymphedema of the extremity is likely to occur.

Postoperative Complications

Skin necrosis is preventable if care is taken in preparing the skin flaps and if unnecessarily extensive dissection of the skin flaps is avoided.

Reference

Holmes EC, Mosely S, Morton D, Clark W et al. (1977) A rational approach to the surgical management of melanoma. Ann Surg 186:481

Head and Neck

91 Parotidectomy

Concept: How Much Gland to Remove for a Parotid Tumor

In designing an operation for the removal of benign tumors of the parotid gland, two important facts must be noted. First, although over 75% of parotid tumors are benign, the vast majority of these benign tumors are mixed tumors (pleomorphic adenomas). Simple enucleation of a mixed tumor is followed by a high recurrence rate. Often the *recurrent* mixed tumor will become malignant. Consequently, a wide margin of normal salivary gland must be excised around the benign mixed tumor. Second, although the parotid gland is not anatomically a truly bilobed structure, for purposes of surgical anatomy it may be considered to have a superficial and deep lobe with the branches of the facial nerve passing between these two structures. Consequently, it is feasible to excise the superficial lobe with preservation of the branches of the facial nerve. This dissection will be indicated for most patients who have mixed tumors of the parotid gland. A few mixed tumors will arise in the deep lobe of the gland. In these cases, perform a superficial parotid lobectomy in order to identify each of the facial nerve branches. Then, with preservation of the facial nerve, remove the deep lobe. The Warthin tumor (papillary cystadenoma lymphomatosum) does not require a margin of normal parotid tissue and may be enucleated. However, in most cases the surgeon will not be able to make a positive diagnosis of a Warthin's tumor preoperatively so that most of these tumors will also require exposure of the facial nerve and a partial superficial lobectomy. Small mixed tumors may similarly require a dissection of the facial nerve only in the region of the tumor. Then the tumor may be resected with a good margin of parotid tissue by doing a partial superficial lobectomy.

Malignant tumors of the parotid gland, unless unusually small in size, should be removed by total parotidectomy with excision of that portion of the facial nerve lying within the parotid gland. The nerve may be reconstructed by using microsurgery to insert a nerve graft, which is often taken from the auriculotemporal nerve.

Indications

Tumors of parotid gland

Chronic sialadenitis or calculi of the parotid ducts

Pitfalls and Danger Points

Damage to facial nerve and its branches

Failure to excise a mixed tumor with a sufficient margin of normal parotid tissue

509

Operative Strategy

Locating and Preserving the Facial Nerve

Some surgeons prefer to locate the major trunk of the facial nerve by first identifying a peripheral branch such as the marginal mandibular branch. Then they trace this nerve backward toward its junction with the cervical facial branch and finally to the main facial trunk. However, most authorities prefer to identify the main trunk of the facial nerve posterior to the parotid gland as the initial step in the nerve dissection. Before it enters the parotid gland, the main facial nerve is a large structure, often measuring 2 mm in diameter. Once this main trunk is identified, the key to dissection technique is to use either a fine, blunt-tipped Jones scissors or a mosquito hemostat. The closed hemostat tip is inserted in the plane immediately anterior to the nerve. After the surgeon gently opens the hemostat, the assistant will cut the loose fibrous tissue that attaches the nerve to the overlying parotid gland. Never divide any parotid tissue before identifying the facial nerve and its branches.

If the proper plane of dissection is maintained, bleeding is rarely a problem. Most bleeding vessels will consist of small veins. These will generally stop with application of gauze pressure. An important part of the dissection technique is for the surgeon to apply pressure on the tissue posterior to the nerve with gauze while the assistant applies tension to the superficial lobe of the parotid gland using either Allis clamps or small retractors. An occasional small vein will have to be clamped with a small mosquito hemostat and tied with a fine absorbable ligature. Electrocautery may be used for hemostasis in areas of the dissection away from the facial nerve and its branches.

Using a nerve stimulator has not generally been found useful in this dissection.

The surgeon should have sufficient familiarity with the appearance of the facial nerve so that he can make a positive visual identification. Occasionally some fibers of questionable nature attach to the facial nerve branches. These may be tested by gently pinching the fiber. Then look at the cheek for muscle twitching. This, of course, requires that the entire cheek and the corner of the eye be exposed when the surgical field is draped.

The key to successful nerve preservation is early identification of the main facial trunk. The facial nerve emerges from the skull through the stylomastoid foramen. This is situated just anterior to the mastoid process and just below the external auditory canal. Beahrs emphasizes that if the surgeon will place the tip of his index finger over the mastoid process with the fingertip aimed toward the nose, the middle of his finger will be pointing to the facial trunk which will emerge about 0.5 cm anterior to the center of the fingertip and perhaps 1 cm deep to the external surface of the mastoid process. An idea of the depth at which the nerve will emerge can be gained by identifying the posterior digastric muscle and tracing it toward its insertion deep to the mastoid process. The nerve will cross at a level equivalent to the surface of the digastric muscle. In other words, dissect along the anterior surface of the sternomastoid muscle and the mastoid process posterior to the parotid gland. There will be no vital structure in this plane crossing superficial to the main trunk of the facial nerve.

There is a tiny arterial branch (posterior auricular artery) crossing just superficial to the facial trunk. If the exposure is not adequate for accurate clamping and ligating, simple pressure will stop bleeding from this vessel if it has been transected. Consequently, focus intense attention on an area about 1 cm in diameter just anterior to the mastoid process and about 1 cm deep to its surface. This is where the facial trunk will be found unless there is a tumor in the deep portion of the parotid gland that has displaced the nerve to a more superficial plane. The cephalad margin of this 1 cm area of intense attention may be considered to be the fissure between the external auditory canal and the superior portion of the mastoid process.

Another point of caution in avoiding nerve damage is the elevation of the skin flap along the inferior border of the parotid. Avoid elevating the caudal portion of the flap beyond the anterior edge of the parotid gland before the facial nerve dissection because the marginal mandibular branch of the facial nerve emerges from the parotid gland together with the posterior facial vein with which the nerve may be in contact. This is the smallest branch of the facial nerve and the easiest to injure since it is quite superficial at this point. Damage to this nerve will cause weakness in the area of the lateral portion of the lower lip.

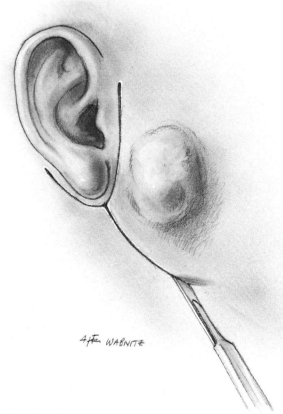

Fig. 91–1.

Operative Technique

Incision and Exposure

Although many incisions have been devised for this operation, we prefer the one illustrated in **Fig. 91–1.** It starts in a skin crease just anterior to the tragus and continues in the form of a "Y" as shown. Continue the posterior limb of the incision over the mastoid process in a caudal direction roughly parallel to the underlying sternomastoid muscle down to a point about 1 cm below the angle of the mandible. Do not make the angle of the "Y" too acute. Carry the incision through the platysma muscle. Obtain hemostasis with accurate electrocoagulation. Apply small rake retractors to the anterior skin flap and strongly elevate the tissue in the plane just deep to the platysma. As soon as the surface of the parotid gland is exposed, continue the dissection with a small Metzenbaum scissors. Some of the fibrous tissue attaching the parotid gland to the overlying tissue will resemble tiny nerve fibers. There are no facial nerve fibers superficial to the parotid gland. Therefore each of these fibers may be rapidly divided. If a total superficial lobectomy is planned, continue the dissection in a cephalad direction to the level of the zygomatic process and anteriorly to the anterior margin of the parotid gland. Do not continue the dissection beyond the anterior and inferior margins of the gland as the small facial nerve branches may inadvertently be injured if this is done prior to identifying the facial nerve.

Elevate the skin flaps and the lobe of the ear in a cephalad posterior direction to expose the underlying sternomastoid muscle, the mastoid process, and the cartilage of the external auditory canal. Elevate the posterior flap to expose 1–2 cm of underlying sternomastoid muscle. Obtain complete hemostasis. Some surgeons prefer to place a few sutures to temporarily attach the skin flaps to the underlying cheek, maintaining exposure of the gland.

511

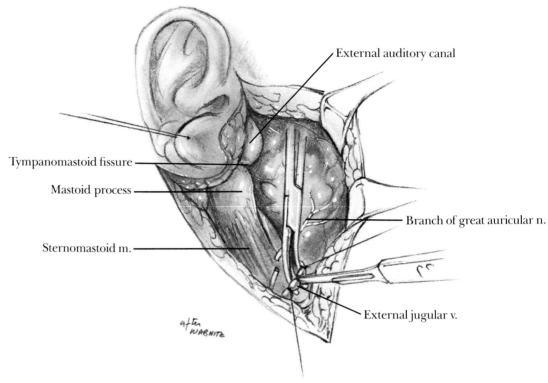

External auditory canal

Tympanomastoid fissure

Mastoid process

Sternomastoid m.

Branch of great auricular n.

External jugular v.

after WARNITZ

Fig. 91–2.

Exposing the Posterior Margin of the Parotid Gland

Identify the great auricular nerve overlying the surface of the sternomastoid muscle about 3–4 cm caudal to the mastoid process. Divide the branch of the great auricular nerve that enters the parotid gland. Adjacent to this nerve will be found the external jugular vein, which is generally also divided and ligated posterior to the parotid gland **(Fig. 91–2).** Now expose the anterior border of the sternomastoid muscle. Continue this dissection in a cephalad direction toward the mastoid process. In dissecting the tissues away from the anterior surface of the mastoid process, some bleeding may occur from branches of the superficial temporal vessels. These may be controlled by accurate clamping or electrocoagulation.

Locating the Facial Nerve

Running from the tympanomastoid fissure to the parotid gland is a fairly dense layer of temporoparotid fascia. Elevate this layer of fascia with a small hemostat or right-angle clamp and divide it **(Fig. 91–3).** Continue the dissection deep along the anterior surface of the mastoid process. Remember that the main trunk of the facial nerve is located in a 1 cm area anterior to the tympanomastoid fissure and the upper half of the mastoid process at 0.5–1.0 cm depth. Try to identify the small arterial branch of the posterior auricular artery in this area. Divide and ligate it. If it has been

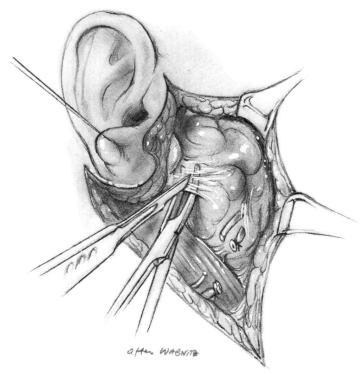

after WABNITZ

Fig. 91–3.

inadvertently divided and accurate clamping cannot be achieved, simply apply pressure for a few minutes and the bleeding will stop. Continue the blunt dissection using a hemostat until the posterior portion of the parotid gland can be retracted away from the mastoid process. Continuing to separate and divide the fibrous tissue in this area will uncover the main trunk of the facial nerve. Although the nerve usually runs in a transverse direction from the mastoid process toward the gland, it sometimes can run obliquely from the upper left portion of the operative field toward the right lower portion as it enters the parotid gland. Some idea of how deep the dissection must be carried to expose the facial nerve can be obtained by observing the depth of the surface of the posterior digastric muscle as it reaches its origin behind the mastoid process. The nerve will be at or just superficial to this level (**Fig. 91–4**).

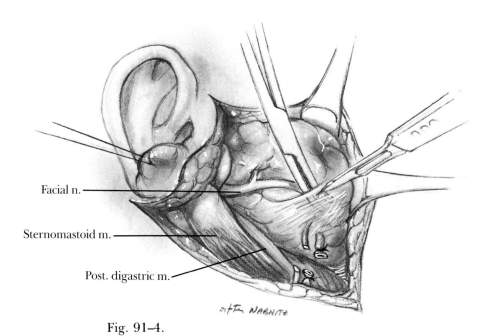

Facial n.

Sternomastoid m.

Post. digastric m.

after WABNITZ

Fig. 91–4.

Dissecting the Facial Nerve Branches

Now apply traction to the superficial lobe of the parotid using either several Allis clamps or retractors. Insert a small hemostat in the plane *just superficial* to the facial nerve. Ask the assistant to divide the fibrous tissue being elevated by the hemostat (see Fig. 91–4). Continue the dissection in this plane until each of the branches of the facial nerve has been separated from the overlying parotid tissue. Pay special attention to the cervical division and its marginal mandibular branch as this will permit elevation of the lowermost portion of the parotid gland. As the dissection reaches the anterior margin of the parotid gland, identify Stensen's duct. Ligate with 3–0 PG and divide the duct (**Fig. 91–5**). After all of the nerve branches have been identified and the duct has been divided, remove the superficial lobe of the gland.

Hemostasis during the nerve dissection can generally be achieved by gauze pressure. At this point in the dissection, carefully identify each bleeding point and clamp it with a mosquito hemostat. Ligate with 4–0 or 5–0 PG. Do not use electrocautery in areas close to the nerve.

Removing Deep Lobe of Parotid Gland (When Indicated)

First, excise the superficial lobe of the parotid as described above. Then, carefully free the lower division of the facial nerve from the underlying tissue. By retracting one or more of these divisions, one can begin to mobilize the deep lobe.

Identify the posterior facial vein. Separate the marginal mandibular nerve branch from the vein. Then divide and ligate the posterior facial vein with 4–0 PG as in **Fig. 91–6**. Now divide the superficial temporal artery and vein as in **Fig. 91–7**. Elevate the lower border of the gland and divide and ligate the external carotid artery. Then divide and ligate the internal maxillary and the transverse facial arteries at the anterior border of the gland, after which the deep lobe may be removed. The

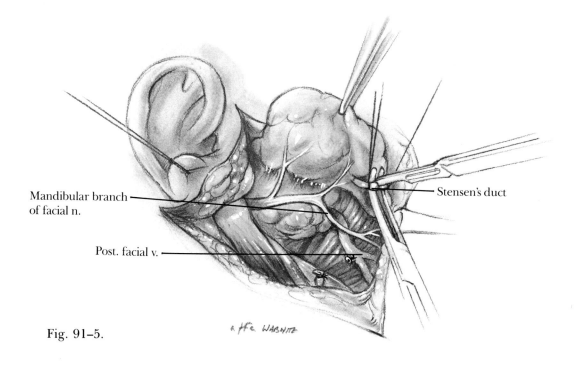

Mandibular branch of facial n.

Post. facial v.

Stensen's duct

Fig. 91–5.

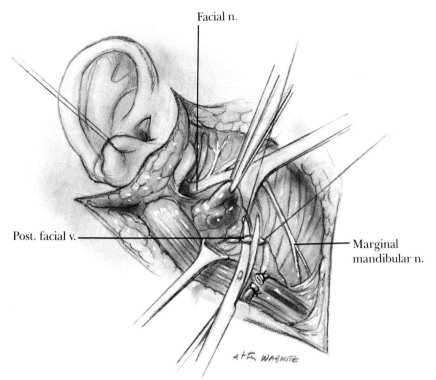

Facial n.

Post. facial v.

Marginal
mandibular n.

Fig. 91–6.

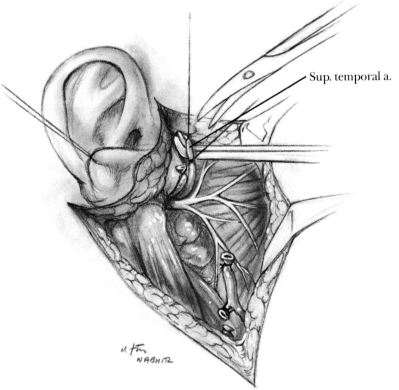

Sup. temporal a.

Fig. 91–7.

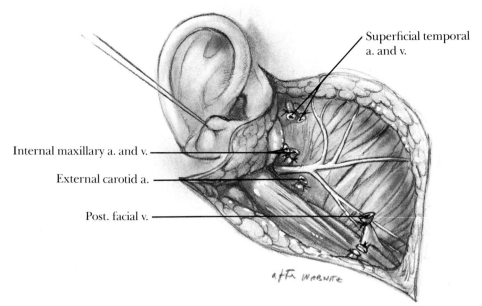

Fig. 91–8.

appearance of the operative field after removing the deep lobe is seen in **Fig. 91–8.**

Drainage and Closure

Place a small Silastic closed-suction drain through a puncture wound posterior to the incision. Close the incision using interrupted 5–0 PG sutures to the platysma and subcutaneous fat. Close the skin with interrupted 5–0 nylon sutures.

Postoperative Care

Leave the closed suction drain in place until the drainage has essentially ceased (3–4 days).

Postoperative Complications

Gustatory sweating, or Frey's syndrome, manifested by the occurrence of almost painful sweating in the skin of the operative area while eating, may occur to some extent in as many as 25% of patients. This is believed to be due to the regrowth of parasympathetic motor nerve fibers of the auriculotemporal nerve into cutaneous nerve fibers of the skin flap. This crossed innervation of the sweat glands produces uncomfortable gustatory sweating. Loré states that this may be prevented by removing a section of the auriculotemporal nerve during surgery of the parotid gland.

Facial weakness due to nerve damage

Hematoma

A salivary fistula may appear when a significant portion of the parotid gland had been left intact. This complication will generally correct itself with expectant treatment.

Infection

References

Beahrs OH (1977) Parotidectomy. Surg Clin North Am 57:477

Loré JM (1962) An atlas of head and neck surgery, Saunders, Philadelphia

Woods JE (1983) Parotidectomy: points of technique for brief and safe operation. Am J Surg 145:678

92 Thyroidectomy

Concept: Which Diseases of the Thyroid Require Operation

Hyperthyroidism

Diffuse Toxic Goiter

Most patients with diffuse hyperthyroidism or Grave's disease are now treated with radioactive iodine. This method has the advantage of simplicity and safety, although a longer period of time is required to correct the hyperthyroidism than is necessary with surgery. Operating on a toxic thyroid gland is more difficult than excising a solitary adenoma. The gland is larger and more vascular, especially if the patient has been prepared with propylthiouracil or methimazole. A recent advance in this area has been the use of propanolol for the preoperative preparation of a toxic patient. When an adequate dose has been administered, the symptoms of hyperthyroidism disappear quite rapidly and the thyroid gland is less vascular than is the case after the more traditional preparatory medications. Nevertheless, even a highly skilled thyroid surgeon experiences a 5% morbidity rate, including laryngeal nerve damage (less than 1%) and permanent hypoparathyroidism (less than 1%). Transient postoperative hypoparathyroidism may occur in an additional 5%–10% of cases.

Earlier fears that radioiodine therapy would be followed by the late development of thyroid cancer, leukemia, or genetic damage have not been confirmed in long-term followup studies of over 25,000 patients. It has been noted, however, that when radioiodine is administered to patients under age 30, a number of them in later decades do develop benign thyroid tumors (Dobyns, Sheline, and Workman).

In summary, there are three options from which one may select the best method to manage a patient with toxic diffuse goiter. A young, reliable patient with only mild enlargement of the thyroid gland and mild elevation of the serum T-4 level may anticipate a 40%–50% long-term remission rate on thiocarbamide (propylthiouracil or methimazole) therapy. Other categories of patients with Grave's disease can anticipate remissions with this therapy in *fewer* than 40% of cases. Treatment with radioactive iodine is simple, effective, and in patients over age 30 it appears to be quite safe, although at least half of the treated patients will develop permanent hypothyroidism during the subsequent two decades. In pregnant women, using radioactive iodine is contraindicated; and in patients younger than 30, some observers feel that there has been an inadequate period of followup observation to determine the ultimate safety of radioactive iodine treatment. Surgery, in expert hands, is safe and effective but does have the small risk of recurrent nerve damage and hypoparathyroidism. Postoperative permanent hypothyroidism may be somewhat less common than is the case after radioactive iodine treatment.

Nodular Toxic Goiter

Patients with hypermetabolism secondary to nodular toxic goiter do not respond as well to thiocarbamide or radioactive iodine therapy as do patients with diffuse toxic goiter. Consequently, there is a stronger argument to advise surgical treatment in the case of patients with nodular toxic goiter.

Autonomous Hyperfunctioning Adenoma

Some patients with a solitary nodule in the thyroid gland can be demonstrated on scintiscan to have a hyperfunctioning adenoma. The scan in these patients will show a hot nodule with diminished function in the remainder of the thyroid tissue, which indicates that the adenoma is autonomous in its hyperactivity. The circulating level of thyroid-stimulating hormone (TSH) will be diminished. Surgical therapy in a patient of this type requires only that the entire adenoma be excised. Some endocrinologists treat this type of patient with radioactive iodine.

Nontoxic Solitary Thyroid Nodule

Differential Diagnosis

A *family history* suggestive of multiple endocrine neoplasia, type 2a, (MEN-2a; medullary thyroid cancer, pheochromocytoma, and parathyroid adenoma) indicates that the patient may have medullary thyroid cancer. Patients with medullary thyroid cancer of familial origin will have an elevation of their serum thyrocalcitonin levels. If the patient has a borderline thyrocalcitonin level, repeat the test after stimulation with pentagastrin. Also study the patient for the possible presence of a pheochromocytoma or a parathyroid adenoma. Elevation of the serum thyrocalcitonin level, even if pentagastrin stimulation is required, indicates that the patient is suffering from medullary thyroid cancer and total thyroidectomy is indicated.

In pursuing the *past history* of a patient with a thyroid nodule, inquire carefully whether he or she was exposed to radiation therapy of the neck during childhood. About one-third of exposed patients were found to develop thyroid nodules, of which one-third were malignant (Becker, Economou, and Southwick). These nodules should all be excised and biopsied.

If, on *physical examination,* a thyroid nodule is hard, or there appears to be fixation to surrounding structures, or there is paralysis of a vocal cord, the nodule has a high likelihood of being malignant and surgery is indicated purely on physical findings, although some surgeons would perform a preoperative needle aspiration also. The palpation of cervical lymphadenopathy is also highly suggestive of malignancy in a patient who harbors a solitary thyroid nodule. If there is a history of rapid recent growth of the nodule, this also increases the likelihood of malignancy.

Age and *sex* are also important factors in deciding the likelihood that a given nodule is malignant. Benign solitary nodules are rare in patients under age 20 and in children. Therefore, in patients younger than 20 years of age all nodules are presumed to be malignant until ruled out by a proper biopsy. Benign solitary nodules are uncommon in the male sex while such nodules are common in women. Therefore, a solitary thyroid nodule in a man should arouse suspicion of cancer. Those patients who do not have the indications for surgery mentioned above will require further diagnostic study.

If a skilled cytologist is available to read the smears, needle aspiration of the thyroid nodule for *cytological study* can be a valuable test. Several experts (Block; Rosen, Wallace, Strawbridge, and Walfish) use aspiration cytology as the prime diagnostic tool in differentiating malignant from benign thyroid nodules. Of course, this test does require an experienced thyroid cytologist before the method achieves reliability. There are additional important considerations in the use of aspiration cytology. For instance, a follicular adenoma cannot be differentiated from follicular carcinoma by this method. Also, lesions that are partly cystic or that contain degenerating tissue give rise to difficulty in interpretation. However, when the cytologist unequivocally reports the presence of cancer, prompt operation is indicated. Clearly benign lesions can be treated by continued observation. The large number of solitary nodules that are caused by benign cystic lesions may be cured by simple aspiration. If any residual mass remains after aspiration, further diagnostic studies or open biopsy is necessary. When the expertise to interpret aspiration cytology specimens is not available, then patients with a solitary thyroid nodule should be submitted to a thyroid scintiscan.

Those patients categorized as indeterminate by aspiration cytology should be subjected to a *thyroid scintiscan*. Patients whose nodules show a normal or high radioiodine uptake have a low incidence of carcinoma. This group of patients is usually treated by a 3-month trial of suppression with thyroid hormone. Blum and Rothschild administer 25 micrograms of L-triiodothyronine four times a day. This therapy is contraindicated in patients with cardiac disease or advanced age. Medication is continued for a period of 3 months unless adverse symptoms occur. The adequacy of the suppressive therapy is determined by measuring the serum level of TSH, which should be very low. If after 3 months of adequate TSH suppression, a nodule fails to shrink as much as 50% in diameter, surgery is recommended. If successful shrinkage has been achieved, these authors recommend lifelong suppression with L-thyroxine 0.2 mg–0.3 mg daily. An objective method of measuring and recording the changes in the size of a thyroid nodule is sonography.

Thyroid sonography can identify solitary thyroid nodules over 0.5 cm in size, and can identify simple cysts, solid tumors, and other solid lesions that have undergone hemorrhagic degeneration. Simple cystic nodules are treated by aspiration. If the mass disappears completely after aspiration, continued observation is the only further treatment required. Solid, cold nodules require operation, although some physicians treat these nodules by means of thyroid suppression if no other high-risk factors of cancer are present.

Block, Daily, and Robb believe that obtaining a *core biopsy* with a cutting needle (like the Travenol Tru-Cut) in nodules greater than 2 cm in diameter can be a valuable supplement to thin-needle aspiration cytology. These authors advise operation for most of the indeterminate cases.

Surgical Management

Surgical management of thyroid nodules is greatly enhanced by the availability of cryostat frozen-section histopathology and a pathologist experienced in thyroid disease. Lesions that appear grossly to be benign need only be excised locally with a rim of adjacent normal thyroid tissue and submitted for frozen-section examination. Larger or deeper nodules may require subtotal or total thyroid lobectomy for complete excision after visualization of the recurrent laryngeal nerve and parathyroid glands.

If the frozen-section examination discloses that the nodule is malignant, perform the operation that is appropriate to the specific malignancy, as discussed under "Thyroid Cancer" below. In addition to excising the thyroid nodule for diagnosis, also identify and palpate the lymph nodes both in the jugular chain and, even more important, the paratracheal nodes in the superior mediastinum. Biopsy any of these nodes that appear to be suspicious.

A patient with a history of radiation therapy to the neck in infancy, who has a benign nodule by frozen-section examination, should probably have near-total thyroidectomy (Block) or total thyroidectomy (Paloyan).

Multinodular Goiter

A nonsymptomatic, nontoxic multinodular goiter does not generally require surgery unless one can palpate a suspicious hard nodule in the gland or one obtains a positive biopsy. On the other hand, nodular goiter can produce annoying symptoms due to pressure partially occluding the trachea. Some patients are unwilling to accept the unsightly appearance that a large goiter presents. All of these represent adequate reasons for subtotal thyroidectomy. Patients who have a toxic nodular goiter do not respond well to radioactive iodine and toxicity constitutes an indication for thyroidectomy.

Thyroid Cancer

Papillary and Mixed Papillary-Follicular Carcinoma

Follicular thyroid carcinoma that contains an element of papillary tumor behaves clinically in a manner quite similar to that of pure papillary carcinoma. For this reason treatment of pure papillary or mixed papillary-follicular tumors is identical. Although many physicians feel that papillary thyroid cancer is a relatively benign disease that does not require early detection or radical treatment, Cady, Sedgewick, Meissner, Wool, and associates (1979) report that of the patients who developed papillary cancer after age 50, 29% died of this disease. Of 441 patients with papillary and mixed papillary-follicular thyroid cancer treated at the Lahey Clinic from 1931 to 1970, 12% died of this cancer. At the same time, 190 patients were treated for follicular thyroid cancer and 25% died of this disease. It is fascinating to note that among patients who were suffering from papillary cancer, those who had cervical node metastases enjoyed better prognoses than those who had no node involvement. Also, none of the 16 patients who had 10 or more metastatic nodes died of thyroid cancer after a followup period of at least 15 years. These authors emphasized that relatively few of their patients with papillary cancer over age 50 had cervical node metastases.

On the other hand, Woolner, Beahrs, and Black demonstrated that patients who had occult (less than 1.5 cm in diameter) papillary tumors experienced a 20-year survival curve no different from that of the normal population. Papillary tumors, small enough to be confined completely within the capsule of the thyroid gland, also did not greatly affect the patient survivorship curve compared with normal persons of comparable age and sex. The papillary group of thyroid cancers constitutes the most common type and predominates in children and young adults. It is twice as common in women as in men. Clark, White, and Russell reported that 90% of patients with papillary cancer in one lobe of the thyroid had evidence of microscopic multicentric papillary cancer when the thyroid gland was studied by serial microscopic sections of the entire gland following total bilateral thyroidectomy. However, Tollefson, Shah, and Huvos reported that only 5.7% of 298 patients who had undergone unilateral lobectomy for papillary cancer developed recurrent cancer in the opposite lobe during followup periods of 5–35 years. About half of the patients with recurrence died of metastatic disease.

Because the presence of microscopic cancer did not lead to clinical disease very often, Tollefson and his associates felt that total thyroidectomy for all papillary cancers would lead to an unacceptable number of serious complications. They did not do a total contralateral lobectomy unless there was palpable evidence of bilateral cancer. In reviewing total thyroidectomies performed at Memorial (Sloane-Kettering) Hospital, Tollefson and associates reported a 29% incidence of permanent hypoparathyroidism following total thyroidectomy for cancer. They advocated total lobectomy and removal of the thyroid isthmus as the primary treatment for unilateral papillary cancer. Other surgeons (Attie; Block; Clark; and Mazzaferri, Young, Oertel, Kemmerer et al.) feel that total thyroidectomy for papillary cancers larger than 1.5 cm is the most effective treatment, providing that the surgeon is experienced and has the technical skill to avoid nerve and parathyroid injuries. The surgeon's skill and experience are extremely important considerations in deciding to perform a total thyroidectomy. If the patient has evidence of bilateral disease on clinical examination, total thyroidectomy and appropriate cervical lymph node dissection are indicated as the primary operation, and the patient should be referred to a surgeon who can do this type of operation safely. Total thyroidectomy also has the advantage of permitting later treatment of distant metastases with large doses of radioactive iodine. The patient with unilateral papillary cancer following external radiation therapy in childhood is also a suitable candidate for total thyroidectomy in the hands of an expert. Complications like permanent hypoparathyroidism or vocal cord paralysis following total thyroidectomy by an expert surgeon should occur in less than 2% of cases (Attie; Clark).

Follicular Carcinoma

Follicular cancer of the thyroid also is more common in women than men. This category of disease constitutes about 20% of all thyroid cancer. Patients who develop the disease prior to age 40 appear to have a good prognosis. However, over 60% in the study of Cady and associates (1979) were over 40, and 36% of these patients died of thyroid cancer. Distant metastases are the common cause of death in these patients.

Encapsulated, small, well-differentiated follicular carcinoma that shows no significant degree of blood vessel invasion has a good prognosis, and patients with this disease may be treated by unilateral lobectomy if the opposite lobe is normal to palpation.

The aggressive follicular carcinoma with a high degree of blood vessel invasion is also a relatively slow-growing tumor, but 80% of patients with angioinvasive follicular tumors in the study reported by Woolner and associates were dead within 20 years. For these patients Block recommends a total or near-total thyroidectomy. One reason for performing a total thyroidectomy is that it facilitates the use of therapeutic dosages of radioactive iodine to treat distant metastases, should they develop at a later date. Wanebo, Andrews, and Kaiser were not impressed with the efficacy of radioactive iodine in improving patient survival, while Cady, Sedgewick, Meissner, Brookwalter, and associates (1976) felt that it was beneficial when given to patients in the low-risk category, but not in the older, high-risk category of patients. Actually, there is inadequate data to determine the value of using ^{131}I radiotherapy. Also, randomized followup studies comparing total thyroidectomy with subtotal thyroidectomy or lobectomy in follicular cancer patients have not been reported. For truly angioinvasive follicular carcinoma, we would perform a near-total or total thyroidectomy.

Another subdivision of follicular cancer is the Hürthle cell cancer. These tumors resemble follicular cancer in their behavior and are treated in a similar fashion.

Cady and associates (1976) found that thyroid suppression by means of administering thyroid hormone postoperatively did not improve the prognosis in follicular cancer, while such therapy was indeed demonstrated to have a beneficial effect on survival following papillary and mixed cancers. Also, therapeutic external radiation administered because the surgeon suspected that residual cancer had been left behind had no effect on survival. Nor did prophylactic adjuvant radiotherapy improve survival, either in papillary or follicular cancer.

Medullary Carcinoma
Seven percent of thyroid carcinomas are medullary in type. These may be either sporadic or hereditary. The sporadic type appears to be more common than the hereditary. While the sporadic type may be unilateral in distribution, the hereditary type is always multicentric and involves both lobes. The average age at which the diagnosis is made is over 40 in the sporadic type and under 40 in the hereditary. Medullary cancer is an aggressive tumor with frequent lymph node and distant metastases. In Woolner's report, patients with medullary cancer who had negative lymph nodes tended to have a survival curve not greatly lower than that of a comparable normal population, while 60% of those with positive nodes died within 10 years.

Elevation of the serum calcitonin level, stimulated by pentagastrin when necessary, is characteristic of medullary carcinoma. Families of patients with hereditary medullary thyroid cancer should have semiannual serum calcitonin determinations in order to detect the cancer at an early stage, often even before a nodule can be palpated. It is important to study all patients suspected of having the hereditary form of medullary thyroid cancer for the presence of a pheochromocytoma (MEN-2 syndrome). The MEN-2a syndrome also includes hyperparathyroidism, while patients with the MEN-2b syndrome invariably have multiple mucosal neuromas. If the patient has a pheochromocytoma, this lesion (often bilateral in MEN-2 cases) will have to be removed prior to thyroidectomy. If the patient suffers from hyperparathyroidism, it will be necessary to explore the parathyroid glands and evaluate their pathology while performing the thyroidectomy.

Total thyroidectomy is recommended for patients with medullary thyroid cancer. The middle third of the jugular lymph node chain should routinely be explored and biopsied to determine the presence of metastatic lymph nodes, as should the paratracheal nodes in the superior mediastinum. If nodes are involved, a neck dissection is indicated in addition to total thyroidectomy.

Anaplastic Carcinoma
Constituting about 5%–10% of all thyroid cancers, anaplastic carcinoma is a very aggressive tumor occuring primarily during the sixth and seventh decades of life. When it is first detected, the tumor has generally already shown invasion of the larynx or trachea and overlying muscles as well as metastatic lymph nodes and distant metastases. This disease is almost invariably fatal, often due to respiratory obstruction. The tumor should be resected, if possible, to avoid tracheal obstruction.

Indications

Diffuse toxic goiter in young patients (under age 30), in pregnant women, or by patient preference

Toxic nodular goiter

Selected solitary thyroid nodules (see discussion above)

Suspicious nodules in multinodular goiter

Thyroid carcinoma

Preoperative Care

In patients with Grave's disease of mild or moderate severity, it may be possible to prepare the patient by administering Lugol's iodine solution, 10 drops three times a day for a week or 10 days. In more severe cases, give an adequate amount of propylthiouracil, beginning with a dose of 100 mg three times a day. In some patients larger doses must be given for many weeks, although generally 8 weeks of propylthiouracil treatment is adequate. During the last 10–14 days give the patient Lugol's solution 5–10 drops three times a day together with the propylthiouracil. Recently a third method of preparing the toxic patient for surgery has been introduced. Propanolol is administered in sufficient quantities to reduce the pulse rate to normal. Frequently no more than one week of preoperative propanolol treatment is necessary. Continue the drug during and after the operation for 7–10 days. Although this method appears to be effective in most patients, occasional cases of postoperative thyroid storm have been reported with propanolol management.

For patients with a thyroid nodule, preoperative management may include aspiration cytology, thyroid scan, thyroid sonogram, and thyroid suppression therapy as discussed under "Concept."

A patient suspected of having medullary carcinoma of the thyroid should have preoperative studies to detect a pheochromocytoma or a parathyroid adenoma.

Pitfalls and Danger Points

Trauma to or inadvertent excision of parathyroid glands

Trauma to or inadvertent laceration of recurrent laryngeal or external laryngeal nerves

Inadequate preoperative preparation of the toxic patient resulting in postoperative thyroid storm

Inadequate surgery for the more aggressive thyroid cancers

Operative Strategy

Preserving Parathyroid Glands

Preventing damage to the parathyroid glands requires the surgeon to achieve thorough familiarity with the anatomical location and appearance of these structures. Wearing telescopic lenses with about 2.5 times magnification can be helpful in identifying both the parathyroid glands and the recurrent nerve. If the surgeon will take the time to identify the parathyroid glands in every thyroid operation, he will soon find that this maneuver can be accomplished with progressively more efficiency. The inferior parathyroid gland is frequently found in the fat that surrounds the inferior thyroid artery at the point where

523

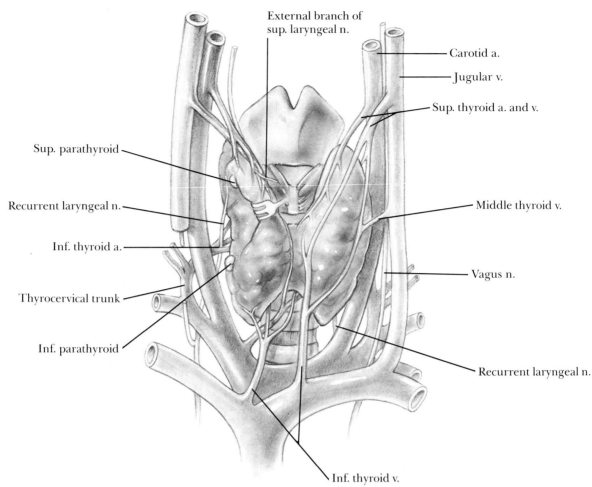

External branch of
sup. laryngeal n.

Carotid a.

Jugular v.

Sup. thyroid a. and v.

Sup. parathyroid

Recurrent laryngeal n.

Inf. thyroid a.

Thyrocervical trunk

Inf. parathyroid

Middle thyroid v.

Vagus n.

Recurrent laryngeal n.

Inf. thyroid v.

Fig. 92–1

it divides into several branches **(Fig. 92–1)**. Normally, the inferior gland is anteromedial to the recurrent laryngeal nerve while the superior parathyroid is posterolateral to the nerve **(Fig. 92–2)**. With the thyroid gland retracted anteriorly, both parathyroids may assume an anteromedial position relative to the nerve **(Fig. 92–3)**. The superior gland is generally situated on the posterior surface of the upper third of the thyroid gland, fairly close to the cricoid cartilage. Frequently, the parathyroids are loosely surrounded by fat and have a red-brown color. Measuring only about 5–8 mm in maximum diameter, the average gland weighs about 30 mg.

One method of protecting the parathyroid glands is to preserve the posterior

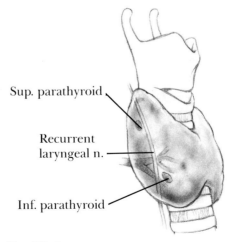

Sup. parathyroid

Recurrent
laryngeal n.

Inf. parathyroid

Fig. 92–2

524

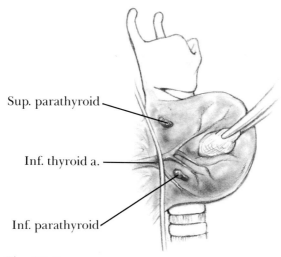

Sup. parathyroid

Inf. thyroid a.

Inf. parathyroid

Fig. 92–3

capsule of the thyroid gland by incising the thyroid along the line sketched in Fig. 92–11. Also, divide the branches of the inferior thyroid artery at a point distal to the origin of the blood supply to the parathyroids. Some surgeons feel that ligating the inferior thyroid artery lateral to the thyroid gland may impair the blood supply to the parathyroid glands, although this contention has never been proved.

When a total lobectomy is performed, the only means of insuring the preservation of the parathyroid glands is to positively identify the inferior and the superior gland. Then dissect each gland carefully away from the thyroid without impairing its blood supply.

If a parathyroid gland has been inadvertently excised, and this error is recognized during the operation, it is possible to slice the gland into particles measuring 1 mm by 1 mm and then to transplant these fragments into pockets made in the muscles of the neck or of the forearm (Wells, Ross, Dale, and Gray).

Preserving the Recurrent Laryngeal Nerve

The recurrent laryngeal nerve ascends slightly lateral to the tracheoesophageal groove. At the level of the inferior thyroid artery, the nerve almost always makes contact with this vessel, passing either directly under or over the artery. Sometimes the nerve passes between the branches of the inferior thyroid vessel. Above the level of the artery, the nerve ascends to enter the larynx between the cricoid cartilage and the inferior cornu of the thyroid cartilage. In this area the nerve lies in close proximity to the posterior capsule of the thyroid gland. It may divide into two or more branches prior to entering the larynx. On rare occasions the recurrent nerve does not recur, but it travels from the vagus directly medially to enter the larynx near the superior thyroid vessels or at a slightly lower level relative to the thyroid gland.

For most surgeons, the best way of locating the recurrent laryngeal nerve is to trace the inferior thyroid artery from the point where it emerges behind the carotid artery to the point where it crosses over or under the recurrent nerve. Using the inferior thyroid artery as a guide, locate the recurrent nerve immediately deep to or superficial to this artery and carefully dissect the nerve in a cephalad direction until it reaches the cricothyroid membrane just below the inferior cornu of the thyroid cartilage. Remember that the nerve may divide into two or more branches in the area cephalad to the inferior thyroid artery. Once the nerve has been exposed throughout its course behind the thyroid gland, it is a simple matter to avoid damaging it.

Preserving the Superior Laryngeal Nerve

The internal branch of the superior laryngeal nerve penetrates the thyrohyoid membrane and is the sensory nerve of the larynx, while the external branch controls the cricothyroid muscle. Although it is possible to damage both branches of the superior laryngeal nerve by passing a mass ligature around the superior thyroid artery and vein above the superior pole of the thyroid, the external branch is the one most often injured. Transection of the external branch impairs the patient's ability to voice high-pitched sounds. Since the external branch may be intertwined with branches of the superior thyroid artery and vein (see Fig. 92–1), avoiding damage to this nerve requires that each branch of the superior thyroid vessels be isolated, ligated, and divided individually at the point where it enters the thyroid gland. If the superior thyroid artery and vein are dissected *above* the superior pole of the thyroid, it will be necessary to identify and preserve the superior laryngeal nerve and its branches. This step is not necessary if the terminal branches of the superior thyroid vessels are individually isolated and ligated.

Operative Technique

Incision and Exposure

Place a small pillow or other support beneath the patient's shoulders in order to extend the head and neck. It is helpful, also, to elevate the upper half of the operating table so that the patient assumes a semisitting position. Make a slightly curved incision transversely in the neck at a level 2–3 fingerbreadths above the sternal notch **(Fig. 92–4).** The incision should extend just beyond the anterior border of the ster-

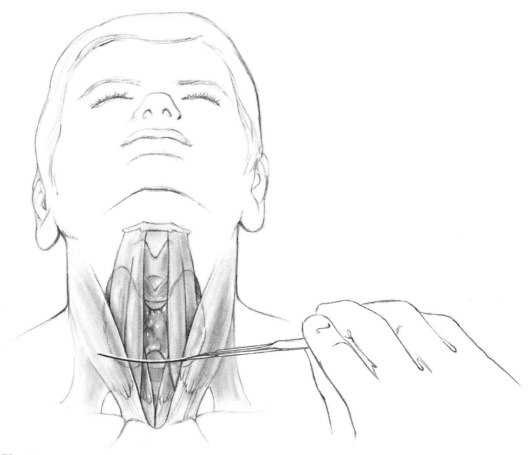

Fig. 92–4

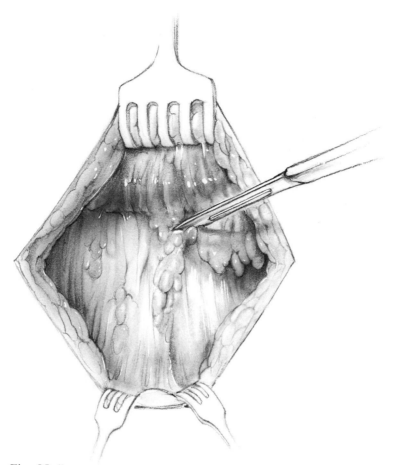

Fig. 92–5

nomastoid muscle on each side. In patients who have large goiters a longer incision will be necessary. Carry the incision down to the platysma muscle. This muscle will be easier to identify in the lateral portions of the incision. When the longtitudinal fibers of this muscle are seen, transect them with precision because the upper flap will be dissected in a plane along the deep aspect of the platysma. There is a thin layer of fat deep to this muscle. If the plane of dissection is carried down to the cervical fascia, a number of veins will be encountered that will produce unnecessary bleed-

ing. Leaving a thin layer of fat on these veins will avoid this problem. Continue the dissection along the deep surface of the platysma muscle in a cephalad direction by using both sharp and blunt maneuvers until a point 1–2 cm above the notch of the thyroid cartilage has been reached in the midline of the dissection (Fig. 92–5).

527

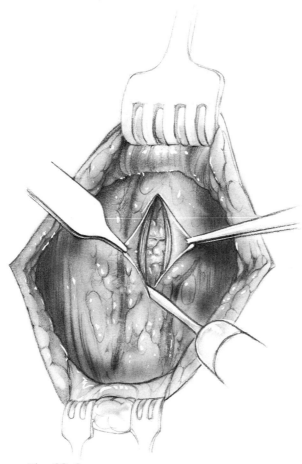

Fig. 92–6

Once this has been accomplished, elevate the lateral portions of the flap. Adequate exposure requires wide dissection of this musculocutaneous flap. Achieve hemostasis, primarily with electrocoagulation. Also elevate the inferior flap for a distance of about 2 cm.

Now palpate the prominence of the thyroid cartilage in order to identify the midline. Make an incision through the cervical fascia in the midline (**Fig. 92–6**) and extend the incision in the fascia to expose the full length of the strap muscles. Elevate the sternohyoid muscle in the midline. Then elevate the sternothyroid muscle and dissect the thyroid capsule away from it on both sides. This will permit an adequate digital exploration of the entire thyroid gland. In most cases retracting the strap muscles laterally while the thyroid lobe is retracted in the opposite direction will provide good exposure for a thyroidectomy. If the gland is unusually large or the exposure is inadequate, do not hesitate to transect the sternohyoid and sternothyroid muscles. Transect them in their upper thirds (**Fig. 92–7**) as their innervation enters from below.

Identifying the Inferior Thyroid Artery, Recurrent Laryngeal Nerve, and Inferior Parathyroid Gland

Retract the strap muscles firmly with a small Richardson retractor while forcefully drawing thyroid gland in a medial direction using either a peanut sponge (**Fig. 92–8**) or a gauze square held in the assistant's fingers. A layer of thin fibrous and areolar tissue is now divided in layers, either by using Metzenbaum scissors or dissecting bluntly with a hemostat. A variable distribution of one or more middle thyroid veins may be encountered along the anterolateral margin of the thyroid. Divide these

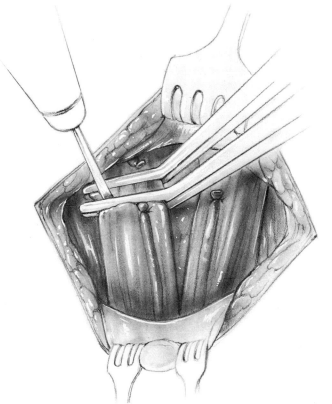

Fig. 92–7

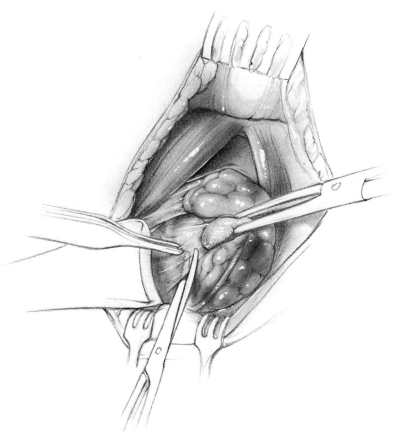

Fig. 92–8

529

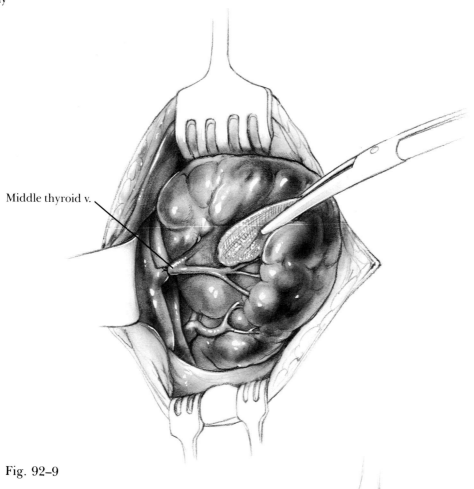

Middle thyroid v.

Fig. 92–9

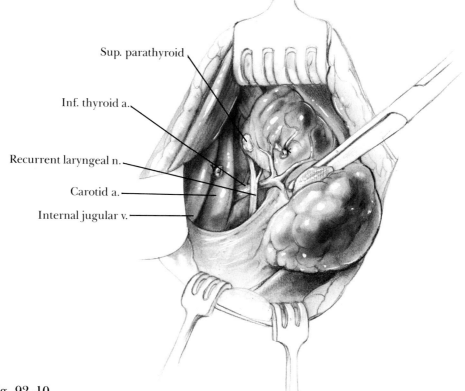

Sup. parathyroid

Inf. thyroid a.

Recurrent laryngeal n.

Carotid a.

Internal jugular v.

Fig. 92–10

veins between ligatures **(Fig. 92–9)**. This will permit further elevation of the lower portion of the thyroid lobe.

Identify the carotid artery. Carry the dissection through the fibrous tissue along the medial surface of the carotid artery down to the level of the prevertebral fascia. Now retract the carotid artery laterally. Dissection medial to this vessel will reveal the inferior thyroid artery passing deep to the carotid toward the junction of the middle and lower thirds of the thyroid gland **(Fig. 92–10)**. Once the inferior thyroid artery has been identified, encircle it with a Vesseloop. Apply mild traction to the artery and follow the anterior surface of this structure in a medial direction by blunt dissection with a Metzenbaum scissors.

Before this vessel enters the thyroid gland, it will either pass directly beneath or cross directly over the recurrent laryngeal nerve. Make use of the inferior thyroid artery as a guide to the nerve. If the nerve is not immediately seen, dissect the loose fibrous tissue at a point just inferior to the artery near the groove between the trachea and the esophagus in order to identify the recurrent nerve. Once the nerve is identified, use a small hemostat to delineate the plane just superficial to the nerve. Continue this plane of dissection in a cephalad direction up to the inferior cornu of the thyroid cartilage, the point near which the nerve enters the larynx. Be aware that the nerve may divide into two or more branches along its course from the level of the inferior thyroid artery to that of the larynx.

Now identify the inferior parathyroid gland, generally located close to the point where the inferior thyroid artery divides into its branches **(Fig. 92–11)**. Divide each of these branches of the inferior thyroid artery between ligatures on a line medial to the parathyroid gland so that the blood supply to the parathyroid is not impaired.

Once the recurrent nerve has been identified, proceed to dissect out the lower pole of the thyroid lobe. One or more inferior thyroid veins will be encountered in this location. Divide and ligate each of these veins and liberate the inferior pole.

Dissecting the Superior Pole and Superior Parathyroid Gland

Identify the upper portion of the thyroid isthmus. If a fingerlike projection of thyroid tissue can be identified extending from the region of the isthmus in a cephalad direction, this represents the pyramidal lobe of the thyroid. If a thyroidectomy is being performed for Grave's disease, it is important to remove the pyramidal lobe. Otherwise, postoperatively, it may become markedly hypertrophied and cause a serious cosmetic deformity overlying the thyroid cartilage.

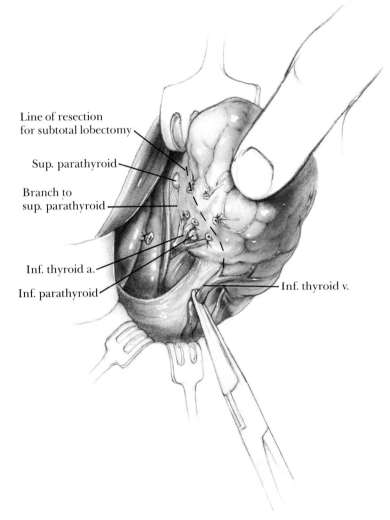

Line of resection for subtotal lobectomy

Sup. parathyroid

Branch to sup. parathyroid

Inf. thyroid a.

Inf. parathyroid

Inf. thyroid v.

Fig. 92–11

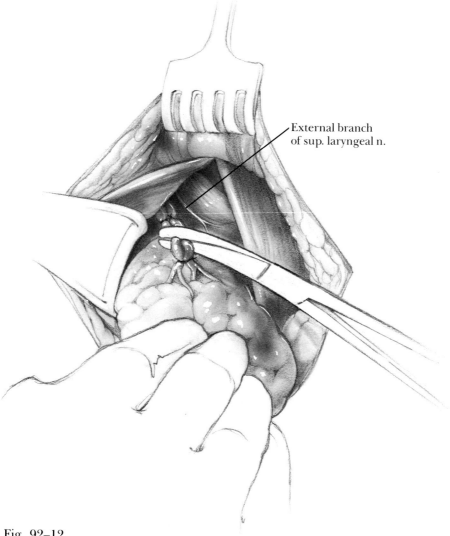

External branch
of sup. laryngeal n.

Fig. 92–12

With a retractor drawing the upper portion of the strap muscles in a cephalad direction, use a peanut sponge dissector to sweep the upper pole of the thyroid away from the larynx. This will separate the upper pole from the external branch of the superior laryngeal nerve, which is closely applied to the cricothyroid muscle at this level. Also free the lateral portion of the superior pole by blunt dissection. There may be one or two small veins entering the posterior portion of the upper pole. Be careful to identify and occlude these branches if encountered. Then identify the terminal branches of the superior thyroid artery and vein. Ligate each of these with two 2–0 cotton ligatures and then divide each of these vessels between the ligatures **(Fig. 92–12).** After these vessels have been ligated and divided, the superior pole of the thyroid will be completely liberated and can be lifted out of the neck. Now search along the posterior surface of the upper third of the thyroid lobe for the superior parathyroid gland. Its usual location is sketched in Fig. 92–11. Dissect the gland away from the thyroid into the neck.

It should be remembered that if any difficulty is encountered in exposing the recurrent laryngeal nerve, the inferior thyroid artery, or the inferior parathyroid gland, do not hesitate to perform the superior pole dissection earlier in the operation in order to improve exposure of the posterior aspect of the thyroid gland.

At this point the surgeon must decide whether to perform a subtotal or a total thyroid lobectomy. Generally, if the patient has what obviously appears to be a localized benign tumor, perform a subtotal thyroid lobectomy and obtain an immediate frozen section, if possible. If the frozen section should prove malignant, a total lobectomy is indicated as discussed above. For larger tumors that are suspicious of malignancy, a total thyroid lobectomy should be carried out.

Subtotal Thyroid Lobectomy

If a subtotal resection of the lobe is the operation elected, free the upper pole completely and divide the lobe along the line of resection as outlined in Fig. 92–11. At this level of dissection both parathyroid glands and the recurrent nerve, all of which

have been previously identified, may be left in their normal locations. Divide the remaining gland between hemostats until the anterior surface of the trachea has been reached. At this point transect the isthmus as described below. Some surgeons feel that the lateral margin of the residual segment of thyroid should be sutured to the trachea, although this step is not essential.

For patients undergoing bilateral subtotal thyroidectomy for Grave's disease, leave no more than 2–4 grams of thyroid tissue on each side.

Total Thyroid Lobectomy

Before considering a total lobectomy, be certain that you have positively identified the recurrent nerve as well as the superior and the inferior parathyroid glands. After these structures have been dissected away from the thyroid, one can proceed with the total lobectomy. The gland is firmly attached to the two upper tracheal rings by dense fibrous tissue that constitutes the ligament of Berry **(Fig. 92–13)**. The upper

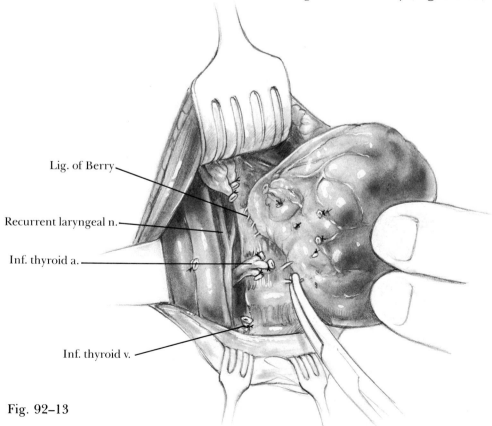

Lig. of Berry

Recurrent laryngeal n.

Inf. thyroid a.

Inf. thyroid v.

Fig. 92–13

portion of the recurrent laryngeal nerve passes very close to the point where this ligament attaches to the trachea. Also, very often there is a small artery passing very close to the recurrent nerve in this ligament. Be careful to control this vessel without injuring the nerve, before dividing the ligament. After this ligament has been freed, the thyroid lobe can easily be liberated from the trachea by clamping and dividing several small blood vessels until the isthmus has been elevated. The isthmus may be divided serially between hemostats or by a single application of the TA-55 stapling device containing 3.5 mm staples as seen in **Fig. 92–14.** Then divide the isthmus with a scalpel leaving the left lobe

of the thyroid in place as seen in **Fig. 92–15.**

As you irrigate the operative field with saline and obtain *complete* hemostasis by ligatures and electrocoagulation, always keep in view the recurrent nerve and the parathyroid glands.

Partial Thyroid Lobectomy

On some occasions, what appears to be an obviously benign lesion will occupy a small portion of the thyroid gland. Under these conditions, local excision or partial lobectomy may be indicated. The stapling

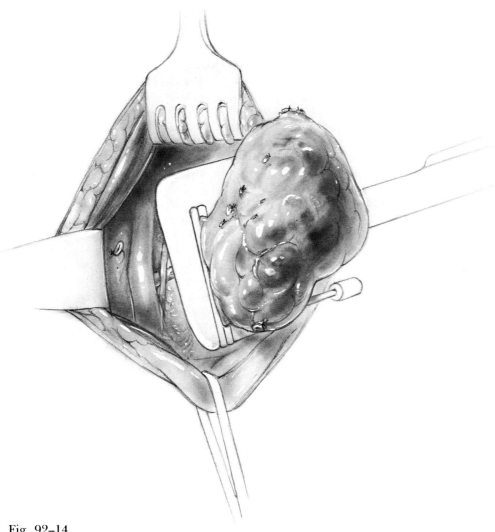

Fig. 92–14

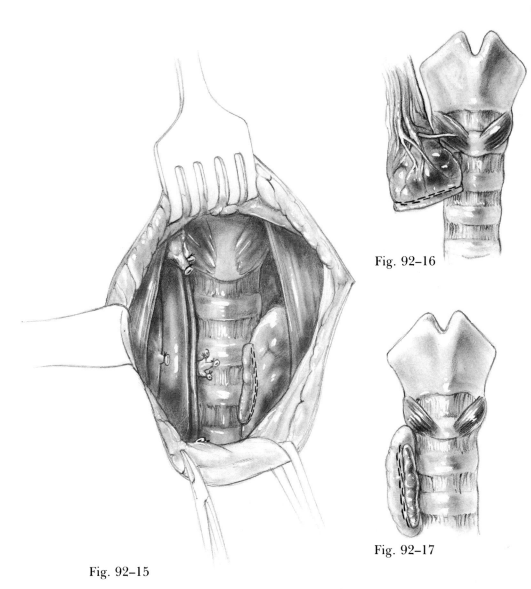

Fig. 92–16

Fig. 92–17

Fig. 92–15

device is sometimes useful under these conditions. **Fig. 92–16** illustrates removal of the lower half of the right thyroid lobe, a stapling device having been used first to close and control bleeding from the remaining segment of thyroid. Remember that *identification* and *preservation* of the recurrent nerve must be achieved early in the dissection. If the gland is fairly thick, use 4.8 mm staples.

For benign lesions of the isthmus, one can dissect the isthmus away from the trachea and apply the stapling device to the junction between the isthmus and the adjacent thyroid lobes **(Fig. 92–17)**.

Closure

In the unusual situation where the strap muscles have been transected, resuture these two muscles by means of interrupted mattress sutures of 2–0 PG as illustrated

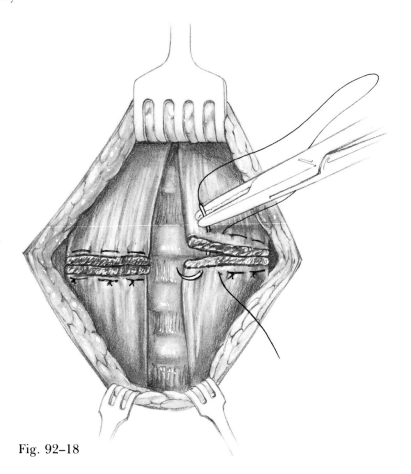

Fig. 92–18

in **Fig. 92–18.** In other cases, simply suture the right and left strap muscles together loosely with interrupted 4–0 PG sutures. We rarely drain thyroidectomy cases. Hemostasis should be *perfect* before the operation is terminated. It is not safe to depend on a drain to evacuate blood clots.

After the strap muscles have been reapproximated, suture the divided platysma muscle together using interrupted 5–0 Vicryl. Close the skin by means of carefully applied skin staples **(Figs. 92–19 and 92–20)** or interrupted fine nylon.

Postoperative Care

In patients with Grave's disease, carefully monitor vital signs in order to detect early evidence of a *thyroid storm.* Those patients, who were prepared for operation with pro-panolol, will require treatment with this medication for 7–10 days following operation.

Carefully observe the patient's neck for signs of swelling or ecchymosis. Active *bleeding* in the bed of the excised thyroid gland can rapidly compress the trachea and cause respiratory obstruction, especially if the bleeding is due to a major artery. Under rare circumstances, it may be necessary to remove all of the sutures in the skin and the strap muscles in order to release the blood clot at the patient's bedside. In most cases, evacuate the blood clot in the operating room. After the removal of a very large goiter, one may occasionally observe the gradual swelling of the tissues of the neck due to slow venous bleeding that infiltrates the tissues and may produce respiratory distress by laryngeal edema. This type of patient requires orotracheal intubation as well as evacuation of the clot

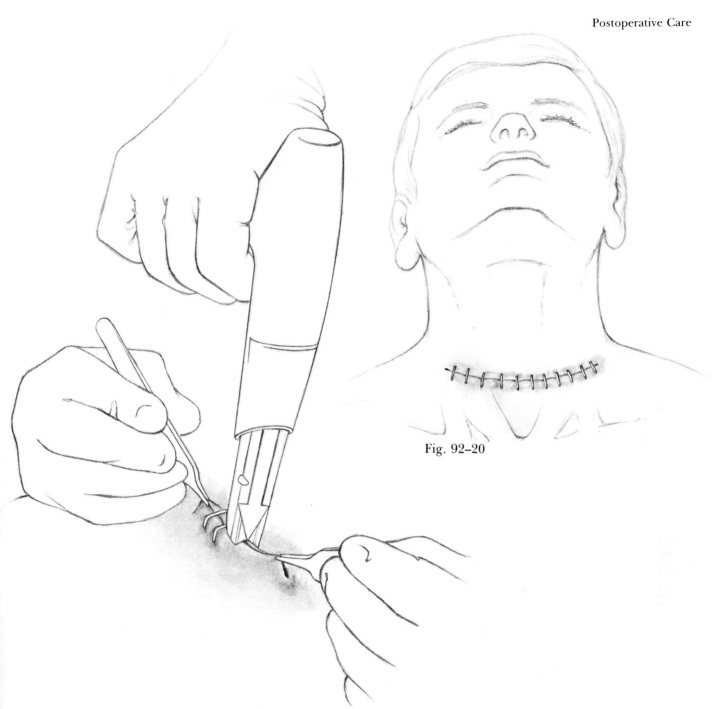

Fig. 92–20

Fig. 92–19

in the operating room. It is extremely rare that an exploration or a tracheostomy must be done at the patient's bedside.

Following bilateral thyroid lobectomy, check for *hypocalcemia* by measuring the serum calcium level until the patient is discharged. Observe for the signs of par-

esthesia of the extremities or face, symptoms that generally appear when the calcium drops below a level of 7–8 mg/dl. Treat the symptoms with intravenous calcium gluconate, 1 gram of a 10% solution several times a day. Give oral calcium lactate tablets, 4–12 grams per day, as required to maintain the serum calcium level. If calcium alone does not control the symptoms, administer vitamin D, 50,000–100,000 units a day by mouth. The milder forms of hypocalcemia following thyroid surgery will probably be transient because it is caused by minor trauma to the parathyroid glands. Severe postoperative hypoparathyroidism is often permanent in nature.

The patient who has undergone trauma or laceration of both recurrent laryngeal nerves may develop a complete *airway obstruction* requiring prompt endotracheal intubation and then tracheotomy. This complication should be extremely rare.

Postoperative Complications

Hematoma with possible tracheal compression and respiratory distress may occur.

There may be *injury to the recurrent laryngeal nerve.* If unilateral, this generally produces some degree of hoarseness and weakness of voice. As mentioned above, bilateral recurrent nerve damage causes bilateral vocal cord paralysis and marked narrowing of the glottis with respiratory obstruction, which often requires immediate tracheotomy. The airway may later be improved by an arytenoidectomy. Postoperative hoarseness may be also due to transient vocal cord edema or vocal cord injury due to the endotracheal tube used for anesthesia.

External laryngeal nerve injury may result in the patient being unable to utter high-pitched sounds.

Hypoparathyroidism, transient or permanent, results from inadvertent removal or trauma to several of the parathyroid glands. If during operation it is noted that one or more parathyroid glands have been removed, slice these into segments 1 mm by 1 mm each. Then transplant them into a muscle of the forearm or the neck. If the fragments are sufficiently small, satisfactory function may develop. Transient hypoparathyroidism lasting as long as several months may result from manipulation of the parathyroid glands without permanent damage.

Thyroid storm may develop following thyroidectomy for Grave's disease, especially if the preoperative preparation has not been adequate. This condition is characterized by fever, severe tachycardia, mental confusion, delirium, and restlessness. Rarely seen in the present era, thyroid storm may be treated by adequate doses of propylthiouracil and intravenous sodium iodide, as well as propanolol, 2 mg intravenously, with electrocardiographic control, followed by 10–40 mg by mouth several times a day. A patient with a high fever should be placed on a hypothermic blanket.

Hypothyroidism may occur following bilateral subtotal thyroidectomy. Although many surgeons believe that after an interval of 1–2 years following thyroidectomy the thyroid hormone secretion continues at a stable rate, other observers contend that, like radioactive iodine, thyroidectomy may induce hypothyroidism many years after operation. Consequently, these patients should be checked for thyroid function at intervals of 1–2 years for an indefinite period of time.

References

Attie JN (1979) Feasibility of total thyroidectomy in the treatment of thyroid carcinoma. Am J Surg 138:555

Becker FO, Economou SG, Southwick HW (1975) Adult thyroid cancer after head and neck irradiation in infancy and childhood. Ann Intern Med 83:347

Block MA (1983) Surgery of thyroid nodules and malignancy. Curr Probl Surg 20:137

Block MA, Dailey GE, Robb JA (1983) Thyroid nodules indeterminate by needle biopsy. Am J Surg 146:72

Blum M, Rothschild M (1980) Improved non-operative diagnosis of the solitary "cold" thyroid nodule: surgical selection based on risk factors and three months of suppression. JAMA 243:242

Cady B, Sedgewick CE, Meissner WA, Brookwalter Jr et al. (1976) Changing clinical pathology, therapeutic, and survival patterns in differentiated thyroid carcinoma. Ann Surg 184:541

Cady B, Sedgewick CE, Meissner WA, Wool MS et al. (1979) Risk factor analysis in differentiated thyroid cancer. Cancer 43:810

Clark OH (1982) Total thyroidectomy: the treatment of choice for patients with differentiated thyroid cancer. Ann Surg 196:361

Clark RL, White SC, Russell WD (1959) Total thyroidectomy for cancer of the thyroid: significance of intraglandular dissemination. Ann Surg 149:858

Dobyns BM, Sheline GE, Workman JB (1974) Malignant and benign neoplasms of the thyroid in patients treated for hyperthyroidism: a report of the cooperative thyrotoxicosis therapy follow-up study. J Clin Endocrin 38:976

Mazzaferri EL, Young RL, Oertel JE, Kemmerer WT et al. (1977) Papillary thyroid carcinoma: the impact of therapy in 576 patients. Medicine 56:171

Paloyan E (1977) Operation for the irradiated gland for possible thyroid carcinoma: criteria, technique, and results, in DeGroot LJ, (ed.), Radiation—associated thyroid carcinoma, New York, Grune and Stratton

Rosen IR, Wallace C, Strawbridge HG, Walfish PG (1981) Reevaluation of needle aspiration cytology in detection of thyroid cancer. Surgery 90:747

Tollefson HR, Shah JP, Huvos AG (1972) Papillary carcinoma of the thyroid: recurrence in the thyroid gland after initial surgical treatment. Am J Surg 124:97

Wanebo HJ, Andrews W, Kaiser DL (1981) Thyroid cancer: some basic considerations. Am J Surg 142:472

Wells SA Jr. Ross AJ, Dale JK, Gray RS (1979) Transplantation of the parathyroid glands: current status. Surg Clin North Am 59:167

Woolner LB, Beahrs OH, Black BM (1968) Thyroid carcinoma: general considerations and follow-up data on 1,181 cases, in Young S, Inman DR (eds.), Thyroid neoplasia, London, Academic Press

93 Cricothyroidotomy

Concept: Which Kind of Emergency Airway

When a hospitalized patient requires the establishment of an airway in the upper respiratory tract under emergency conditions, the first priority is to achieve endotracheal intubation, generally through the mouth, with a laryngoscope. In situations where endotracheal intubation cannot be established with great rapidity, an immediate cricothyroidotomy or tracheotomy is indicated. Of these two procedures, we agree with Boyd, Romita, Conlan, Fink, and associates that cricothyroidotomy has many advantages over tracheotomy under emergency conditions. The cricothyroid membrane is situated directly under the skin with no intervening tissues, such as muscle and the thyroid isthmus, which are encountered during tracheotomy. Cricothyroidotomy is easily learned and can be performed very rapidly with minimal risk. It involves an incision in the membrane between the lower border of the thyroid cartilage and the cricoid cartilage for purposes of tracheal intubation. Utilized under proper conditions, it has been demonstrated to be safe in a series of 655 cases reported by Brantigan and Grow (1976) and in another series of 147 cases reported by Boyd and associates.

Although the older literature contains many warnings that cricothyroidotomy is followed by many complications such as glottic or subglottic stenosis, both Boyd and associates and Brantigan and Grow (1982) did not encounter this complication when cricothyroidotomy was the initial procedure used for upper airway obstruction. On the other hand, patients who have been maintained on mechanical ventilation with endotracheal intubation for more than 7 days and who have then undergone cricothyroidotomy, have sustained an unacceptable incidence of subglottic stenosis. Presumably, prolonged intubation with secondary ulceration and inflammation of the larynx, followed by cricothyroidotomy, combine to cause permanent damage to the subglottic region. Patients with acute inflammation of the epiglottis or vocal cords due to infection or external trauma also should not undergo cricothyroidotomy, except possibly as a temporary lifesaving measure. On the other hand, Boyd and associates and Brantigan and Grow (1982) have found that maintaining a patient on a mechanical ventilator for many weeks following intubation via cricothyroidotomy appears to produce no permanent damage, provided the patient was not orally intubated for more than 7 days prior to the cricothyroidotomy.

Indications

Establishing an emergency airway when oral or nasal endotracheal intubation cannot be achieved

Under elective conditions the cricothyroid route is suitable for tracheal intubation, provided (1) the patient has not been orally or nasally intubated for a period of more than 7 days and (2) there is no preexisting infection or external trauma of the larynx.

540

Preoperative Care

Like tracheotomy, cricothyroidotomy is simpler to perform in a patient who has already been orally intubated. However, many cricothyroidotomy procedures are performed under emergency conditions where no preoperative preparation is possible.

Pitfalls and Danger Points

Making Erroneous Incision in Thyrohyoid Membrane

A dangerous error, occasionally performed by a neophyte under conditions of excitement, is to make the incision *above* the thyroid cartilage in the thyrohyoid membrane instead of *below* the thyroid cartilage in the cricothyroid region. This erroneous incision may result in serious damage to the structures of the larynx. In learning to do this operation, remember that the incision is made at the lower border of the thyroid cartilage between the thyroid and the cricoid cartilages.

Failure to Control Subcutaneous Bleeding

Occasionally a vein in the subcutaneous space is transected. The veins should be either ligated or electrocoagulated; otherwise, postoperative bleeding may occur.

Operative Strategy

Because cricothyroidotomy is often performed in an emergency situation, local infiltration of the skin over the cricothyroid membrane is the anesthetic usually employed. In desperate situations, of course, no anesthesia is necessary.

Since the most dangerous error is making the incision in the wrong place, the surgeon should avoid this error by grasping the lateral margins of the thyroid cartilage between the thumb and the middle finger of his left hand, using the tip of his index finger to palpate the space between the lower margin of the thyroid cartilage and the upper margin of the cricoid. With this maneuver, one can pinpoint accurately the proper site for the incision. Under conditions of desperate emergency in the field without instruments, it is possible to perform this procedure with a sharp penknife by inserting the tip of the blade through the skin and the cricothyroid membrane with one motion. Then twist the blade 70°–90° to provide a temporary airway until some type of tube can be inserted into the trachea.

Operative Technique

Incision

Place a folded sheet under the patient's shoulders to elevate them 4–8 cm above the table level. This extends the neck somewhat. After the usual skin preparation, grasp the lateral margin of the thyroid cartilage between the thumb and the middle finger of the left hand. Palpate the cricothyroid space accurately with the tip of the index finger. Then infiltrate the line of the incision with local anesthesia. Make a transverse incision in the cricothyroid space, about 2 cm in length. Carry the incision down to the cricothyroid membrane. Occlude any bleeding points with ligatures or electrocoagulation. Use a scalpel with a No. 15 blade to stab the cricothyroid

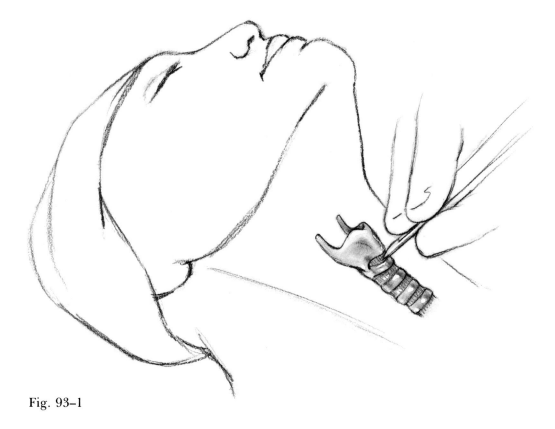

Fig. 93–1

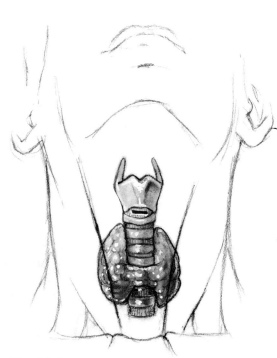

Fig. 93–2

membrane (**Figs. 93–1** and **93–2**). Enlarge the stab wound with a small hemostat or a Trousseau dilator, if available. Then insert a heavy Mayo scissors into the incision and spread the tissues transversely (**Fig. 93–3**) until the opening is sufficiently large to insert a low-pressure cuff tracheotomy tube, generally 8 mm in diameter (**Fig. 93–4**). Fix the tube in place and maintain it in the same manner as employed for intubation through the traditional tracheotomy incision. Closure of the skin wound is generally not necessary.

Postoperative Care

(See Chap. 94.)

Postoperative Complications

Peristomal bleeding
Transient hoarseness
Infection, cellutitis

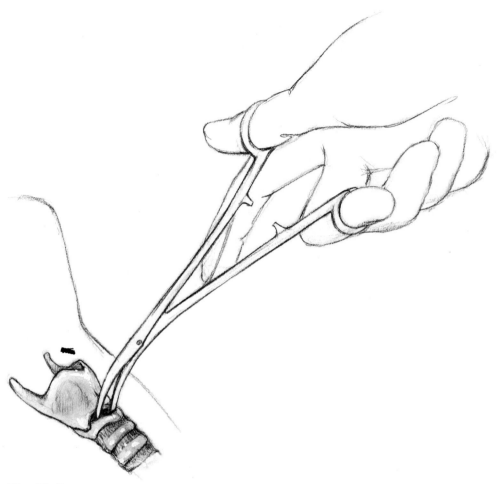

Fig. 93–3

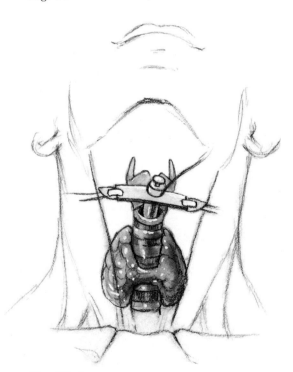

Fig. 93–4

Subglottic stenosis has not been seen unless the patient had undergone preoperative endotracheal intubation for more than 7 days or had an inflammatory condition of the larynx prior to operation.

References

Boyd AD, Romita M, Conlan A, Fink S et al. (1979) A clinical evaluation of cricothyroidotomy. Surg Gynecol Obstet 149:365

Brantigan CO, Grow JB (1976) Cricothyroidotomy: elective use in respiratory problems requiring tracheotomy. J Thorac Cardiovasc Surg 71:72

Brantigan CO, Grow JB (1982) Subglottic stenosis after cricothyroidotomy. Surgery 91:217

94 Tracheotomy

Concept: When to Do a Tracheotomy

As mentioned in Chap. 93, tracheotomy is not the optimal operation for use in emergency situations in the absence of adequate light, instruments, and suction apparatus. Under these conditions, orotracheal intubation or cricothyroidotomy are far better procedures.

At one time tracheotomy was frequently employed in patients with pulmonary disease in order to improve respiratory function by reducing the dead space and by providing a direct route to the trachea to facilitate aspiration of excessive bronchial secretions. At present, improved methods of pulmonary physiotherapy have reduced the necessity to perform tracheotomy to facilitate tracheal suctioning; efficient nursing management of orotracheal tubes in patients on mechanical ventilators has made it unnecessary to perform a tracheotomy in these patients if their need for assisted ventilation does not exceed 1–3 weeks' duration. This requires meticulous suctioning of the trachea and the use of a low-pressure cuff on the endotracheal tube. As a result of all these developments, the present primary usefulness of the tracheotomy arises in patients who require it for the *long-term* maintenance of an airway.

Indications

Organic upper airway obstruction
Radical oropharyngeal or thyroid surgery

Severe laryngeal trauma
Long-term ventilatory support

Preoperative Care

Pass an oral or nasal endotracheal tube preoperatively whenever possible.

Pitfalls and Danger Points

Injury during surgery to cricoid or first tracheal ring
Inadequate hemostasis
Asphyxia

Operative Strategy

Because most tracheotomy operations are performed with the orotracheal or nasotracheal tube in place, inhalation anesthesia is the agent most commonly employed. Local anesthesia is also quite satisfactory in most patients.

With an indwelling endotracheal tube in place, the risk of anoxia during tracheotomy is virtually eliminated. If for some reason an endotracheal tube is not in place, be certain the hemostasis is adequate prior to opening the trachea. Otherwise, blood may pour into the tracheal stoma, obstructing the airway. An adequate suction apparatus should always be available during tracheotomy. This is one reason why a cricothyroidotomy is a better operation

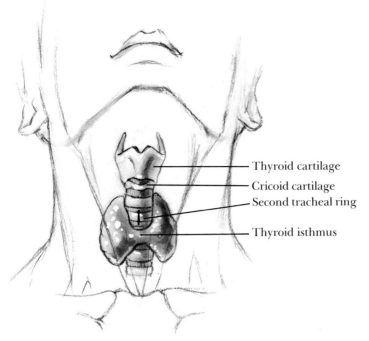

Thyroid cartilage
Cricoid cartilage
Second tracheal ring
Thyroid isthmus

Fig. 94–1

during an emergency situation when an endotracheal tube has not been passed.

If the incision in the trachea is made in the area of the first ring or the cricoid cartilage, there is great risk that a subglottic stenosis will occur after the tracheotomy tube has been removed. It should be recognized that the opening in the trachea, made by the tracheotomy tube, heals by cicatrization, incurring the risk that a mild narrowing of the trachea will occur at the site of

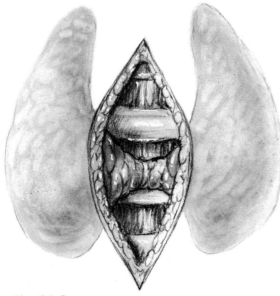

Fig. 94–2

the tracheotomy. If this occurs in the subglottic region, corrective therapy will be extremely difficult. For this reason, take every precaution to avoid incising or injuring the first ring or cricoid cartilage.

A very low tracheotomy incision, for instance in the 4th ring, may also entail an unnecessary risk for the patient. This is true because inserting a tracheotomy tube low down in the trachea may cause erosion of the innominate artery due to pressure exerted by the tip of the tube. This complication has on occasion resulted in massive hemorrhage into the trachea with prompt asphyxiation of the patient. This risk is especially applicable in children where the innominate artery is relatively close to the tracheotomy site.

Operative Technique

Endotracheal Tube

Virtually all patients should have an endotracheal tube in place prior to undergoing tracheotomy.

Incision and Exposure

Although some surgeons believe that a horizontal incision produces a better scar, the generally preferred incision is a vertical one beginning at the level of the cricoid and continuing in a caudal direction for about 4–5 cm. Carry the incision through the subcutaneous fat and the platysma muscle directly over the midline of the trachea, exposing the sternohyoid muscles. Achieve complete hemostasis with electrocautery and PG ligatures. Now elevate the strap muscles and make a vertical incision down the midline separating these two muscles. Carry the incision down to the upper trachea and expose and divide the capsule of the thyroid gland. Clamp, divide, and ligate all veins in this vicinity. Identify the thyroid isthmus. This bridge of tissue crosses the trachea generally in the vicinity of the 3rd tracheal ring (**Fig. 94–1 and 94–2**).

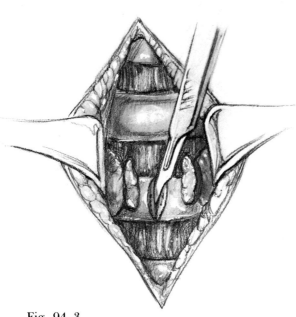

Fig. 94–3

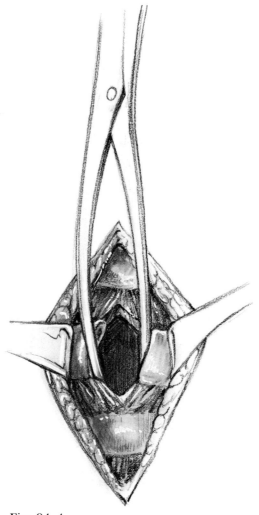

Fig. 94–4

Identifying the Tracheal Rings

Clearly visualize the cricoid cartilage and the first tracheal ring. Preserve these two structures from injury. Occasionally it may be possible to retract the thyroid isthmus in a cephalad direction to expose the 2nd and 3rd tracheal rings. However, in most cases, it will be necessary to elevate the thyroid isthmus from the trachea by sliding Metzenbaum scissors beneath the isthmus and elevating it. Then divide the isthmus between clamps and insert suture-ligatures to maintain complete hemostasis. This will clearly reveal the identity of the 2nd and 3rd tracheal rings (**Fig. 94–3**).

Opening the Trachea

Check that hemostasis is complete. Also, check that the suction apparatus is functioning.

In some cases incising only the 2nd ring will provide an adequate tracheotomy opening, but generally it will be necessary to incise both the 2nd and 3rd rings. This procedure is facilitated by inserting a single hook retractor to elevate the upper portion of the 2nd ring. Insert a scalpel with a No. 15 blade to incise the membrane transversely just above the 2nd ring. Then

divide the 2nd ring with the scalpel (Fig. 94–3) and also the 3rd ring if necessary. Never divide the 1st ring or the cricoid cartilage.

Inserting Tracheotomy Tube

Retract the edges of the trachea by inserting either a hemostat, two small hook retractors, or a Trousseau 3-prong retractor (**Fig. 94–4**). Since most tracheotomy operations will require the insertion of a tube with a large balloon cuff for mechanical ventilation, be certain to apply a water soluble lubricant to the tip of the tracheotomy tube and cuff. Then insert the tube

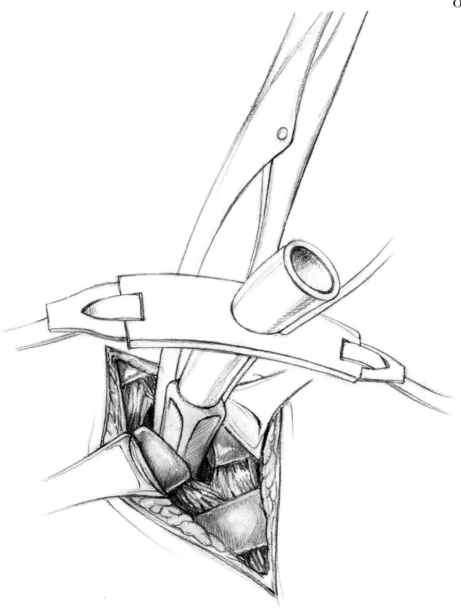

Fig. 94–5

into the tracheal incision **(Fig. 94–5)** while the anesthesiologist extracts the nasotracheal tube. Insert a suction catheter into the tracheotomy tube and aspirate mucous from the bronchial tree. Attach an oxygen line to the tracheotomy tube if necessary.

Closure

Reapproximate the sternohyoid muscles in the midline with interrupted 4–0 PG sutures. Insert several additional sutures to reapproximate the platysma muscle. Then close the skin *loosely* with interrupted 4–0 nylon sutures. Suture the tracheotomy tube to the skin in two places. As soon as practicable, tie the cotton tapes together in the back of the patient's neck to guarantee fixation of the tracheotomy tube.

547

Postoperative Care

Humidified air is necessary to prevent crusting of secretions and eventual obstruction of the tracheotomy tube.

Use light-weight swivel connectors to attach the tracheotomy tube to the ventilator to avoid unnecessary pressure on the trachea at the stoma.

If the tracheotomy tube has to be changed 1–2 weeks postoperatively, be certain to have instruments available for instant endotracheal intubation or emergency cricothyroidotomy if difficulty is encountered in reinserting a tracheotomy tube. Remember, the track between the skin and the tracheal stoma will not be established for a variable number of days after the operation. Therefore, locating the tracheal stoma deep in the neck may sometimes be extremely difficult. This is a procedure not to be performed by an inexperienced resident.

To improve the exposure of the trachea in the neck, hyperextend the patient's head by placing a rolled-up sheet under his shoulders. In order to help maintain the track of the tracheotomy tube, place the patient in a recumbent position with a sheet or sand bag beneath the shoulders. This will extend the head and neck, bringing the tracheal stoma closer to the skin incision. Only with the patient in this position should the old tracheotomy tube be removed and replaced. Never attempt this maneuver during the first two postoperative weeks with the patient in a sitting position.

Postoperative Complications

Hemorrhage following tracheotomy may occur as a result of the surgeon having failed to ligate the bleeding points in the wound. This will become manifest by bleeding around the tracheotomy tube. A far more serious hemorrhage may occur late in the postoperative period, the result of either the tip of the tracheotomy tube or the balloon cuff eroding through the anterior wall of the trachea into the innominate artery. This is a life-threatening complication manifested by arterial bleeding into the trachea. Emergency management of this condition depends on temporarily controlling the bleeding by inflating the balloon cuff. If inflating the cuff around the tracheotomy tube does not promptly control the bleeding, then remove it and immediately insert an orotracheal tube. Inflating the cuff of the orotracheal tube may then occlude the fistula from the trachea to the innominate artery. Emergency resection of the innominate artery with suture of both ends may be necessary for definitive repair of the fistula with resection also of the damaged trachea in some cases.

Subcutaneous emphysema may be avoided if the tissues are not sutured too snugly against the tracheotomy tube. There may be some air leakage between the trachea and the tracheotomy tube. If this air has access to the outside, subcutaneous emphysema will not occur.

Wound infection

Pneumothorax (rare)

Accidental displacement of tracheotomy tube

Stenosis may occur sometime after the tracheotomy tube has been removed. This complication may take place either at the tracheal stoma or in the area of the trachea occluded by the balloon cuff. Strictures at the stoma level may be minimized by making the incision in the trachea as small as possible. Constrictions lower in the trachea have been virtually eliminated by the large-volume, low-pressure balloon cuffs. If a patient who has undergone a period of mechanical ventilation with a tracheal tube ever develops signs of an upper airway obstruction (stridor or wheezing or shortness of breath), a stricture of the trachea should be strongly suspected.

A lateral X ray of the neck will disclose an upper tracheal stricture, while an oblique chest X ray should identify lower tracheal lesions. Tracheal resection and anastomosis may be necessary for serious strictures. A granuloma may be resected through a bronchoscope.

Miscellaneous

95 Ileoanal Anastomosis with Ileal Reservoir Following Total Colectomy and Mucosal Proctectomy

Concept: Currently Available Operations for Ulcerative Colitis and Familial Polyposis

Total Colectomy with Abdomino-perineal Proctosigmoidectomy and Permanent Ileostomy

This combination of operations will certainly accomplish complete removal of the diseased colonic mucosa. The threat that carcinoma may develop postoperatively in the colon is eliminated at the cost of removing all of the colon and rectum. The patient must live henceforth with a permanent ileostomy. Although many patients may make a good adjustment to life with a permanent ileostomy, the ileostomy does engender late surgical and psychosocial complications.

Kock Continent Ileostomy

While the Kock operation, with its various modifications, may eliminate the need for the patient constantly to wear an appliance, the operation is accompanied by many complications, and in several large series of such procedures as many as 30% of the patients have required reoperation for one cause or another. Even when the Kock ileostomy functions perfectly, it requires the patient to insert a catheter of some type into the ileostomy four times a day in order to empty the pouch.

Subtotal Colectomy with Ileoproctostomy

Although anastomosing the terminal ileum to the rectum following subtotal colectomy for ulcerative colitis has never achieved any popularity in the United States, it is an operation frequently performed in the United Kingdom, especially by Aylett. It is suitable in less than half the patients undergoing colectomy for ulcerative colitis. The recurrence of colitis is often severe enough to require dismantling the ileoproctostomy. Also, the remnant of rectum is subject to the development of carcinoma over a period of years. For this reason the operation is not a satisfactory solution to the problem of treating ulcerative colitis by surgical means.

Total Colectomy and Mucosal Proctectomy with End-to-End Ileoanal Anastomosis

In 1947 Ravitch and Sabiston (also Ravitch 1948) postulated that removing all of the rectal mucosa but preserving the wall of the rectum, followed by an ileoanal anastomosis, might preserve fecal continence subsequent to total colectomy. Although Ravitch and Handelsman subsequently reported nine successful results in patients with ulcerative colitis and familial polyposis, the operation did not achieve acceptance because of its complexity and because it was followed by many complications. However, because of their familiarity with the Soave operation, pediatric surgeons like Martin and LeCoultre and like Telander and Perrault have re-

553

ported satisfactory results with this operation in children and young adults. Telander's group initiated a program of balloon catheter dilatations of the distal ileum 2 weeks following operation. They felt that the dilatations accelerated the adaptation of the ileum into a successful reservoir more rapidly than was ordinarily the case. Nevertheless, 4 of Telander's 14 patients, who were followed for more than 1 year, continued to have fecal staining nightly. Also the average daily number of stools exceeded six, and 2 patients of the 14 were converted to permanent ileostomies. For this reason considerable interest was directed to the addition of an ileal reservoir to the operation under discussion.

Total Colectomy, Mucosal Proctectomy, Ileal Reservoir, and Ileoanal Anastomosis

Martin and LeCoultre performed 19 operations without a reservoir, and Martin and Fischer reported 18 patients who underwent the same operation with the addition of an "S" reservoir similar to the one reported by Parks, Nicholls, and Belliveau. Martin and Fischer found that the patients who were given a reservoir have had significantly fewer bowel movements. Their patients sustained no complications related to the reservoir except for mild temporary stasis in two cases. They emphasized that the reservoir should be brought down to within 1 cm of the end-to-end ileoanal anastomosis, unlike Parks's reservoir, which remains about 5 cm above the anastomosis. Parks and associates noted that in a large number of their early cases, catheterization of the reservoir was required in the early postoperative period to assure complete emptying.

Utsunomiya, Iwama, Imajo, Matuso, and associates introduced the concept of a "J" shaped ileal reservoir, the elbow of which was anastomosed to the anus. This brings the pouch itself inside the cuff of rectal muscularis. These authors found that patients with the "J" pouch achieved

satisfactory bowel function sooner than did those undergoing different types of sphincter-saving colectomies. Pemberton, Heppell, Beart, Dozois, and associates, after reviewing the literature together with their own experiences, came to the conclusion that it was advisable to construct

"an ileal reservoir in order to achieve increased capacity of the ileum more rapidly and reliably and, therefore, reduce or eliminate overflow incontinence, nocturnal soiling and perineal excoriation. If a patient is to be continent after undergoing ileoanal anastomosis and not merely possess an anal ileostomy, reservoir capacity as well as sphincteric preservation must be provided."

These authors prefer the "J" pouch. It should be noted that even in the absence of an ileal reservoir, Heppel, Kelley, Phillips, Beart, and colleagues found that the resting pressures and squeeze pressures of the anal sphincter subsequent to mucosal proctectomy and ileoanostomy were similar to those in healthy control patients. These authors concluded that, although the sphincter function seemed to be good, the maximum capacity of the ileum was far less than that of normal rectum. Taylor, Beart, Dozois, Kelly, and associates compared 50 patients following straight ileoanal anastomoses with 74 patients subjected to "J" pouch-anal anastomoses. The patients with pouches experienced less diarrhea, better continence, and an improved quality of life in this study.

Our operation of choice at this time is mucosal proctectomy combined with a "J" shaped ileal reservoir and anastomosis between the elbow of the reservoir and the anus.

One-, Two-, or Three-Stage Operation

In well-nourished patients who do not have much disease in the distal rectum, a total colectomy, mucosal proctectomy, and ileoanostomy may be performed at one sitting, provided the possibility of Crohn's disease has been eliminated. Martin and Fischer advocate a 4- to 6-week period of total parenteral alimentation, systemic steroids, steroid enemas, and systemic antibiotics. Meanwhile, nothing is given by mouth. Of the 27 patients treated by this regimen, 26 healed almost all the inflammation and ulcerations in their rectums. Then, a total colectomy, mucosal proctectomy, and ileoanostomy were performed. Rothenberger, Vermeulen, Christenson, Balcos, and associates as well as other surgeons prefer to pursue a different strategy in the acutely ill or malnourished patients. They treat these patients by means of a three-stage procedure, the first stage of which is an ileostomy, subtotal colectomy with mucous fistula or a Hartmann pouch. Then, nutritional rehabilitation is combined with steroid enemas, systemic steroids, or antibiotics as necessary prior to the second-stage operation, which consists of mucosal proctectomy, reservoir construction, ileoanostomy, and a diverting temporary loop ileostomy. The third stage, generally performed 3 months later, consists of closing the loop ileostomy.

In general, we prefer the three-stage sequence of procedures for the malnourished patient. At the present stage of development, we still prefer with respect to these operations to routinely perform a temporary diverting loop ileostomy because it is extremely important to avoid infection in the area of the ileoanostomy. So much depends on the proprioceptive nerves in the puborectalis and levator ani muscles that permitting an anastomotic leak to develop into a cuff abscess may produce sufficient fibrosis to eliminate the function of these nerve endings. Consequently, until we learn more about these procedures, it is wise to take precautions that will minimize the incidence of cuff or pelvic abscesses.

Indications

Colectomy, mucosal proctectomy, and ileostomy are indicated in ulcerative colitis when the complications or intractability of the disease or the threat of cancer requires surgery, provided there is no advanced ulceration of the lower rectum.

Familial polyposis

Contraindications

Crohn's disease

Perianal fistulas

Advanced disease of the lower rectum

Preoperative Care

Inflammation and ulcerations of the lower rectum must be treated preoperatively. If the patient has had a subtotal colectomy and ileostomy, steroid enemas (Proctocort)—and sometimes systemic steroids and antibiotics—may be helpful.

Nutritional rehabilitation when necessary

Perioperative antibiotics

Nasogastric tube

Foley catheter in bladder

Endoscopy of ileum via the ileostomy when Crohn's disease is suspected after subtotal colectomy

If one-stage colectomy and ileoanostomy is anticipated, appropriate mechanical and antibiotic bowel preparation is indicated.

Pitfalls and Danger Points

Performing an inadequate mucosectomy, which may produce a cuff abscess and possibly lead later to carcinoma

555

Establishing inadequate pelvic, reservoir, or anastomotic hemostasis, which may result in postoperative hemorrhage

Injuring the nervi erigentes or the hypogastric nerves so that either sexual impotence or retrograde ejaculation results

Failing to properly diagnose Crohn's disease with development of Crohn's ileitis in the reservoir

Using improper technique in closing temporary loop ileostomy which in turn leads to postoperative leakage or obstruction

Operative Strategy

Mucosectomy

Both Rothenberger and associates and Sullivan and Garnjobst recommend starting the operation by placing the patient in the prone jackknife position in order to excise the distal 5–6 cm of rectal mucosa transanally. This dissection is expedited by injecting a solution of epinephrine (1:200,000) into the submucosal plane. If the rectum is so badly diseased that mucosectomy cannot be reasonably accomplished, the remainder of the operation is contraindicated.

Some of the earlier authors reporting on muscosal proctectomy felt that it was necessary to dissect the mucosa away from the rectal muscularis for a distance of perhaps 8–10 cm above the dentate line. This is not necessary. Good fecal continence can be maintained if the mucosa is dissected away from the rectum up to a point no more than 1–2 cm above the puborectalis, the upper end of the anal canal. This amount of dissection can generally be accomplished transanally with less difficulty in the adult patient than from the abdominal approach, although mucosectomy by the abdominal approach (as described by Soave) is also an acceptable method. Com-

plete hemostasis in the region of the retained rectum must by attained. Generally, careful electrocoagulation will accomplish this end.

Frozen-section histological examination of the excised mucosa may be helpful in ruling out Crohn's disease.

Abdominal Dissection

Division of Ileum
In performing the colectomy, transect the ileum just proximal to its junction with the ileocecal valve in order to preserve the reabsorptive functions of the distal ileum. If a previous ileostomy is being taken down, again preserve as much terminal ileum as possible.

Rectal Dissection
In dissecting the rectum away from the sacrum, keep the dissection immediately adjacent to the rectal wall. Divide the mesenteric vessels near the point where they enter the rectum and leave the major portion of the "mesentery" behind. In this way the hypogastric nerves will be preserved.

Similarly, when the lateral ligaments are divided, make the point of division as close to the rectum as possible in order to avoid dividing the parasympathetic nerves essential for normal male sexual function. Anteriorly, the dissection proceeds close to the rectal wall posterior to the seminal vesicles and Denonvillier's fascia down to the distal end of the prostate.

Division of Waldeyer's Fascia
In the adult patient it will not be possible to expose the levator diaphragm unless the fascia of Waldeyer is divided by sharp dissection. This layer of dense fascia is attached to the anterior surface of the sacrum and coccyx and attaches to the posterior wall of the rectum. Unless it is divided just anterior to the tip of the coccyx, it will not be possible to expose the lower rectum down to the level of the puborectalis muscle.

Temporary Loop Ileostomy

Described by Turnbull and Weakly (see Chap. 35), the loop ileostomy will completely divert the fecal stream, yet it is a simple ileostomy to close without requiring the resection and anastomosis of the ileum. Since several authors have reported complications, such as stricture and leakage, following closure of the temporary ileostomy, it behooves the surgeon to perform this operation carefully. If the tissues are not unduly traumatized in freeing the ileostomy from the abdominal wall, closure of this ileal stoma should have a low complication rate.

Ileoanostomy

In order to facilitate anastomosing the ileum or the ileal reservoir to the anus, it is helpful to flex the thighs on the abdomen to a greater extent than is usually the case when the patient is placed in the lithotomy position for a two-team abdominoperineal operation. Be certain that the rectal mucosa has been divided close to the dentate line. Otherwise, it will be necessary to insert sutures high up in the anal canal where transanal manipulation of the needle will be extremely difficult. Also, it is important to remove all of the diseased mucosa in this operation to eliminate the possibility of the patient developing a rectal carcinoma at a later date.

One method of achieving exposure with this anastomosis is to insert the bivalve Parks retractor with the large blades into the rectum. Then draw the ileum down, between the open blades of the retractor, to the dentate line. Insert two sutures between the ileum and the anterior wall of the anus. Insert two more sutures between the ileum and the posterior portion of the dentate line. Now, remove the

Parks retractor. Remove the large blades from the retractor and replace them with the small blades. Then carefully insert the blades of the Parks retractor into the lumen of the ileum and open the retractor slowly.

With the Parks retractor blades in place, continue to approximate the ileum to the dentate line with 12–15 interrupted sutures of 5–0 Vicryl. This will require that the retractor be loosened and rotated from time to time to provide exposure of the entire circumference of the anastomosis. Be certain to include the underlying internal sphincter muscle together with the epithelial layer of the anal canal when inserting these sutures.

An alternative and more effective method of exposing the anastomosis is to use a Gelpi retractor with one arm inserted into the tissues immediately distal to the dentate line at about 2 o'clock while the second arm of this retractor is placed at 8 o'clock. A second Gelpi retractor is inserted into the anus with one arm at 5 o'clock and the second at 11 o'clock. If the patient is properly relaxed, these two retractors should assure visibility of the whole circumference of the cut end of the anorectal mucosa at the dentate line. Then draw the ileum down into the anal canal and complete the anastomosis.

Constructing the Ileal Reservoir

We prefer a J-loop ileal reservoir that is constructed by making a side-to-side anastomosis in the distal segment of the ileum. We do not include the elbow of the J-loop in the staple line so that there is no possibility of impairing the blood supply to the ileoanal anastomosis. The terminal end of the ileum is occluded with staples.

Although it is possible to establish an ileoanal anastomosis by using an EEA stapler, we prefer to suture this anastomosis because there is some risk of sacrificing too much anoderm and internal sphincter muscle when the stapling device is used.

Operative Technique—Mucosal Proctectomy, Ileal Reservoir, and Endoerectal Ileoanal Anastomosis

Mucosal Proctectomy Combined with Total Colectomy

When the mucosa of the distal rectum is devoid of visible ulcerations and significant inflammation, mucosal proctectomy may be performed at the same time as total colectomy. In these cases perform the colectomy as described in Chap. 32. Be certain to divide the mesentery of the rectosigmoid close to the bowel wall in order to avoid damaging the hypogastric and the parasympathetic nerves. Also, divide the branches of the ileocolic vessels close to the cecum to preserve the blood supply of the terminal ileum. It is important to transect the ileum within 1–2 cm of the ileocecal valve. Preserving as much ileum as possible will salvage some of the important absorptive functions of this organ.

In transecting the terminal ileum, use a GIA stapler and lightly electrocoagulate the everted mucosa. Mobilize the entire colon down to the peritoneal reflection, following the procedures illustrated in Figs. 32–1 to 32–7. Divide the specimen with a GIA stapler at the sigmoid level.

Before proceeding with the mucosal proctectomy, perform multiple frozen-section histological examinations of the colon specimen to rule out the possibility that the patient may be suffering from Crohn's disease. If there is a question that the patient may have Crohn's disease, one may perform an ileostomy and a mucous fistula and wait for permanent histological sections rather than proceed to immediate mucosal proctectomy.

Divide the rectosigmoid mesentery close to the bowel wall to avoid interrupting the hypogastric nerves (see Fig. 36–1). Divide the lateral ligaments close to the rectum and divide Denonvillier's fascia proximal to the upper border of the pros-tate. If the dissection is kept *close to the anterior and lateral rectal walls* in men, the incidence of sexual impotence following surgery will be minimized. After dividing Waldeyer's fascia (see Fig. 30–8), expose the puborectalis portion of the levator diaphragm (see Fig. 30–23).

At this time, transect the anterior surface of the rectal layer of muscularis in a transverse direction down to the mucosa. Make this incision in the rectal wall about 2–4 cm above the puborectalis muscle. Now dissect the muscular layer away from the mucosa. Injecting a solution of 1:200,000 epinephrine between the mucosa and muscularis expedites this dissection. After the muscle has been separated from 1–2 cm of mucosa anteriorly, extend the incision in the muscularis layer circumferentially around the rectum. Use a Metzenbaum scissors and a peanut sponge dissector in this step. Achieve complete hemostasis by accurate electrocoagulation. Continue the mucosal dissection until the middle of the anal canal has been reached. Divide the mucosal cylinder at this point, remove the specimen, and leave an empty cuff of muscle about 4 cm in length above the puborectalis, which marks the proximal extent of the anal canal. If any mucosa has been left in the anal canal proximal to the dentate line, it will be removed transanally later in the operation.

Alternatively, one may perform the rectal mucosectomy prior to opening the abdomen. This method is described in the next section of this chapter.

Mucosal Proctectomy by the Perineal Approach

We agree with the suggestion of Sullivan and Garnjobst that the rectal mucosal dissection is best performed as the initial step in the operation, whether or not the procedure is combined with a simultaneous total colectomy. If it is not possible to dissect the mucosa away from the internal sphincter, then perform an ileostomy and abdominoperineal total proctectomy instead of an ileoanostomy.

Performing the mucosal proctectomy with the patient in the prone position affords better exposure than is available in the lithotomy position. After inducing endotracheal anesthesia, turn the patient face down and elevate the hips either by flexing the operating table or by placing a pillow under the hips. Also place a small pillow under the feet and spread the buttocks apart by applying adhesive tape to the skin and attaching the tape to the sides of the operating table. Gently dilate the anus until it admits three fingers. Obtain exposure by using either a large Hill-Ferguson, a

narrow Deaver, or a bivalve Pratt (or Parks) retractor. Inject a solution of 1:200,000 epinephrine in saline in the plane just deep to the mucosa, immediately proximal to the dentate line around the circumference of the anal canal (**Fig. 95–1**). Now make a circumferential incision in the transitional epithelium immediately cephalad to the dentate line. Using a Metzenbaum scissors, elevate the mucosa and submucosa for a distance of 1–2 cm circumferentially from the underlying circular fibers of the

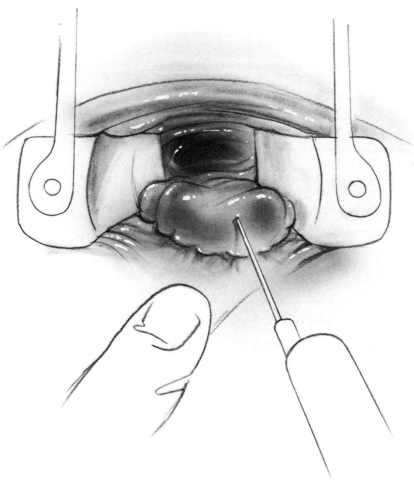

Fig. 95–1

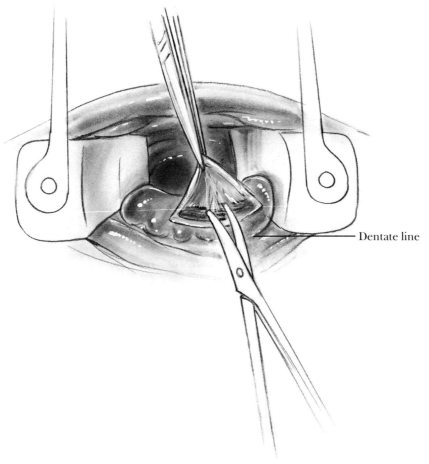

Dentate line

Fig. 95–2

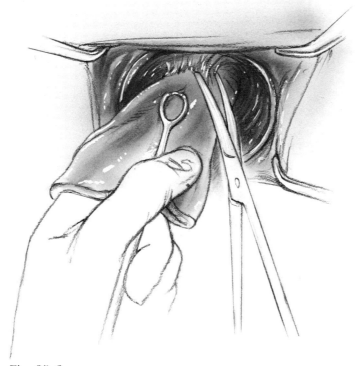

Fig. 95–3

internal sphincter muscle **(Fig. 95–2).** Apply several Allis clamps to the cut end of the mucosa. Maintain hemostasis by accurate electrocoagulation. It is helpful to roll up two 10 × 20-cm moist gauze sponges and to insert this roll into the rectum. This step facilitates the dissection between mucosa and muscle. Continue the dissection to a point 6–8 cm above the anal verge **(Fig. 95–3).** As the dissection continues cephalad, exposure is obtained by inserting two narrow Deaver retractors that the assistant holds in varying positions appropriate to the area being dissected.

After an adequate tube of mucosa has been dissected, insert a purse string near the apex of the dissected mucosal tube and amputate the mucosa distal to the purse-string suture. Submit this specimen to the pathologist for frozen-section histological examination to identify any hitherto undiagnosed cases of Crohn's disease. Insert into the denuded rectum a loose gauze pack that has been moistened with an epinephrine solution. Reposition the patient on his back with the lower extremities elevated on Lloyd-Davies stirrups (see Figs. 31–1a and 31–1b).

Abdominal Incision and Exposure

In patients who have undergone a previous subtotal colectomy with a mucous fistula and an ileostomy, reopen the previous long vertical incision, free all of the adhesions between the small bowel and the peritoneum, and liberate the mucous fistula from the abdominal wall. Divide the mesentery between Kelly hemostats along a line close to the posterior wall of the sigmoid and rectosigmoid until the peritoneal reflection is reached. Incise the peritoneal reflection to the right and to the left of the rectum. Continue the dissection downward and free the vascular and areolar tissue from the wall of the rectum. Then elevate the rectum out of the presacral space and in-cise the peritoneum of the rectovesical or rectouterine pouch (see Fig. 31–7). Keep the dissection close to the rectal wall, especially in males, to avoid the nervi erigentes and the hypogastric nerves. Pay special attention to dividing the lateral ligaments close to the rectum; also avoid the parasympathetic plexus between the prostate and the rectum.

Now, with a long-handled scalpel incise Waldeyer's fascia (see Fig. 31–8) between the tip of the coccyx and the posterior wall of the rectum. Enlarge this incision with a long Metzenbaum scissors. In the male, incise Denonvillier's fascia on (see Fig. 31–9) the anterior wall of the rectum proximal to the prostate and the seminal vesicles. Separate prostate from rectum. These last two maneuvers will permit exposure of the levator diaphragm. Palpating the rectum at this time should enable the surgeon to detect the level at which the purse-string suture was placed in the mucosa during the first phase of this operation. If this purse-string suture is not palpable, ask the assistant to place a finger in the rectum from the perineal approach to help identify the apex of the previous mucosal dissection. Now transect the rectum with the elctrocoagulator and remove the specimen. Remove the gauze packing that was previously placed in the rectal stump and inspect the muscular cylinder, which is all that remains of the rectum. This consists of the circular muscle of the internal sphincter surrounded by the longitudinal muscle of the rectum. All of the mucosa has been removed down to the dentate line. Check for complete hemostasis.

Constructing the Ileal Reservoir

In patients, who have had a previous ileostomy, carefully dissect the ileum away from the abdominal wall. Preserve as much ileum as possible. Apply a TA-55 stapler across a healthy portion of the terminal ileum. Fire the stapler and amputate the scarred portion of the ileostomy. Lightly electrocoagulate the everted mucosa and remove the stapling device. Now liberate the mesentery of the ileum from its attachment to the abdominal parieties. Determine whether the mesentery is long enough that the distal ileum may be brought down to the anal canal after a J-shaped reservoir has been constructed, about 12 cm in length. In an obese man who has a deep pelvis the mesentery of the ileum may not permit the elbow of the reservoir to reach the anus. In some cases, freeing the small bowel mesentery from its posterior attachments (see Figs 20–1 and 20–2) will sufficiently elongate the mesentery so that the ileal reservoir will reach the anal canal *without tension.* If this maneuver is not successful, transilluminate the

mesentery and determine whether dividing certain mesenteric blood vessels may permit the mesentery to stretch while at the same time an adequate blood flow to the marginal arcades is preserved (**Figs. 95–4 and 95–5**). If this is not the case, construction of an ileoanal reservoir will have to be abandoned in favor of a permanent ileostomy.

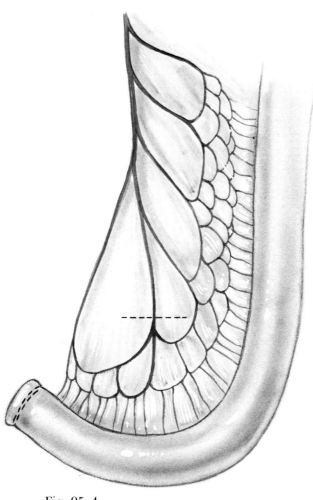

Fig. 95–4

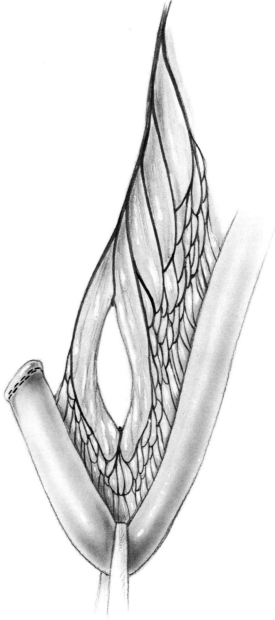

Fig. 95–5

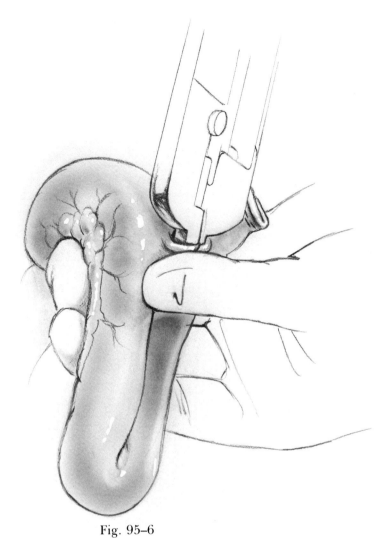

Fig. 95–6

Be certain that the blood supply to the terminal ileum will remain vigorous and that there will be no tension on the ileoanal anastomosis. Take great care to isolate and ligate each vessel in the ileal mesentery individually, especially if the mesentery is thickened from scar tissue or obesity. Several cases have been reported of postoperative hemorrhage from divided mesenteric vessels as well as of a large hematoma of the mesentery producing ileal ischemia.

Now align the distal ileum in the shape of a U, each limb of which measures about 16–18 cm. Create a side-to-side anastomosis between the antimesenteric aspects of the ascending and descending limbs of this U. Make a transverse stab wound 6 cm proximal to the staple line of the terminal ileum. Make a second transverse stab wound in the descending limb of ileum just opposite the first stab wound. Insert a GIA stapler in a cephalad direction, one fork in the descending limb and one fork in the ascending limb of jejunum. Remember that this anastomosis is created on the antimesenteric borders of both limbs of jejunum. Fire the GIA stapler. This will create a 4–5 cm side-to-side anastomosis. Withdraw the stapling device and inspect the staple line for bleeding. Electrocoagulate bleeding points cautiously. Then reinsert the device into the same two stab wounds but direct the GIA in a caudal direction **(Fig. 95–6).** Lock the device and fire the staples. Remove the GIA and inspect for bleeding. Now make two additional transverse stab incisions in the ileum 8 cm distal to the two initial stab wounds

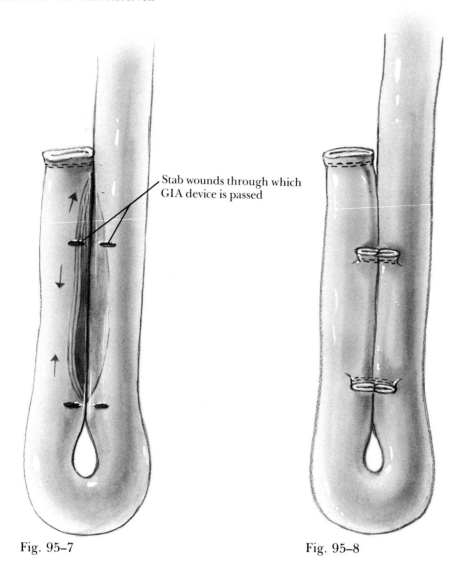

Stab wounds through which GIA device is passed

Fig. 95–7   Fig. 95–8

(Fig. 95–7). Insert a freshly reloaded GIA device, one fork in the descending and one fork in the ascending jejunum with the GIA pointed in a cephalad direction. Lock the GIA into a position that will permit the device to engage the previous anastomotic staple lines. Fire the staples and remove the GIA device. Inspect the staple line via the stab wounds and electrocoagulate the bleeding points. The patient should now have a completed side-to-side stapled anastomosis about 12 cm in length. If it is desired to lengthen the anastomosis somewhat, insert a reloaded GIA device through the distal stab wounds and point the device in a caudal direction grasping about 2–3 cm of tissue and fire the staples. Under no conditions should the staple line be continued distally to the end of the reservoir since this step would not leave any free antimesenteric wall of ileum for the ileoanal anastomosis. For this reason, leave an intact circular loop of ileum distal to the side-to-side anastomosis.

The ileal reservoir is now complete except for the two remaining defects through which the GIA stapling device was previously inserted. Apply Allis clamps to approximate, in a transverse direction, the walls of the ileum in preparation for the transverse application of a TA-55 stapling device that will accomplish an everted closure of the defect. Be certain that the superior and inferior terminations of the previous staple lines are included in the TA-55 device before firing the staples. Also, avoid the error of trying to fire the TA-55 when the two terminations of the previous staple lines are in exact apposition (see Figs. 27–18 to 27–20). After the TA-55 has been fired, lightly electrocoagulate the everted mucosa and carefully inspect the staple line to be sure of proper "B" formation. Then repeat this procedure to close the defect of the distal stab wounds **(Fig. 95–8)**.

Alternatively, sutures may be used to construct the side-to-side anastomosis. Make longitudinal incisions 12 cm in length on the antimesentric borders of both the ascending and descending limbs of the ileum. Achieve hemostasis with the electrocoagulator. Insert interrupted sutures to approximate the bowel walls at the proximal and distal margins of the anastomosis with 3–0 Vicryl. Insert another suture at the midpoint between these two. Then use a straight atraumatic intestinal needle with 3–0 Vicryl starting at the apex of the posterior portion of the anastomosis and use a continuous locked suture encompassing all the layers of the bowel. Accomplish closure of the anterior layer of the anastomosis by means of a continuous seromucosal or Lembert (see Figs. B–16 and B–17) suture. Rothenberger and associates use a single layer of continuous suture to complete the entire anastomosis.

Carefully inspect all aspects of the side-to-side anastomosis, both front and back, to be certain that there are no defects or technical errors.

Ileoanal Anastomosis

Before passing the elbow of the ileal reservoir down through the anus, recheck the position of the pelvis and the buttocks on the operating table. The perineum should project beyond the edge of the table. The simplest method of exposing the dentate line for the anastomossis is to insert two Gelpi retractors, one at right angles to the other. The prongs of the retractors should be inserted fairly close to the dentate line so that the transected anorectal junction can be seen. Insert the first Gelpi retractor in the axis between 2 and 8 o'clock and the second between 5 and 11 o'clock. If exposure, for some reason, is not adequate, it may be helpful to readjust the stirrups so that the thighs are flexed upon the abdomen. This position makes more convenient the application of retractors to the anus.

Insert two long Babcock clamps through the anus and grasp the dependent portion of the ileal reservoir. Bring this segment of ileum into the anal canal. Be certain that the bowel has not been twisted during this maneuver and that the mesentery lies flat and *that it will not exert significant tension* on the anastomosis to be constructed. Make a longitudinal incision along the dependent border of the ileal

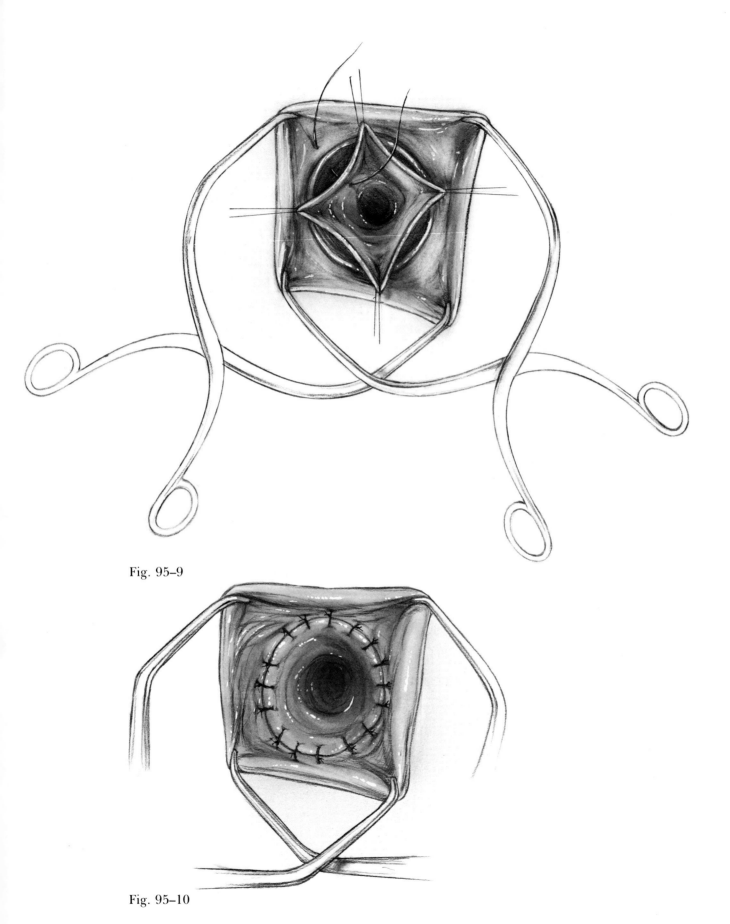

Fig. 95–9

Fig. 95–10

reservoir. Electrocoagulate the bleeding points. Apply traction sutures to the incised ileum, one to each quadrant **(Fig. 95–9)**. Construct a one-layer anastomosis between the ileum and the dentate line of the anus. Be sure to include in each stitch a 4-mm bite of underlying internal sphincter muscle as well as anal epithelium. Use atraumatic 4–0 Vicryl sutures (Fig. 95–9).

If the anal canal is deep, using a double-curved Stratte needle-holder (see Fig. D–14) is helpful. Insert the first four sutures at 12, 6, 3, and 9 o'clock. Then continue to insert sutures by the method of successive bisection (see Figs. B–22 and B–23). The resulting ileoanal anastomosis should be widely patent **(Fig. 95–10)**. If desired, the ileal reservoir may now be inflated with a methylene blue solution to check for possible defects in the reservoir staple or suture lines. **Fig. 95–11** illustrates the completed anastomosis.

Loop Ileostomy

Until more experience has accumulated to demonstrate that this step is not necessary, we believe that all of these patients should have a temporary diverting loop ileostomy similar to that described by Turnbull and Weakley (see Chap. 35). If the patient has a defect in the abdominal wall that remains from the dismantling of a previous ileostomy, it is generally possible to use the same site for the loop ileostomy. Insert a large Babcock clamp through the opening in the abdominal wall and grasp the antimesenteric aspect of a segment of ileum proximal to the ileal reservoir. Select a segment of ileum that will not exert any tension whatever on the ileal reservoir. Draw the loop of ileum through the opening in the abdominal wall **(Fig. 95–12)**. Position the ileum so that the afferent or proximal limb of ileum enters the stoma from its cephalad aspect and the distal ileum leaves the stoma at its inferior aspect. In order

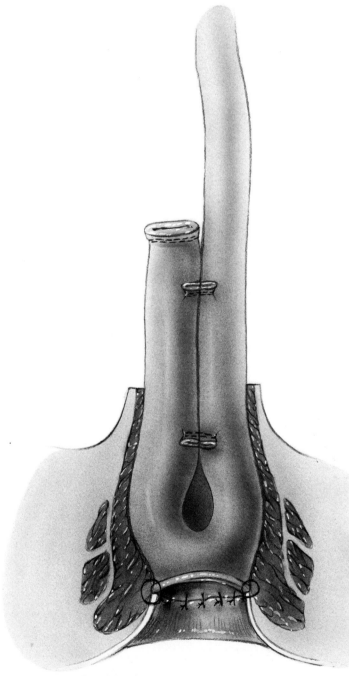

Fig. 95–11

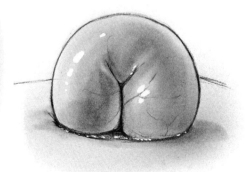

Fig. 95–12

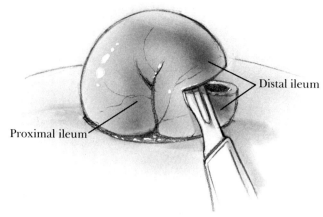

Fig. 95–13

to insure that the proximal stoma will dominate the distal stoma and completely divert the fecal stream, transect the anterior half of the ileum at a point 2-cm distal to the apex of the loop **(Fig. 95–13)**. Then evert the ileostomy **(Fig. 95–14)**. Insert interrupted atraumatic sutures of 4–0 Vicryl to approximate the full thickness of the ileum to the subcuticular portion of the skin. The end result should demonstrate a dominant proximal stoma that compresses the distal stoma **(Fig. 95–15)**. We do not suture the ileum to the peritoneum or fascia.

In order to minimze the contamination of the abdominal cavity, it is possible to deliver the loop of ileum through the abdominal wall, then pass a small catheter around the ileum and through the mesentery in order to maintain the position of the ileum. The actual division of the ileum and suturing of the ileostomy may be post-poned until the abdominal incision has been completely closed. After suturing the ileum to the subcutis, remove the catheter.

Drainage and Closure

Intermittently throughout the construction of the ileal reservoir and the perineal anastomosis, we irrigate the operative field with a dilute antibiotic solution. This step is repeated during the closure of the abdominal wall.

With respect to draining the operative site, a number of authors insert a tube drain between the rectal cuff and the ileal reservoir because a hematoma or infection in this area may produce fibrosis and impair fecal continence. We do not believe that this step will compensate for imperfect hemostasis. Consequently, at this point in the operation, make every effort to achieve complete hemostasis in the rectal cuff and in the pelvis. Insert one or two Jackson-Pratt silicone closed-suction drains through puncture wounds in the abdominal wall down to the rectal cuff. Some authors believe it is important to place a layer of sutures between the proximal cut end of the rectal cuff and the ileal reservoir. Although we do not believe that these sutures will compensate for an inadequate ileoanal anastomosis, they may help prevent tension on the anastomosis.

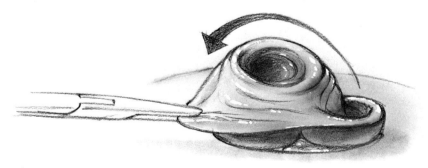

Fig. 95–14

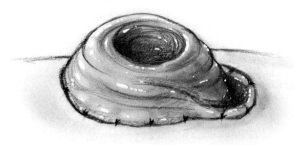

Fig. 95–15

Close the abdominal wall with interrupted 1 PDS or nonabsorbable sutures by the modified Smead-Jones technique described in Chap. 5. Close the skin with interrupted fine nylon or skin staples. Then mature the loop ileostomy as described above if this step has not already been done.

Postoperative Care

Continue perioperative antibiotics for 24 hours.

Continue nasogastric suction until the ileostomy begins to function.

Remove the closed-suction drains from the pelvis between the 4th and 6th postoperative day, depending on the volume of drainage. Inject 25 mg kanamycin in 25 ml saline into the drainage catheters every 6 hours.

Until the loop ileostomy is closed, perform weekly or biweekly digital examinations of the anastomosis in order to prevent the development of a stricture.

About 8 weeks following operation, if there has been uneventful healing without any evidence of hematoma or sepsis in the pelvis, perform a barium enema to visualize the ileal reservoir. Rule out anastomotic defects by direct inspection and palpation. If both these procedures are negative, close the loop ileostomy.

Following closure of the loop ileostomy, administer medications such as Lomotil, Immodium, codeine, or Metamucil, which will probably be required to help solidify the consistency of the bowel movements for a period of weeks.

Postoperative Complications

An abscess may occur in the rectal cuff or the pelvis. This complication has been reported in the early postoperative period but, remarkably enough, it has also been noted 2 and 6 months postoperatively in other cases. If the loop ileostomy is still in place, most cuff abscesses may be treated by drainage directly through the anastomosis. Pelvic abscesses may require laparotomy for drainage. With proper precautions postoperative sepsis should be rare.

Hematoma in pelvis or in reservoir

Anastomotic dehiscence or stricture

Wound infection

Urinary tract infection

Excessive number of stools

Fecal incontinence

"Pouchitis" rarely occurs following the "J" pouch, but in the "S" pouch described by Parks, Nicholls, and Belliveau, where stagnation is more common, bacterial overgrowth produces an enteritis. This condition may require metronidazole combined with frequent catheterization of the pouch by the patient.

Acute intestinal obstruction due to adhesions

References

Aylette SO (1966) Three hundred cases of diffuse ulcerative colitis treated by total colectomy and ileorectal anastomosis. Br Med J 1:1001

Heppel J, Kelley KA, Phillips SF, Beart RW Jr et al. (1982) Physiologic aspects of continence after colectomy, mucosal proctectomy, and endorectal ileo-anal anastomosis. Ann Surg 195:435

Martin LW, Fischer JE, (1982) Preservation of anorectal continence following total colectomy. Ann Surg 196:700

Martin LW, LeCoultre C (1978) Technical considerations in performing total colectomy and Soave endorectal anastomosis for ulcerative colitis. J Pediatr Surg 13:762

Parks AG, Nicholls RJ, Belliveau P (1980) Proctocolectomy with ileal reservoir and anal anastomosis. Br J Surg 67:533

Pemberton JH, Hepell J, Beart RW Jr, Dozois RR, et al. (1982) Endorectal ileoanal anastomosis. Surg Gynecol Obstet 155:417

Ravitch MM (1948) Anal ileostomy with sphincter preservation in patients requiring total colectomy for benign conditions. Surgery 24:170

Ravitch MM, Handelsman JC (1951) One stage resection of entire colon and rectum for ulcerative colitis and polypoid adenomatosis. Bull Johns Hopkins Hosp 88:59

Ravitch MM, Sabiston DC (1947) Anal ileostomy with preservation of the sphincter. Surg Gynecol Obstet 84:1095

Rothenberger DA, Vermeulen FD, Christenson CE, Balcos EG et al. (1983) Restorative proctocolectomy with ileal reservoir and ileoanal anastomosis. Am J Surg 145:82

Soave F (1964) A new technique for treatment of Hirschprung's disease. Surgery 56: 56:1007

Sullivan ES, Garnjobst WM (1982) Advantage of initial transanal mucosal stripping in ileo-anal pull-through procedures. Dis Colon Rectum 25:170

Taylor BM, Beart RW Jr, Dozois RR, Kelly KA et al. (1983) Straight ileoanal anastomosis v. ileal pouch-anal anastomosis after colectomy and mucosal proctectomy. Arch Surg 118:696

Telander RL, Perrault J (1981) Colectomy with rectal mucosectomy and ileoanal anastomosis in young patients. Arch Surg 116:623

Utsunomiya J, Iwama T, Imajo M, Matuso S et al. (1980) Total colectomy, mucosal proctectomy, and ileoanal anastomosis. Dis Colon Rectum 23:459

96 Drainage of Subphrenic Abscess

Concept: Etiology and Modern Management of Subphrenic Abscess

Etiology

Although subphrenic abscesses may arise from primary infections of the biliary tract, the appendix, or the colon, in the great majority of cases subphrenic sepsis follows a previous abdominal operation. In DeCosse, Poulin, Fox, and Condon's study of 52 patients in whom subphrenic sepsis followed previous surgery, 22 of them developed abscesses subsequent to operations on the stomach and 11 of them, abscesses after biliary tract surgery. Other causes of subphrenic abscesses included surgery for trauma in 7 patients and colon operations in another 7 cases. These authors felt that postoperative bleeding was a common contributing cause in their series of subphrenic abscesses, many of which were, in fact, infected hematomas. Inadvertent splenectomy was another postoperative complication associated with left-sided subphrenic sepsis following gastric surgery.

Diagnosis

Clinical Assessment
Only about two-thirds of the patients with subphrenic abscesses demonstrate a typical clinical picture of fever, localized pain or tenderness, leukocytosis, and ipsilateral pleural effusion on chest X ray. In the *early* stages, many patients manifest few of the above manifestations. Consequently, recent advances in radiographic and other types of body imaging have been most welcome.

Nuclear, Sonographic, and CT Scanning Assessments
Although the liver-lung nuclear scan and sonography have been of some value in identifying subphrenic sepsis, the fourth generation 2-second CT scanning devices are proving to be by far the most accurate method of identifying an abdominal abscess. The accuracy of computed tomography is so impressive, that it is probably cost effective to perform this study on any patient who has an unexplained persistent fever following abdominal surgery.

Surgical Approach

Posterior (12th-Rib Excision) Approach
At one time, removing the 12th rib and entering the "subphrenic" space from the posterior approach was popular. However, anatomical studies by Boyd, and by DeCosse and associates demonstrated that the bare area of the right lobe of the liver is located on its posterior surface. For this reason, there is no significant space caudal to the bare area between the right lobe of the liver and the diaphragm. The only space that can be approached efficiently via the bed of the 12th rib is the right *subhepatic* space. In order to drain a right suprahepatic subphrenic abscess through the bed of the 12th rib, the surgeon would have to divide the triangular ligament and penetrate the bare area of the liver. Exposure from the 12th rib approach is hardly

adequate for this dissection. Consequently, only a right posterior subhepatic abscess can properly be approached through the bed of the 12th rib. In the report of De-Cosse and associates, failure to achieve adequate drainage was noted in 12 of the 15 cases in which the posterior approach was used to the subphrenic space.

For purposes of this discussion, we have adopted the classification of Boyd with a slight modification. On the right side there is a single suprahepatic subphrenic space and a right infrahepatic space. On the left there is a subphrenic space. The left infrahepatic space can be divided into two spaces: the posterior infrahepatic space, which constitutes the lesser sac; and the left anterior infrahepatic space, which is situated anterior to the stomach.

Lateral and Subcostal Extraperitoneal Approach

DeCosse and associates modified the subcostal extraperitoneal approach of Clairmont and Ranzi by extending it in a lateral direction as far as the tip of the 11th rib. The layers of the abdominal wall are divided down to the peritoneum. Then the surgeon's hand dissects the peritoneum away from the diaphragm until the abscess is reached. The lateral extraperitoneal approach may also be used in the treatment of a right posterior infrahepatic abscess. DeCosse and associates were successful in draining left subphrenic as well as left posterior infrahepatic abscesses in the lesser sac through the subcostal or lateral extraperitoneal approach. The lesser sac abscesses were reached by dissecting the peritoneum away from the upper pole of the kidney. The right suprahepatic subphrenic abscess is easily approached through an anterior (subcostal) extraperitoneal approach. An abscess in the left anterior infrahepatic space is best approached by performing a laparotomy.

Laparotomy

Halasz as well as Dineen and McSherry advocated draining subphrenic abscesses by a transperitoneal route. Although it is true that, thanks to modern antibiotics, there is no great risk of spreading the infection by draining an abscess transperitoneally instead of extraserously, no one can doubt that exploring the abdomen 2–3 weeks following major surgery is more difficult and more hazardous than is draining the abscess by an extraserous route. Prior to the achievement of diagnostic accuracy with computed tomography, there was a considerable risk that the patient might have an abscess in more than one location. Under these conditions, an extraperitoneal operation might overlook the second or third abscess. When a CT scan demonstrates a *solitary* right or left subphrenic abscess, or a right posterior infrahepatic abscess, we prefer to attempt drainage by the extraserous approach because the operation is safe and relatively simple. If this procedure fails to eliminate the signs of sepsis, a laparotomy should be performed. In patients suspected of having a lesser sac abscess, a peripancreatic, or a left anterior infrahepatic abscess and in those suspected of having an anastomotic leak with multiple intermesenteric abscesses, laparotomy is mandatory.

Percutaneous Catheter Drainage of Subphrenic Abscess

With the aid of a 2-second CT scanning device and ultrasonography, Johnson, Gerzof, Robbins, and Nabseth were successful in draining 89% of subphrenic or other abdominal abscesses by means of catheters inserted via the percutaneous route. Their indications for using percutaneous drainage included: (1) a well-established unilocular fluid collection having the various CT and ultrasound signs of an abscess; (2) a safe percutaneous access route; (3) a joint evaluation by the surgical and radiology services, and (4) an immediate operative backup for any complication or failure. Percutaneous drainage was considered to be especially indicated if, in addition to meeting the above criteria, the patient was an exceptionally poor surgical risk. These procedures were performed by the department of radiology. All patients were observed for a minimum of 6 months to detect recurrent abscesses. In the same institution, 12 patients underwent surgical drainage for subphrenic abscess. Of these, 4 patients suffered from inadequate drainage; all told, 5 patients died of sepsis.

These authors stated that computed tomography "has become our method of choice to identify and follow . . . intraabdominal sepsis." It should be emphasized that abscesses having many loculations at this time are not considered suitable for this technique. In many cases, it will also be an inadequate method of curing an abscess that communicates with the intestinal or biliary tract. Similar successful results were described by Mandel, Boyd, Jaques, Mandell, and associates who reported on 24 of their own patients and also collected reports of 252 cases from the world literature.

If computed tomography detects a subphrenic abscess in its early stages, before the abscess wall has become fibrotic and rigid, drainage by surgery or percutaneous catheter will permit the abscess to collapse. Consequently, the drain or catheter may be removed at a relatively early date. Otherwise, when the abscess wall is rigid, drainage must be continued for several weeks until the CT scan or a Hypaque sinogram X ray demonstrates that the abscess cavity has disappeared. As experience develops with the new rapid scanning technique of computed tomography, it is probable that a large percentage of subphrenic and intra-abdominal abscesses will be successfully treated by percutaneous catheter drainage.

Indications

It is true, that in the early stages of the development of a subphrenic abscess, there probably is a stage of cellulitis that can successfully be treated with antibiotics. However, in the vast majority of patients who have symptoms of sepsis, it is too late for treatment by antibiotics alone by the time the diagnosis of a subphrenic abscess is made. Prompt institution of drainage is thus indicated, either by the percutaneous route or by surgery.

Preoperative Care

Therapeutic doses of appropriate antibiotics should be administered. Until the culture report is available, we believe the patient should receive an aminoglycoside, clindamycin, and ampicillin intravenously because in most cases the causative organisms will respond to these agents. Other antibiotic regimens, that include various combinations of a third or fourth generation cephalosporin and metronidazole may also prove to be acceptable.

Whereas the older diagnostic workup for a subphrenic abscess depended on the abdominal and chest X ray together with a liver-lung nuclear scan, at this time the best single diagnostic procedure to localize a subphrenic abscess is computed tomography using rapid scan.

Nasogastric tube

In patients nutritionally depleted by chronic sepsis, initiate total parenteral nutrition, but do not delay operation on this account.

Pitfalls and Danger Points

Failure to locate and adequately drain all loculations and multiple abscesses

Injuring the spleen, liver, or hollow viscus

Operative Strategy

Extraserous Approach

Dissection in the extraserous preperitoneal or retroperitoneal plane is generally simple if the surgeon enters the proper plane by incising the transversalis fascia but not the peritoneum. The incision should be made long enough to admit the surgeon's hand. Then blunt dissection will separate the peritoneum from the undersurface of the diaphragm until an area of induration is reached. This represents the abscess. Generally blunt dissection with a finger will permit entry into the abscess. Although DeCosse and associates have successfully drained abscesses in the posterior right subhepatic space and in the lesser sac by the extraserous approach, we usually prefer a laparotomy to accomplish drainage of these two spaces.

When an extraserous approach has failed to reveal an abscess, it is generally simple to lengthen the incision in the abdominal wall transversely, converting it to a subcostal incision. Then incise the peritoneum and continue the exploration for the abscess transperitoneally. Alternatively, a second vertical incision may be made in the midline of the abdomen for further exploration.

Laparotomy

When the transperitoneal approach has been elected, we prefer a midline incision, especially if there is any suspicion of an anastomotic leak or an abscess located within the folds of the small bowel mesentery. If the exploration of the subphrenic, subhepatic, and lesser sac spaces does not reveal the source of the patient's sepsis, it may be necessary to free the entire small bowel and the pelvis in order to positively rule out an abdominal abscess.

Operative Technique— Extraserous Subcostal Drainage of Right Subphrenic Abscess

Incision and Exposure

Make a 10–12 cm incision, beginning near the tip of the right 11th rib and continue medially parallel to the costal margin. Carry the incision through the external oblique muscle and aponeurosis **(Fig. 96–1)**. Generally, the internal oblique muscle **(Fig. 96–2)** can be separated along the line of its fibers. It will usually be necessary to divide the 9th intercostal nerve. Then transect the transversus muscle with the electrocautery. If necessary, the incision may be continued through the lateral quarter of the rectus muscle.

Identify the transversalis fascia and carefully divide it with a scalpel **(Fig. 96–3)** revealing the underlying peritoneal membrane. Use a gauze sponge on a sponge-holder to dissect the peritoneum

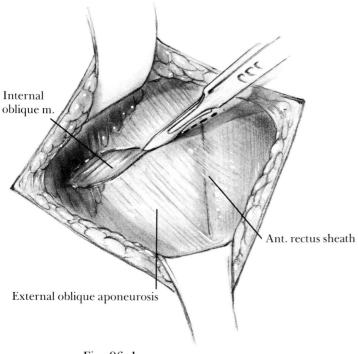

Internal oblique m.

Ant. rectus sheath

External oblique aponeurosis

Fig. 96–1

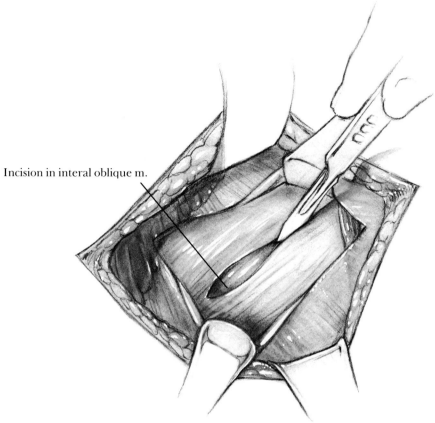

Incision in interal oblique m.

Fig. 96–2

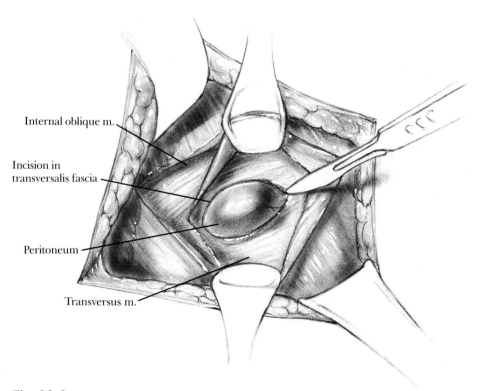

Internal oblique m.

Incision in transversalis fascia

Peritoneum

Transversus m.

Fig. 96–3

away from the transversalis fascia. Continue the dissection upward by inserting the hand to further separate the peritoneum from the undersurface of the diaphragm until the dome of the liver is reached **(Fig. 96–4)**.

A right posterior infrahepatic abscess can be reached by the extraserous approach if the peritoneum is dissected laterally **(Fig. 96–5)** until the fat overlying Gerota's fascia is encountered. This is swept away from the posterolateral peritoneal envelope. The abscess will then be encountered medial and superior to the upper pole of the right kidney. On the left side a posterior infrahepatic or lesser sac abscess can be approached in a similar fashion by dissecting the posterolateral peritoneum away from the fat over Gerota's capsule. The abscess will be encountered medial to the upper pole of the left kidney.

Drainage and Closure

After exposing an area of induration in one of the subphrenic spaces, the abscess may be entered by inserting a fingertip or the tip of a blunt Kelly Hemostat. Open the abscess cavity widely and irrigate out the purulent material after obtaining a sample for routine and anaerobic cultures **(Fig. 96–6)**.

If an abscess has been drained in its early stages before its walls have become rigid, evacuating the pus will permit the abscess cavity to collapse and disappear. In cases of this type it is necessary to insert only a single large sump drain and a single large latex drain. These drains may be

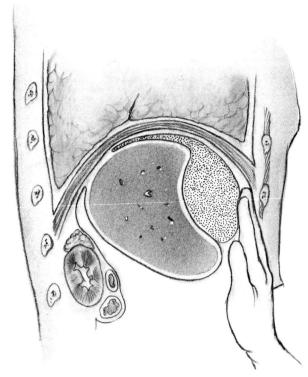

Fig. 96–4

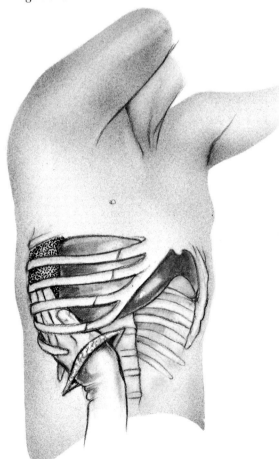

Fig. 96–5

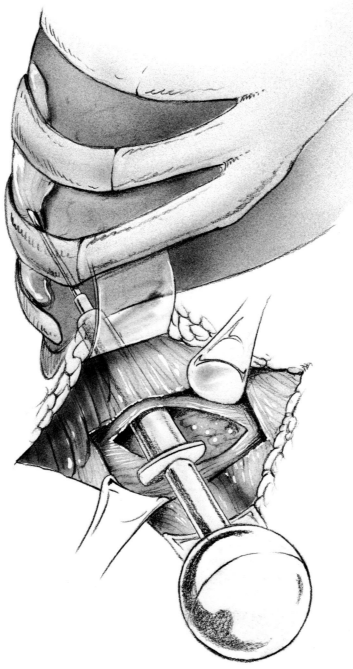

Fig. 96–6

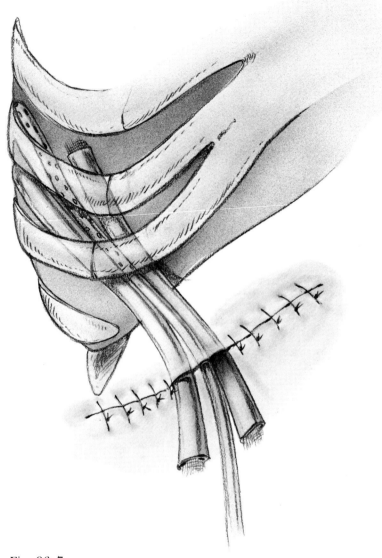

Fig. 96–7

brought out through the incision (**Fig. 96–7**) (or through a stab wound). Close the remainder of the abdominal wall incision so that one finger may be inserted into the abdominal cavity alongside the drains. Although many surgeons prefer to sew the skin closed after this operation, we believe that the skin and the subcutaneous tissue should be lightly packed with a strip of moistened gauze and left unsutured. Several untied interrupted nylon skin sutures may be inserted, in anticipation of a delayed secondary closure at the bedside 4–7 days following operation. If the patient has a large subphrenic abscess with rigid walls that do not collapse after evacuating the pus, insert two sump drains and 3–4 large latex drains, anticipating that the drains may have to be left in for a number of weeks before the abscess cavity collapses or fills with granulation tissue.

578

Operative Technique—Laparotomy for Subphrenic and Abdominal Abscesses

Incision and Exposure

When draining an accurately localized right infrahepatic abscess a right lateral subcostal incision is suitable. Left anterior infrahepatic and lesser sac abscesses, suprahepatic abscesses and most other abdominal abscesses are better drained through midline incisions. If the patient has had a recent operation through a midline incision, try to enter the abdomen by extending the previous midline incision into a virginal area of the abdominal wall so that one is less likely to encounter densely adherent bowel when opening the peritoneum. After the abdomen is opened, identify the falciform ligament and peritoneum. Dissect these two structures away from all the underlying bowel and omentum, first on the right side and then on the left. After this has been accomplished, pass a hand over the liver to explore the suprahepatic and then the infrahepatic spaces.

Divide the avascular portion of the gastrohepatic ligament and enter the lesser sac behind the lesser curvature of the stomach. If this approach has been obliterated by previous surgery or adhesions, enter the lesser sac by dividing the omentum along the greater curvature and expose the posterior wall of the stomach and the anterior surface of the pancreas. Identify the right and left paracolic spaces and expose the pelvic cavity since both are likely locations of abscesses, especially in patients suffering ruptured appendicitis or diverticulitis. Finally, if it is necessary to rule out the possibility of an interloop abscess, the surgeon will have to patiently free the entire length of small intestine and its mesentery.

Drainage and Closure

When a long midline incision has been used, drains should be brought out through suitable stab wounds. Although large sump drains are suitable for subphrenic abscesses, there is a considerable risk of creating a colocutaneous or enterocutaneous fistula if a large plastic drain remains in contract with a segment of bowel for period of time exceeding 2 weeks. Consequently, it may be preferrable to use soft Silastic sump drains or latex Penrose drains rather than a more rigid type of drain.

Close the midline incision by the modified Smead-Jones technique (Chap. 5) using No. 1 PDS or 2–0 stainless steel wire sutures to the abdominal wall. Insert vertical mattress sutures of 3–0 interrupted nylon about 2 cm apart into the skin but do not tie any of these sutures for 4–8 days.

Postoperative Care

Continue therapeutic doses of suitable antibiotics, guided by Gram stain studies taken in the operating room and by bacterial culture results. Antibiotics will be required for a minimum of 7–10 days in patients undergoing surgery for a subphrenic abscess.

If early feeding cannot be tolerated by the patient, initiate total parenteral nutrition.

If the abscess cavity was not rigid and its walls collapsed after the pus was evacuated, remove the drains after 10–14 days. If there is any question about a risidual cavity, inject sterile Hypaque or other iodinated aqueous contrast medium through the sump drain to perform a sinogram X ray. If there is any cavity remaining, leave at least one of the drains in place until the cavity has been eliminated, as demonstrated by an X-ray study.

If the patient has a large abscess cavity with rigid walls, and thick pus, consider the advantages of irrigating the abscess daily through one of the sump catheters with a dilute antibiotic solution.

Postoperative Complications

Residual or recurrent abscess

Overlooked abscess

Colocutaneous or enterocutaneous fistula

Hematoma secondary to hepatic or splenic operative trauma

References

DeCosse JJ, Poulin TL, Fox PS, Condon RE, (1974) Subphrenic abscesses. Surg Gynecol Obstet 138:841

Boyd DP (1966) The subphrenic spaces and the emperor's new robes. N Engl J Med 275:911

Clairmont P, Ranzi E (1905) Kasuistischer Beitrag zür operativen Behandlung des subphrenischen Abszesses. Wien Klin Wochenschr 18:653

Dineen P, McSherry CK (1962) Subdiaphragmatic abscess. Ann Surg 155:506

Halasz NA (1970) Subphrenic abscess. JAMA 214:724

Johnson WC, Gerzof SG, Robbins AH, Nabseth DC, (1981) Treatment of abdominal abscesses. Ann Surg 194:510

Mandel SR, Boyd D, Jaques PF, Mandell V et al. (1983) Drainage of hepatic, intraabdominal, and mediastinal abscesses guided by computerized axial tomography; successful alternative to open drainage. AM J Surg 145:120

Appendix

E. Glossary

Angiocath Intravenous Catheter Placement Unit. A plastic catheter introduced over a needle.

Deseret
Sandy, Utah 84070

Adaptic Non-Adhering Dressing.

J & J Products
New Brunswick, New Jersey 08903

Biopsy needle, Travenol/Tru-Cut

Travenol Lab
Deerfield, Illinois 60015

Burhenne Soft Steerable Catheter System. A device for extracting retained common bile duct stones via the drain tract remaining after removing the T-tube.

Medi Tech Division
Cooper Scientific
372 Main Street
Watertown, Mass. 02172

Catheter, Cholangiogram, Taut

Taut
2571 Kaneville Court
Geneva, Illinois 60134

Contrast media, radiographic

1. Conray; iothalamate meglumine. Aqueous radiopaque iodinated medium useful in cholangiography.
2. Gastrografin; diatrizoate meglumine and diatrizoate sodium solution. Aqueous radiopaque iodinated medium for radiographic visualization of the gastrointestinal tract.

Drugs

1. Immodium; loperamide hydrochloride; Janssen
2. Lomotil; diphenoxylate hydrochloride; Searle
3. Metamucil; psyllium hydrophilic mucilloid; Searle
4. Senokot-S; senna concentrate and docusate sodium; Purdue Frederick

Elastic sleeve. Sleeve made to order according to measurements of the individual patient's arm circumference at various levels.

Jobst
Box 653
Toledo, Ohio 43694

Gelfoam. Absorbable gelatin sponge, useful to induce hemostasis by direct contact with a bleeding surface.

Upjohn
Kalamazoo, Michigan 49001

Hemorrhoid Banding Instrument, McGivney Type. An effective device to apply a tight rubber band to internal hemorrhoids.

Ford Dixon
P.O. Box 35704
Dallas, Texas 75235

Mesh, polypropylene. Plastic mesh useful in repair of large hernias.

1. Marlex Mesh
   Bard Implants Div.
   Box M
   Billerica, Mass. 01821
2. Prolene Mesh
   Ethicon
   Somerville, New Jersey 08876

Pump, Infusion, Pressure. A pump that compresses a 1-liter bag of saline solution during choledochoscopy.

Sorenson Research
P.O. Box 15588
Salt Lake City, Utah 84115

Steri-Strip. Sterile paper adhesive tape.

Surgical Products Div. 3M
St. Paul, Minnesota 55144

Suture material

1. PDS. Polydiaxanone, synthetic monofilament absorbable suture; slowest rate of absorption of currently available suture materials.
2. Vicryl. Polyglactin, synthetic absorbable suture material.

Ethicon
Somerville, New Jersey 08876

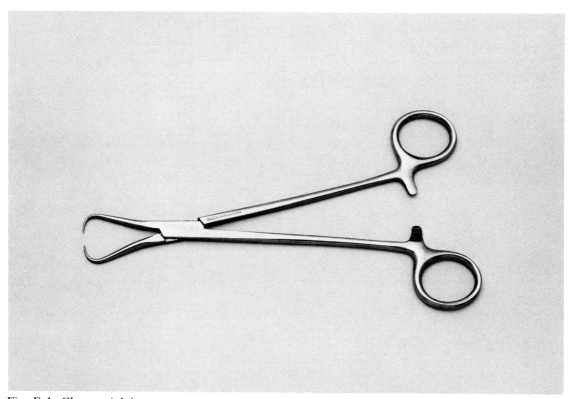

Fig. E-1. Clamp, Adair

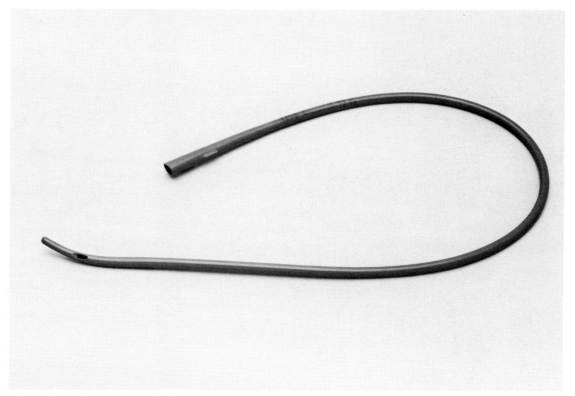

Fig. E-2. Catheter, Coudé-tip

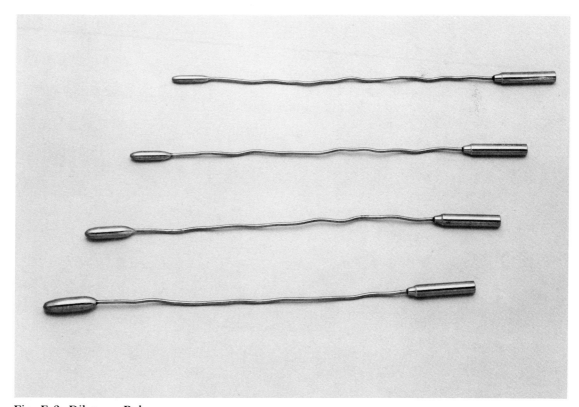

Fig. E-3. Dilators, Bakes

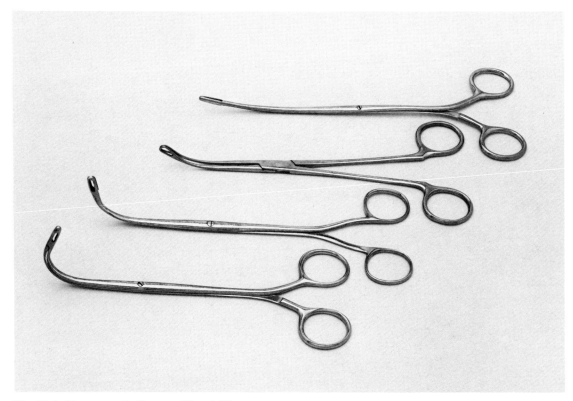

Fig. E-4. Forceps, Gallstone (Randall)

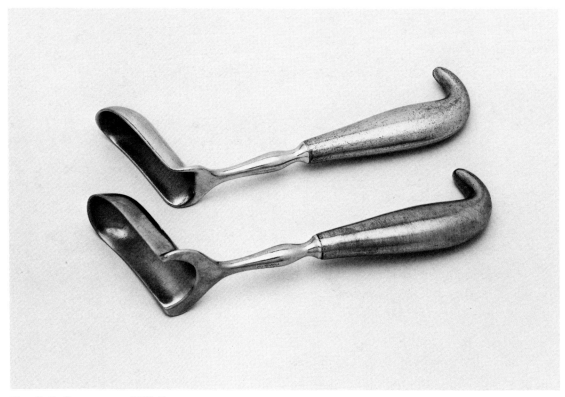

Fig. E-5. Retractors, Hill-Ferguson

586

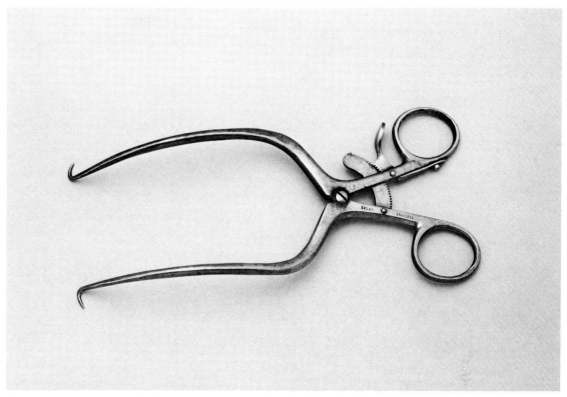

Fig. E-6. Retractor, Gelpi

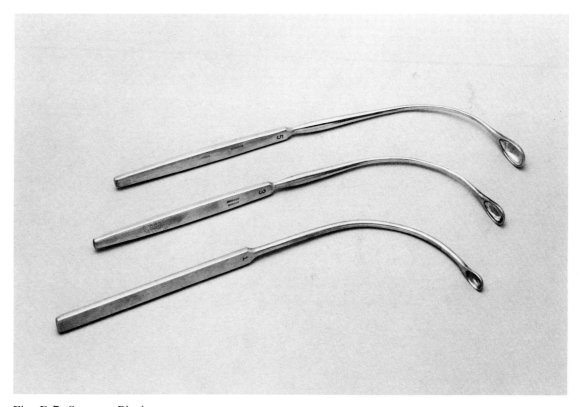

Fig. E-7. Scoops, Pituitary

Index